OPERATIVE SURGERY

THE ABDOMEN AND RECTUM

BY

DR. MARTIN KIRSCHNER

ORDINARIUS PROFESSOR OF SURGERY AND DIRECTOR OF THE SURGICAL CLINIC
AT THE UNIVERSITY OF TÜBINGEN, (GERMANY)

AUTHORIZED TRANSLATION
BY

I. S. RAVDIN, B.S., M.D.

J. WILLIAM WHITE PROFESSOR OF RESEARCH SURGERY
UNIVERSITY OF PENNSYLVANIA: SURGEON,
UNIVERSITY HOSPITAL, PHILADELPHIA

With 395 Illustrations, Mostly Colored

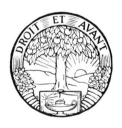

PHILADELPHIA AND LONDON
J. B. LIPPINCOTT COMPANY

PRINTED IN THE UNITED STATES OF AMERICA

EDITOR'S PREFACE

The first volume of the American edition of Professor Martin Kirschner's Operative Surgery was published in 1931. The plan was to follow this immediately with the second volume, but the German edition of the second volume was delayed for reasons which the author explains in his preface. The enthusiastic reception which was accorded the first volume has made the editing of the present volume a welcome task. The second volume covers the field of abdominal surgery including the rectum. As in the first volume Professor Kirschner has been meticulous in the inclusion of every detail of the operations which he discusses. Every important point is illustrated with the same skill and precision which distinguished the first volume. Most of the illustrations are in color.

The text represents the German viewpoint in regard to the problems which are daily met in the surgical clinic. It must be accepted as such although occasionally we may disagree with the classification or technique. The editor has taken the same liberty which he took in translating the first volume in that, while he has carefully and faithfully construed the author's ideas he has, at the same time, avoided a literal translation.

The editor has had the capable assistance of Dr. Richard Kern in the translation. Dr. Elizabeth Glenn Ravdin has been of invaluable assistance in the preparation of the American text. Without her help the volume would have been still further delayed. To both he is deeply grateful for the time and patience which they have given to the work. To the publishers many thanks are due for their patience during many delays.

I. S. RAVDIN

May 1933

FOREWORD

Four years have passed since the appearance of the first volume of my Operative Surgery, which discussed General and Special Considerations. The second volume has been unduly delayed, contrary to my own expectations and those of my readers. During this time numerous subscribers to the first volume and a few book dealers have registered complaints because of the long wait for the continuation of the work. I am taking the opportunity of the appearance of the present volume to present my reasons and apologies.

For several years, as a result of the unexpected change of the field of my professional activities from Königsberg to Tübingen in the Fall of 1927, the practical and clinical side of my work had to be emphasized at the expense of my scientific and literary endeavors. Aside from the fact that in the Surgical Clinic at Tübingen with its 265 beds I found considerably more clinical material than in the Königsberg Clinic, it became necessary to devote more time to the practical work of the clinic, because of the exchange of a clinic organization which had functioned smoothly for years for one that was new to me; and because of the replacement of nearly all my assistants, to whom I have been accustomed for years, by new co-workers. For the clinician, if he would not disregard the qualities required of a true surgeon as stated in the first volume of my Operative Surgery, belongs in the first place to his patients, his students and his assistants. His other activities must take second place.

Moreover, in apportioning the time which remains to him for scientific work, the head of a University clinic, if he feels any call to take an active part in the advancement of science, must not wholly suppress for years his own investigation of new problems, which attract him in his specialty, in favor of a textbook. Whether my experiments of recent years along these lines will sufficiently excuse me with the subscribers to my Operative Surgery, I shall not venture to decide.

A further diversion of my efforts from the book lay in rearranging the first volume for an American edition which has appeared in the meantime and for a Spanish edition which is about to appear. At a time when German science and German texts are struggling for recognition in the world, I felt that for patriotic reasons I could not withdraw from this duty.

The fact that both translations of the first volume were undertaken by the foreign publishers without regard to the time of completion of the whole work confirms the view which I have constantly maintained, namely, that the first volume represents a complete unit in itself. It does not unconditionally or immediately require a continuation in the form of a "Special Operative Surgery" any more than does a "Textbook of General Surgery". This, in my opinion, most effectively disarms the critics of the delay in the appearance of the "Special Sections".

As an additional extenuating circumstance I wish to plead another severe, though recent drain on my time, the assumption of the Rectorship of the

University of Tübingen. In my opinion, the pursuit of literary work does not justify even the incumbent of a chair of surgery, burdened as he is by his time-consuming operative work, to refuse the highest position of honor which the University can bestow.

To all of these hindrances there was added an extraordinary development, lying outside the narrower limits of my calling, a development that was unforeseen in the working program of my life and which made unusual demands upon my time, the erection of the new surgical clinic of the University of Tübingen. Such a project means a serious and far-reaching responsibility for the director of the Clinic. It involves the expenditure of huge sums of money that are doubly valuable in the present time of need—a matter of over 5 million marks in this instance. The conformation of the new clinic will be a determining factor for many generations in the fate of thousands of persons and in numerous conditions; in the fate of the patients; in the education of students and the post-graduate instruction of physicians; in the activities of employes, of the male and female nursing staffs and of the deaconesses; in the training of assistants; in the selection of future heads of the clinic and in their activities; in the whole scientific life of the clinic and consequently in its relation to the rest of the scientific world, at home and abroad, and in its share in the advances of surgical science.

If in the planning of such a structure one does not limit the cooperation and the responsibility of the director of the clinic merely to the theoretical statement of his requirements and wishes and to the inspection of the plans subsequently submitted to him by the architect, but grants him the right and the duty of actually planning the building independently and after his own designs, as I attempted to describe in my article on "The Erection of the New Surgical Clinic of the University of Tübingen" in "Chirurg.," 1929-30, then one can form some idea of the burden imposed upon me by the building of the clinic, of the enforced diversion of my thoughts to construction problems and of the estrangement of my mental processes from surgical questions.

It is difficult to commit to paper the details of a gastric operation while the riveting of the steel framework of the new clinic is hammering into the consciousness of the writer that from minute to minute there is growing under his responsibility an unalterable structure. It requires a violent change of thought to fix one's attention with the artist on the details of an operative procedure while on the next table the plan of the new operating room lay-out or of the new Roentgenologic Institute must be drawn with the architects and building specialists down to the last electrical outlet. Perhaps the new 12-story Surgical Clinic at Tübingen which has come under roof at the same time that this volume appears will be a work of atonement that permits me to hope for pardon at the hands of the impatient and not always friendly subscribers to my textbook.

Under the combined pressure of these numerous circumstances, and in order not to delay further the already unduly belated book, I was compelled with a heavy heart to give up my original plan of writing the whole work with a single collaborator as a unified joint production. Such a change became all the more necessary when my separation from my collaborator on the first volume, entailed by my removal to Tübingen, made impossible the further close collaboration which such a work requires.

Furthermore, in working up some of the "Grenzgebiete," I discovered that I frequently lacked the detailed knowledge which is indispensable for an inclusive presentation of the subject. At the same time, I felt that I dared not omit important neighboring fields from my Operative Surgery which plans to be a faithful adviser in all fields of surgical procedure. In a time when textbooks on gynecology discuss stomach resection and the operations on the biliary tract, and when the operative works of otolaryngologists devote considerable space to brain surgery and the operations on the thyroid, the representatives of these fields could justly make a charge of deprecation of their art against an Operative Surgery which did not include a correspondingly broad treatment of the operations of their specialties.

I therefore decided to give over extensive fields to independent elaboration. I am happy to have found in Messrs. Guleke of Jena, Kleinschmidt of Wiesbaden, Lautenschläger and Wagner of Berlin distinguished and well-known collaborators who will insure a pleasant surprise for the subscribers to the first volume who are awaiting the continuation of the work.

Through this division of the material among several writers it will be possible to produce the whole of the Special Sections in a short time.

The publisher, in spite of the present low economic status of our country and of the whole world, has placed no restrictions on the format of text or illustrations of the second volume of my Operative Surgery, so that the book can appear in a worthy and acceptable form. The work thereby testifies to the firm and unswerving faith in the future and in the rehabilitation of the German People.

MARTIN KIRSCHNER

Tübingen

CONTENTS

OPERATIVE SURGERY

THE ABDOMEN AND RECTUM

CHAPTER I

THE ABDOMINAL INCISION (LAPAROTOMY)

The caution which for many years influenced surgeons in their attitude toward abdominal operations has been greatly lessened by the improved technique of abdominal surgery, the relatively low mortality, the knowledge of the tolerance of the abdominal cavity to operative insult, and the resulting temptation to establish diagnoses by exploratory laparotomy. It should however always be borne in mind that for every laparotomy the indications must be carefully considered, for a patient whose abdominal wall has once been the site of an incision is left in most instances with a damage that is permanent, even though it may be slight.

A. THE PREPARATION AND POSITION OF THE PATIENT

When the nature of the disease permits waiting for several days, the preparation of the patient for an abdominal operation differs but little from the preparation for other surgical procedures. It follows the general principles set forth in Volume I, page 6. The limitation of food and the emptying of the digestive tract may be emphasized somewhat more strongly, but not excessively. When the intestines are well emptied the exposure and the replacement of the abdominal viscera are facilitated; there is less danger of injuring the bowel, and lesser demands are placed on the suture lines. However, in the presence of even a partial obstruction of the intestine, especial caution must be observed in the use of cathartics, since "whipping up" the gut segment proximal to the stenosis may lead to serious consequences.

If the operation is not to be started in the early morning, but more than three hours after awakening, then a cup of coffee or tea and some toast may be permitted as a breakfast before the operation.

In operations on the stomach, when there is no immediate danger of hemorrhage or perforation, the stomach should be carefully lavaged on the evening before the operation and again one-half an hour before the operation. Some surgeons intubate and empty the stomach even in the presence of gastric perforation; but here I believe lavage is contraindicated. Even simple emptying under these condition is contraindicated because the gagging which this procedure entails may cause additional gastric contents to be forced out into the peritoneal cavity. (This does not mean that a Jutte or similar tube should not be kept in the stomach after operation. I. S. R.)

If the nature of the illness demands immediate operation, and the patient has been vomiting, then, aside from the preparatory measures of a general nature described in Volume I, thorough gastric lavage should be practised (and a small tube, Jutte or otherwise, left in the stomach. I. S. R.). I even advise lavage before abdominal operations if the patient has eaten shortly before.

The artificial emptying of the stomach meets the danger that during operation aspiration of vomitus may occur, an event which may lead to death by suffocation or to aspiration pneumonia. With such possibilities in mind, a word of caution is not amiss in regard to the use of the Trendelenburg position or its modified form in such cases.

In order to facilitate the emptying of the large bowel, a rectal tube is kept inserted in the rectum during all laparotomies.

Since the abdominal cavity is usually opened anteriorly, the usual position of patients for an abdominal operation is on the back. The structures in the midportion of the body cavity between the diaphragm and the sacral promontory can be elevated by a lordotic curvature of the corresponding portion of the spine, which is effected by placing a roll under the lumbar region, preferably in the form of a pneumatic cushion which can be inflated (Vol. I, Fig. 23). Since this position is uncomfortable or painful for the conscious patient, the air cushion is not inflated until after anaesthesia has begun. One must not forget to deflate the pillow before replacing eventrated abdominal viscera or before beginning to suture the abdominal wall.

The position of the body has a material influence upon the position in the opened abdomen of the individual abdominal viscera, especially of the loops of small intestine hanging by their long mesentery. After opening the peritoneal cavity, we make extensive use of the possibility of shifting the position of the abdominal contents, at times to bring the diseased organ as close as possible to the incision, or to remove troublesome intestines, especially the small bowel, from the operative field. In placing the patient in position, the region of the organ to be attacked should form the point of highest elevation of the abdomen. According to the investigations of my former assistant Grube (German Surgical Congress, 1927), no danger is thereby entailed that localizing purulent collections will gravitate and contaminate other parts of the abdominal cavity while the abdomen remains closed.

In operations above the umbilicus, especially for lesions of the gall bladder and stomach, I place the patient with the upper part of the body elevated (low-pelvis position). In deep anaesthesia the pull of the weight of the liver on the comparatively relaxed diaphragm and liver attachments often permits that organ to emerge appreciably from beneath the costal margin, and the small intestine sinks into the true pelvis. Usually in operations below the umbilicus, and always in pelvic operations, I employ the Trendelenburg position. In every operation in which the Trendelenburg position is even remotely to be considered, I strap the patient securely to the table with his knees flexed at a right angle. It is a routine measure, therefore, in all incisions which open the abdomen below the umbilicus, including hernia and appendix operations. With a steep Trendelenburg position the fold of peritoneum, reflected from the bladder wall to the inner surface of the anterior abdominal wall, glides upward toward the umbilicus under certain circumstances, a matter of several centimeters when the bladder is full. In this position it is easier to reach the bladder extraperitoneally than with the patient in the horizontal position. The former position is, therefore, always preferred in approaching the bladder. For the technique, dangers and contraindications of the Trendelenburg position and its modified form, see Volume I, page 61.

The advantages of the girdle-type of spinal anaesthesia which I now employ (Surgery, Gynecology, and Obstetrics, 1931), and which requires an uninterrupted Trendelenburg position so that the caudal end of the dural sac shall be filled by an air bubble, are so decided in abdominal operations as compared with other forms of anaesthesia that the Trendelenburg position is frequently given preference over positions which might be considered for other reasons.

I also make extensive use of the displacement of the viscera by turning the patient on the long axis of the body (right lateral position, left lateral position), for example in operations on the appendix, gall bladder, stomach, and spleen. For this purpose, of course, a table is required that can be rotated on its long axis. Usually the lateral position is combined with a high- or low-pelvis position, so that the body lies obliquely in two planes. In operations in the posterolateral aspect of the abdomen, for example those on the spleen, the patient may be placed directly on his side to advantage (kidney operation position). In this position both arms are securely fastened to the same side of the operating table.

During a laparotomy the surgeon usually stands at the right of the patient. Opposite him, as a rule, stands the first assistant; at the left of the latter and toward the feet of the patient is the instrument passer with the instrument table. The second assistant is usually at the left of the surgeon. When the surgeon is operating on a patient in the Trendelenburg position, he usually stands at the left of the patient, the first assistant at the right, the instrument passer shifts to the head and the second assistant to the foot of the patient beside the operator. In operations on structures just beneath the costal margin, the surgeon may also find the position on the opposite side of the lesion advantageous.

Marking of the skin incision and protection of the operative field by covers is done according to the directions given in Volume I, page 266. The skin is painted with a tannin-alcohol solution and the line of the incision is marked with a dye. In order to prevent contact between the abdominal viscera, the skin and the substances used to disinfect it, I paint the skin surrounding the site for incision for some distance with Mastisol and fix to this surface a large piece of sterile transparent rubber dam. The sterile covers are applied over the rubber dam in the following manner: (1) the part of the body caudad to the incision is covered by a large sterile sheet; (2) the part of the body cephalad to the incision is covered with a large sterile sheet, the upper end of which is fastened with clamps to a frame, so as to form a kind of tent which excludes the patient's head and the anaesthetist from the operative field; (3) and (4), both sides are covered, with small sheets. (I find it very convenient to further safeguard the operative field with four sterile towels after the sheets have been applied. I. S. R.). The incision is then made through the sterile rubber dam which lies exposed in the center of the operative field.

In order to permit thorough examination of, and easy approach to a lesion within the abdominal cavity, the incision should be adequate and the edges of the wound well retracted. This is accomplished by the insertion of retractors which are held by the assistants. Not only does a balanced pull on the retractors open the wound in the desired shape and direction, but by making unequal traction the wound may, up to a certain point, be displaced over parts of the abdominal cavity at some distance from the original position of the incision. If the intestines protrude into the wound and thus interfere with the view or with the approach to the depths of the abdominal cavity, they are held back by retractors. The insertion of gauze pads, as later described, facilitates this task, and prevents injury to the structures. A self-retaining retractor (Vol. I, Fig. 51) is of great value, especially for midline incisions. The power and uniformity of its action cannot be equalled by any assistant.

B. GENERAL PRINCIPLES OF INCISION AND SUTURE OF THE ABDOMINAL WALL

An abdominal incision must meet three requirements. (1) The incision should lead directly to the operative site, and should afford a good view of and easy access to the focus of disease. (2) The incision should permit of enlargement without difficulty, so that through it adjacent lesions can be reached in those cases in which the location and extent of the disease prove to be different from what was expected. (3) Such closure of the incision should be possible as to protect against postoperative prolapse or hernia. This last requirement is especially difficult to fulfill. Opinions as to the most suitable means to this end are at present still divided.

The following points are particularly to be observed:

(a) The larger nerves of the abdominal muscles must not be divided. Just as the muscles of the extremities degenerate after the interruption of their nervous connection with the spinal cord, so also are the abdominal muscles damaged by the division of their nerve supply. This leads to weakness of the abdominal wall and thus to the formation of a hernia. The nerves of the abdominal muscles have in general the same direction as do the muscles to which they belong, so that incisions carried parallel to the muscle fibers do the least harm. Only the nerves of the recti do not run parallel to the muscle fibers. They enter the recti from behind and at first course parallel to the ribs and then turn downward and medialward. If the nerves to the recti are to be spared they must be exposed individually or the muscle fibers should be divided transversely. Fortunately cutting one or two adjacent nerves of the recti does not tend to cause any appreciable harm, so that if necessary this can be done.

(b) As a rule the abdominal muscles and their aponeuroses should not be divided at right angles to their direction and line of pull, but parallel to their fibers. It is still better to separate the fibers in their course by blunt dissection. If the muscle substance or the aponeurosis is cut transversely, the stumps retract, are difficult to reunite by suture and tend to tear apart after suture when the abdominal wall is put on tension. The resulting gap will be filled in by scar tissue which has little power of resistance. (The upper abdominal transverse incision which divides the rectus has however proven very satisfactory in my hands provided the rectus sheath is adequately reunited. I. S. R.). On the other hand, when the separation is made parallel to the

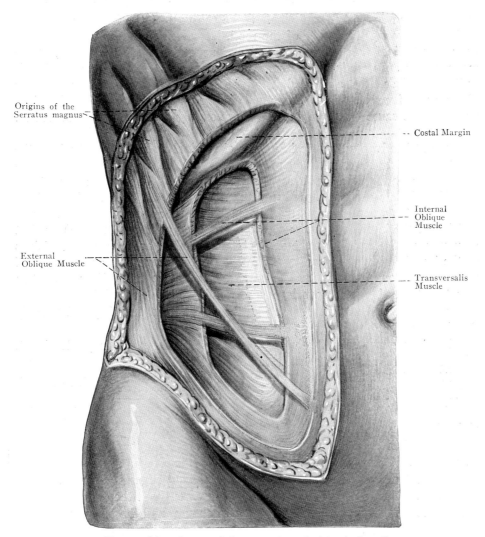

Origins of the
Serratus magnus

Costal Margin

Internal
Oblique
Muscle

External
Oblique Muscle

Transversalis
Muscle

FIG. 1. Musculature of the anterolateral abdominal wall.

direction of the fibers, the opening, as a rule, tends to close automatically as a result of the elasticity of the muscle fibers, and the firmness of the closure increases as the muscle contracts.

In the lateral regions of the abdomen the muscles in the main run transversely to the body axis; the external oblique from behind forward and downward, the internal oblique fans out from the anterior superior spine, while the transversalis runs almost wholly transversely. (Fig. 1.)

The anterior midportion of the abdomen is bounded by the two recti which run parallel to the long axis of the body. The lineae transversae in the muscle substance fuse the muscle with the anterior rectus sheath, so that the division of this muscle at one point merely permits the separation of the muscle bundles between two such lineae, while the portions beyond the two adjacent lineae are not affected.

The two recti are sheathed in the aponeuroses of the lateral abdominal muscles which fuse in the midline. Since the pull of the lateral muscles is said to be stronger than that of the recti, lateral traction also preponderates over longitudinal traction in the midportions of the abdominal wall. This means that transverse incisions tend to cause only a slight gaping while longitudinal incisions effect a marked gaping of the wound with a greater tendency to postoperative separation. (It should also be noted that transverse incisions on the whole cause less injury to the nerve supply of the abdominal muscles. I. S. R.)

(c) It is advantageous to incise the abdominal wall at a point where the greatest possible number of layers are superimposed, and to arrange the incision of these layers in such a way that the suture lines and scars of the individual layers are not directly in apposition, but are displaced one from the other. This displacement may be effected either by making the lines of incision of the individual layers cross one another (gridiron incision) so that scar falls upon scar only at the one point of crossing, or by parallel incisions of the individual layers, each incision being made to one side or the other of the preceding one (curtain incision), in which case the suture lines are not in direct contact. A similar security is obtained if we incise the abdominal layers in a single plane, but overlap the individual layers in suturing and thereby double the number of layers.

In the transversalis fascia a transverse line of tension is predominant. The peritoneum lacks a clearly defined line of elastic tension.

Lines of cleavage in the skin of the abdominal wall (Fig. 352, page 351, Vol. I) need not be considered seriously in abdominal incisions.

(d) Smooth wound healing is an essential factor in obtaining a dependable abdominal scar. This requires that healing of the wound should not be complicated by infection. The wound must therefore be kept as free of bacteria as possible. Many surgeons therefore after completion of the abdominal incision, fasten gauze pads or rubber dam to the cut edges of the peritoneum, so that the abdominal wall wound is protected throughout the operation. The covering is continuous with the parietal peritoneum, and the peritoneal cavity opens in the center. With such complete enclosure of the abdominal wound, eventrated viscera do not come in contact with the skin so that they can not be infected by skin bacteria nor irritated by chemical substances used for skin disinfection. (It is very important that the subcutaneous fat should not be subjected to undue trauma. I. S. R.)

The universal protection of the wound does not seem to me theoretically correct. If in the course of a laparotomy any infectious material gets into the operative field, it is almost impossible to prevent the contamination of the wound by such an inadequate mode of covering. The bacteria will find their way through the compresses and around the rubber dam, in spite of the most careful protection. If a wound is contaminated with bacteria to any great extent, it is pretty much a matter of indifference whether a few germs more or less gain access to the exposed tissues. Only the prevention of contact of viscera with the skin surface seems to me to be of value, although the disadvantages of such contact are minimized by the routine use of the tannin-alcohol solution instead of tincture of iodine. Furthermore, I prevent such contact by fixing rubber dam to the skin with Mastisol before applying the sterile sheets. If this is not done it is sufficient to bring the large sheets, or additional towels, up to the line of incision, and to fix them to the edges of the

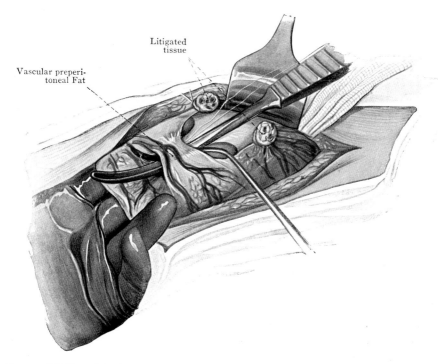

Fig. 2. Midline abdominal incision. Division of vascular portions of preperitoneal fat between double ligatures.

wound with towel clips after the incision is made. The laparotomy wound itself then requires no further covering.

Another important prerequisite for smooth healing of an abdominal wound is careful hemostasis, for postoperative hematomas favor infection and thus retard the healing of a wound. (The gentle handling of the tissues, the inclusion of only minute amounts of tissue when tying ligatures, and the prevention of strangling tissues when inserting sutures are also of importance in the prevention of wound complications. I. S. R.).

It is advisable to carry out hemostasis as far as possible by catching and ligating divided vessels before opening the peritoneum, both to guard the peritoneal cavity against the entrance of blood, and to avoid interfering with the approach to the interior of the abdomen by dangling hemostats. In the preperitoneal fat fair sized blood vessels at times cross the field of approach.

They should be picked up on an aneurysm needle and divided between two ligatures (Fig. 2).

Every drain or tampon that passes through an abdominal wound endangers its strength. On the one hand, infection of the wound may result. On the other, the opening which remains in the wall after the removal of the drain or tampon can only be closed by the process of granulation, which is followed by scar tissue of a low degree of resistance. The subsequent formation of a hernia in the scar is thereby favored.

(e) After completion of the intra-abdominal procedure, the abdominal wound must be closed carefully. Abdominal wall suture is preceded by the

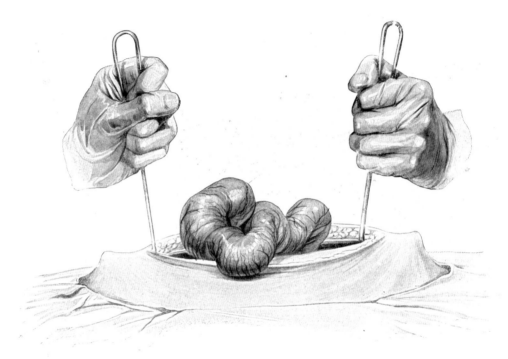

Fig. 3.   Reposition of the viscera. Upward traction with hook retractors inserted in the angles of the wound causes the viscera to drop back into the enlarged abdominal cavity.

replacement of abdominal viscera which were purposely or accidentally eventrated. This step is materially facilitated by the complete relaxation of the abdominal muscles, as occurs in deep general or in spinal anaesthesia, while severe straining can make both the operation difficult and dependable wound closure almost impossible. When general anaesthesia is used it is therefore the duty of the anaesthetist to increase the depth of the anaesthesia at the proper time.

To replace the viscera, the anterior abdominal wall, which through gravity and muscle tone tends to approach the vertebral column, is lifted and in this way the peritoneal cavity approaches a spherical shape, thus increasing its capacity. To accomplish this the assistants elevate the sides of the abdominal wound, each with a rounded abdominal retractor, or the angles of the wound are elevated with narrow hook retractors. This should be done cautiously

(Fig. 3). During this maneuver, the eventrated viscera frequently fall back of their own accord into the peritoneal cavity, or with some assistance from the operator.

If difficulties in replacing the viscera arise as a result of severe straining or because of undue distension of the intestines, the surgeon must replace the viscera in a systematic way. While the assistants pull the retractors steadily upward, the operator proceeds with both hands to place one loop of bowel after another back into the abdominal cavity. In doing this he must take care that a loop once replaced does not again come out of the wound. Preferably

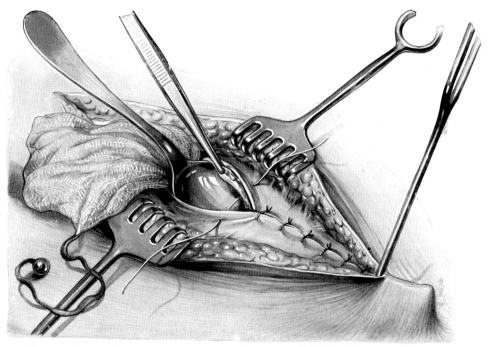

FIG. 4. Suture of the abdominal wall. By elevating the lower angle of the wound with a hooked retractor the abdominal cavity is enlarged to receive the viscera. The latter are prevented from protruding against the suture line by means of a spoon and a moist gauze pad. The union of the abdominal wall is effected by interrupted sutures which include all layers of the abdominal wall except the skin.

the first assistant retracts the abdominal walls, the second assistant guards the opening against the further escape of viscera, while the operator attends to the replacement. In order to retain the viscera while the wound is being closed, and to guard them against needle pricks and against inclusion in the suture of the wall, a moist gauze pad is spread out in a fan shape over them and projects through the angle of the wound last to be closed, through which it is withdrawn bit by bit as closure progresses (Fig. 4). The insertion of a tablespoon and later of a smaller spoon will help or sometimes completely suffice to hold back the omentum and intestines. Care should be taken to prevent any omentum from being caught in the suture line since it has a decided tendency to become attached at this point.

Normally, the closure of an abdominal incision consists in the careful suture of each individual layer of the abdominal wall. The meticulous execution of the closure is of great importance in the prevention of postoperative prolapse or ventral hernia. One therefore sutures muscle layer to muscle layer, fascial layer to fascial layer, and finally the skin. Since I am of the opinion that the peritoneum separately does not have any great tensile

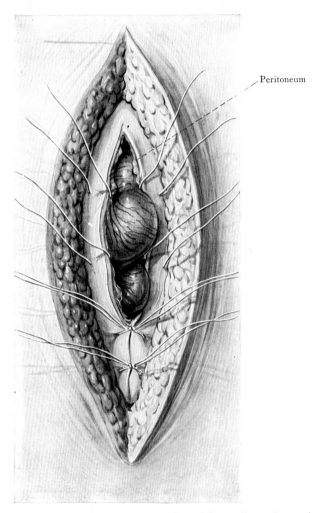

Peritoneum

FIG. 5. Difficult abdominal wall suture because of straining. Since closure in the usual manner is impossible, each side of the wound is provided with a number of double sutures which include all layers except the skin. These sutures are tied in pairs.

strength, but actually tears in most instances when sutured alone, I do not practice separate suture of the peritoneum but include with it the transversalis fascia and the deepest muscle layer. Only when the transversalis fascia is well developed, as for example in the region of the posterior rectus sheath above the semilunar line of Douglas, is it and the peritoneum sutured without inclusion of muscle.

In some instances the attempt to suture each layer individually fails because the sutures cut through. In other cases the time lost in individual layer suture is not justified or is detrimental; for example, if the patient, because of the severity of his illness, cannot live until an incisional hernia develops, or if the operation must be terminated with the greatest possible speed because of the condition of the patient. In these exceptional cases we dispense with the suture of the individual layers, and merely introduce a series of interrupted silk sutures which include all layers except the skin. (The use of through and through silver wire sutures for this type of closure is also advantageous. I. S. R.) In order to speed up the closure of the abdominal wall the individual sutures may be placed fairly far apart (2 or 3 cm.). After the completion of this first row of sutures the gaps remaining between each pair of sutures are closed by interrupted sutures (intermediate sutures) which grasp only the most superficial fascial layers.

In these cases however the skin wound is also closed separately, a procedure which with the use of skin clamps entails no great loss of time. It should be remembered however that this type of closure is not the ideal which the surgeon should seek to obtain.

If there is a marked disproportion between the capacity of the abdominal cavity and the volume of the viscera and especially if the patient is straining, this simple method of suture will often fail in effecting the closure desired. In such difficult situations I often resort to the following method (Fig. 5). With a large curved needle long heavy silk sutures are passed through all the layers of one wound edge with the exception of the skin, and pulled half way through. A similar suture is passed through the corresponding point of the opposite wound edge, and in this manner both wound edges are provided with a number of pairs of sutures at intervals of 2 to 4 cm. After all the sutures have been inserted, the abdominal wall is lifted by traction on the sutures, and then each opposing pair of double sutures are tied together, beginning at one angle of the wound. A few intervening sutures are placed in the aponeuroses and fascia and finally the skin sutures are introduced. Instead of silk sutures one can also use wire in an emergency, by piercing all layers including the skin and twisting together the paired loop ends.

If at the outset it appears desirable to reinforce the simple abdominal wall suture, the reinforcement is effected by means of one or more tension sutures (Vol. I, Fig. 85), or preferably, by wire plate sutures (Fig. 6). The needle enters the skin several centimeters from the one wound edge, pierces the remaining layers of the abdominal wall, and emerges in the wound edge just at the free margin of the peritoneum, and is then passed through the other wound edge in the reverse order. One or more sutures are applied at intervals in this manner. The abdominal wall, with the exception of the skin, is then united in the usual manner by interrupted sutures. In so doing, care must be taken to see that an interrupted suture passes **beneath** each wire suture, because otherwise there would exist the danger that a portion of gut would be included when the wire is subsequently drawn taut. As soon as the abdominal wound exclusive of the skin has been closed, the wire sutures are tightened and secured as described in Vol. I, page 92. The skin edges are then sutured.

Complete primary closure of the abdominal cavity after a laparotomy should always be practised unless definite contraindications exist. Only if an active source of infection remains, or if the line of suture of a hollow viscus is uncertain, or if a bleeding area has been packed, is the abdominal wound left sufficiently open to permit the egress of drains or tampons. The fact that peritonitis is discovered on opening the abdomen, or that soiling of the peritoneum occurred during the operation, is in itself no absolute indication for drainage, so long as it is possible to close the source of infection with certainty before the closure of the abdominal wound. (Whether drainage is or is not essential in the individual case must be left to the operator's experience and judgment. I. S. R.). Drainage entails a number of dangers and disadvantages.

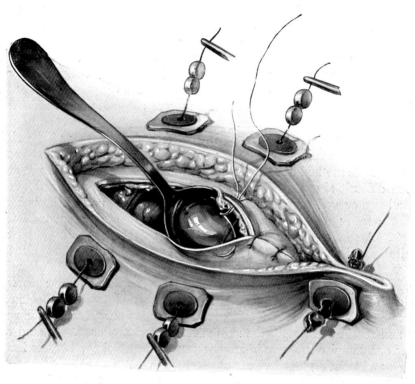

FIG. 6.   Wire tension sutures.   Several wire sutures are passed through all the layers of the abdominal wall and are provided with metal discs and lead shot but are not made taut.   The abdominal wound is closed by interrupted silk sutures through all layers except the skin, after which the wire tension sutures are made taut and fastened.   Error in illustration: The interrupted silk suture must be passed **beneath, not above** the wire suture, since otherwise there is danger that a viscus may be caught when the wire is eventually pulled tight.

The resultant defect in the wound can only heal secondarily by granulation and therefore frequently gives rise to the development of ventral herniation. There is the additional danger of infection of the whole wound, which again can predispose to incisional hernia. Drains are frequently the cause of postoperative intestinal obstruction. The proximity of a drain or tampon furthermore materially increases the likelihood of the breakdown of an insecure suture line of a hollow viscus. These facts have acted in the direction of a more and more restricted use of drainage and tamponade of the peritoneal cavity. If drainage cannot be avoided, its extent is restricted as far as possible, and the objects used are removed as soon as feasible. Further details concerning drainage and tamponade will be discussed in the section on suppurative peritonitis.

The natural approach to the abdominal cavity is through its anterior wall. The incisions are made in the midline or to the side, depending upon the position of the diseased organ.   The farther the incisions extend to the side, the more are they likely to involve the posterior abdominal wall.   The approach through the posterior wall, however, is greatly limited by the costal margin and the crest of the ilium.   It is nevertheless often possible to gain an adequate view of and access to the interior of the abdomen from behind and the side by carefully utilizing the space here available, as in the diagonal kidney incision.   The posterior incision, lumbar laparotomy (Haertel) is rarely used as a routine measure but is reserved for drainage, for the evacuation of abscesses located posteriorly, and very occasionally for laparotomies in case of a mistake in the diagnosis.   The technique of this incision has been described under operations on the kidney.   (In such instances the editor feels that closure of the posterior incision followed by an anterior incision correctly placed is much more advisable.   I. S. R.)

C. THE MEDIAN LONGITUDINAL INCISION

One of the most important prerequisites of an abdominal incision, as already emphasized, is that it should lead directly to the suspected site of disease.   Since several abdominal organs, whose location in different individuals is fairly similar, require operative treatment with particular frequency, and since the disease processes for the most part require fairly similar operative measures, a number of constantly recurring "typical" incisions have been developed.

Also for those intra-abdominal conditions whose origin we are unable to diagnose prior to the laparotomy, or those which are not confined to any closely delimited region, a number of characteristic incisions are in use.   They are based above all upon good exposure and the possibility of enlargement. The incision which best meets these requirements, the incision which gives the best access to all the organs situated near the midline of the abdomen (stomach, pancreas, transverse colon, small intestine, female genitalia, rectum) and which therefore is most generally used, is the longitudinal incision in the midline.

The skin is divided exactly in the midline, which is usually easily discernible by the pigmentation present in this area.   As soon as the skin edges gape, pronged retractors are inserted into the right and the left wound edge, and these are pulled outward and upward so that the skin and the subcutaneous fatty tissue are lifted off the subjacent connective tissue (Vol. I, Fig. 46).   The subcutaneous connective tissue and the fibrous expanse of the linea alba can then be split with a single cut to the full extent of the skin incision.   By means of marked lateral and upward pull on the retractors the aponeurosis is forced against the scalpel, while the slack peritoneum avoids the scalpel and thereby escapes the danger of being divided at the same time. The operator and the assistant each grasp the exposed peritoneum with a toothed forceps and elevate it.   As soon as a small opening is made in the peritoneum between the two forceps, air rushes into the abdominal cavity and the peritoneum can be lifted off the viscera as they move back and forth with respiration, permitting incision of the peritoneum without injury to the viscera. (The intraperitoneal pressure is, under ordinary conditions, subatmospheric. I. S. R.) Bleeding vessels are caught and ligated as the incision is made. The incision is everywhere extended down into the peritoneum.

Many operators immediately grasp the edges of the peritoneum with Mikulicz forceps at intervals of about 5 cm., in order to prevent its alleged tendency to retract, a measure which to me seems unnecessary. The attached forceps often impede the access to the wound and I have never had any difficulty in finding the peritoneal edges at the time of closure.

It is advisable to exercise care from the beginning in the permanent control of bleeding from the cut abdominal wall, lest blood continue to trickle into the open cavity during the entire operation.

The median longitudinal incision permits the opening of the abdominal cavity from the ensiform process to the symphysis. If the umbilicus falls within the range of the incision, I purposely cut right through its center in order later to eliminate the umbilical hernia present in so many persons. Before closure of the abdomen, the skin of the umbilicus must be separated for some distance from the aponeurosis by sharp dissection. Most operators, however, curve the incision around the umbilicus, 1 cm. to the left if the site of the disease is more to the left, a similar distance to the right if the lesion is chiefly to the right of the umbilicus.

I routinely maintain the separation of the edges of the median abdominal incision by means of the self-retaining retractor illustrated on page 76 of Volume I. I can scarcely imagine serene abdominal surgery without the use of this aid which I have long since found indispensable.

In case of uncertainty as to the site of the disease, only a small incision is made at first in the region of the suspected focus of disease. After one has become oriented as to its location, the incision is enlarged in the required direction of the midline or by a transverse incision.

If, after opening the abdomen, it becomes evident that the lesion is not sufficiently accessible from the median incision, then a transverse incision can be made at any desired point; or if need be, to both sides. The transverse incision is carried successively through skin, anterior rectus sheath, rectus muscle, posterior rectus sheath, transversalis fascia, and peritoneum. If the transverse incision does not suffice, it may be extended beyond the outer border of the rectus through the lateral abdominal muscles, which are preferably to be divided parallel to the course of their fibers.

Under ordinary circumstances I close the median longitudinal incision in the following manner (Fig. 4). The peritoneum, the transversalis fascia, and the aponeurosis are jointly united by interrupted sutures, alternating as a rule two catgut sutures with one silk suture. After the abdomen has been closed, the outer layers of the aponeurosis and then the fascia are sutured with interrupted catgut sutures so placed that each suture lies between a pair of deep sutures. The skin wound is then closed. In certain instances the suture of the median incision is strengthened by using only silk as the suture material or by wire tension sutures in the manner described on page 11.

If the median incision was enlarged by a transverse incision, then this is closed first. In so doing, care must be taken that the tips of the right-angled abdominal wall flaps are brought into exact apposition. Not until after the closure of the transverse incision is the median incision sutured. In the closure of transverse incisions, tier or layer suture is preferred. The transversely divided recti cannot of course be sutured separately, since the sutures will cut out of the muscle tissue. Aside from the skin, one can therefore suture only two or at most three layers, posterior rectus sheath with transversalis fascia and peritoneum, and anterior rectus sheath with muscle and occasionally the

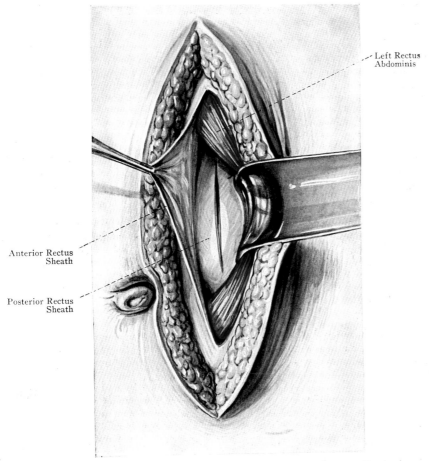

Left Rectus
Abdominis

Anterior Rectus
Sheath

Posterior Rectus
Sheath

FIG. 7. Paramedian rectus incision. The anterior sheath of the left rectus has been opened, the muscle has been retracted outward, the posterior rectus sheath has been incised.

superficial fascia. The V-sutures which have been recommended for suturing the recti possess no advantage over the usual interrupted sutures.

Experience has shown that occasionally postoperative prolapse or postoperative ventral hernia develops after the median longitudinal incision. This fact is not surprising if we bear in mind the prerequisites previously enumerated as necessary for the security of abdominal wall suture.

To be sure, the condition that the minimum of nerve fibers be injured is fulfilled by the midline incision. But this incision divides the attachments of the lateral abdominal muscles, for the linea alba is nothing more than the fusion and the insertion of the aponeuroses of these muscles. After the closure of this aponeurotic layer, both suture line and scar are placed under very unfavorable mechanical conditions. This state of affairs is all the more disadvantageous since only a single strong resistant layer is present in the midline.

When it is necessary to open the abdomen near the midline, we can try to avoid the disadvantages of the midline incision in one of three ways:

(a) by a parallel, lateral displacement of the incision and the use of "curtain" incisions at a point where the abdominal wall has more layers;

(b) by abandoning longitudinal incisions in favor of those dividing all layers transversely to the body axis;

(c) by gridiron incisions which divide the individual layers of the wall in different directions and parallel to their respective lines of tension.

D. THE PARAMEDIAN RECTUS INCISION (LENNANDER)

The skin, subcutaneous connective tissue and the anterior rectus sheath are divided 1½ to 2 cm. from the medial border of the right or left rectus. The 2 cm.-wide strip of the anterior rectus sheath to the medial side of the

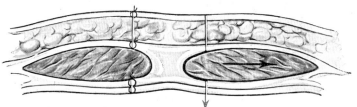

Fig. 8. Diagrammatic cross-section through the central portion of the anterior abdominal wall, showing course and suture of the paramedian rectus incision.

incision is separated from the subjacent muscle until the free edge of the latter appears. This requires dissection at the lineae transversae. The medial edge of the rectus is freed from its bed for a short distance and is drawn outward by means of a retractor. The exposed posterior rectus sheath and the peritoneum are divided about 2 cm. laterally from the medial border of the rectus sheath (Fig. 7).

The wound is sutured in three layers: (1) joint suture of the peritoneum and posterior rectus sheath, replacement of the muscle which returns of its own accord to its old bed over this suture line; (2) suture of the anterior rectus sheath; (3) skin suture (Fig. 8).

E. THE LATERAL RECTUS INCISION (LENNANDER)
THE WAVE INCISION (KEHR)

The lateral rectus incision is performed according to practically the same technique as the paramedian incision, except that the approach to the abdominal cavity is at the lateral instead of the medial border of the rectus muscle. The skin and the anterior rectus sheath are incised about 2 cm. within the lateral margin of the rectus. In muscular individuals we can recognize the contour of the recti under the skin or can feel their edges. Otherwise, one must remember that in diastasis of the recti their lateral margins are quite far out to the side, and that these lateral margins curve decidedly outward from the symphysis to the costal border, so that they are much farther from the midline in the upper half of the abdomen than in the lower.

We incise the skin along the surmised position of the lateral border of the rectus and then expose the aponeurosis until the outer border of the rectus sheath comes into view. The rectus sheath is incised 1 cm. medial to its

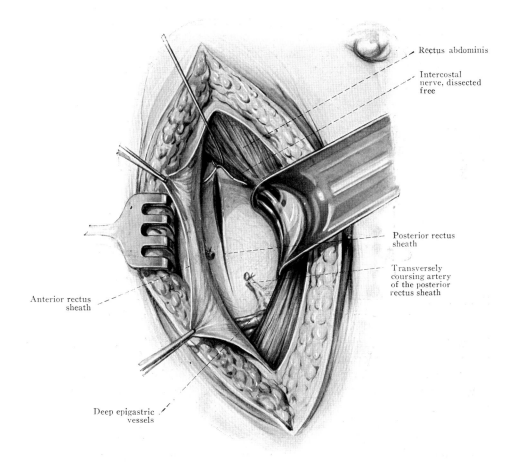

Rectus abdominis

Intercostal
nerve, dissected
free

Posterior rectus
sheath

Transversely
coursing artery
of the posterior
rectus sheath

Anterior rectus
sheath

Deep epigastric
vessels

FIG. 9. Lateral rectus incision. The anterior rectus sheath has been opened and the rectus muscle retracted medially. An intercostal nerve has been dissected free in the upper angle of the wound and held aside by a nerve retractor. An artery running transversely has been doubly ligated and cut. The posterior rectus sheath has been incised.

lateral border throughout the extent of the skin incision (Fig. 10a). The centimeter-wide lateral strip of the anterior rectus sheath is separated outward from the subjacent muscle, using dissection at the lineae transversae. After the lateral edge of the muscle has been exposed, the muscle is freed from the posterior rectus sheath, beginning at the lateral edge. In so doing, the inter-costal nerves which enter the muscle from behind and their accompanying vessels come into view as they pass diagonally medially and downward. The vessels are ligated while the nerves should be spared if possible. With this in view they are freed and drawn upward or downward beyond the confines of the incision by means of a nerve retractor or a thread (Fig. 9). Such displacement of the nerves is of course possible for only a limited distance. In very long incisions, one or two nerves must be sacrificed, which is not usually a matter of great significance. The posterior rectus sheath which has been exposed in this manner, the transversalis fascia and the peritoneum are divided 1 or 2 cm. within the lateral edge of the rectus sheath.

The closure of the wound is attempted in a three tier suture. Since the posterior rectus sheath is absent below the semilunar line of Douglas, the sutures may have a tendency to cut through the transversalis fascia and the peritoneum. Under these circumstances one should not tarry long, but use through and through sutures which catch the anterior rectus sheath, the outer edge of the rectus muscle, the transversalis fascia and the peritoneum on the one side and the same layers with the exception of the muscle on the other. Over this suture line the anterior rectus sheath is again sutured separately. The skin is then sutured.

If it becomes necessary to extend the incision downward to near the pubis, the deep epigastric vessels will be encountered as they course from lateral and

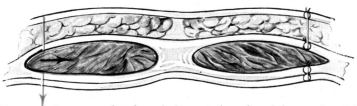

FIG. 10a. Diagrammatic cross-section through the central portion of the anterior abdominal wall showing the course and the suture of a lateral rectus incision.

below to medial and above on the transversalis fascia. The artery and two veins are carefully freed, doubly ligated and divided.

The costal margin-lateral rectus incision. If the incision must be extended upward farther than the costal margin, then as soon as it approaches the costal margin it is deviated toward the midline and is continued parallel to, and at a distance of 1 to 2 cm. from the costal arch, if need be, as far as the ensiform process. In so doing, the skin, the anterior rectus sheath, the rectus itself and the posterior rectus sheath with the peritoneum are divided (Fig. 10b). With the formation of an obtuse angle the incision thus becomes the medial part of a costal margin incision. I prefer this incision in gallbladder operations. At times it may suffice to mobilize the muscle without dividing it and to pull it aside.

If the rectus muscle is divided, then in closing the wound the rectus sheaths must be carefully sutured. The muscle itself is not sutured, since the sutures will tend to cut through anyway.

If the incision is extended laterally, one divides the skin and splits the three transverse muscles here encountered in the direction of the course of their fibers.

I do not advise the "direct" lateral rectus incision which divides the skin and the tendinous pararectal line in the same plane without opening the rectus sheath. It divides all the intercostal nerves leading to the rectus muscle in the region of the incision and it affords no overlapping of layers in the subsequent suture.

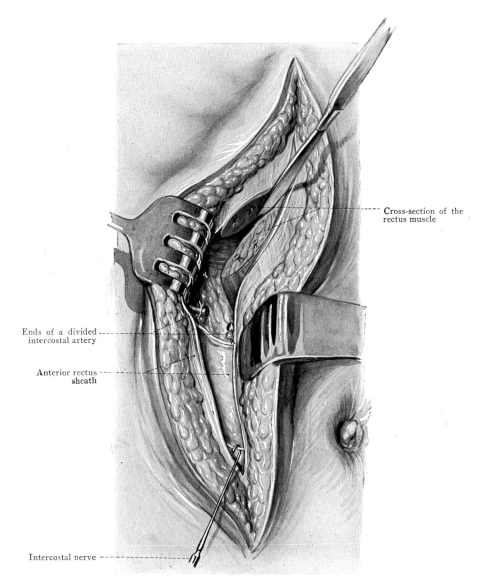

Cross-section of the rectus muscle

Ends of a divided
intercostal artery

Anterior rectus
sheath

Intercostal nerve

FIG. 10b. Combined costal margin and lateral rectus incision. The incision runs from the xiphoid process, parallel to and at a distance of 1 cm. from the costal margin, to the lateral border of the rectus and then downward for some distance along the edge of the rectus. The anterior sheath of the rectus is split, the lateral border of the rectus is exposed, the muscle is separated from its posterior sheath after dividing an intercostal vessel and retracting two intercostal nerves. The rectus muscle is cut across close to its attachment to the costal margin.

The Wave Incision (Kehr). A combination of the lateral rectus incision with the supra-umbilical midline incision by cutting across the rectus diagonally constitutes the wave incision of Kehr or Z-incision. It divides the abdominal wall in the midline from the ensiform process about half way to the umbilicus, then turns diagonally outward as far as the lateral border

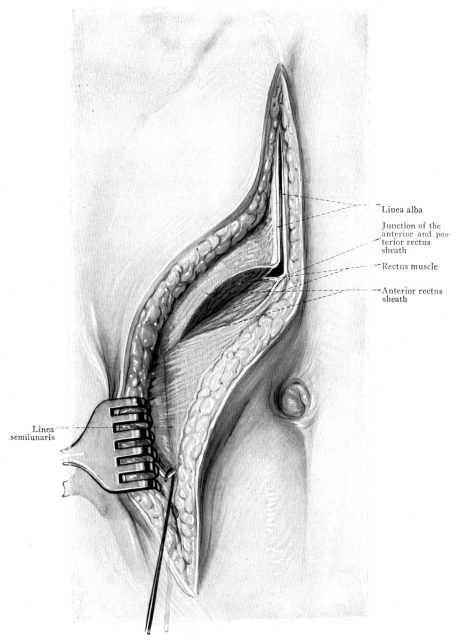

Linea alba

Junction of the anterior and posterior rectus sheath

Rectus muscle

Anterior rectus sheath

Linea semilunaris

FIG. 11. Kehr incision. The incision extends in the midline from the xiphoid process to a point midway between xiphoid and umbilicus, passes diagonally across the rectus muscle to its lateral border and ends as a lateral rectus incision. The linea alba and the anterior rectus sheath have been incised.

of the rectus (usually the right), dividing the rectus and its sheath, and then continues for a variable distance as a lateral rectus incision (Fig. 11). It was recommended by Kehr as the best incision for gall bladder operations but has recently lost much of its popularity.

F. THE MEDIAN TRANSVERSE INCISION (SPRENGEL, HEUSSNER)
THE FISH-HOOK INCISION (KIRSCHNER)

The Median Transverse Incision. Based on the assumption that the longitudinal pull of the recti is materially weaker and less important than the horizontal pull of the lateral abdominal muscles, this incision shows no consideration for the recti but divides them at right angles to the course of their fibers. The skin is divided from the lateral edge of one rectus to the lateral edge of the other, and all the subjacent layers are divided in the direction and to the full extent of the skin incision. The structures divided are the anterior rectus sheath, rectus muscle, posterior rectus sheath and peritoneum on each side, and the aponeurosis of the linea alba with the peritoneum in the middle. If the incision is inadequate, it can be extended laterally beyond the lateral edges of the recti by splitting the oblique abdominal muscles as far as possible in the course of their fibers.

The individual layers of the abdominal wall are sutured separately as far as possible. However, since suture of muscle alone is not satisfactory, it is generally necessary to include the muscle and the anterior rectus sheath in the same suture. In spite of its theoretical advantages, the transverse incision has not as yet succeeded in being generally adopted.

The Fish-Hook Incision. The fish-hook incision proposed by me may be considered a variation of the median transverse incision. It is serviceable when the operation involves the thoracic and abdominal cavities at the same time;—thoraco-laparotomy. The patient lies in the semi-right-lateral position with the head elevated. A positive-pressure apparatus is kept at hand. The line of the skin incision in thorax and abdomen is marked with a dye. The incision begins at a point one-third of the distance down from the ensiform to the umbilicus, passes diagonally outward across the left rectus to the left costal margin which it meets a little above the point where the seventh intercostal space is closed by the costal margin. The incision is continued in the direction of this intercostal space to the region of the angle of the rib and the lower angle of the scapula. The whole incision is thereby given the shape of a fish-hook, the shank of which lies over the thorax, and whose barbed end is in the region of the abdomen. The abdominal cavity is opened by deepening that part of the incision, in doing which the left rectus is divided.

The soft tissues of the seventh intercostal space are also divided layer by layer in the full extent of the skin incision until the transparent parietal pleura is everywhere exposed. Before the pleura is opened positive intratracheal pressure is started. With the insertion of a rib-spreader into the seventh intercostal space this space is spread as much as possible. Its further spread is prevented, aside from the attachment of the ribs to the spine, by their attachment to the costal margin in front. This obstacle is removed by inserting a blunt instrument beneath that part of the costal margin which bounds the seventh interspace in front and separates it from the abdominal incision. In

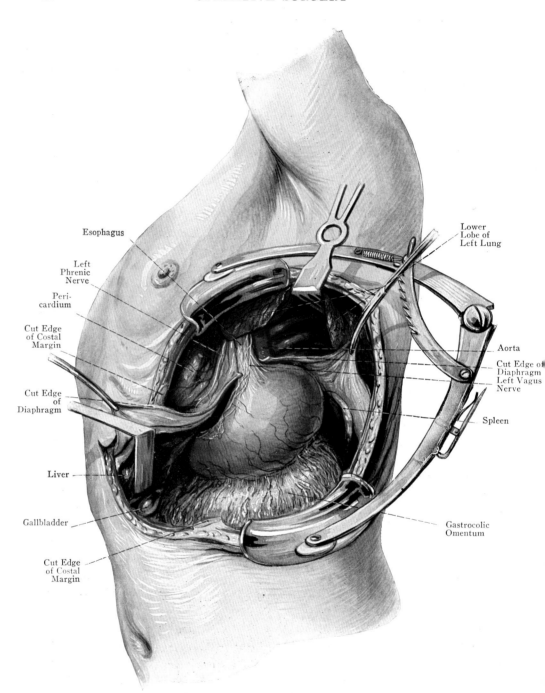

Esophagus

Left
Phrenic
Nerve

Peri-
cardium

Cut Edge
of Costal
Margin

Cut Edge
of
Diaphragm

Liver

Gallbladder

Cut Edge
of Costal
Margin

Lower
Lobe of
Left Lung

Aorta

Cut Edge of
Diaphragm
Left Vagus
Nerve

Spleen

Gastrocolic
Omentum

FIG. 12. Kirschner incision. Thoracolaparotomy. A transverse abdominal incision dividing the left rectus has been continued through the 7th intercostal space into the thorax, dividing the costal arch in the line of the incision. The diaphragm is split radially as far as the esophageal foramen, so that a wide approach to the lower left thoracic and the upper left abdominal cavity is afforded.

so doing the insertion of the diaphragm at this point is freed from the costal margin by blunt dissection. The costal margin is then divided with a costotome. This completes the free communication between the thoracic and the abdominal incision. The division of the costal cartilage closing the seventh intercostal space is to be regarded as the key to the thoracotomy.

The seventh interspace now gapes to a surprising degree if the rib-spreader is opened wide and it affords an excellent view into the left thoracic cavity, the upper abdominal cavity and to both sides of the diaphragm separating these two cavities. If the diaphragm is now divided in a radial direction as far as the esophageal foramen (Fig. 12), an excellent approach to the thoracic and abdominal cavities is provided, permitting almost unrestricted access to the lower segment of the esophagus, the cardia and the upper portion of the stomach.

If necessary the short limb of the fish-hook incision can be extended as far as the right costal margin by dividing the right rectus. This materially widens the approach to the upper abdomen.

If in dividing the soft tissues of the seventh interspace one avoids opening the parietal pleura but frees it from the inner surface of the chest wall by blunt dissection in a manner similar to that later described for the insertion of an extrapleural pack, this incision after cutting the costal arch affords an excellent approach to the highest part of the left upper abdomen, especially to the fundus of the stomach, the abdominal esophagus and the under surface of the left diaphragm. In such a case the incision need be carried only a short distance along the thoracic wall.

G. THE MEDIAN GRIDIRON INCISION (TRANSVERSE APONEUROSIS INCISION OF PFANNENSTIEL)

In a gridiron incision every structure as it is encountered is either divided in its line of cleavage or is pushed aside uninjured. The suprapubic aponeurosis incision is used with preference by some gynecologists for the approach to the pelvis. The median gridiron incision can, however, be used at any other level in the midline of the abdomen.

The skin, the subcutaneous tissues and the full breadth of the right and left anterior rectus sheaths are divided by a transverse incision, which in the suprapubic area is made two fingers' breadth above the symphysis. The two cut edges are freed upward and downward as extensively as possible from the fleshy substance of the recti and, under certain circumstances, from the pyramidalis muscles. This is done as a single aponeurotic flap (Fig. 13), in that the aponeurosis in the midline (linea alba) is split by sharp dissection into a reflected anterior layer and a residual posterior layer. The exposed recti are freed from the transversalis fascia by blunt dissection from the midline to right and left and are retracted lateralward with blunt muscle retractors (Fig. 14). The broad expanse of the transversalis fascia, which now presents, is opened together with the peritoneum in the midline.

In closing the wound, the layers are sutured separately in the line of their division.

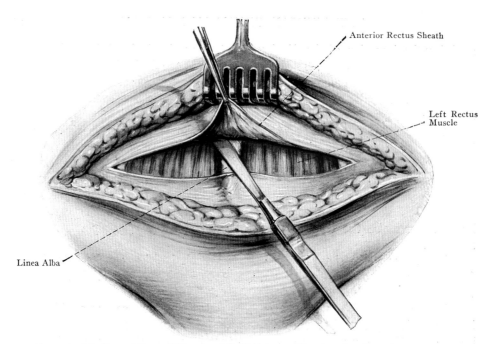

Anterior Rectus Sheath

Left Rectus Muscle

Linea Alba

FIG. 13. Median gridiron (Pfannenstiel) incision. The anterior rectus sheath is opened transversely above the symphysis. Its upper segment is dissected free from the two recti muscles and from the linea alba.

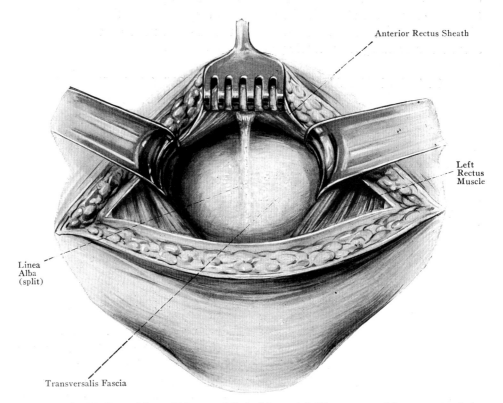

Anterior Rectus Sheath

Left Rectus Muscle

Linea Alba (split)

Transversalis Fascia

FIG. 14. Median gridiron (Pfannenstiel) incision. (2) The upper and lower parts of the anterior rectus sheath have been dissected free, both recti muscles have been drawn outward by retractors. The transversalis fascia and the posterior layer of the linea alba, which has been split in the frontal plane, are exposed.

H. THE LATERAL GRIDIRON INCISION
(McBURNEY-SPRENGEL)

The right lateral gridiron incision is used especially in operations for disease of the appendix. It affords convenient access to the cecum, and in the left hypogastrium, to the sigmoid.

The skin incision is made in the direction of the fibers of the external oblique muscle, bearing in mind that in the hypogastrium this muscle drops steeply at an acute angle to Poupart's (inguinal) ligament. The incision

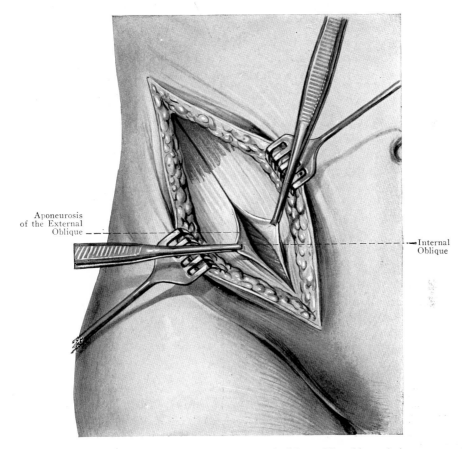

Aponeurosis of the External Oblique

Internal Oblique

FIG. 15. Lateral gridiron (McBurney-Sprengel) incision. The skin and the aponeurosis of the external oblique muscle have been divided, the latter along the course of its fibers, and the muscle substance of the internal oblique is exposed.

should not be made at too great a distance from the anterior superior iliac spine, but only 1 to 3 cm. to its medial side, with about one-third of the incision above, and two-thirds below this point. The length of the skin incision depends upon the extent of the disease process to be attacked and upon the thickness of the abdominal wall. In general, one cannot warn enough against skimping in the length of the skin incision (beware of the buttonhole incision). As a rule the incision should be not less than 6 cm. long.

After dividing the subcutaneous connective tissue, the course of the fibers of the external oblique can be recognized (Fig. 15). As a rule, the region of the incision includes the transition of the muscular portion into the aponeurosis, so that in cutting the muscle in the direction of its fibers to the full extent of the skin incision we cut partly through muscle (where several blood vessels must be ligated) and partly through aponeurosis. The margins of the divided external oblique are grasped with tissue forceps (Fig. 16) and separated from the internal oblique beneath, by means of both blunt and sharp

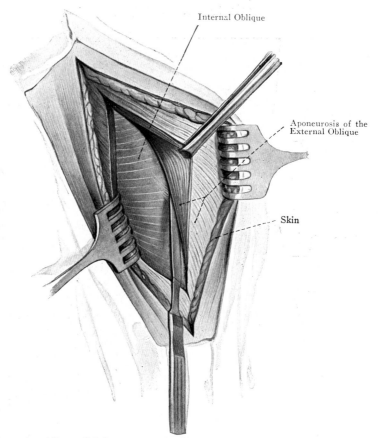

Internal Oblique

Aponeurosis of the External Oblique

Skin

Fig. 16. Lateral gridiron (McBurney-Sprengel) incision. (2) The aponeurosis of the external oblique is separated from the muscle substance of the internal oblique by sharp dissection.

dissection. It is important to carry out this separation quite extensively so that to the medial side the semilunar line of Spigelius appears, which for the time being limits the dissection. The freed edges of the external oblique are then pulled aside by pronged retractors so that the wound is wide open, and the horizontal fibers of the internal oblique are exposed for a considerable distance. This muscle is then split at the midpoint of the external wound and parallel to the direction of the muscle fibers (Fig. 17). The transversalis muscle beneath, whose fibers run in nearly the same direction, is split at the same time. This splitting is best begun with a knife at a point close to the line of Spigelius in the aponeurotic portion of the muscle between two toothed forceps with which the aponeurosis has been picked up. The knife is carried from the medial toward the lateral side of the incision. A branch of the circumflex iliac artery is often divided and must be ligated. The further separation of the muscle fibers can be effected by gentle blunt dissection with two forceps. As soon as the transversalis fascia is exposed for a sufficient distance, it is picked up with two tissue forceps (Fig. 18) and is incised in the direction

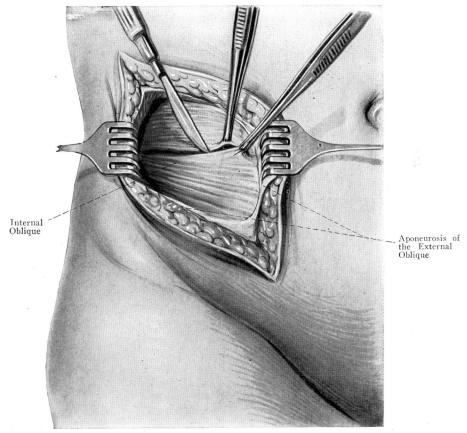

Internal
Oblique

Aponeurosis of
the External
Oblique

Fig. 17. Lateral gridiron (McBurney-Sprengel) incision. (3) The aponeurosis of the external oblique has been retracted and the internal oblique and transversalis muscles are split with the knife in the direction of their fibers.

of the internal oblique and transversalis muscles. This exposes the peritoneum which is then picked up with two forceps and cut between them in the same or in the opposite direction. Into the resultant opening are placed two blunt retractors, the two hooked retractors being removed. Forceful retraction produces a large rectangular wound (Fig. 19).

Enlarging the Incision. If the opening so made is not adequate, it may be enlarged in the following manner: A transverse incision is made in the aponeurosis of the external oblique on the medial side of the wound, at the level and in the direction of the line of incision in the internal oblique, enlarging the skin incision if necessary. The incision at first is carried only a short distance medially to the lateral edge of the rectus, but if need be it can be extended to the linea alba or even to the lateral edge of the rectus of the opposite side. At the semilunar line of Spigelius the aponeurosis of the external oblique, which here becomes the anterior rectus sheath, is dissected free both upward and downward for some distance with the knife, so that a part of the anterior surface of the rectus muscle is exposed. The muscle is freed from its bed and is retracted toward the midline (Fig. 20). The transversalis

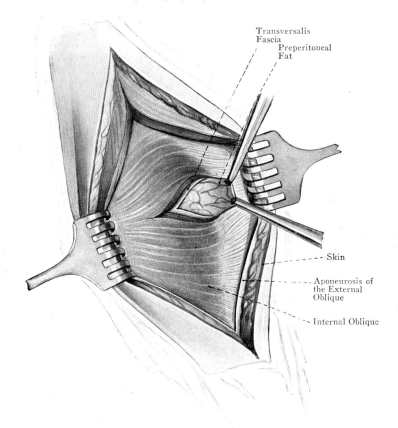

Fig. 18. Lateral gridiron (McBurney-Sprengel) incision. (4) The internal oblique and transversalis muscles and the transversalis fascia have been split in the direction of their fibers. The preperitoneal fat appears in the opening.

fascia and the peritoneum may now be opened further by extending the original incisions. The retractor holding the rectus muscle is now made to include the peritoneum as well.

Should this opening still be too small, the rectus itself may be divided, and the incision extended through all layers to the midline. In an emergency the incision may be extended to the lateral edge of the opposite rectus. (The incision may also be enlarged by cutting across the fibers of the internal oblique and transversalis in the direction of the symphysis pubis or upward toward the costal margin. When this is done it is possible to gain access to the pelvis especially on the right side or to the ascending colon as far as the hepatic flexure. I. S. R.)

Closure of the Incision. I suture the gridiron incision in three layers, using as a rule catgut, except for the skin where clips are usually used. To facilitate the insertion of the deep sutures, pronged retractors are inserted at the midpoints of the lateral and the medial cut margins of the external oblique muscle (Fig. 21) and the wound in the aponeurosis is separated widely. By means of blunt retractors inserted in the angles of the wound, the abdominal wall is forcibly elevated. This causes the viscera to drop into

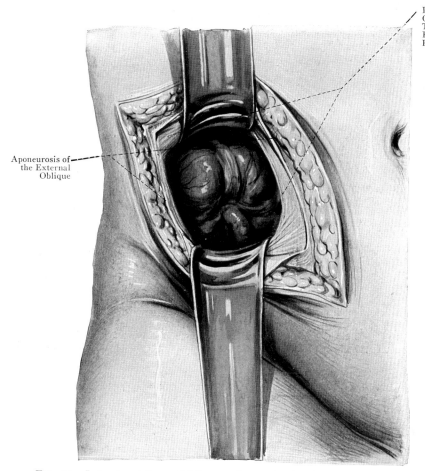

Internal
Oblique,
Transversalis
Fascia and
Peritoneum

Aponeurosis of
the External
Oblique

FIG. 19. Lateral gridiron (McBurney-Sprengel) incision. (5) All the layers of the abdominal wall have been divided and the wound is held open by retractors. The cecum and appendix are exposed.

the abdomen and the wound edges are exposed for suture. If in spite of these measures the viscera continue to protrude, a small spoon is inserted between the viscera and the parietal peritoneum. The deepest suture layer consists of interrupted sutures of #1 catgut and is carried from the medial toward the lateral angle of the wound. The first suture layer includes the peritoneum, transversalis fascia and internal oblique muscle. (If the peritoneum has been opened in the direction of the external oblique fibers the

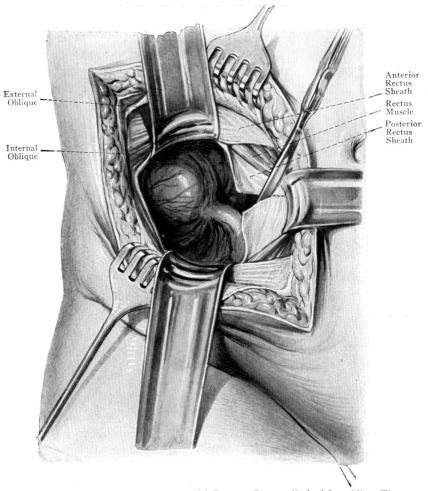

External
Oblique

Internal
Oblique

Anterior
Rectus
Sheath

Rectus
Muscle

Posterior
Rectus
Sheath

FIG. 20. Enlarging a lateral gridiron (McBurney-Sprengel) incision (6). The anterior
and the posterior rectus sheaths are incised transversely and the rectus muscle is retracted toward
the midline.

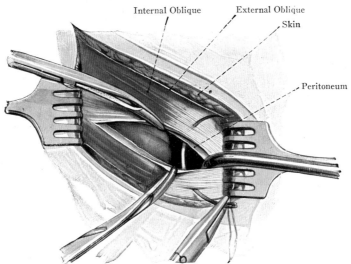

Internal Oblique   External Oblique

Skin

Peritoneum

FIG. 21. Suture of the lateral gridiron (McBurney-Sprengel) incision. (7) The inner
angle of the wound is elevated by means of a hooked retractor, the aponeurosis of the external
oblique is retracted on each side with a sharp hooked retractor. The peritoneum, the transversalis
fascia and the transversalis and internal oblique muscles are sutured jointly.

internal oblique muscle should not be included, the muscle being closed as a separate layer. I. S. R.)

The second suture layer reunites the external oblique. The third suture layer is that of the skin. Since all the layers of the abdominal wall are divided in the direction of their fibers, their edges fall nicely together, almost of their own accord, even if the patient strains.

I. THE COSTAL MARGIN INCISION. REFLECTION OF THE COSTAL MARGIN

The Costal Margin Incision. In operations on organs that lie beneath or near the costal margin (cardia or fundus of the stomach, liver, biliary tract,

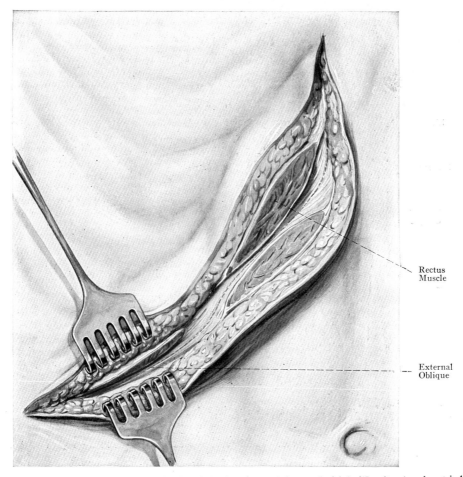

Rectus
Muscle

External
Oblique

FIG. 22. Costal margin incision. The incision, beginning at the xiphoid process and carried parallel to and below the right costal margin, has divided the skin, the anterior rectus sheath, the rectus muscle and, in part, the external oblique muscle. The posterior rectus sheath and the internal oblique muscle are exposed.

spleen), the abdomen may be opened to advantage by a curved incision along the costal arch. The incision is carried parallel to and at a distance of 1 to 2 cm. from the costal margin (Fig. 22). It may be started at the base of the ensiform process or lower, and can be carried into the flank as far as desired. If the incision approaches the midline of the abdomen, the attachment of the rectus muscle is divided more or less extensively close to the costal arch. Toward the side the oblique abdominal muscles are also divided

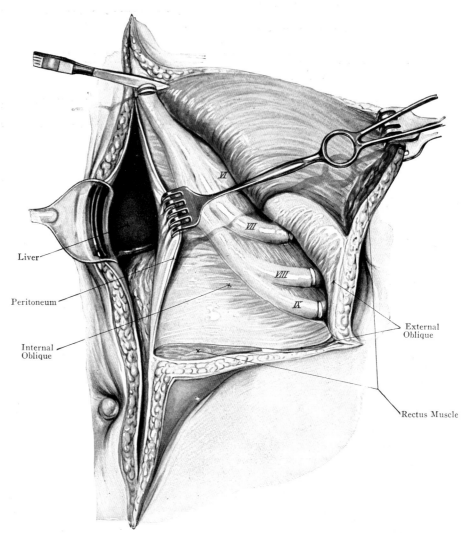

Liver

Peritoneum

Internal Oblique

External Oblique

Rectus Muscle

FIG. 23. Reflection of the left costal margin. A median laparotomy incision has been enlarged above the umbilicus by a transverse incision dividing the rectus and external oblique muscles. The upper right-angled flap of soft tissue has been dissected free, so that the anterior surfaces of the lower ribs lie exposed. The individual ribs are divided in the region of their cartilages.

by layers in the line of the incision, the division being made in the direction of the fibers as far as this is possible.

The incision is sutured in layers.

Reflection of the Costal Margin. If the operation involves an area very close to the diaphragm, the costal margin incision may be combined with actual reflection of the lower costal arch on one side. The procedure as advised by Marwedel is usually carried out as an emergency measure. The costal margin incision is at first carried only as deep as the posterior rectus sheath and through the external oblique which is attached to the ventral edge of the costal margin. The rounded muscle flap so outlined is reflected upward and outward and is dissected away from the costal margin (Fig. 23)

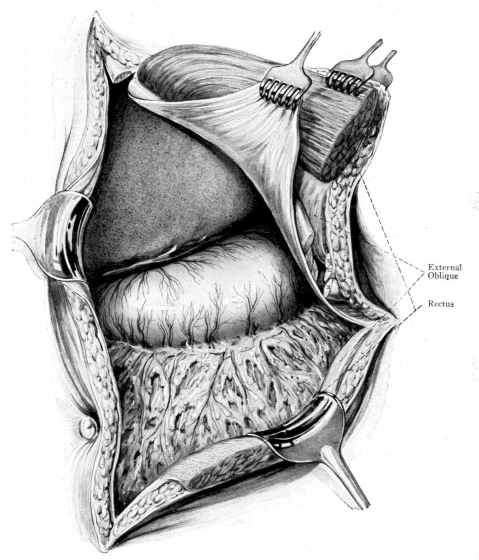

External
Oblique

Rectus

Fig. 24. Reflection of the left costal margin. (2) After the division of the ribs, the transverse incision is continued through the posterior rectus sheath and outward through the internal oblique and transversalis muscles and the peritoneum. The edges of the abdominal wound have been separated by retractors. Liver, stomach, transverse colon and greater omentum are exposed.

until the cartilages of the 6th to 9th ribs are exposed in their full extent. These cartilages are first divided close to the sternum where they are fused into a common cartilaginous plate, and again far out to the side. This division is carried out by gradually deepening the incision as far as the posterior perichondrium and excising a wedge-shaped piece. After carrying the incision in the soft parts through the peritoneum, the mobilized costal margin may be reflected lateralward and upward (Fig. 24). If this reflection is difficult, it is advisable that the costal cartilages, which were exposed in the manner described, be removed subperichondrially and extrapleurally in their full extent.

If, as is often the case, the abdomen has already been opened by a midline incision before the reflection of the costal margin and this incision has been extended to one side of the ensiform process as far as its base, then, if the left costal margin is to be reflected, a horizontal incision is made, perpendicular to the midline incision and tangent to the lower border of the left costal margin. This secondary incision reaches the costal arch at the ninth rib. It divides all the layers of the abdominal wall except the posterior rectus sheath and the internal oblique. The right-angled superficial flap of soft tissue thus outlined is dissected upward and to the left, the exposed cartilages of the 6th to 9th ribs are divided in the manner described, and finally the transverse incision is carried through all the layers of the abdominal wall.

In closing the incision, the soft parts are sutured in layers, without suture of the divided cartilages.

J. THE ISOLATION OF THE LESION DURING THE OPERATION

After opening the abdominal cavity, one of the chief concerns is to prevent contamination of the peritoneum or the spread of an existing infection to previously uninvolved parts of the abdomen. Such a contamination is probable from two major sources. In the first place, following the intentional or an accidental opening of a hollow viscus (stomach, intestine, gall bladder or urinary bladder) infectious contents may escape and flow into the open abdominal cavity. In the second place, by the freeing of encapsulating adhesions the pus of a localized suppurative process in the abdomen may be disseminated and relatively free parts of the abdominal cavity may thus become infected. Therefore, before opening any hollow viscus, or before freeing adhesions which might encapsulate a collection of pus, the area must be well isolated from the remainder of the abdominal cavity and the neighboring viscera.

The packing off of the operative field from the remainder of the abdominal cavity is, however, necessary for an additional reason. The various organs of the abdominal cavity, especially the loops of small intestine, possess a considerable degree of mobility, so that they are apt to fall into the operative field repeatedly during breathing, and particularly when the patient strains. If the operation is to be done in a clear, well visualized field, its site must be blocked off from the other abdominal organs.

The suitable position of the patient as described in Volume I is the first measure to be considered. The patient is turned on his horizontal and his long axis in such a way that undesired viscera tend to gravitate out of the operative field. This may also be aided by "extraperitonealizing" the organs to be attacked.

If the mobility of the organ permits, an attempt is made to deliver it through the abdominal incision. This is possible, however, with only a few particularly mobile organs. The most useful measure in isolating the operative field against the surrounding organs is the use of moist pads. For temporary walling-off of the abdominal cavity gauze pads and rolls described in Vol. I, pages 234 and 235, are used. In order to guard against the well-known danger of a sponge "forgotten in the abdomen" the precautions noted there are

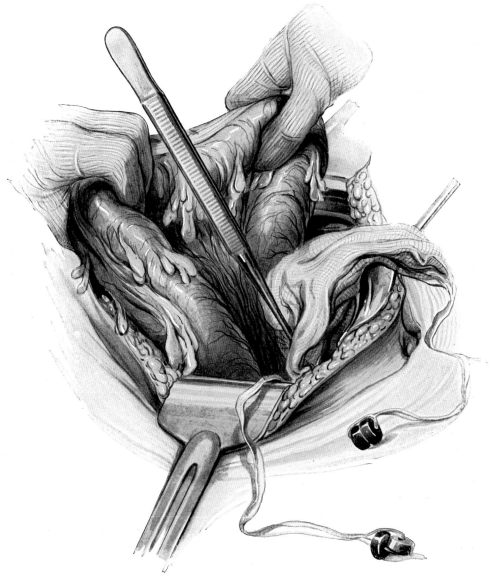

Fig. 25. Walling off the general abdominal cavity. The edges of the abdominal incision have been elevated with retractors, while the hands of an assistant hold up the viscus which is the site of operation: the transverse colon. The other viscera are being pushed back with moist compresses with the aid of an anatomic forceps.

carefully followed. Only rarely may smaller pieces of gauze or gauze sponges be introduced into the abdominal cavity even for temporary tamponade. Should this be necessary for urgent reasons in an unusual case, the small pads are secured at once by long clamps or one assistant is made solely responsible for the counting and removal of each piece. Unsecured objects are only too easily overlooked, especially when the laparotomy must be concluded hastily because of some emergency. The history of foreign bodies forgotten in the abdominal cavity is an extensive and tragic one and carries an eloquent warning. It is a matter of scant comfort and little gain if a radiopaque ring or marker discloses a forgotten pad in a subsequent roentgenogram.

The walling-off of the general abdominal cavity must be done carefully and systematically. The focus of disease is surrounded with a funnel of compresses, open only at the top, toward the operator. The abdominal walls are retracted and elevated so that the focus of disease is brought into view (Fig. 25). The surgeon grasps a gauze pad or roll at one corner with a long forceps and introduces it into the bottom of the wound, pushing back the surrounding viscera with the greatest gentleness, and continues in this manner until a complete wall of gauze has been formed around the operative field. The introduction of the moist pads, as well as their subsequent removal, must be carried out with the greatest gentleness, in order to avoid injuring the surface of the viscera, which might result in bleeding, irritation, and adhesions. If clefts or spaces are encountered in the course of walling-off, as for example the subphrenic space or the foramen of Winslow, their entrances are likewise blocked with gauze pads.

The gauze pads remain in place until the completion of the intraperitoneal part of the operation, or they may be reinforced or replaced by fresh ones during the operation, if they become soiled.

K. THE AFTER-TREATMENT OF LAPAROTOMY PATIENTS

The rules for the after-treatment of laparotomy patients were discussed in the volume on General Considerations.

Postoperative pain should be relieved immediately. In this regard, care is necessary in the use of morphine because of its paralyzing effect on peristalsis. (Recently some question has arisen as to whether morphine actually does paralyze peristalsis. I. S. R.) Eukodol is less harmful in this respect, but causes vomiting in many patients. The use of spinal anaesthesia with nupercain frequently saves the patient from any severe postoperative pain because of the long duration of its analgesic action. (I have recently used Dilaudid with excellent results especially in restlessness. Pitressin frequently will give relief from "gas" pains. I. S. R.)

Postoperative pain may also be materially lessened or abolished by the injection of the parietal peritoneum in the region of the abdominal wound from within with nupercain solution just before closure of the wound. This can be carried out in a few seconds by means of a high-pressure local-anaesthesia apparatus such as I have recommended. (Nupercain is a powerful anesthetic and should be used very sparingly. I. S. R.)

Except in peritonitis the suppression of peristalsis by opiates as formerly practiced has been discarded in my clinic in favor of the stimulation of intestinal activity. There is no need even after intestinal suture of putting the intestinal tract completely at rest, for experience has shown that intestinal sutures when properly applied in normal tissue possess adequate holding power. It is our rule, except after operations on the large bowel, that every laparotomy patient receives a low enema of 50 to 100 cc. of glycerin and water, in equal parts, every morning beginning with the second day after operation if spontaneous evacuation does not occur. If gas is not passed spontaneously, a soft rectal tube is inserted for a few hours, a procedure which is more sparing and just as effective as stretching the rectal sphincter at the end of a laparotomy which some have advised. If these measures are not successful, we employ high enemata of soap and water. If this treatment fails, I do not hesitate, even in the presence of entero-anastomoses, to give cathartics by mouth on the second day. Hypodermatic injections of pituitrin (1 cc. two or three times a day) are an excellent means of stimulating peristalsis. Hypodermatic injections of physostigmin are also useful for this purpose. If these substances are not effective when used subcutaneously, they are given intravenously, pituitrin especially in the manner advised by A. Mayer. A solution of 5 ampoules in 1 liter of normal saline is allowed to flow very slowly into a vein until a bowel movement occurs. Heating of the abdominal wall is usually well tolerated. It warms patients who are chilled and in collapse, and often stimulates peristalsis appreciably.

I see no justification for the routine use of castor oil immediately and at intervals after operation ("castor-oil treatment of laparotomy patients") as has frequently been advised in gastro-intestinal cases, especially after operations on the large intestine. I believe that a healthy individual would have his sense of well-being decidedly impaired by such a practice, let alone a laparotomized patient.

In spite of these measures, serious manifestations of ileus may develop after a laparotomy, with abdominal distension, hiccough and, finally, vomiting. The chief problem then is to determine whether the condition is merely functional or whether it is due to some more tangible cause. If there exists a mechanical obstruction the patient must be reopened at once. The abdomen must also be reopened when peritonitis develops and there is the prospect that the source of infection can be isolated or removed. The manifestations and the treatment of postoperative acute dilatation of the stomach and of arterio-mesenteric intestinal obstruction are described in Vol. I, page 48. Attention is again called to the advantages, there described, of continuous drainage of the stomach by an indwelling tube with suction attached. This may be effected by means of a small tube (duodenal tube, Jutte tube) passed through the mouth or the nose.

The dependability of intestinal sutures would of itself give us a free hand in the matter of food intake after operation. Nevertheless, bearing in mind postoperative vomiting, it is wise to restrict fluid ingestion in the first few days and to give water preferably by bowel or parenterally. It is our practice to give every laparotomy patient a rectal drip, except after rectal or colon operations.

Furthermore, as a rule, no solid food should be given to a patient in the first week after a gastric resection, but there is no reason why after the first few days he should not be given moderate portions of liquids, and, after this a soft diet in small amounts. Patients with suture or anastomosis involving the small or large intestine, should avoid all heavy foods with bulky residue, but they may take liquids as early as the day after operation. The early administration of fluids and nourishment to greatly weakened patients can be a life-saving measure.

The great value of the free administration of fluids (saline and glucose) by intravenous infusion and of blood transfusion to seriously dehydrated patients should be borne in mind. The technique of these procedures was discussed in the first volume.

Morphine should be used very sparingly in patients after an abdominal operation; the drug seems to favor the occurrence of postoperative gastric or intestinal atony. Eukodol is to be preferred if narcotics cannot be avoided.

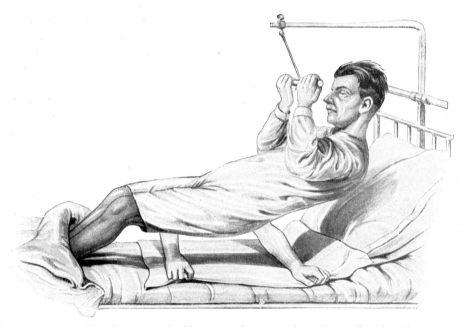

FIG. 26. Overhead bar by means of which the patient can raise and exercise himself and assist the nurse in arranging the bedding.

(I find myself unable to agree with the preceding statements. Morphine has a definite place in abdominal surgery. I. S. R.)

The postoperative measures described in Volume I, pages 41-48, for the prevention of complications involving the respiratory tract and of thrombosis and embolism are to be applied with particular care after abdominal operations. Increased attention should be paid especially to changing the position of the patient and to the early use of breathing exercises. A "gallows" (Fig. 26) attached to the head of the bed is especially serviceable since by means of this the patient can change his position himself very soon after the operation and can use it for certain indicated exercises. In addition, the "gallows" renders a welcome service to the nursing staff by making possible the active cooperation of the patient during rearrangement of the bedding.

L. POSTOPERATIVE INTESTINAL PROLAPSE. THE REOPENING OF THE ABDOMINAL CAVITY

Without any visible error at the time of closure of the abdominal wall, the closure may not hold and intestinal prolapse may occur at any time within two or even three weeks after the operation. Cachectic patients, especially those with extensive carcinomata and attendant ascites, patients who have had gastric operations and patients with excessive cough are most liable to this unpleasant and serious complication. Frequently an infection of the wound is the actual cause of the giving way of the suture line. The complication occurs most often in midline laparotomy wounds. It may occur without alarming manifestations. The patients in whom this has taken place may not suffer pain. They become conscious of the wound dressings becoming wet or they may actually see intestinal loops protruding from beneath the dressing. If the eventration is covered by a fairly large dressing, the coils of intestine may lie unnoticed for some time. On removing the dressing one usually finds a few distended loops of small intestine or the transverse colon protruding from the wound. The deeper layers of the wound have frequently separated to a greater extent than the skin, so that the coils of intestine are also partly contained in a subcutaneous pouch. (The patient should be given morphine as soon as the condition is observed so as to prevent straining or coughing which will cause further prolapse. I. S. R.)

The first care should be to prevent further prolapse of viscera. For this purpose a sterile cover should immediately be spread over the abdomen. This is covered with sterile gauze and reinforced with broad strips of adhesive tape tightly applied, horizontally from back to back. All preparations for laparotomy are made at once and the patient is taken to the operating room, with care to avoid jarring. Without removing the bands supporting the abdomen, the patient is anesthetised. For this purpose intravenous avertin anesthesia is unexcelled because of the absence of any excitation. In fact, no other form of anesthesia even approaches it in value in such cases.

As soon as the abdominal wall has been exposed, the region of the wound is quickly disinfected and surrounded by sterile covers. The protruding intestine is cleansed by irrigation with normal salt solution, and without further attempts at disinfection is replaced by lifting of the abdominal wall and pushing back the loops. The abdominal wall is closed tightly with large wire tension sutures (Vol. I, page 92) which include all layers of the wall. After the application of a dressing the abdominal wound is supported by wide strips of adhesive plaster which run horizontally from back to back.

The prognosis of this accident is surprisingly good, in most cases the convalescence is not even stormy.

Reopening the Abdomen. If a postoperative complication necessitates the reopening of a laparotomy wound, the patient is taken to the operating room and the area prepared as previously described. The sutures are removed layer by layer and the wound edges are retracted. The necessary operative procedure is then carried out in a systematic manner. I believe that the closure of such a reopened abdominal wound is best effected by wire tension sutures.

If infection with suppuration of the abdominal wound develops after operation, drainage should be established as soon as this complication is recognized. Aside from the general dangers of an undrained purulent collection, there is the additional potential danger of rupture into the abdominal cavity. (Furthermore a deep infection undoubtedly causes the omentum to become attached along the site of the wound as recently shown by Muller and Rademaker. I. S. R.) Pain localized to the wound, a rise of temperature not attributable to other causes, or localized peritoneal irritation raises the suspicion of an infection of the abdominal wound and demands its inspection. If the local examination confirms this suspicion, several skin sutures should be removed and, if pus does not appear spontaneously, a narrow forceps should be inserted at one point between the fascial sutures and beneath the fascia. If pus escapes drainage should be established.

Whether in such instances one should immediately open the whole skin incision and also a part of the fascia, depends on the extent of the findings. As a rule it is sufficient to make one or two small openings to insure adequate drainage. If, however, the gravity of the findings necessitates the opening of the entire skin wound, an attempt to conserve, at least provisionally, all or at least some of the deeper sutures should be made, lest the entire suture line separate and prolapse of the intestines occur. Furthermore if not necessary it is not justifiable to expose the patient to the likelihood of a postoperative hernia.

If marked manifestations of infection gradually subside after a partial opening of the wound, it is permissible to temporize. However, rapid and complete healing of the wound may not occur. Stitch abscesses commonly develop which will close only after the expulsion or removal of the non-absorbed suture material. Such stitch abscesses may make their appearance weeks or months after primary healing of the wound.

Since the spontaneous expulsion of such sutures often takes a long time, or may never occur spontaneously, their artificial removal is frequently advisable. This, however, should be undertaken only after satisfactory organic union of the wound has occurred when the sutures are no longer serving any function. This may be assumed after two to three weeks.

If it is impossible to "fish" out the sutures in the manner described in Vol. I, page 118, the scar should be incised under local anaesthesia in the region of the abscess and the suture searched for and withdrawn. If all of the sutures involved have been removed, the wound as a rule heals in a few days.

The situation is quite a different one when after a laparotomy there develops a fistula in connection with a hollow viscus, as for instance a cecal fistula after operations for gangrenous appendicitis. The extirpation of such intestinal fistulae is described elsewhere.

CHAPTER II

GENERAL OPERATIVE PROCEDURES ON THE GASTRO-INTESTINAL CANAL

A. THE GENERAL TECHNIQUE OF INCISION AND DIVISION OF THE GASTRO-INTESTINAL CANAL

The operative treatment of the numerous diseases of the gastro-intestinal canal consists fundamentally in the combination of a few fairly uniform constantly recurring individual procedures. It is usually a matter of opening the intestinal tract at a certain point, of closing an existing or an artificially made opening, of anastomosing two segments, of removing a part of the gastro-intestinal canal, or of bringing a segment of intestine in communication with the exterior. Each of these problems, in whichever part of the intestinal tract it may present itself, is solved with a similar technique.

Since the contents of the gastro-intestinal canal are highly infectious, incision through the intestinal wall opens an almost limitless source of infection in the very midst of the operative field which until then had been guarded with the greatest effort and the most circumstantial detail against contamination. The contents of the intestinal tract are progressively more infectious the nearer they are to the anal end of the gut. In this respect, gastric contents are the least infectious, while rectal contents are the most infectious of any portion of the gastro-intestinal tract. In case of obstruction the virulence of the bacteria is materially increased. The opening of the intestine is all the more dangerous since the serous-covered intestine and serous-lined abdominal cavity are particularly susceptible to infection. We must therefore meet this danger with special measures.

The most important point is that every incision of the intestinal tract be dependably closed, or that an opening, purposely remaining, which connects two intestinal segments or one segment with the cutaneous surface of the abdominal wall, be securely sealed from the general peritoneal cavity, so that no source of infection shall remain within the abdomen.

In addition, care must be taken to avoid dissemination of infectious material during the operation. Therefore the stomach or the loop of intestine before being opened should be most carefully walled off from surrounding structures by moist pads, in addition to the protection of the operative field by covers as already described. The pads are intended to absorb any leakage of intestinal contents. They are laid snugly around the operative field and are fastened together with clamps. In order to prevent the escape of intestinal contents in larger amounts, the intestinal segments are milked empty and as a rule closed by means of clamps which are applied before opening the intestine. The incision is then made in a viscus that is and remains practically empty. The intestinal clamps must on the one hand exert sufficient pressure

41

to hold the walls of the bowel in firm apposition and to control the blood flow along the line of incision, and on the other hand they must be so gently applied as not to injure the wall or mesentery. The control of bleeding by the clamps is desirable in incisions of the intestinal tract because escaping blood can materially disturb the view and because the blood from the incised intestine aids the spread of infection.

In attempting to achieve the required gentleness of action on the part of the clamps, there is always the danger that a long clamp will not compress the thick-walled stomach sufficiently at its free end or that a part of the stomach will slip out of the clamp. To prevent such undesirable occurrences, many elaborate devices and auxiliary instruments have been recommended. I have always been satisfied to use simple clamps with a weak spring, whose blades are covered with rubber so as to hold the slippery stomach or intestine, and whose free ends may be tied together in case of necessity. In tying together the ends of a clamp, care must be taken that they are pressed together tightly by an assistant while the knot is being tied.

I must warn against the use of non-flexible clamps, for material damage of the intestine may result. The stomach is injured less easily in this manner than is the intestine. The development of jejunal ulcer is in part attributed to damage of the mucosa by clamp pressure. The majority of the clamps obtainable on the market are usually too stiff. When the viscus is to be removed, as is the case in gastric or intestinal resections, it is permissible, of course, to use a stiff springed clamp or a large Kocher forceps.

If the opening in the bowel is to be small, if it can be kept wholly and constantly in view, and if no further search need be made through the opening, for example, in making an entero-anastomosis, the clamps are applied to the stomach and the intestine parallel to the long axis. To insure dependable control of the blood supply, the clamp should grasp only the wall and not the mesentery as well, since the large vessels of the latter are not sufficiently compressed by gentle clamps. In more extensive operations or in end to end anastomosis the clamp grasps the whole breadth of the stomach or intestine transversely on each side of the operative site.

In order to save the intestine from unnecessary trauma and to give it the necessary freedom to mold itself to the sutures, the clamps should be removed as soon as the opened viscus has been closed by the first row of sutures, unless the clamps are needed to hold the viscus in the proper position.

Even the most careful protective covering does not relieve the surgeon and his assistants from the responsibility of catching and sponging away every drop of intestinal content that appears in the open segment. This should be done before it reaches the pads. For this purpose I greatly prefer the use of suction obtained by means of an electrically driven pump (Fig. 160). Lateral fenestrations in the tip prevent the intestinal wall from being sucked in.

If it is found impossible to clamp off the segment before opening it, and if the constant exuding of intestinal contents threatens visibility and asepsis (as may be the case, for example, when the duodenum is opened in operations on the Papilla of Vater), the lumen of the opened viscus should be blocked off proximally and distally by means of gauze tampons. It must, however, be an invariable rule never to insert such tampons unattached. They must always be tied firmly to long tapes or silk threads or at least held firmly by forceps. I have found it most convenient to attach the tampons intended for the proximal and distal segments to the two ends of a long silk thread (Fig. 27) and to allow the intervening loop to hang out of the abdominal wound after the tampons have been inserted. In this way they cannot be forgotten. Sponges forgotten in the intestinal canal play the same role as do gauze pads or other objects left behind in the abdominal cavity. The danger of leaving the tampons within the intestine is all the greater because they may be carried along unnoticed during the operation by peristalsis.

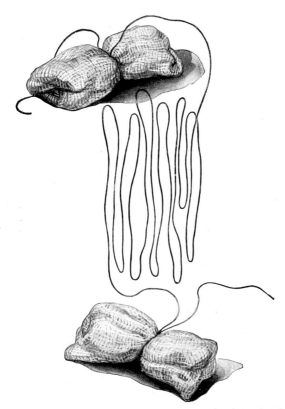

FIG. 27. Gauze tampons tied to the ends of a long thread, for insertion into the two ends of an opened intestine.

The stomach or intestine may be incised with a knife, scissors, cautery or electrosurgical knife.

The cautery or electrosurgical knife has the advantage over the ordinary cutting instruments in that the incision is made almost bloodlessly. This not only affords the advantage of better visibility but also of greater cleanliness. The danger that secondary hemorrhage might occur as a result of failure to ligate the vessels which have been divided can be met by careful suture of the mucosa. The electrosurgical knife possesses a further advantage over the cautery in causing a materially lesser degree of tissue damage. It is for this reason that I prefer that the incision of the intestinal wall be made by the former. Its use has brought about a veritable transformation in gastro-intestinal surgery, since the application of clamps for hemostasis is now often unnecessary.

It must be remembered in procedures involving the incision and subsequent suture of the wall of stomach or intestine that every closing suture entails the expenditure of a portion of the wall and therefore easily leads to a narrowing of the lumen. This danger is minimal in the larger portions of the stomach as compared with the narrower intestine.

To avoid such a constriction it is generally the rule when possible to open the intestine in its long axis and to suture the incision transversely. This rule is however obviously not applicable in case of very long incisions, nor does adherence to the rule necessarily guard against all encroachment on the lumen. In fact, it occasionally leads to a relative stenosis because of the resultant bulging of the suture line. If stenosis results from opening and suture of a gastro-intestinal segment, such an obstruction must be immediately short-circuited. This is accomplished by an anastomosis between the afferent and the efferent loops. If there exists a choice a section of intestine as devoid of blood vessels as possible should be selected as the site for an incision of its wall.

The incision is simple when it is for the purpose of removing a foreign body which is easily palpable through the gut wall, for example, a swallowed denture or a gall stone. Here the incision is made down to the foreign body as it is held firmly against the intestinal wall and it is made just large enough to allow the foreign body to be squeezed through it (Fig. 77).

When a fairly long incision must be made in a given direction, for example, the opening of stomach or intestine in making an anastomosis, it will be found useful to trace the line of incision superficially on the serosa with the knife, or with the cautery and only then to carry the incision through all the layers. This is because the gut easily changes its shape and because its musculature usually contracts on being grasped and cut, so that the line of incision may thus be distorted. After the line of incision has been marked on the serosa, a fold of intestine at one end of this line is picked up between two tissue forceps and a small opening is made into its lumen (Fig. 76). Through this opening a narrow grooved director is inserted (Fig. 114), by means of which the anterior wall is lifted away from the posterior wall in the line of incision as marked on the serosa. The incision of the intestine is then completed in the outlined direction with the electrosurgical knife or with one of the other instruments mentioned before, using the grooved director as a guide (Fig. 28).

In complete transsection of the stomach or the intestine, the first step is to free the part from its mesentery sufficiently to permit of the application of clamps and to provide ends which can be easily sutured. However, I wish to warn against excessive ligation and division of mesenteric vessels lest the vitality of the segments be disturbed. Depending on the diameter of the viscus, it should be freed for a distance of 2 to 4 cm. The technique of the ligation of the mesentery will be described with that of intestinal resection on page 267.

Before transsecting the stomach or intestine every precaution must be taken against the escape of intestinal contents and of blood. A simple and satisfactory method of accomplishing this is by the application of intestinal clamps. If the transsected portion is to be removed, the clamps can be applied very firmly, as is the case with Billroth clamps. The clamps applied to parts which are to remain should be applied gently (spring clamps) so as not to injure the viscus.

Division of a portion of the gastro-intestinal tract, and its isolation and closure are procedures which frequently are not strictly separate and suc-

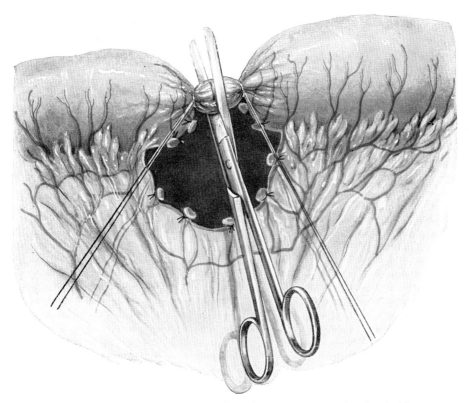

Fig. 28. Transverse division of the intestine. A segment of intestine, freed of its mesentery and emptied as far as possible by "milking," has been tied tightly with two ligatures a short distance apart. The bowel is divided between the ligatures with a scissors.

cessive, but often overlap. Consequently they can not be discussed wholly apart from each other.

Transsection of the intestine is performed in its simplest form by dividing the gut with scissors, knife, or the electrosurgical knife between two ligatures placed a short distance apart (Fig. 28). The segment to be divided is first milked empty of its contents, freed from its mesentery and then doubly ligated.

Before division of broad intestinal segments, especially the stomach, the line of division may first be crushed with an enterotribe, for example the crushing clamp of Payr (Fig. 29). This crushes and divides muscle and mucosa and closes the blood vessels, leaving only the serosal layers adherent to each other. Before removal of the enterotribe, the end that is to remain can be closed by a through-and-through suture while the segment to be removed is cut off close to the clamp (Fig. 29). A crushing clamp is however by no means necessary.

The best, cleanest and most rapid procedure for division of the intestine is that effected by means of the suture instrument of Petz (Figs. 48, 49, 66, 102, 109). The line of division is crushed by an enterotribe and in the region of the resultant furrow a double row of metal clips is applied which effectively

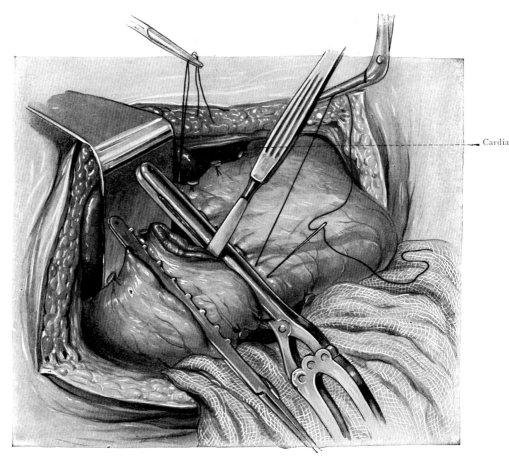

Cardia

FIG. 29. Transverse division of the stomach with the aid of the enterotribe. The gastric segment proximal to the line of division has been closed with an enterotribe, the distal segment with a spring clamp. The stomach has been closed proximal to the enterotribe by means of a through-and-through suture and is being divided distal to the enterotribe with the knife.

controls intestinal contents and hemorrhage. After the removal of the instrument the crushed zone is cut across between the rows of clips with a straight scissors or a scalpel. I consider the use of the Petz instrument the most satisfactory procedure. It has given gastro-intestinal surgery a new aspect.

The two ends resulting from the transsection of the intestine or stomach, in spite of the measures taken to prevent the gross escape of intestinal contents, are nevertheless not safe. Moreover, if they are allowed to remain in the abdomen without further attention, they will reopen in a few days, since the suture does not provide serosal approximation.   Therefore, if the cut ends are not to be removed from the body immediately, they must be taken care of both temporarily and permanently.

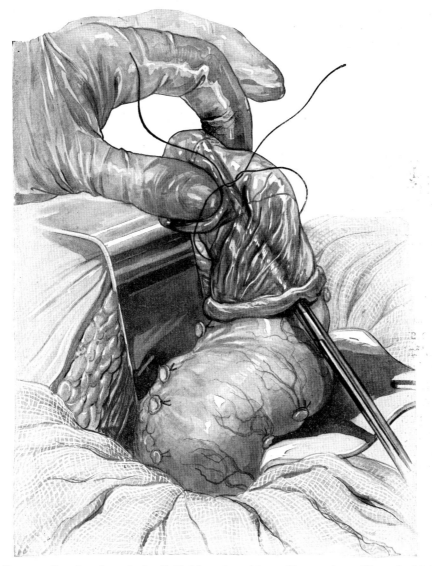

FIG. 30.   Covering the end of a divided intestine with a rubber condom.   The end of intestine has been grasped with a smooth forceps.   A condom is pulled over the viscus and is tied tightly with a ligature, the forceps being removed at the same time.

The immediate dissemination of bacteria is prevented by carefully enclosing the stump in a very thick pad (Fig. 122) or a rubber condom.   This is prevented from slipping off the stumps by Kocher clamps, towel clips or by tying with a silk thread.   Since the protection offered by a cloth compress against the escape of infected fluid is only relative and of short duration, I find it better to tie a small rubber bag over the intestinal stump.   For this purpose a condom is most suitable because it is waterproof and pliable. The intestinal stump is grasped by the end and as nearly in its long axis as possible with one or two Billroth or Moynihan forceps (Fig. 30) so that the condom may be pulled over the end of the gut and the supporting forceps. A silk thread is tied loosely around the base of the condom. The gut is then grasped through the condom near its end, the Billroth forceps is carefully withdrawn and the silk thread is tied tightly around the condom and the gut. If the divided viscus is to remain in the body, the end must be securely closed in the manner described in the next section.

Painting the exposed mucosa with tincture of iodine or other disinfectants in an attempt at sterilization is of small and very doubtful value. No diminution of bacteria of any particular significance is achieved thereby.

All instruments used during the division of the gastro-intestinal tract must be considered infected and must be replaced by clean instruments immediately after the completion of this infectious procedure (Vol. I, page 275). All those taking part in the operation cleanse their hands at this point or put on clean gloves.

B. THE GENERAL TECHNIQUE OF THE CLOSURE OF OPENINGS IN THE GASTRO-INTESTINAL CANAL

In view of the highly infectious contents of the gastro-intestinal canal and the great susceptibility of the abdominal cavity to infection, every opening made in the gastro-intestinal canal must be closed promptly and carefully. The sutures must afford a closure that will prevent the leakage of intestinal contents permanently as well as at the time of operation. To permit a continuing focus of infection to remain in the abdomen predicates peritonitis. Closure may be effected by oversewing a lateral opening; by terminal suture of a divided segment; by the anastomosis of openings in two segments, or by the permanent communication with the body surface of a gastric or intestinal opening by means of a fistula.

There are certain difficulties involved in obtaining satisfactory suture of the stomach and the intestine. The sutures are constantly in contact with the infectious intestinal contents, yet infection is the most important factor working against stability of sutures and primary healing. Furthermore, the intestinal contents place a definite mechanical strain on the suture line, since gas, fluids, or solid feces are forced against it, and may cause distension of the adjacent loops. Changes of position of the intestines incident to peristalsis may also exert considerable tension on the sutures joining two segments. The mechanical demands placed upon a suture line in this manner may be very great in the presence of active gastric and intestinal contractions. As a result of the combined action of these factors, intestinal sutures are subjected to strains of considerable proportions.

In spite of these unfavorable conditions, gastric and intestinal sutures in actual practice are usually dependable. This can be explained by the fact that the gastro-intestinal wall is pliable and resilient and therefore, in a mechanical sense, represents a very suitable material for suture, and above all, by the fact that when the serous surfaces are brought accurately into close apposition by suture they rapidly adhere. This union takes place all the more quickly and completely because of the irritation of the serous surfaces induced by the infectious intestinal contents. Therefore, the security of a gastro-intestinal suture is actually very great (Vol. I, page 82) and within 5 or 6 days the serous surfaces are usually firmly united (Vol. I, page 92).

In every intestinal suture certain end-results are desired; first, by carefully and closely applied sutures to effect a primary tight closure of the gut lumen; second, by a broad apposition of serous surfaces to bring about organic union as soon as possible; third, to control bleeding of the incised intestinal

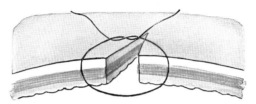

a.   Albert Suture through all layers.

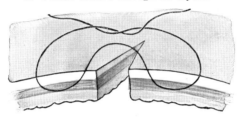

b.   Lembert Invaginating Suture.

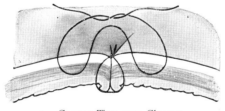

c.   Czerny Two-row Closure.

FIG. 31.   The Czerny two-row closure consists of (a) the Albert suture and (b) the Lembert serosa-muscularis suture.

wall, and fourth, to approximate neatly the cut edges of the mucosa, in order to prevent a subsequent cicatricial stenosis.

There are many methods which, in the main, meet these requirements. Any one of the customary procedures will give good results in skilled hands, an example of the triumph of system, care, and pedantic attention to orderly detail. For the surgical practitioner a single procedure will usually suffice, but he should master it completely.

The closure of every gastro-intestinal opening, of every terminal opening, of every lateral opening and of every anastomatic opening is effected under ordinary circumstances according to the fundamental principles of **double-row suture** (Fig. 31c) as introduced by **Czerny** in 1877.

(a) **The first row of the Czerny suture, the through-and-through** three-layer suture (Fig. 31a) (Albert suture), grasps serosa, muscularis, mucosa of one wound edge, and mucosa, muscularis, serosa of the other. The wound margins of the mucosa are pierced as close as possible to the edge and are thus displaced toward the interior, while the serosa is grasped about 3 mm. from the edge. This three-layer suture effects the mechanical holding of the wound edges, prevents the escape of intestinal contents, controls bleeding, and achieves excellent apposition and infolding of the edges of the mucosa.

While in most suture procedures the two wound edges are properly approximated without difficulty, the coaptation of the wound edges by the

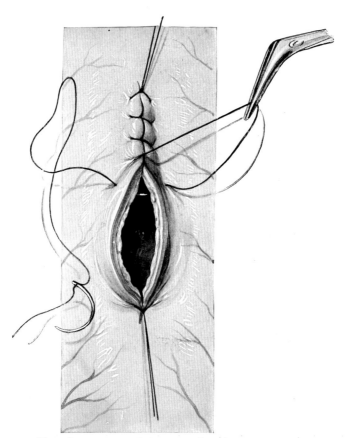

Fig. 32. Three-layer suture of the gastro-intestinal wall. Furrier's suture.

three-layer suture encounters difficulties both in the closure of lateral or terminal gastro-intestinal openings and in the anterior three-layer suture in entero-anastomosis, because the mucosa has a decided tendency to evert. To obviate these difficulties there are in use a number of procedures, none of which is wholly satisfactory. Consequently, and in contrast to other sutures, an unusual degree of attention must be given in this procedure to the infolding of the everting mucosa. The following suture procedures are in general use:

(1) The Furrier's Suture (Fig. 32). The suture is passed through the serosa-mucosa of one side, the mucosa-serosa of the other side, and drawn

taut. The everting mucosa must be pushed back with a dissecting forceps before pulling each suture taut.

(2) **The Mikulicz Suture (Fig. 33).** The suture is passed in the reverse order from the Furrier's Suture, but it is drawn taut on the inside of the gut instead of the outside, that is, through the mucosa-serosa of one side, serosa-mucosa of the other side, and then drawn taut. In this procedure

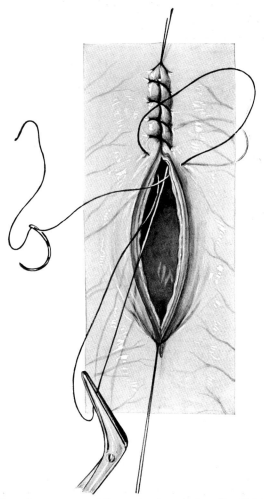

FIG. 33. Three-layer suture of the gastro-intestinal wall. Mikulicz suture.

the serosal surfaces are for the most part excellently approximated with infolding of the mucosa. However, in terminating the suture the Furrier's suture must be used for the last few stitches, since the suture can no longer be drawn taut nor tied from within the lumen inside the gut when the opening has become very small.

(3) **The Schmieden Suture (Fig. 34).** The suture is passed through the mucosa-serosa of one side, pulled taut, passed through the mucosa-serosa of the other side, and drawn taut. If the stitches are close together, the mucosa is infolded very well as a rule. However, mucosa always comes to be

partly against serosa, so that the suture line, at least theoretically, is less secure.

(4) **The U or Connel Suture (Fig. 35).** The suture is passed about half a centimeter from and parallel to the wound edge on each side, passing through all layers of the gut wall and grasping a fold of a few millimeters in each stitch, in the following order: serosa-mucosa-mucosa-serosa of one side, drawn taut, serosa-mucosa-mucosa-serosa of the other side, drawn taut. With close stitching, the wound edges are nicely approximated. The dependability or hemostasis with this suture is possibly not all that might be desired.

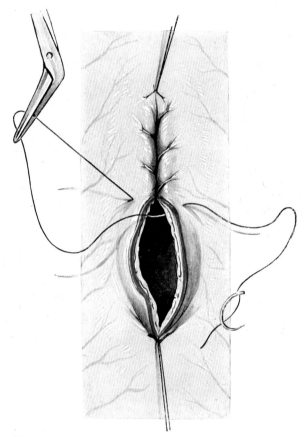

FIG. 34. Three-layer suture of the gastro-intestinal wall. Schmieden suture.

With the exception of the Schmieden suture, which can only be carried out as a continuous suture, these sutures may be applied as continuous sutures, or as interrupted sutures. They can all be used in terminal or lateral closure of the gut or in entero-anastomosis.

(b) **The second suture row of the Czerny suture (Fig. 31b).** The superficial two-layer sero-muscular suture (Lembert suture, 1826), is applied about 2-5 mm. away from the first suture row. The individual sutures include only serosa and muscularis, grasping on each side a sero-muscular fold in the order serosa-muscularis-serosa. (The classical Lembert suture is placed at right angles to the line of division of the gut while the Cushing suture is placed parallel to it. I. S. R.) In tying these sutures, the first suture line is buried. In general, the stitches of the second suture line are also passed perpendicular to the line of incision (transverse suture), the needle entering about 6 mm. and emerging about 3 mm. from the first suture line. Under certain circumstances, however, the stitches may be passed parallel to

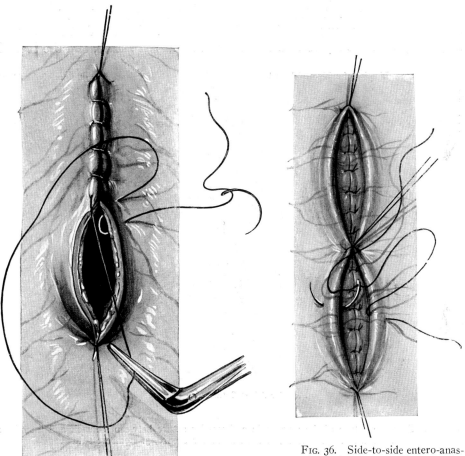

FIG. 35. Continuous three-layer suture of the gastro-intestinal wall. U-suture.

FIG. 36. Side-to-side entero-anas-tomosis: 4th stage. The anterior sero-muscular suture is applied by means of interrupted sutures between the traction sutures.

the line of incision (parallel suture), the needle entering and emerging about ½ cm. from the first suture line. By means of the Lembert suture together with the preceding Albert suture there is effected a broad apposition of serous surfaces which seals the wound dependably. In addition, this suture affords a firm mechanical closure.

The Lembert suture, if very carefully and closely applied, can, in case of inadequacy or absence of the Albert suture, take over the whole task of the latter in an emergency. But such a single-row suture (used routinely by Bier) is not sufficiently secure to make it possible to recommend closure with only a single-row suture as a routine procedure. In my opinion it is justified only in an emergency when there is an extreme lack of time.

On the other hand, a two-row suture is so dependable that I see no reason to replace it under ordinary circumstances with a three-row suture, such as some operators (von Eiselsberg) use routinely. Such a three-row suture may be carried out in different ways: The first suture row includes only the mucosa, the second grasps both muscularis and serosa, the third is a Lembert suture of the serosa (Fig. 37). This method effects particularly dependable hemostasis and a particularly snug apposition of the mucosa. Or, the first suture row may grasp all three layers in the manner of an Albert suture, and the second

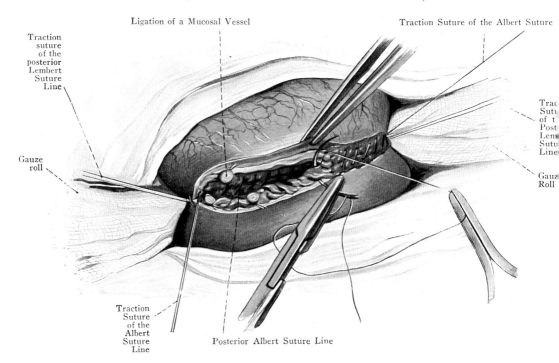

FIG. 37. Separate suture of the mucosa in a three-tier suture between stomach and intestine: 1. Suture of the mucosa, 2. Sero-muscular suture, 3. Lembert suture.

and third each a sero-muscular fold in the form of a Lembert suture. In this way very broad serous surfaces are approximated and the ends are firmly sealed, but there is usually too great an infolding of the gut ends. This latter form of the three-row suture is nothing more or less than the usual two-row suture with an additional reinforcement by an outer Lembert sero-muscular suture. A three-row suture is often used as a supplementary suture if there is some doubt as to the firmness of the routinely applied two-row suture and reinforcement is desired. A few stitches over the two-row suture can be applied in a more or less connected sequence and the three-row suture is completed.

Intestinal sutures may be either interrupted or continuous. Interrupted sutures are more dependable (Vol. I, page 82) because if a suture cuts through or breaks, the remaining sutures are not endangered and because the tension of the individual sutures is independent of the state of contraction of the gut at the moment. The interrupted sutures are applied in such a manner that each suture halves the distance between two traction sutures; each newly

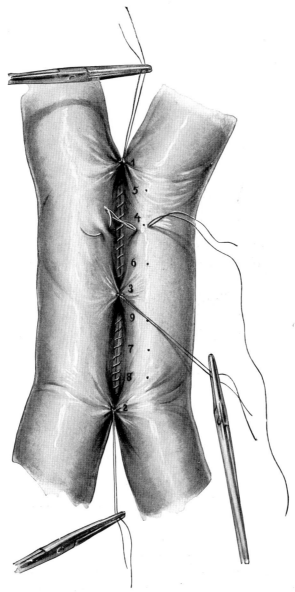

FIG. 38. The direction and subdivisions of an intestinal suture line are established by means of traction sutures. The numbers indicate the order in which the interrupted sutures are applied, each subsequent suture halving the distance between two traction sutures.

applied suture is in turn used as a traction suture as long as an additional suture seems necessary between it and the next suture (Fig. 38).

The continuous suture can be applied more rapidly, and, if it is kept taut and remains so, effects tighter closure and better hemostasis. The response of a continuous suture in contrast to an interrupted suture line to the changing conditions of tension in the gut may result in imperfect approximation of the sutured surfaces and therefore this type of suture is less dependable. Personally under ordinary circumstances I place an inner continuous Albert and an outer interrupted Lembert suture. When any question as to effectiveness arises both suture rows are carried out as interrupted sutures.

Several years ago I changed from a continuous to an interrupted Lembert suture, and since then my results have noticeably improved. Previously I

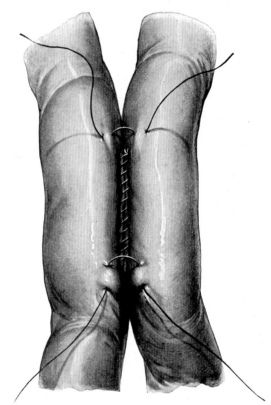

Fig. 39. The direction of the anterior Lembert suture line is established by the application of a traction suture at each end of the intended line of suture.

attributed disturbances in the patient's convalescence to excessive sensitiveness on the part of the patient, gastro-intestinal hemorrhage, intestinal paralysis, gastric atony, the after-effects of anaesthesia, thrombotic processes, and the spread of infection during the operation which I now believe may have often been due to small leaks along the line of suture.

As suture material, silk, linen, or catgut of the smallest size can be used. I use catgut for the inner suture (inner continuous catgut suture) because unabsorbed sutures projecting into the intestinal lumen may produce ulceration. I use linen for the outer serosal suture (outer interrupted linen suture) because catgut does not hug the eye of the needle very snugly and therefore tears disproportionately large holes as it is passed through the wall of the intestine (unless one uses the expensive atraumatic catgut needles) and because it is not dependable for this purpose on account of the rapidity with which it is absorbed.

The sutures are carried through the tissues either with small full curved needles grasped with a needle holder, or with long, straight or slightly curved needles grasped with the fingers. The needles are either triangular or round in cross-section. Each type has its adherents. I use a needle holder because I do not like the direct contact of the intestinal mucosa and contents with the fingers, and because it seems to me that with the use of a needle holder the needles are handled with greater safety and accuracy. I prefer round needles

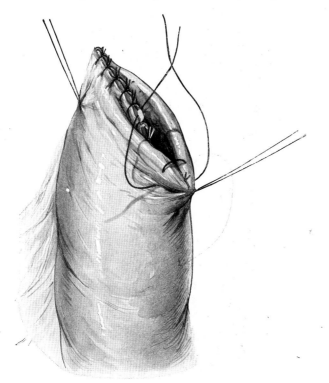

FIG. 40. Terminal closure of a divided intestine by means of furrier's Albert sutures and by Lembert sutures.

because the resulting round hole is closed more closely by the suture material, and because the round needles, in contrast to cutting needles, do not endanger the integrity of a previously placed suture with which the needle might come in contact as it is reinserted.

My personal technique is therefore usually: **Two-row suture with round needles and needleholder, the inner suture a continuous one with catgut, the outer an interrupted suture with linen.**

Every intestinal suture row, no matter where it is applied or which layers of the intestine it includes, is begun with two knotted sutures, carefully approximating the corresponding layers of the gut wall, one at the beginning and one at the end of the intended suture line (Fig. 39). The ends of the suture are left long and caught with hemostats. These act as end traction sutures. By making traction on them the direction and length of the intended suture line are clearly indicated and the layers to be united are caused to lie side by side. It is scarcely possible with this aid to misplace the intervening sutures. The direction of suture should always be toward the operator, and the suture may be either continuous or interrupted as above described. With the two-row suture as described, every opening in the gastro-intestinal canal can be closed, whether the opening be lateral or terminal.

The Closure of a Lateral Intestinal Opening. In a lateral wound there are first applied two catgut sutures grasping all three layers, one at

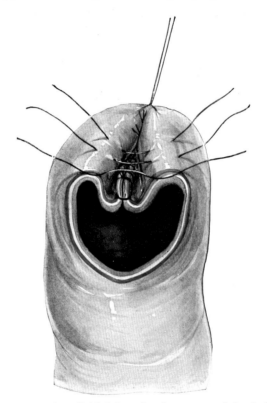

FIG. 41. Terminal closure of a divided intestine by means of furrier's Albert suture and by Lembert sutures. Diagrammatic.

each end of the opening to be closed. While the end traction sutures are held taut (Figs. 31-34), one end of the suture farthest from the operator is used for a continuous suture, or interrupted sutures are applied. The ends of the resultant three-layer suture (Albert suture) are now in turn pulled toward the middle of the suture line by means of the catgut end traction sutures while a single linen Lembert suture is applied beyond each end of the suture line. These linen sutures are now used as end traction sutures and the catgut sutures are cut short. While traction is made on the linen end sutures the intervening space is closed either with a continuous Lembert suture or preferably with interrupted sutures (Fig. 36) with resultant burial of the three-layer catgut suture. If interrupted sutures are used, their sequence involves a constant halving of the space between sutures in the manner already described (Fig. 38).

If the closure is of only a small lateral opening, the first three-layer suture may be replaced by a simple purse string of the opening. The little projecting

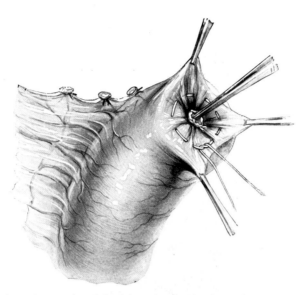

Fig. 42.   Terminal closure of a divided intestine by ligation and a purse-string suture.

tip which results is buried by interrupted sutures, by a second purse-string suture or a cross-stitch suture (Figs. 44 and 45) as later described under terminal closure. I personally do not use these last two types of suture, but,

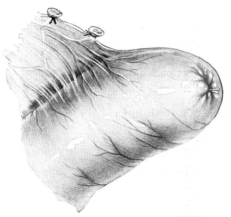

Fig. 43.   End closed by purse-string suture.

even when only a small ligated tip is to be buried, I use a few standard Lembert interrupted sutures.

The Closure of a Terminal Intestinal Opening is carried out in the following manner: If the ends of the intestine were not immediately closed in the manner described under the technique of division by ligation or by the use of the Petz instrument, it is first closed with silk or catgut interrupted sutures applied in the form of an Albert suture catching all three layers on both sides of the wound (Figs. 40 and 41). This primary closure is further reinforced by an invaginating interrupted Lembert suture. This is done by first applying two interrupted sutures through two folds of the intestinal wall on opposite sides and at a distance of ½ to 2 cm. from the first line of closure (Fig. 40). While these sutures are being pulled tight, the projecting stump is invaginated into the gut lumen, like the finger of a glove, with the help of a dissecting forceps. The resultant serosal funnel is then closed by interrupted silk or linen sutures (Figs. 40 and 41).

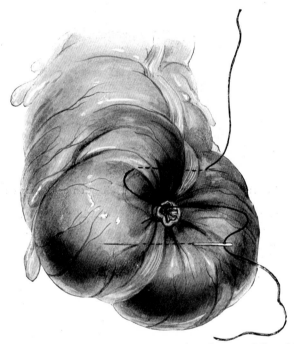

FIG. 44. Cross-stitch suture. The intestinal wall is pierced tangentially with a straight needle and thread on both sides of and at a short distance from the ligated appendiceal stump.

A terminal opening may also be invaginated by means of a purse-string or a cross-stitch suture just as in the closure of lateral openings, provided that the end of the gut has been made fairly small by means of a circular ligature. In a purse-string suture, a continuous silk or linen suture is passed in a complete circle around the site of primary closure. Each stitch picks up a sero-muscular fold (Fig. 42). The site of primary closure is invaginated into the circle of the purse-string and is buried by pulling tight and tying the ends of the suture (Fig. 43).

Closure by cross-stitch suture is carried out in the following manner: At some distance from the Albert suture of the segment a suture is passed on one side by a stitch through serosa and muscle from right to left, and then in a similar manner on the other side of the gut end from right to left (Fig. 44).

If the ends of the thread are now crossed and tied over the center of the first suture line (Fig. 45), the gut wall is brought together over the free tip and buries it.

The Moynihan clamp is useful in terminal closure, especially of the duodenum. The intestine is grasped transversely with this instrument and is then divided as close as possible to the clamp. Beginning at one end (Fig. 46), the operator passes a needle carrying a linen or silk suture through a fold of serosa and muscularis on one side of the gut a short distance below the clamp, then carries the suture over the clamp and takes a similar stitch in the gut on the other side, then back again over the clamp to take a stitch on the first side, and so on in a continuous suture until the other end of the wound is reached. The suture is drawn only moderately taut at first. While an assistant slightly opens the clamp and cautiously withdraws it (Fig. 47), the operator pulls taut

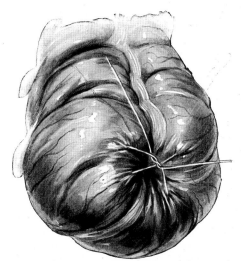

Fig. 45. Cross-stitch suture. The stump is buried by tying the thread.

the two ends of the suture. This brings the gut walls together and folds in the cut edge of the gut. Without tying the ends of the suture, the operator applies a second continuous Lembert suture over the first, using one end of the first suture. This in turn buries the first suture line. Finally, the two ends of the suture are tied. (It is important first to suture the mucosa and sub-mucosa with continuous or with interrupted catgut sutures before placing the sutures just described. I. S. R.)

In the closure of terminal openings of segments which, like the duodenum, the ascending and descending colon and the upper part of the rectum, are not completely covered with peritoneum, there arise difficulties in that serous surfaces are not everywhere apposed to serous surfaces unless special measures are taken. This difficulty may be obviated by infolding in the long axis the part of the intestine devoid of peritoneum by means of long sero-muscular sutures. The portion of the intestine which is now completely covered by serosa is invaginated and oversewed. In this way segments of intestine which are not covered on all sides by peritoneum may be closed dependably and it is not necessary to extend resections to more distant portions of the bowel which are completely covered with peritoneum.

The Suture Apparatus of Petz. Every intestinal suture is made up of a number of recurring individual procedures which are quite similar, and whose uniformity could better be achieved by machine than by the human hand. It was obvious, therefore, that someone should attempt to devise some type of sewing machine for suture of the wall of the gastro-intestinal canal. These attempts have finally led to the construction of the excellent gastro-intestinal suture apparatus of Petz (Fig. 48), with which terminal openings and, if there is adequate material, also lateral openings in the gastro-intestinal

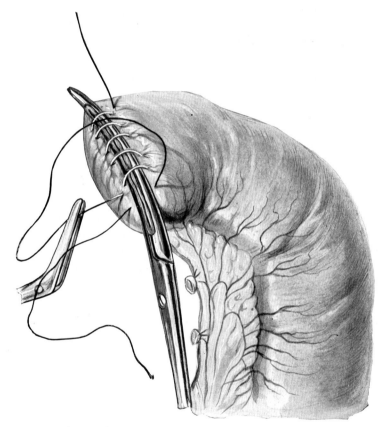

FIG. 46. Terminal closure of an end of the small intestine by means of the Moynihan clamp. The clamp is oversewed with a running suture.

canal can be closed with speed, safety and cleanliness. The apparatus consists of a large clamp which grasps the section of gut to be closed, and crushes it in the line of transsection by an enterotribe. The crushing action can be increased by means of a lock attached to the ends of the arms of the clamp. Small metal clips are expelled from a magazine at the turn of a wheel in such a way that the crushed part of gut in the grasp of the clamp is closed by the clips in two parallel rows a few millimeters apart. When the intestine is divided between the rows of clips (Fig. 49), each free end is found tightly closed by a row of clips in the manner of an Albert suture. If the part is to remain in the body, the suture line must be buried by an additional Lembert suture.

The advantages of the Petz suture machine are speed, visibility, cleanliness, and absolute dependability, since the escape of intestinal contents is completely prevented, and hemorrhage almost completely so, and since the closure is quite tight. The advantages are so great, that I use this apparatus

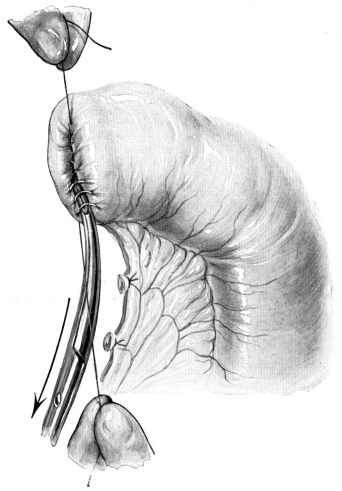

FIG. 47. As the Moynihan clamp is removed, the running suture is pulled tight, so that the cut edge of the stump is closed and buried.

routinely in every terminal closure and also in every lateral closure when there is sufficient tissue. Moreover, in end-to-end or end-to-side anastomoses, the transsection of the gut may be carried out with the Petz apparatus. In completing the anastomosis, the line of clips is excised (Fig. 66).

When an entero-anastomosis is to be performed at the site of a terminal or a lateral opening in an intestinal segment, the closure of the intestinal opening is effected by the joint suture of the two gut segments, as described in the following section.

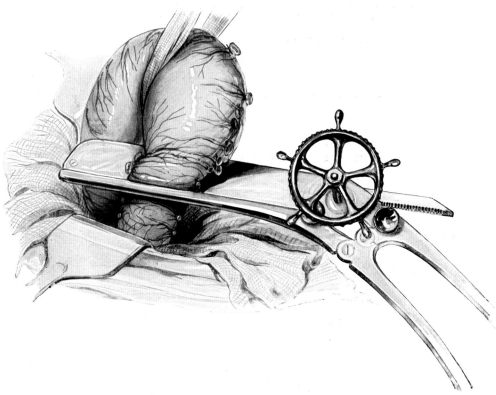

Fig. 48. Closure and crushing of the duodenum by means of the Petz suture instrument. The gut is crushed by the clamp and when the wheel is turned a double row of wire clips is placed.

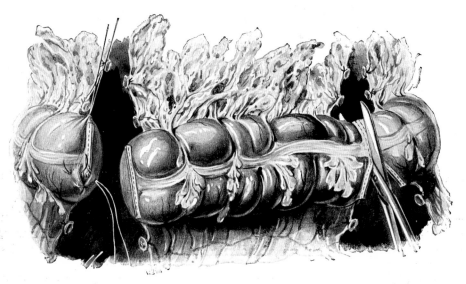

Fig. 49. Division and closure of the transverse colon which has been closed by a double row of clips by the Petz suture instrument. On the right the bowel is being divided with the scissors. On the left it has been divided and the proximal end is being closed with interrupted Lembert sutures.

C. ANASTOMOSIS BETWEEN TWO SEGMENTS OF THE GASTRO-INTESTINAL CANAL

The establishment of an anastomosis between two parts of the gastro-intestinal canal becomes necessary (1) when there is partial or complete interruption of the normal channel by operative intervention or by a pathological condition that is irremovable (stenosis, an inflammatory lesion, a benign or malignant tumor, kinking or adhesions, intussusception, the closure of a perforation); or, (2) when a diseased segment of the bowel must, for therapeutic reasons, be side tracked permanently or temporarily. The difficulty in anastomosis lies in making an opening large enough, and in making the connection dependably tight.

There are the following types of anastomosis:

(1) A lateral opening in one segment is joined to a lateral opening in the other segment (side-to-side anastomosis).

(2) The open end of one segment is joined to the open end of the other segment (end-to-end anastomosis).

(3) The open end of the proximal segment is joined to a lateral opening in the distal segment (end-to-side anastomosis); or vice versa, a lateral opening in the proximal segment is joined to the open end of the distal segment (side-to-end anastomosis).

A fundamental condition in making an anastomosis between two segments of the gastro-intestinal canal is that the sutures must not be under any tension.

In anastomosing the stomach and the intestine it frequently happens that after opening the viscus the thinner wall of the intestine tends to stretch much more than the more resistant gastric wall. As a result, if segments of apparently equal length of each viscus are sutured side-to-side before being opened, after their opening the intestinal incision may seem to be too large. This difficulty can be avoided by using a somewhat shorter segment of intestine than of stomach in applying the first Lembert suture so that the intestine is under some tension for the moment, while the segment of gastric wall appears too large. After incision of the viscera this difference disappears.

1. SIDE-TO-SIDE ANASTOMOSIS

This anastomosis may always be carried out if enough tissue is available, and especially when there has been no resection of a segment of intestine, as for example when a diseased portion has been left in the body, and is to be short-circuited. Side-to-side anastomosis is technically simple and dependable and in practice meets all functional demands. It does not, however, reproduce normal anatomic and physiologic conditions as completely as does end-to-end anastomosis and it takes longer to perform than does an axial anastomosis of two ends. Experimental investigations of my former assistant, Melzer (German Surgical Congress, 1926) have also shown that the resumption of peristalsis after a lateral anastomosis is somewhat delayed when compared with end-to-end anastomosis. In actual practice, however, these theoretical disadvantages are of little importance.

(a) **The Position of the Gastro-intestinal Segments.** Side-to-side anastomosis is usually carried out in the direction of peristalsis (Fig. 50), although the antiperistaltic direction (Fig. 51) may be selected without serious consequences. The two segments to be joined are placed side by side for a

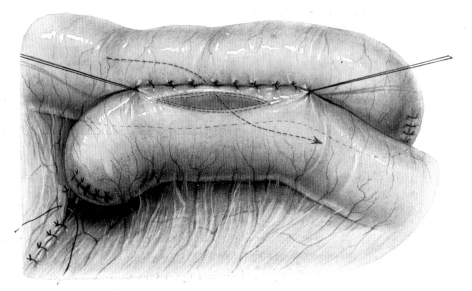

Fig. 50. Side-to-side entero-enterostomy in an isoperistaltic direction.

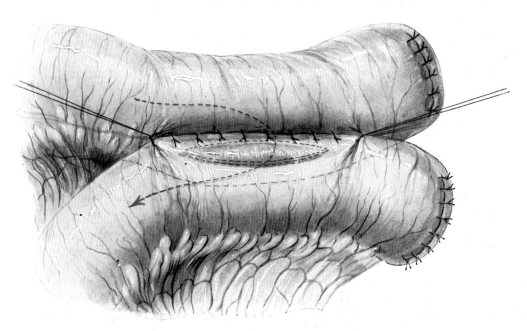

Fig. 51. Side-to-side entero-enterostomy in an antiperistaltic direction.

considerable distance, some 10 to 15 centimeters. If the intestine is full, a longitudinal fold 8 to 10 cm. long in one or both segments may be clamped off with a straight spring clamp (Fig. 54). In the small intestine the side opposite the mesenteric attachment is used, and in the large bowel, a section as free as possible of epiploic appendages. In the intestine, especially the large intestine, a longitudinal fold is picked up with two forceps to facilitate the application of the clamp (Fig. 52). The segments may also be milked empty and blocked

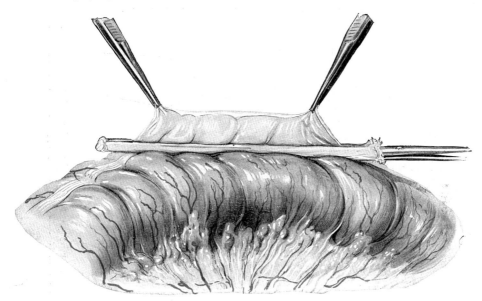

FIG. 52. Application of cloth covered spring clamp to the large bowel for lateral anastomosis. The wall of the intestine has been picked up with two surgical forceps.

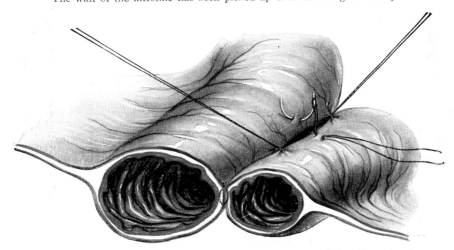

FIG. 53. Side-to-side entero-enterostomy, first step (diagrammatic). Posterior interrupted serosa-muscularis sutures.

off by applying clamps across the gut (Fig. 61). When the intestine is not unduly distended, the application of clamps can be dispensed with in most cases, for clamps always inflict a certain amount of damage on the intestinal wall, and the escape of intestinal contents can practically be prevented by sponging and aspirating, while the use of the electrosurgical knife to a large extent prevents bleeding.

A moist gauze roll is placed between the two segments, and the surrounding field is protected by moist compresses passed beneath the clamps and held together by suitable (Allis) forceps.

(b) **The Posterior Lembert Suture (Figs. 53 and 54).** The segments, placed side-by-side, are now joined for a distance of from 4 to 8 cm. by inter-

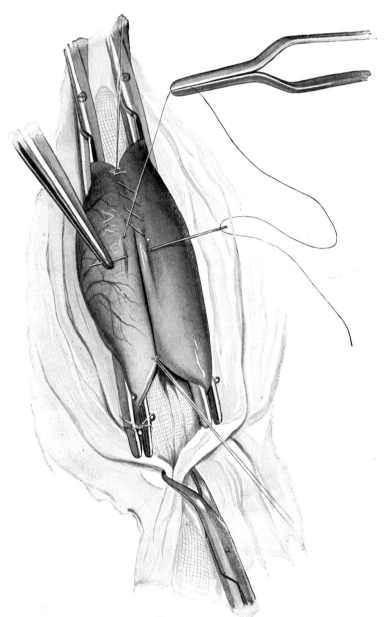

FIG. 54. Side-to-side entero-enterostomy, first step. The two intestinal segments have been clamped, two end traction sutures have been placed and between these the posterior sero-muscular suture is being applied as a continuous suture with a straight needle held in the fingers.

rupted Lembert sutures of silk or linen. In the small intestine the suture is not applied to the free margin of the gut directly opposite the mesenteric attachment, but an appreciable distance back toward the mesentery, because the several suture lines gradually take up a considerable part of the intestinal wall. The suture begins according to the familiar technique with two knotted traction sutures placed at the beginning and at the end of the intended first line of suture. By making traction on the long ends of these two sutures, the line to be incised is well marked and the posterior interrupted sutures can easily be placed.

(c) **Opening of the Intestinal Segments.** After the suture ends have been cut short (with the exception of the two traction sutures) and gauze sponges have been introduced under the suture line, one from each end, both segments of the intestine are opened at a distance of ½ cm. from the first suture line in the manner described on page 51. I prefer to do this with the electrosurgical knife after inserting a grooved director into the lumen of the gut (Fig. 114). Each of the two outer wound edges is drawn outward by means of an Allis forceps or a traction suture applied at the midpoint.

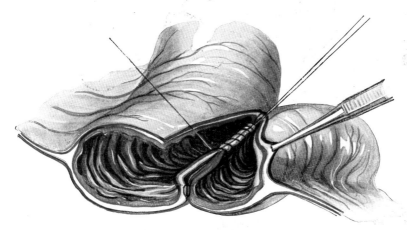

Fig. 55. Side-to-side entero-enterostomy, second step (diagrammatic). Continuous posterior three-layer suture after the opening of both intestinal loops.

(d) **The Posterior Albert Suture (Fig. 55).** This is applied as a continuous catgut suture. It is begun with two end traction sutures. Each end-suture is applied exactly in the angle of the wound, that is, the needle is passed in the long axis of the gut from within outward in the one segment of gut, and from without inward in the long axis of the other segment. In the wound angle farthest away from the operator, the suture is tied so that the knot comes in the middle of the suture, which must be long, and both ends are left long. With one of these ends a continuous suture is next run toward the traction suture at the opposite angle of the wound. The suture passes through all the layers of the gut wall, the direction being mucosa-muscularis-serosa in one segment and serosa-muscularis-mucosa in the other. The mucosa is included as scantily as possible in the suture, the serosa to a breadth of about a quarter of a centimeter, so that the distance of this suture line is about ¼ of a centimeter from the posterior Lembert suture. Care must be taken that each stitch grasps all six layers of the two gut walls, verifying this separately at each serosal and mucosal layer. When the thread of this running suture reaches the other traction suture, they are tied together. One end is cut short, the other end is left long and by means of a needle is passed through the one gut wall from within outward and is then used as a traction suture.

(e) The Anterior Albert Suture (Figs. 56 and 57). This suture is by far the most difficult, since material difficulties are encountered in burying

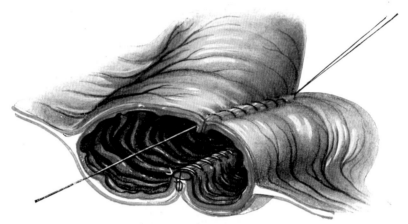

FIG. 56. Side-to-side entero-enterostomy, third step (diagrammatic). The anterior three-layer suture is being applied as a running suture according to Mikulicz.

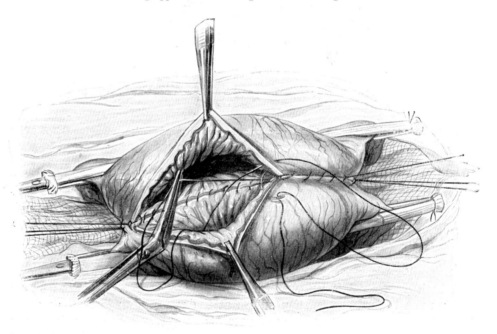

FIG. 57. Side-to-side entero-enterostomy, third step. The anterior three-layer suture is being applied as a continuous suture between two traction sutures according to Mikulicz.

securely the everting edges of the mucosa and in joining the serosal edges without a gap. To obviate these difficulties the various suture procedures described on page 48, are used. I generally use the invertible suture of Mikulicz, as described on page 51. (The Connell suture (page 52) is extensively used in the English speaking countries. I. S. R.)

After the forceps or traction sutures with which the intestinal openings have been kept apart have been removed, the second long end of the catgut suture at the angle of the wound farthest from the operator is passed through the intestinal walls in the order mucosa-muscularis-serosa of one segment and serosa-muscularis-mucosa of the other, and is then drawn taut. In this order a continuous suture is run so that the thread is always drawn taut within the lumens of the segments (Mikulicz suture). With a dissecting forceps the mucosa is pushed in as the suture is drawn taut. Special difficulty is encountered at the end of the suture where the remaining opening in the intestines has become so small that the needle can no longer be inserted from within under guidance of the eye. In the last one or two stitches the order of procedure is therefore changed. The suture is drawn taut for the first time as it emerges from the serosal surface, is continued in the manner of the furrier's suture, and finally tied to the other end of the catgut suture that had previously

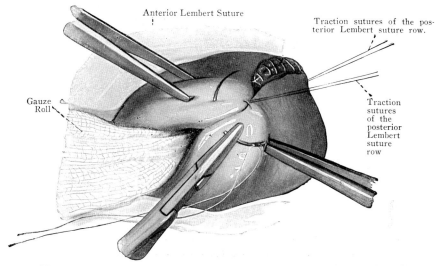

Anterior Lembert Suture

Traction sutures of the posterior Lembert suture row.

Gauze Roll

Traction sutures of the posterior Lembert suture row

FIG. 58. Side-to-side entero-enterostomy, preparation for the fourth step. Application of the end traction sutures of the anterior Lembert suture row behind and beyond the end traction sutures of the posterior Lembert suture row.

been passed through the gut wall from within outward. The ends of the catgut suture are cut short.

It is possible to apply the anterior Albert suture row throughout its course in the form of a furrier's suture as previously described, or the Schmieden or the U- or Connell suture may be used. The difficulty in properly turning in the mucosa in the anterior Albert suture is particularly great in the closure of the last angle of the wound. The difficulty at this point can be avoided by beginning the anterior Albert suture successively at each angle of the wound so that the suture ends at about the middle of the anterior suture line instead of in an angle of the wound.

Instead of always beginning the posterior and the anterior Albert sutures with the ends of the same thread at the wound angle farthest from the operator, it is possible to complete the whole suture by suturing continuously with the one end of the thread. That is, the posterior Albert suture row is inserted from one wound angle to the other and then continued as the anterior Albert suture row back to the starting point. I do not consider this a good procedure because the surgeon has to sew away from himself in one row of sutures, whereas, if he uses one end of the thread from the far angle of the wound for the posterior and the other for the anterior row, he can sew both rows toward himself.

(f) **The Anterior Lembert Suture (Figs. 58 and 59).** Since the intestines are completely closed with the completion of the anterior Albert suture, the anterior Lembert suture is in itself an entirely aseptic operation. Before beginning it, therefore, fresh covers are applied, gloves are changed and clean instruments laid out. Intestinal clamps are removed unless they serve to hold the bowel in a more convenient position.

The two end-traction sutures of the posterior Lembert suture may also be used as traction sutures for the anterior Lembert suture. I prefer, however, to apply two fresh traction sutures about half a centimeter beyond the

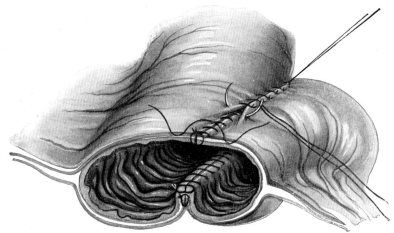

Fig. 59. Side-to-side entero-enterostomy, fourth step (diagrammatic). The anterior sero-muscular (Lembert) suture is being applied in the form of interrupted sutures between two traction sutures.

ends of the posterior Lembert suture line (Fig. 58). After these new sutures have been placed, the old traction sutures divided and the new traction sutures made taut, the anterior Lembert suture is applied with interrupted linen sutures in the usual manner. It should be at least half a centimeter away from the anterior Albert suture. Of course, the anterior Lembert suture row may also be carried out as a continuous suture.

The portions of the two intestines nearest the anastomosis may be fastened together for an additional short distance with a few interrupted sutures. A looping of the mesentery which may have resulted from the anastomosis and which might lead to a strangulated internal hernia is closed by a few interrupted sutures to prevent free loops of gut from slipping through it. During these procedures the anastomosis itself may be handled conveniently by means of the roll of gauze which was placed beneath it before starting the suture and on which the anastomosis now lies. At the end of the operation the gauze roll is cut short on one side of the anastomosis and is withdrawn from the other side.

Lateral anastomosis between two segments is always carried out in the manner described, whether loops of the small or large intestine are united with one another or a loop of the small intestine is united with the stomach. The anastomosis of the common bile duct or of the gall bladder to a portion of the gastro-intestinal canal may also be carried out according to the same technical principles.

Since the taeniae are the strongest portions of the wall of the colon and since they are a dependable guide as to the long axis of the bowel, they are used by preference in the application of the first line of suture. Epiploic appendages which are in the way are first excised.

Button Anastomosis. In addition to the method of intestinal suture just described, an anastomosis between two gut segments may be made by means of the Murphy button. The button consists of two parts, the male and the female sections. The male section is inserted into the female section and the two pressed together, forming a tight unit with an open passage-way in its axis. The male section is inserted into one segment of the intestine while the female section is inserted into the other. The sections of the button are locked together so that the two gut segments are joined to each other and the intestinal passage is established by means of the hollow axis. However, in joining the two halves of the button which have been inserted in the intestine, one smooth metal disc is not pressed against another smooth metal disc, but these discs hold between them the two intestinal walls and the serous surfaces are held in contact with each other. The metal discs exert a marked pressure in the central zones, whereas the pressure at the periphery is less. For this reason the gently apposed serous surfaces at the periphery unite, and the organic union of the two segments is thus effected, while the strongly compressed intestinal walls in the central zone gradually become necrotic and slough off. Because of this, the button is loosened, becomes free in the lumen of the intestine, and should be evacuated through the normal channel in from eight to ten days. Changes of position of the button can be followed by the Roentgen ray. When the button slips out of the anastomosis, there is left a wide passage between the lumens of the two segments. (A number of interrupted Lembert sutures should be placed around the site of junction of the two segments. I. S. R.)

The advantages of the button over suture are that the anastomosis may be more quickly performed, and that the button often makes possible an anastomosis in cases in which there is scarcely sufficient room for a suture anastomosis. Opposed to these advantages there are, however, serious disadvantages. The narrow canal of the button may become obstructed by food or feces; perforation may result at the button anastomosis, or the sloughed-off button may not be passed with the feces, but may have to be removed surgically. Suture anastomosis is therefore the routine procedure, while button anastomosis is today but rarely used and only when there are specific indications for its use. The use of the button in the large bowel is usually contra-indicated because of the degree of inspissation of the feces which obtains in that part of the intestine.

The Technique of Lateral Button Anastomosis (Fig. 60). The central canal of each half of the button is lightly plugged with gauze. The wall of each half is grasped with a hemostat. A hole is cut in one segment of the intestine of such a size that when its edges are stretched apart to the utmost by three Kocher hemostats one-half of the button, held obliquely, can just be forced through it. The button is pushed into one angle of the slit in the gut and the slit is narrowed by Lembert sutures to such an extent that it encloses the neck of the button under tension. In the same way the other half of the button is fastened into the other intestinal segment. The heavy male portion should lie in the proximal segment, since it is hoped, often in vain, that this through gravity will favor the dropping of the button into the distal limb and its more ready passage to the anus. The hemostats and the gauze plugs are now removed. Both halves are grasped through the intestinal wall with the fingers, are fitted into each other and are tightly pressed together. A few Lembert sutures are placed around the button anastomosis.

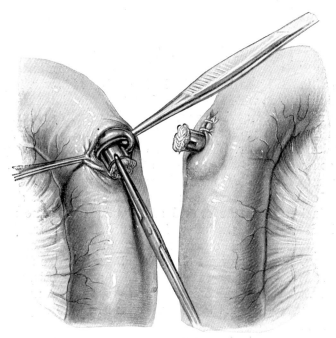

Fig. 60. Side-to-side entero-enterostomy with the Murphy button. One half of the button has been introduced into a slit in the right-hand intestinal segment and the slit closed snugly around it. The other half of the button is being inserted into the intestine on the left.

2. End-to-End Anastomosis

End-to-end anastomosis has the advantage over side-to-side anastomosis in that less gut is necessary. It can therefore be carried out in intestinal segments which cannot be placed side by side for any considerable distance. Peristalsis is less affected than in lateral anastomosis, since the circular muscle of the intestine is not cut across.

End-to-end anastomosis does not require an absolute equality in the size of the lumens of the segments to be united, since an inequality may largely be obviated by placing the sutures a bit farther apart in the wider segment than in the narrower one. In this way the difference in caliber may be distributed evenly over all the sutures. The larger lumen is thus fitted to the smaller one by a sort of puckering. For example, the large cross-section of the stomach can be satisfactorily anastomosed with the small cross-section of the duodenum end-to-end. Frequently one can enlarge the caliber of the narrower segment by dividing it diagonally. If the discrepancy in the size of the two openings is too great, it is advisable partially to close the larger opening and to anastomose the smaller lumen to the resultant residual opening. The technique to be followed is described and illustrated in detail under resection of the stomach on page 163.

End-to-end anastomosis between two parts of the gastro-intestinal canal is often carried out most conveniently when the segment to be resected is still

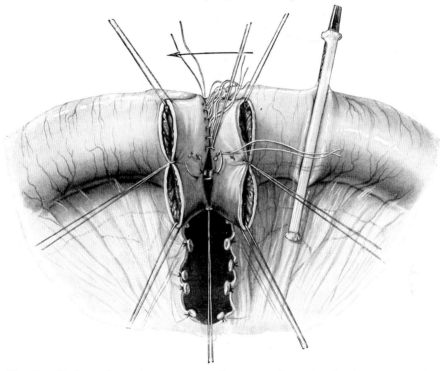

FIG. 61. End-to-end entero-enterostomy, first step. Posterior Lembert suture. Interrupted sutures are being applied between the open intestinal ends which are held apart by traction sutures.

connected with the remaining segments the separation taking place in the course of the anastomosis. This also best prevents the gut segments to be sutured from slipping out of reach, a danger which exists, for instance, in a high resection of the stomach or a low resection of the duodenum. In this procedure the two segments, after they have been freed from their mesenteries and other attachments as far as the site of resection, are placed together so that mesenteric attachment is apposed to mesenteric attachment. The work on the intestinal segments is facilitated if they are grasped with a clamp parallel to the intended site of anastomosis.

The two parts of the intestine are first united by a posterior interrupted linen Lembert suture. The suture is begun with a knotted suture at each end of the suture line (Fig. 61); the ends of the sutures are left long for use as traction sutures. By holding these sutures taut, flat surfaces of both gut segments are brought together so that the posterior Lembert suture can easily be completed between the two traction sutures. The sutures must be carried carefully around the mesenteric attachment if it has not been cut away. The two parts of the intestine are then opened parallel to, and at a distance of 1 cm. from this suture. The openings so made extend for half the circumference of the gut. The wound edges of the segments which are to remain in the body are joined by a running three-layer catgut suture, the posterior Albert suture (Fig. 62). The division of the gut is now completed, permitting the removal of the part to be resected. The newly made wound edges of the intestines are now sutured together by an anterior Albert suture in the form

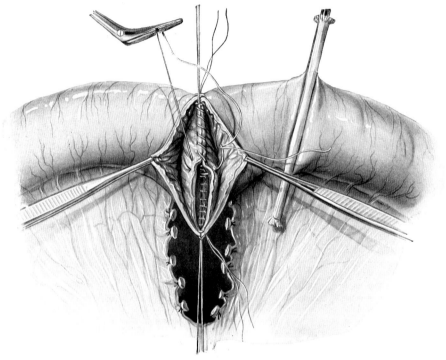

Fig. 62. End-to-end entero-enterostomy, second step. Posterior Albert suture, a continuous suture.

of an anterior running three-layer suture with catgut. I use the invertible suture of Mikulicz (Fig. 63). However, any of the other suture methods previously described may be used. The gut lumens have now been closed. The anterior Lembert suture follows (Fig. 64). It is carried out in the manner above described. Two end-traction sutures are applied half a centimeter beyond the end-sutures of the posterior Lembert suture line and the interrupted sutures which are applied between the end-traction sutures are placed at a distance of about half a centimeter from the anterior Albert suture. The slit in the mesentery is closed with interrupted catgut sutures (Figs. 63 and 64).

Often it is necessary to remove completely the segment to be resected, or to divide one end of the segment before beginning the suture. The task is then that of joining two open ends of intestine, or of joining one open end to an as yet unopened segment. In order to be able to apply the posterior Lembert suture more conveniently, each opening should be provided with three traction sutures, placed close to the cut edges. Each open end is provided with a traction suture at the point of the mesenteric attachment and at the point opposite and a third traction suture is passed through the midpoints of both cut edges lying between the first two traction sutures (Fig. 61). In this manner each end is provided with three traction sutures, the middle one of which holds the walls together at the midpoint, while the other two stretch the opening into a narrow slit. The intestines are now joined by a posterior Lembert suture fully half a centimeter from the cut edges as they

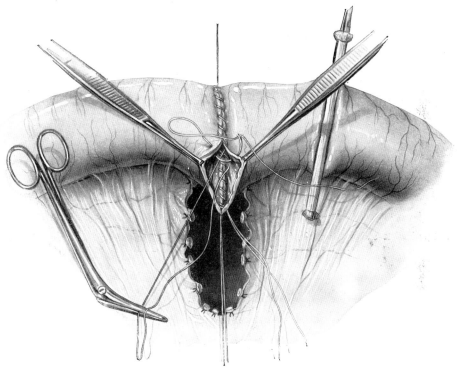

FIG. 63.   End-to-end anastomosis, third step. Anterior Albert continuous suture applied by the method of Mikulicz.

are held taut by the three traction sutures. During this procedure the traction sutures serve to evert the ends of the intestine. The traction sutures may then be removed, and a posterior three-layer running catgut suture is placed (Fig. 62). There follows the anterior three-layer running catgut suture (Fig. 63) and finally the anterior interrupted Lembert suture with silk or linen (Fig. 64).

Even when it is necessary to divide one or both ends of the segment to be removed before beginning an end-to-end anastomosis, it may be advantageous first to close the intestine with the Petz suture instrument and to divide it between the two rows of clips (Fig. 339). The end-to-end anastomosis is then carried out close to the clip suture line, the intestine being opened and divided in stages, with resection of the strip of wound edge bearing the clips.

The Cuff Procedure. Based on the premise that a long cuff-like connection between two intestinal segments should afford greater safety than the end-to-end position just described, there has been advised a cuff-invagination

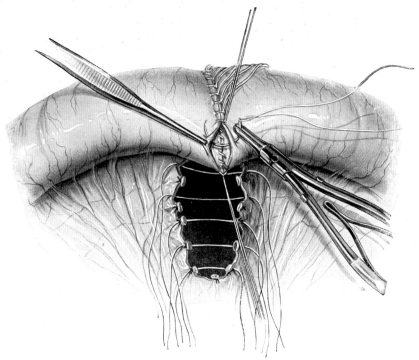

FIG. 64.   End-to-end anastomosis, fourth step.   Anterior Lembert interrupted suture.   The slit in the mesentery is closed by interrupted sutures.

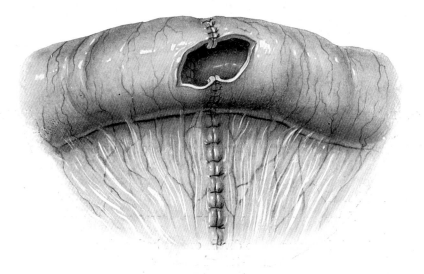

FIG. 65.   End-to-end anastomosis.   A view of and into the completed anastomosis.

type of procedure for entero-enterostomy by Jobert and for gastro-enterostomy by Goepel (Fig. 138). It consists in the removal of the mucosa of the proximal segment for a distance of several centimeters and the application of this inner

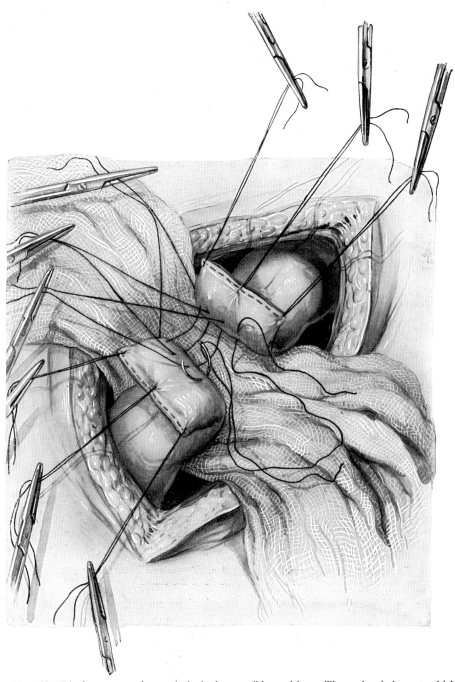

F𝗶𝗀. 66. Placing sutures in a relatively inaccessible position. The ends of the gut which have been closed by Petz clips are joined by interrupted posterior Lembert sutures, the threads of which are not yet tied but are held together, each pair by a hemostat. When all the sutures have been inserted they are tied, one after the other.

wound surface to the serosa of the distal segment over which it is drawn like a cuff and to which it is fastened. This procedure, which entails the use of a considerable amount of tissue, has no advantages over the Czerny double-row suture. It lacks the very property which in our experience gives absolute dependability to intestinal suture—the broad approximation of serosal surfaces.

The Embroidery Suture. The dependability of an intestinal suture depends upon the care with which it is carried out. In relatively inaccessible places, great difficulty may be encountered in accurately placing the individual

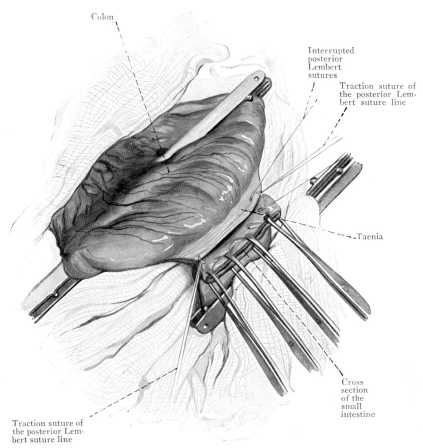

FIG. 67. End-to-side entero-enterostomy, first step. Posterior Lembert suture line grasping on one side a free taenia of the colon.

sutures in the anastomosis of two intestinal segments. This is particularly true if after the application of the first few sutures the gastro-intestinal segments involved block the further approach to the line of suture in the depth of the wound, as, for example, in suturing near the diaphragm in case of total resection of the stomach or in suturing in the depth of the pelvis in case of resection of the sigmoid and rectum. In such instances the application of the sutures, especially of the posterior Lembert suture row, can be facilitated in the following manner:

All the sutures are passed, one after another, and in the proper order, without tying the individual threads (Fig. 66). The two ends of each suture are grasped in a hemostat and brought out of the wound in sequence. Not until all the sutures have been passed are they tied, one after the other.

End-to-end anastomosis by means of the Murphy button—a procedure to be used rarely—is performed as follows: A purse-string suture is placed around each end of intestine. This suture, which barely includes the mucosa, is placed as an overcast suture on the edge of the segment in the direction mucosa-muscularis-serosa, mucosa-muscularis-serosa. The suture begins opposite the mesenteric attachment, overcasts one-half of the circumference

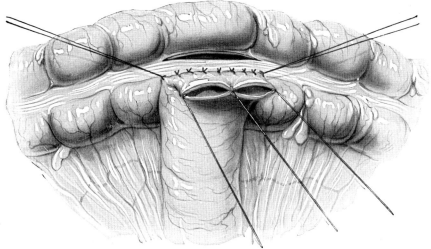

Fig. 68. End-to-side anastomosis. The posterior Lembert suture has been completed. The colon has been opened to correspond with the length and direction of the open end of the small bowel.

of the gut, catches the mesentery with one recurrent stitch and then returns along the other semi-circumference to the point of starting. The ends of the suture emerge on the serosal surface. The halves of the button are then inserted into the two ends and are secured by drawing taut and tying the sutures. The two halves are now pressed together and the anastomosis is secured by a few interrupted Lembert sutures.

3. END-TO-SIDE AND SIDE-TO-END ANASTOMOSIS

Here, too, it is convenient if the end of intestine or stomach to be implanted is not first opened, but is divided during the course of the anastomosis (Figs. 113, 141). In each instance the posterior wall of the segment to be implanted is attached by a row of Lembert sutures to the intestine into which it is to be implanted (Fig. 67). In carrying out the anastomosis the use of clamps will prevent soiling while the suture is being placed. After the segments have been sutured together perpendicular to each other they are opened (in case they are still closed) at a distance of ½ cm. from the line of suture (Fig. 68). The longitudinal incision in the side of the receiving viscus is made somewhat shorter than the opening in the end of the proximal loop. The two intestinal walls are joined by a posterior three-layer running catgut suture (Fig. 69). The anterior wall of the gut to be implanted is then divided, freeing the part to be resected. The anterior three-layer suture (Fig. 70), as a rule in the form of a continuous suture, is placed and then the anterior Lembert suture (Fig. 71), as a rule with interrupted sutures.

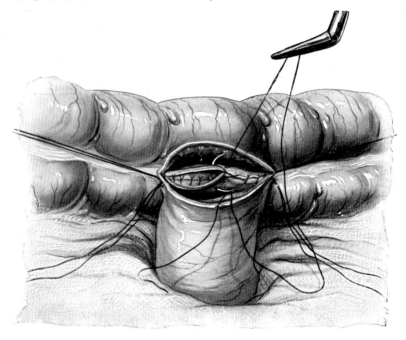

FIG. 69. End-to-side anastomosis, second step. Posterior Albert suture.

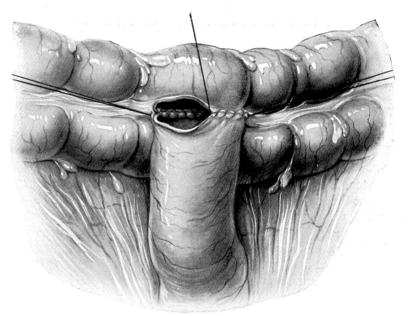

FIG. 70. End-to-side anastomosis. Anterior Albert suture.

If the end of intestine or stomach to be implanted was divided previous to the anastomosis, it is provided with three traction sutures (Figs. 66 and 68), one of which joins the mesenteric attachment to the point just opposite, while the other two are placed at the free corners. Half a centimeter from the cut edge of this viscus a posterior Lembert suture is applied joining it to the side of the recipient intestine and in the long axis of the latter. The latter is then opened at a distance of ½ cm. from this line of suture. The

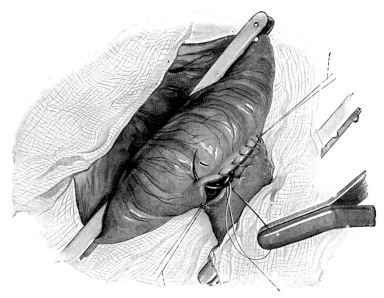

Fig. 71. End-to-side anastomosis, fourth step. Anterior Lembert suture.

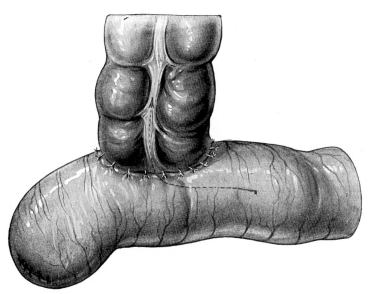

Fig. 72. Side-to-end anastomosis.

three traction sutures are removed and then follow, in the manner described, the posterior three-layer suture, the anterior three-layer suture and the anterior Lembert suture.

In the exceptional use of the Murphy button for end-to-side anastomosis, each viscus is supplied with one-half of the button in the manner described under side-to-side button anastomosis, and end-to-end button anastomosis. The button is closed and the site of anastomosis is oversewed with a few Lembert sutures.

Side-to-end anastomosis is carried out with the same technique. It is employed, for example, in the implantation of a transsected small intestine into the stomach (Fig. 118), more rarely in entero-enterostomy (Fig. 72).

on tension and made accessible. In so doing, it may be advantageous to divide the round ligament of the liver between two ligatures (Fig. 352), since it hinders the displacement of the liver, and then to divide the falciform ligament of the liver. By retracting the right half of the liver, the duodenum can be exposed and inspected as far as the point where it is crossed by the transverse mesocolon.

The duodenum has no free mesentery, and with the exception of its proximal portion nearest the pylorus which is completely surrounded by

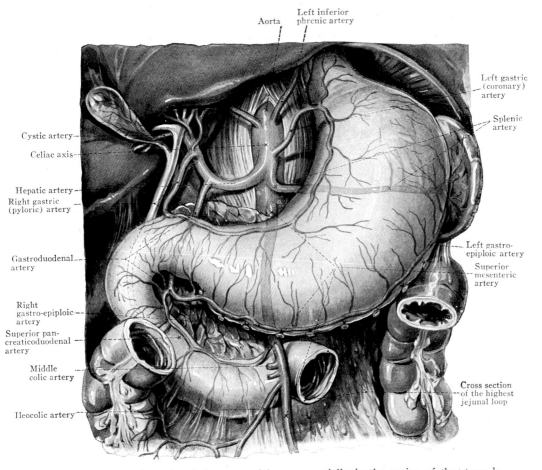

FIG. 73.   The arterial supply of the upper abdomen, especially in the region of the stomach, liver and duodenum.

peritoneum it lies flat against the posterior abdominal wall so that its dorsal surface is not covered by peritoneum. The dividing line between stomach and duodenum is usually clearly marked by a transverse vein, the pyloric vein of Mayo. The duodenum (Fig. 73) may be divided for surgical purposes into a superior portion, a descending portion which lies to the right of the second lumbar vertebra and into which the biliary and pancreatic ducts empty from behind, and an inferior portion which crosses the vertebral column, passes beneath the root of the mesentery to the duodenojejunal flexure and is therefore overlaid and crossed by the superior mesenteric artery and vein. This latter relation is supposedly of significance in the development of arterio-mesenteric ileus.

To inspect the extrahepatic biliary passages and the hepatoduodenal liga-ment (the right free border of the gastrohepatic omentum), the gall bladder is pulled forward with a smooth grasping forceps, the cystic duct is caught and tension is made on it (Fig. 357). The cystic duct passes into the hepato-duodenal ligament which leads to the duodenum. If it is possible without too much trauma to tip the liver up over the right costal margin, the inspec-tion of this region is made easier. Behind the hepatoduodenal ligament the foramen of Winslow leads from right to left and behind the stomach to the lesser peritoneal cavity. By inserting one finger through the foramen and another above it, it is possible to palpate between the fingers the component parts of the hepatoduodenal ligament, especially the common bile duct.

The hepatoduodenal ligament contains vital structures, the common bile duct, the hepatic artery and the portal vein (Figs. 349-351).

The pancreas can be approached at the left of the duodenum, either above the stomach through the gastrohepatic omentum, below the stomach through the gastrocolic omentum, or through the transverse mesocolon, in which case the base of the transverse colon must be elevated.

The blood supply of the stomach is from the celiac axis. The main vessels (Fig. 73) run along the lesser curvature (coronary (gastric) artery, pyloric artery) and along the greater curvature (right and left gastro-epiploic arteries). These two important arterial systems, which run approximately parallel to each other and to the long axis of the stomach, are connected by small transverse vessels which run perpendicular to the long axis of the stomach. In addition the stomach has important vascular connections in the form of the vasa brevia branches of the splenic artery which reach the fundus from behind. As a result of this abundant blood supply the stomach can be freed extensively from its attachments, it can be transsected at the cardia or the pylorus and mobilized without fear of nutritional disturbances from lack of blood supply.

The lymph vessels parallel the blood vessels. They, too, follow the greater and the lesser curvatures. At the attachment of the gastrocolic omentum and especially in the gastrohepatic omentum, are found the most important lymph nodes which usually contain the first metastases in gastric carcinoma. The next most important sites of metastasis lie in the liver, at the hilus of the spleen, and above all in the region of the celiac axis in the retro-peritoneal space.

If the lower abdomen is to be exposed, the transverse colon is grasped and turned upward, together with the greater omentum which is attached to it (Fig. 95). If the entire small intestine is displaced downward toward the pelvis and the transverse mesocolon made tense by traction on the transverse colon, the lower transverse portion of the duodenum can be seen shining through the peritoneum of the posterior abdominal wall. Immediately above it lies the body of the pancreas. Slipping the hand along the under surface of the stretched mesocolon just to the left of the vertebral column, the duodeno-jejunal flexure and the highest loop of jejunum can be reached (Fig. 118).

By making traction on this loop, the most distal portion of the duodenum can be brought into view.

Abdominal Incisions for Operations on the Stomach (see Chapter I). The usual incision for exposing the stomach is the median longitudinal incision from the xiphoid process to the umbilicus or a short distance below it. I carry the incision through the center of the umbilicus, though most surgeons cut around and to the left of it. A paramedian rectus incision may, of course, also be used. If the operation on the stomach extends far beneath

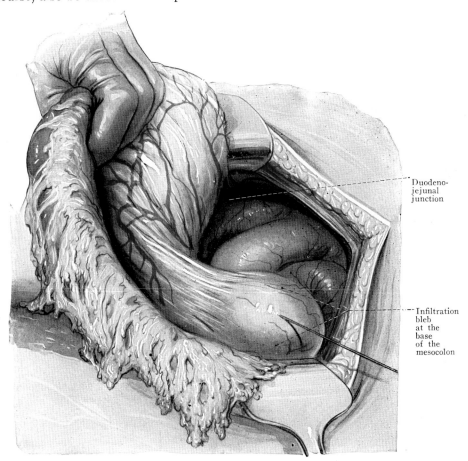

Duodeno-
jejunal
junction

Infiltration
bleb
at the
base
of the
mesocolon

Fig. 74a. Infiltration of the base of the transverse mesocolon with a local anesthetic.

the left costal margin, it is to be remembered that the median incision may be extended to the left of the xiphoid process as far as the body of the sternum and that the removal of the xiphoid process gives still more room. Only exceptionally however is it necessary to enlarge the wound by a transverse incision dividing the left or the right rectus.

In operations which involve the cardia or the fundus of the stomach, or which extend high up on the lesser curvature, a reflection of the left costal margin in the manner previously described and illustrated in Chapter I, may occasionally become necessary.

Anaesthesia. Gastric operations are performed under general anaesthesia by most surgeons because both pain and consciousness are thus lost. Spinal anaesthesia is preferable, however, because of the excellent relaxation of the abdominal walls and the remarkable quietness of the patient. Spinal anaesthesia with injection of air and the anesthetic floating on the spinal fluid as I practice it gives incomparable results and is my routine procedure. Since spinal anaesthesia, especially when a small dose is used, does not with certainty block the pain-conducting sympathetic nerves and vagi, it is necessary to block these nerves individually, after opening the abdomen, and before

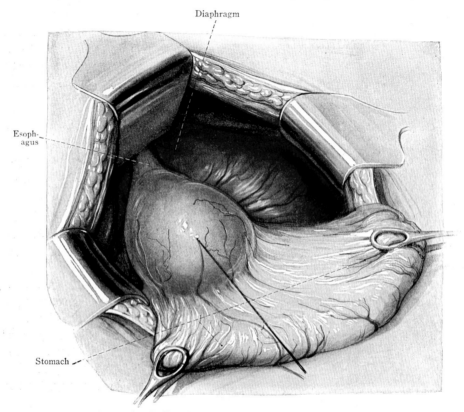

Fig. 74b. Infiltration of the cardia with a local anesthetic.

the patient is subjected to any pain. A complete blocking of these nerve paths is possible only by means of my high-pressure (three atmospheres) local anaesthesia apparatus and can be carried out in a few seconds. Using a $\frac{1}{2}$ per cent novocain, $\frac{1}{40}$ per cent percain solution with adrenalin added, infiltrations in the form of large edematous blebs are carried out (1) in the base of the mesocolon after reflecting the transverse colon upward (Fig. 74a), (2) in the region of the aorta just below the diaphragm after reflecting the colon downward and dividing the gastrohepatic omentum (Vol. I, Fig. 185), and (3) in the region of the cardia while the stomach is pulled downward and forward (Fig. 74b).

If spinal anaesthesia is being used and if a high-pressure local-anaesthesia apparatus is available, the infiltration of the retroperitoneal tissue in the region of the great vessels just below the diaphragm is not carried out with

the aid of touch alone in the manner described in Vol. I, page 199, but the region is clearly exposed and the infiltration is carried out under the safe guidance of the eye. To do this, the stomach is retracted downward and the right lobe of the liver is retracted upward with a large right-angled spatula. The delicate gastrohepatic ligament is divided at a point free of vessels. The caudate lobe of the liver which covers the great vessels is seen through this opening. It is retracted upward with a Kader spatula. The great vessels, the vena cava and the aorta, can now be clearly seen just below the point at which they emerge from the diaphragm. A flexible electric illuminator is valuable in this procedure.

A needle 16 cm. long with a bevel at an angle of 45° is attached to the local anaesthesia apparatus and the tip of the needle is inserted into the loose, extremely delicate tissue over the aorta and about 40 cc. of the standard solution of $\frac{1}{40}$ per cent percain, $\frac{1}{2}$ per cent novocain-adrenalin solution are injected. There is immediately formed a translucent edematous bleb the size of a fist which overlies the vessels and the spine.

Exposure of the site of injection can also be effected by inserting a ground-glass vaginal speculum about 3.5 cm. in diameter and about 15 cm. in length into the opening in the gastrohepatic omentum. The caudate lobe is pushed aside and the end of the speculum is gradually worked close to the great vessels. The injection of the retroperitoneal tissue is then carried out with the aid of a long needle passed through the speculum.

It is absolutely essential in the course of the injection to avoid injuring the peritoneum with repeated needle pricks, for the anesthetic solution will leak from these openings so that the amount remaining in the retroperitoneal tissues will be inadequate for anaesthesia. If the infiltration has been carried out properly, the stomach can be pulled on as much as is necessary without producing the slightest discomfort to the patient.

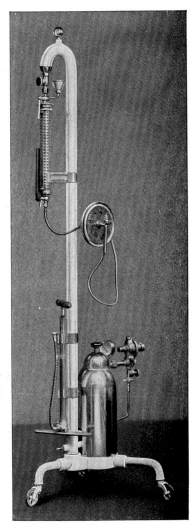

FIG. 75. Kirschner's apparatus for administering local anesthetic solutions under high pressure. The upright part of the stand is a gas chamber in which a pressure of 3 atmospheres is effected by means of the carbon dioxide tank at the base of the apparatus. When the tank is empty, pressure can also be generated by means of the foot pump. The high pressure in the gas chamber forces the anesthetic solution in the glass cylinder through the attached tubing and handle to the injection needle. The rate of flow of the solution through the needle is controlled by pressure on a button in the handle.

If in the course of a long gastric operation the anaesthesia from the spinal anesthetic wears off, severe pain should not be permitted to develop, but the necessary measures should be instituted at the first evidence of discomfort. The self-retaining retractor is removed. First the right and then the left side of the abdominal wound is raised with retractors so that the needle of the high-pressure local-anaesthesia apparatus can be inserted from within the abdomen into the parietal peritoneum. A series of large edematous blebs which elevate the peritoneum and which merge into each other are injected all around the abdominal incision. The anaesthesia so produced persists often for hours. The same procedure is used in case the anaesthesia from an inadequate injection of the spinal anesthetic is unsatisfactory from the beginning. Even if there is no pain during the operation, the prophylactic injection beneath the parietal peritoneum at the end of the operation has the advantage that the patient as a rule experiences little or no after-pain in the region of the wound. (It has been my practice to start an inhalation anesthetic when during the course of an abdominal operation where spinal anaesthesia was used the patient begins to complain of pain. I. S. R.)

Operations on the stomach can be performed under local anaesthesia alone. The procedure is as follows: The line of incision is anesthetized subcutaneously down to the peritoneum (the passage of the needle point through the linea alba can be felt distinctly) by injecting $\frac{1}{2}$ per cent novocain, $\frac{1}{40}$ per cent percain solution with adrenalin. The abdomen is then carefully opened. The abdominal walls are gently elevated, and injected on both sides from the wound. The marginal zone of the parietal peritoneum is injected with particular care from within the abdomen, with the formation of large edematous blebs. With the high-pressure local-anaesthesia apparatus this takes only one or two minutes. After the insertion of the self-retaining retractor, the blocking of the sympathetic and vagus nerves is carried out in the manner described above.

Local anaesthesia with the high-pressure apparatus (Fig. 75) as described by me (Kirschner, Deutsch. Ztschr. f. Chir., Volume 234, Bier Festschrift) is of the greatest assistance for anaesthesia in abdominal operations, because the required injections can be carried out more rapidly, gently, effectively, safely and neatly than with the usual hand syringes. This type of apparatus is superior when local anaesthesia is desired at any site.

In all gastric operations the self-retaining retractor described and illustrated in Vol. I, page 76, will be found especially advantageous. I find it nearly indispensable.

B. INCISION OF THE STOMACH (GASTROTOMY)
THE TREATMENT OF GASTRIC HEMORRHAGE

Gastrotomy is performed for the removal of foreign bodies, tumors, or ulcers; for the inspection or palpation of the interior of the stomach, for the ligation of bleeding gastric vessels, and for the retrograde dilatation of the cardia and retrograde bouginage of the esophagus.

Incision of the Stomach. As a rule the stomach is lavaged before the operation. The abdomen is usually opened by a midline incision. The part of the stomach to be opened is drawn out of the abdominal wound as far as possible. The general abdominal cavity is always carefully walled off by gauze pads. If only a very limited part of the gastric interior is to be inspected and attacked from the opening, that part of the stomach may be shut off from the remainder by two clamps applied across the stomach from the greater to the lesser curvature, one clamp on the cardiac side, the other toward the pylorus (Fig. 76). Portions of the gastrocolic omentum which are

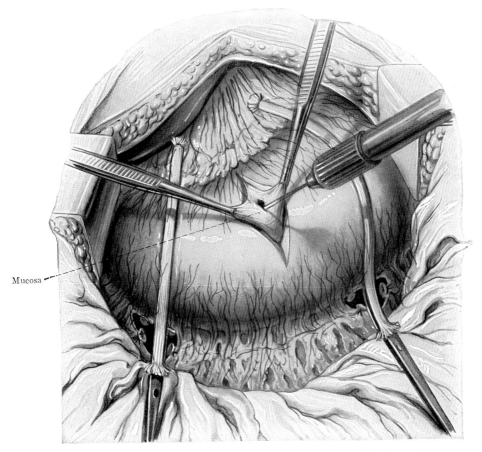

Mucosa

FIG. 76. Gastrotomy. The segment of stomach involved has been closed on each side with a stomach clamp. The incision, made perpendicular to the long axis of the stomach, has divided the serous and muscle coats and is opening the mucosa which is being held with two forceps. The incision is made with an electrosurgical knife.

in the way are divided between ligatures for a short distance close to the stomach. In most instances, however, clamps should not be used.

The direction of choice of the incision corresponds to the course of the vessels—from the lesser toward the greater curvature. Preferably with the electrosurgical knife, the serosa and muscularis are incised for the full length of the intended incision (Fig. 76). The exposed mucosa is lifted up by two forceps and a small incision is made through it. Through the small opening, whose edges are elevated by forceps in order to prevent the escape of gastric contents, there is immediately introduced an aspirating tube which is attached

to an electric suction pump and the stomach is emptied. After enlarging the
opening a little, the aspiration is completed and any material left behind can
be removed with sponges.

Not until then is the opening enlarged to the desired size. Bleeding
vessels are caught and ligated. The wound edges are elevated by means of
Kocher clamps or Allis forceps, or by traction sutures which grasp the edges

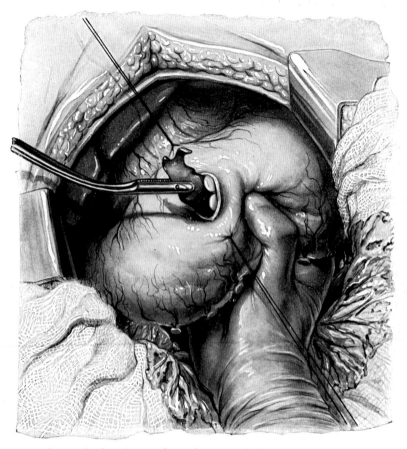

Fig. 77. Removal of a denture from the stomach by gastrotomy. The hand is passed
behind the stomach through an opening in the gastrocolic omentum and presses the denture
against the anterior wall of the stomach, which has been provided with two traction sutures.
The denture is pulled out through a small incision.

of serosa and muscularis, so that any remaining gastric contents cannot escape.
The stomach is once again carefully wiped out with a gauze sponge.

The interior of the stomach can now be palpated and inspected. Inspection is facilitated by careful sponging, by the insertion of large blunt hook
retractors into the gastric wound and by the introduction of a small electric
light or a cystoscope into the gastric interior. If the left hand is placed
behind the stomach through a slit in the gastrocolic omentum, the posterior
wall of the stomach can be brought into the field of vision (Fig. 79).

At the conclusion of the operation the gastric wound is closed in the
line of incision by a continuous three-layer suture of catgut and then by

interrupted Lembert sutures of linen. To facilitate the suture, the gastric incision is put on stretch by means of two end-traction sutures.

If clamps were applied, they are removed and the protecting pads are discarded. The stomach is then dropped back into the peritoneal cavity.

Gastric injuries are taken care of by the same suture technique. In such cases the posterior wall of the stomach must be subjected to careful inspection, since only too often, especially in gun shot wounds, both walls of the stomach are injured.

The abdominal wound is closed without drainage after gastrotomy.

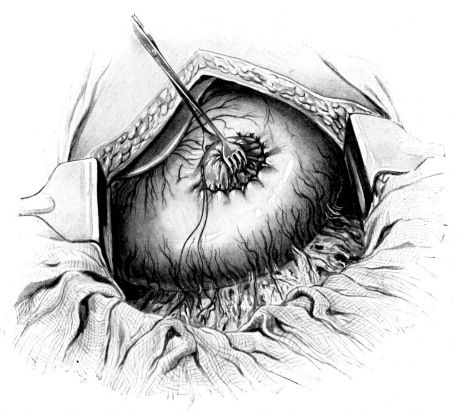

Fig. 78. Encircling a bleeding gastric ulcer from without by overlapping interrupted sutures.

The Removal of Foreign Bodies. If a foreign body is to be removed from the stomach, an attempt should be made to palpate it after opening the abdomen and before opening the stomach. The foreign body is forced against the anterior wall of the stomach, at times with the assistance of a hand passed behind the stomach. A small incision is then made over the foreign body, through which the object is extracted with a forceps (Fig. 77).

The Treatment of Gastric Hemorrhage. Chronic gastric hemorrhage which does not immediately threaten life is dealt with by treating the gastric disease (ulcer, carcinoma) underlying the bleeding according to the principles laid down on page 134.

In the treatment of acute gastric hemorrhage, radical procedures are also to be preferred, notably the resection of the portion of the stomach bearing the lesion. Unfortunately, at times these measures cannot be employed because of the poor condition of the patient as a result of the loss of blood and simpler but also less certain measures must be resorted to, which commonly do not effect a permanent cure. (The editor believes that in acute

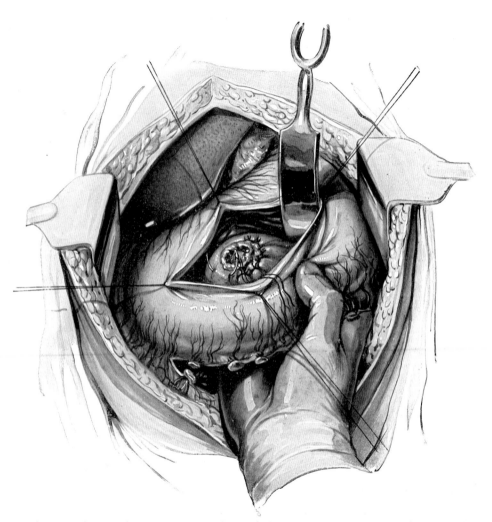

FIG. 79. Surrounding a gastric ulcer from within by overlapping interrupted sutures after opening the stomach. The operator's right or left hand passes behind the stomach through a slit in the gastrocolic omentum, presses the ulcer forward toward the opening in the anterior stomach wall.

gastric or duodenal hemorrhage operation is not primarily indicated. Rest, morphine, and blood transfusion, if the blood pressure drops too low, have in my experience been more satisfactory than primary operation on the stomach or duodenum. Too often primary extensive operative procedures in such cases result in a fatal ending. It has been my practice to palliate acute hemorrhage until the condition of the patient has improved and until the bleeding has stopped. In the hemorrhage associated with certain diseases of the spleen it may be advisable to operate at once but donors should be at hand for transfusion before, during or after operation. I. S. R.)

If, after the exposure of the stomach, the site of the bleeding can be determined from the outside (which is the exception), this point is encircled by a series of sutures applied from without and including all the layers of the gastric wall (Fig. 78). The site of these through-and-through sutures is in turn buried by Lembert sutures. In addition, the large vessels along the gastric curvatures supplying the bleeding point are individually ligated. In most cases the bleeding point can not be determined from the outside, so that it is necessary to open the stomach. But even on internal inspection it may be difficult or impossible to find the source of the hemorrhage. After the stomach has been emptied by suction and by sponging, the bleeding point is sought by a systematic unfolding of the mucosa and with the aid of a light introduced into the stomach or by pushing individual segments of the stomach out through the anterior opening by means of the hand placed behind the stomach. If the bleeding vessel is found on internal inspection, it is controlled by a circle of sutures introduced on the mucosal surface (Fig. 79).

Unfortunately, the source of bleeding is often looked for in vain, and the gastrotomy must be terminated without having accomplished its purpose. Transillumination as advised by Rovsing for the discovery of the bleeding vessel has not proved successful.

Packing the stomach followed by jejunostomy does not give good results in the treatment of gastric hemorrhage and should be condemned.

Attention is called to the fact that hemorrhages recurring at short intervals rarely force one to operate, since they usually stop spontaneously. Nevertheless, there are cases in which operative arrest of bleeding finally seems to be the only hope. A preoperative blood transfusion makes the patient a safe operative risk for the time being.

C. THE ESTABLISHMENT AND CLOSURE OF A GASTRIC FISTULA (GASTROSTOMY—VON HACKER)

Gastrostomy is indicated when the passage of food through the esophagus is blocked, markedly impeded, or attended by danger to the patient. The gastrostomy opening may either remain for life or for a limited time until the disease of the esophagus has cleared up. Gastrostomy is also occasionally used to drain the stomach in case of intense vomiting resulting from paralytic ileus or in case of postoperative dilatation of the stomach. Since patients with a gastric fistula can drink large quantities of fluids at will and without harm, a gastrostomy at the same time serves to relieve the vomiting and the thirst which are so distressing in these conditions. (I believe that the introduction of a Jutte tube will accomplish all of the above advantages without subjecting the patient to operation to accomplish them. I. S. R.)

It is a matter of great importance to the patient from the standpoint of cleanliness that gastric contents shall not escape around the tube. This is controlled primarily by leading the tube which connects the interior of the stomach with the body surface through a long tunnel lined with serosa (canal of Witzel). In consequence of the tendency of irritated peritoneal surfaces to become adherent, the canal tends to become narrower and does not permit any fluid to escape around the tube.

In implanting the tube in the stomach, I prefer the position in which the free inner end is directed toward the cardia to that in which it points toward the pylorus as favored by many surgeons. The location of the end of the tube in the air bubble of the fundus prevents the escape of fluid from the open tube during feeding. The introduction of the food into the proximal segment of the stomach corresponds to the normal conditions, and in some cases of stenosis of the esophagus the direction of the fistula toward the cardia facilitates the subsequent handling of a loop of thread passed through the esophagus and the fistula, or the application of radium to the cardia.

The operation may be performed under local anaesthesia, but the delivery of the stomach usually entails some pain for the patient. The use of avertin anaesthesia is very helpful; the patients tolerate it remarkably well as a rule, in spite of their usually very poor condition. Less taxing is the supplementary blocking of sympathetic and vagus nerves by means of local anaesthesia as above described. (The latter is not necessary if the tissues are handled gently and the abdominal incision is properly placed. I. S. R.) The most comfortable method for the patient is spinal anaesthesia.

I prefer the midline abdominal incision, but it can also be made through the middle of the left rectus according to the old method of von Hacker, or at the outer edge of the left rectus. The incisions are begun just below the costal margin.

After opening the abdomen it is often difficult to find and deliver the stomach, which has frequently become shrunken. To facilitate the search the wound edges are gently elevated with blunt abdominal retractors. In the space between the abdominal wall and the abdominal viscera the anterior wall of the stomach can often be seen and can be identified by its color and vessel arrangement. If the patient coughs the stomach is pushed down and is easier to see. In an emergency, the great omentum may be used as a guide for it will surely lead to the stomach. Traction on the omentum will cause pain if only local anaesthesia of the abdominal walls is being used. The stomach is grasped with intestinal forceps and by gentle traction as large a part of the anterior wall, as near the fundus as possible, is delivered. The highest point of the anterior wall of the stomach which can be brought into the wound is fixed with a traction suture. A second traction suture is applied near the pylorus and in the median longitudinal line of the stomach. By traction on these sutures a straight fold running in the long axis of the stomach is lifted up. At this point the general abdominal cavity is walled off with moist gauze pads.

1. The Establishment of a Gastrostomy with Formation of a Serosal Canal. Witzel's Method

A rubber tube is selected with an external diameter of 8 mm., a caliber of 5 mm., and a length of 50 cm. The length is important because subsequent measurements will always indicate how far the tube extends into the interior of the stomach. This tube is placed upon the fold of gastric wall in such a way that the end toward the cardia extends about 12 cm. beyond the upper traction suture. The end toward the pylorus is clamped. Just on the pyloric side of the upper traction suture two folds of anterior gastric wall are picked up, one on each side of the tube, by introducing an interrupted Lembert suture through serosa and muscularis on each side of the tube (Fig. 80). The two points are at such a distance from each other that when the ends of the suture are tied over the tube, the two folds just meet to form a tunnel which is snug and water-tight around the tube. About 4 to 6 cm. toward the pylorus

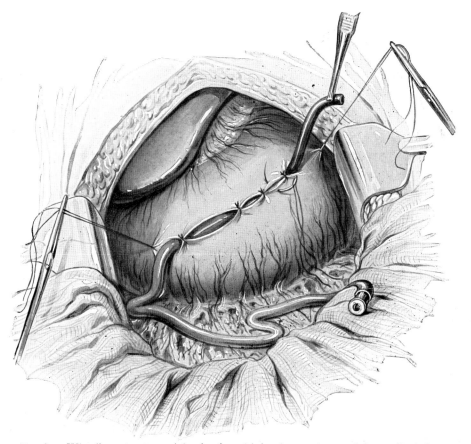

FIG. 80. Witzel's gastrostomy (1). A tube, with its short end toward the cardia, is fastened by means of interrupted sutures to the anterior wall of the stomach between two sero-muscular folds.

a similar short tunnel is formed around the tube by means of a second suture. The portion of the anterior wall of the stomach between these two tunnels is now formed into a continuous tunnel, fitting tightly around the tube, by means of a continuous suture or interrupted sutures which are applied while traction is made on the two end-traction sutures. The rubber tube is thus fixed on the anterior wall of the stomach in a serosal tunnel, about 6 cm. long, which tightly surrounds it. Both ends of the tube project from the tunnel.

The end of the tube toward the cardia is now bent back and the anterior

wall of the stomach is caught close to the point of exit of the tube with two
Lembert stitches that are not tied for the moment. Between these Lembert
sutures and the point of exit of the tube a small opening is made into the
lumen of the stomach. The edges of the hole are immediately caught with
three small Kocher hemostats or Allis forceps (Fig. 81). While the hole is
held open, the free end of the tube is introduced into the stomach by means
of a dissecting forceps. The last-placed Lembert sutures are now immediately
pulled tight and tied, thus covering and burying the opening in the stomach
and the point of entrance of the tube. A few additional sutures secure the

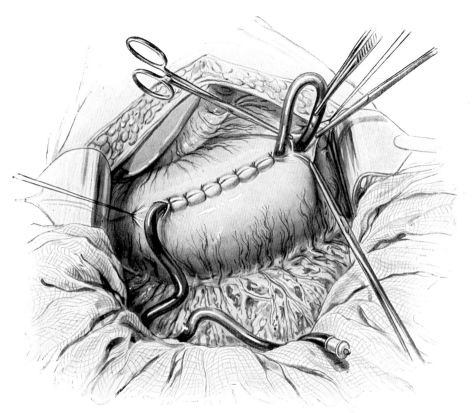

Fig. 81. Witzel's gastrostomy (2). The short end of the tube which is attached to the
anterior surface of the stomach by a Witzel canal is inserted through a small opening into the
interior of the stomach and the area oversewed.

closure of the gastric opening. It is now advisable to inject some fluid through
the tube to assure oneself of its proper position.

A long silk thread is now tied tightly around the long end of the tube close
to its exit from the Witzel canal. The ends of this silk thread are passed from
within outward, each through one of the folds of gastric wall bordering the
point of exit of the tube (Fig. 82).

The tube may be carried out of the abdomen through the laparotomy
wound or through a separate opening. Since the exit of the tube through the
laparotomy wound constitutes a danger to primary wound healing, I consider

it preferable to make a separate opening. The long ends of the silk thread, previously tied around the tube and passed through the two folds of serosa, are now tied firmly by means of a separate thread to the end of the tube bent at right angles. The left side of the abdominal wound is elevated so that the surgeon can get a view of the inner side of the adjacent abdominal wall (Fig. 82). A stab wound is made through the abdominal wall preferably from within outward at a point somewhat to the outer side of the outer border of the left rectus and a little below the costal margin. The tube and the two

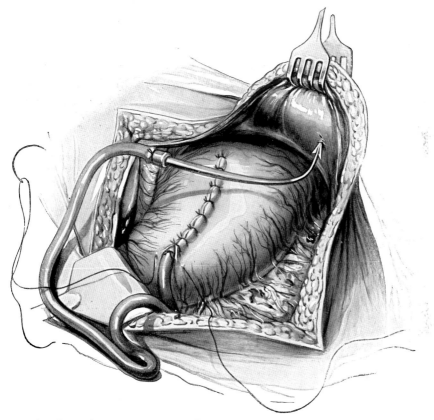

FIG. 82. Witzel's gastrostomy (3). A spearhead has been fastened to the long, free end of the tube, the left border of the abdominal wound is elevated and the spearhead is passed from within outward through all layers of the abdominal wall, drawing the tube through with it.

ends of the long silk thread attached to it are pulled through the opening until the point of exit of the tube out of the stomach lies against the inner surface of the abdominal wall. One end of the long silk thread is now armed with a needle and is passed through the skin close to the fistulous opening, from within outward. The two ends of the thread are tied together, whereby the end of the Witzel canal is pulled tightly against the parietal peritoneum. This apposition is further reinforced from within the abdomen by means of a few interrupted sutures grasping the parietal and the visceral peritoneum.

If the tube is to be carried out through the laparotomy wound, the two ends of the long silk thread, which has been tied around the tube and passed through two folds of gastric wall at the point of exit of the tube, are passed through the parietal peritoneum from within outward, one on each side of the lower angle of the abdominal wound, and tied, so that the end of the Witzel canal is pulled tightly against the parietal peritoneum at the lower end of the incision. A few interrupted sutures may be added for additional security. The suture of the abdominal wall is carried out in the usual way as far as the point of exit of the tube. The tube is then fastened to the skin by a separate suture and the dressing applied in the manner described in Vol. I, page 286.

Should the fistula eventually fail to enclose the tube tightly, then a narrower tube is inserted for a few days, during which the fistula rapidly becomes smaller.

2. The Establishment of a Gastrostomy with Formation of a Submucosal Canal (Marwedel)

Marwedel introduces the tube into the stomach through a canal formed in the submucosa of the gastric wall (Figs. 83 and 84). The stomach is

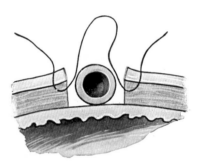

Fig. 83. Gastrostomy of Marwedel. The formation of the canal by suturing the sero-muscular incision. Diagrammatic.

exposed and delivered in the manner described. An incision 5 cm. long is made through the serosa and muscularis down to the submucosa, in the direction chosen for the tube (Fig. 84). A seromuscular flap is dissected free from the intact mucosa for a short distance on each side. A previous injection of adrenalin facilitates the dissection. At the end of the seromuscular incision the tube is introduced into the stomach through a small opening. The serosal wound is then closed over the tube to form a canal. I see no advantage in this procedure over that of Witzel.

3. The Establishment of a Gastrostomy with the Formation of a Circular Canal (Kader)

If there is not sufficient room to apply the tube for some distance to the surface of the stomach, the tube may be carried into the stomach through the center of a purse-string suture through serosa and muscularis, after the manner of Kader (Fig. 85). Over this a second, and sometimes a third purse-string suture is applied. In this manner a canal perpendicular to the gastric wall is formed around the rubber tube (Fig. 86). The stomach around the point of exit of the tube is sutured to the parietal peritoneum with Lembert sutures. (Unless the gastrostomy is to be permanent I do not suture the stomach to the parietal peritoneum. I. S. R.)

The introduction of nourishment can be started on the operating table. Later it is regulated in time and quantity primarily by the "appetite" of the

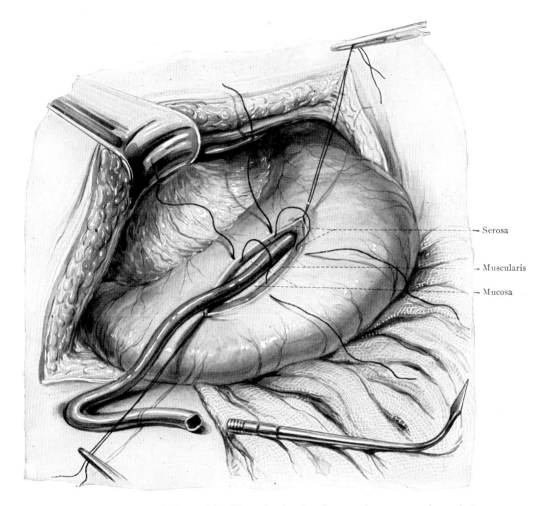

Serosa

Muscularis

Mucosa

FIG. 84. Gastrostomy of Marwedel. The tube is placed upon the outer surface of the mucosa, exposed by an incision through serosa and muscularis, is led through the mucosa into the stomach in the cardiac angle of the wound and is covered by suture of the edges of the sero-muscular incision.

patient. Milk and broths can be given freely. By means of a large glass syringe (Fig. 167) the patient can also be given gruels and puréed foods. The urinary output during artificial feeding should amount to about 1000 or 1500 cc. For a special feeding mixture see the section on jejunostomy, page 216.

It is advisable not to change the tube before the expiration of three weeks, since its replacement may present insurmountable difficulties. If the tube happens to slip out earlier, any attempt to replace it must be made with the greatest caution. All force must be avoided. If the replacement can not be made with the greatest ease, the abdomen should be reopened.

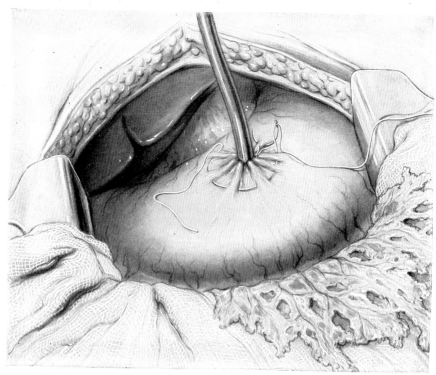

FIG. 85. Kader's gastrostomy. The tube, which has been passed through the anterior wall of the stomach and fastened by a purse-string suture, is being buried and fastened by a second purse-string suture.

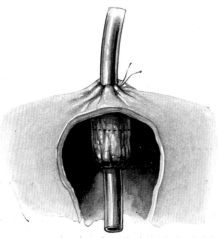

FIG. 86. The position of the tube and the several purse-string sutures in Kader's gastrostomy.

For retrograde bouginage of the esophagus with an endless thread, the patient is made to swallow a shot fastened to the end of a thread (Vol. I, Fig. 59). When the shot has reached the stomach, which can be determined by fluoroscopy, the thread is fished for with a small blunt hook introduced through the gastrostomy (or by direct vision with a gastroscope. I. S. R.). Filling the stomach with water will facilitate the capture of the thread. Sometimes the end of the thread can be flushed out through the fistula with water. If these measures fail, the stomach is filled with clear water, an operating cystoscopic is introduced through the gastrostomy and the thread is caught with a cystoscopic forceps and pulled out.

The thread which has been brought out through the fistula is tied to the end hanging out of the mouth to form an endless loop. It is advisable promptly to insert a second thread in the same manner, so to avoid difficulty in case one thread breaks. The bougies required for this type of bouginage are illustrated on page 80, Vol. I.

4. The Closure of a Gastrostomy

If the fistula is to be closed permanently, the removal of the tube usually suffices to cause the serous canal to close by adhesions. Otherwise, the measures described more in detail under the closure of intestinal fistulae are made use of. They consist essentially in an oval excision of the fistulous opening, a dissection of the tract down to the stomach, the closure of the resultant opening in the stomach by double suture and the suture of the wound of the abdominal wall.

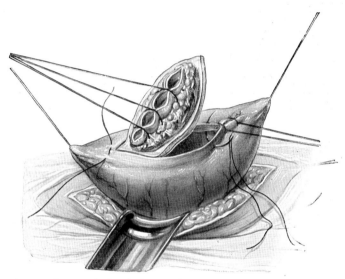

Fig. 87. Closure of a gastric fistula by excision of the fistula and suture of the edges of the wounds of the stomach and of the abdominal wall. The skin was incised around the fistula and sutured with interrupted sutures closing the fistula. The incision was then carried down to the surface of the stomach. The stomach has been elevated by means of traction sutures to prevent the escape of gastric contents. The wound in the gastric wall occasioned by the excision of the fistula is closed by tier suture.

Should this procedure fail, as is the case often in spontaneous gastric fistulae, then the fistula with the tissue immediately surrounding must be excised in the form of a pointed oval mass which includes all layers from the skin to the gastric mucosa. The operation is begun by an oval incision through the skin. The skin is now sewed over the fistulous opening with interrupted sutures to prevent the further escape of gastric contents (Fig. 87). The incision is carried through all the layers of the abdominal wall until the open peritoneal cavity or the surface of the stomach is reached. The stomach is then pulled into the wound. A pointed oval is now excised from the gastric wall, the incision being carried through all the layers of the stomach.

The resultant gastric wound is closed in the usual manner by a double row of sutures. (The suture line may be reinforced with an omental graft. I. S. R.) The stomach is returned to the abdomen and the abdominal wall closed.

5. The Closure of a Duodenal Fistula

An extremely serious complication is the development of a postoperative duodenal fistula. Such fistulae arise most frequently after gastric resections, especially after the Billroth II type of procedure. However, other operations on the duodenum or in the neighborhood of the duodenum may lead to the formation of a fistula. This is particularly the case in operations for the removal of gall stones, if the duodenum has been opened or mobilized, or if a drainage tube exerts pressure on the duodenal wall. The reopening of the duodenal sutures after a gastric resection is based as a rule on a technical defect in the closure, most commonly the result of a lack of normal intestinal wall due to the low position of the lesion (duodenal ulcer). The surface of the duodenum is poor material for suture since its posterior aspect lacks a peritoneal covering. A further handicap for duodenal sutures lies in their digestion by pancreatic juice. Finally, the suture line may give way due to the forceful injection of gastric contents into the proximal limb of the gastro-enterostomy after a gastric resection by the Billroth II method.

If the patient does not die of an acute peritonitis, an external fistula forms, whose connection with the duodenum is soon recognized by the escape of bile-stained foam or by a whitish discharge with a peculiarly musty odor, by the marked redness and maceration of the surrounding skin and by the rapid loss of strength.

Small duodenal fistulae sometimes close spontaneously in a short time. Large duodenal fistulae tend to cause the death of the patient in a short time as a result of the marked loss of fluid, salts and ferments.

Conservative Treatment consists in meticulous care of the skin surrounding the fistulous opening, obstruction of the flow, restriction of food by the normal channels, and the administration of fluid and food by routes which avoid the duodenum.

The fistula must be dressed several times a day. The skin surrounding the opening is thickly coated with a layer of zinc oxide ointment, or with powder, such as powdered animal charcoal. Plugging the fistula with vaseline gauze or applying pressure bandages with elastic tapes as a rule does not check the flow materially, but on the contrary tends to enlarge the opening rapidly. Oral feeding should be restricted as much as possible (fast days) and food is usually limited to dry foods, avoiding liquid foods and drinks ("drying up" the fistula). Fluid requirements are met by giving the patient large quantities of glucose solution by rectal drip and at the same time giving 10 units of insulin three times a day. Continuous intravenous drip may also be used to advantage.

If these measures fail to close the fistula and if it is impossible to maintain the strength of the patient, the only hope lies in prompt surgical closure, the outcome of which is, however, always dubious. (I have found that the introduction into the wound of a small tube which is attached to a suction apparatus keeps the area moderately dry and thus tends to promote healing. Furthermore, the use of gauze dressings or a salve containing small amounts of one of the heavy metals tends to inactivate the ferments which cause superficial erosion. In cases of this type there is a loss of much fluid, base, bicarbonate, calcium and chloride. It is necessary first to prevent dehydration. In order to do this it may be necessary to give intravenously as much as 4000 to 6000 cc. in 24 hours. As a rule sodium chloride suffices, but in several instances we have found it necessary to add calcium. It is conceivable that bicarbonate may become necessary. If feeding becomes important a jejunostomy can be done. Glucose by rectum is of little or no value and since the internal secretions of the pancreas are not lost insulin does not appear to be indicated. I. S. R.)

Operative Treatment involves the closure of the fistula by suture or the shunting of the gastric contents away from the fistulous duodenum, or both procedures.

The simple closure of the fistula by suture fails in most instances. Efforts in this direction have a prospect of success only if it is possible to expose the surface of the duodenum in the region of the fistula far enough into normal tissue, to excise the fistula, and to close the resultant opening in the routine manner with a two-tier Czerny suture.

Shunting the food away from the duodenum is attempted by performing a gastro-enterostomy. Experience has shown, however, that this type of anastomosis fails in many instances effectively to divert the food from the duodenum. It is necessary, therefore, to supplement the gastro-enterostomy at once by an exclusion of the pylorus. Of course, if the duodenal fistula developed after a gastric resection according to the Billroth II method, the pylorus has already been completely excluded. The operations on the stomach should be carried out through a fresh abdominal incision not in contact with the fistula.

The most promising measure is to combine the exclusion of the pylorus and the immediate closure of the fistula in the same operation. In that case the aseptic procedure of exclusion of the pylorus and gastro-enterostomy is carried out first, followed by closure of the fistula. To these are added the non-operative measures previously described.

While on theoretical grounds it would seem likely that a duodenal fistula could be cured by a jejunostomy, practical experience has not confirmed this. If in spite of this experience one wishes to try such measures in the desperately ill, it is necessary to select a point of the small intestine far down for the establishment of the nutritive jejunostomy. As a rule these patients are no longer in a condition to stand the extensive operation of resection of the fistulous segment of the duodenum as described under the treatment of carcinoma of the duodenum.

Unfortunately, all the efforts of the conservative and operative treatment are unsuccessful in a large number of cases, and the patients succumb to a condition which from the beginning must be considered to be of the gravest significance.

D. THE TREATMENT OF STENOSIS OF THE CARDIA

Stenosis of the cardia may be of a malignant nature, that is, caused by a carcinoma, or it may be produced by an essentially benign lesion, such as a scar or spasm.

Attempts at the curative treatment of carcinomatous lesions in this region consist only in the resection of the diseased segment. The treatment of tumors involving the lower esophagus will be discussed under esophageal surgery. If the tumor is limited to the stomach, its removal entails the total extirpation of the stomach or the resection of the cardial half of the stomach as described on page 175.

Even with a benign stenosis the general state of nutrition of the patient is often greatly impaired. For this reason and in view of the magnitude of the operation, a nutritive fistula should first be made. Moreover, the preliminary short-circuiting of the esophagus is recommended since the site of subsequent operation at the cardia is thereby relieved of irritation. I prefer the establishment of a jejunostomy to a gastrostomy, because the jejunal fistula does not impede the approach required for the major operation, nor the movability of the stomach, and because it takes better care of functional rest for, and the mechanical protection of, the stomach after the major operation.

Before operation for stenosis of the cardia, the esophagus, which is usually much dilated and inflamed, and frequently ulcerated, must be carefully lavaged and emptied by suction.

1. Mechanical Dilatation of the Cardia from within the Stomach
(v. Mikulicz)

When conservative treatment of cardiospasm by mechanical dilatation of the cardia through oral bouginage has failed, mechanical dilatation by way of the stomach may be undertaken with greater hope of success. The stomach is delivered, its anterior wall is opened for a considerable extent and its interior is carefully aspirated. The right hand is inserted into the stomach, the cardia is palpated with the index finger and the finger is forced through the opening. If this succeeds, the middle finger is pushed in with it just as one dilates the rectal sphincters. One gradually tries to pass the cardia with three, four or even all five fingers.

Manual dilatation of the cardia is not without danger, since it has repeatedly led to rupture of the esophageal wall with subsequent fatal mediastinitis. Nor is it quite safe to introduce a Korn forceps under guidance of the hand into the cardia, partly dilated by the finger, and then forcibly to withdraw the forceps while it is open.

After the dilatation has been completed, the stomach and the abdominal wound are closed unless one wishes to establish a gastric fistula to insure the food supply and for subsequent dilation by means of an endless thread and retrograde bouginage.

A single mechanical dilatation of a spastic cardia at times leads to permanent cure, although only too frequently the end-result is not satisfactory. It is advisable, however, to supplement the operation by dilatation with bougies.

2. Division of the Cardiac Sphincter from Without
(Cardiomyotomy, Heller)

The excellent results from pyloromyotomy in the pylorospasm of infants suggested the thought to Heller of applying a corresponding operation to the cardia. In this treatment of cardiospasm, however, there are also failures and even fatalities to offset the many successes.

Left Vagus   Mucosa

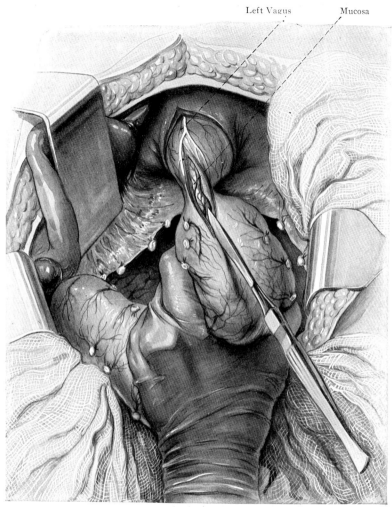

Fig. 88.   Cardioplasty.   The cardia has been freed from the diaphragm and drawn downward. The musculature of the cardia is being incised down to the mucosa in a longitudinal direction.

A midline incision below the ensiform usually suffices and a reflection of the costal margin is not necessary. The operation begins with a mobilization of the cardia, so that a loop of gauze can be passed around the esophagus to draw it into view. In some cases manual traction is sufficient. A longitudinal incision is made into the anterior surface of the lowest portion of the esophagus extending into the first portion of the stomach (Fig. 88). The incision is carried through the serosa and longitudinal muscle of the esophagus and is then cautiously deepened bit by bit through the circular musculature until the mucosa is exposed in the full length of the incision. The mucosa may be recognized by the venous plexus which is adjacent to it. If there is difficulty in judging the proper depth of the incision in dividing the musculature of the cardia, the operator can pass the index finger of the left hand into the stomach and through the cardia and then cut down over the finger. The stomach must be opened for this purpose if it was not opened previously for diagnostic purposes. It is not necessary to apply a patch of omentum over the esophageal incision.

Heller has recently recommended a second similar incision on the posterior wall of the esophagus. This is at times quite difficult and theoretically seems unnecessary, since a stricture which has been divided at one point obviously does not need a second division. This is proved by the excellent results of pyloromyotomy in infants.

3. THE ANASTOMOSIS OF THE STOMACH WITH THE ESOPHAGUS (ESOPHAGOGASTROSTOMY, HEYROVSKY)

As in stenosis of the pylorus in the adult where the surest measure for relief is a shortcircuiting of the constriction by a gastro-enterostomy, so, too, the surest means of dealing with every intractable stenosis of the cardia is esophagogastrostomy. The technical difficulties of this rather dangerous operation are usually somewhat lessened by the fact that the esophagus, as a result of the longstanding stenosis, presents a considerable and frequently saccular dilatation and that the point where the esophagus passes through the diaphragm is displaced toward the cardia.

The saccular dilatation of the esophagus on the other hand entails the danger that its infectious contents may escape during the operation when the esophagus has been opened, contaminating the operative field. The esophagus must therefore be cleansed as well as possible by irrigation immediately before the operation and must be emptied by means of a suction pump attached to a small-bore stomach tube.

The stomach is best exposed by a midline incision, only exceptionally requiring in addition reflection of the left costal margin. The stomach is sufficiently mobilized below the cardia so that a roll of gauze or a rubber tube can be passed around the esophagus, and the latter drawn downward (Fig. 89). The peritoneum which covers the esophagus at its point of exit from the diaphragm and the diaphragm are incised and the lower esophagus is mobilized and carefully drawn out of the esophageal foramen. In so doing, the left vagus must at times be divided. It should be anesthetized previous to division. When a sufficiently long portion of the esophagus has been freed so that it can easily be laid against the dome of the fundus, the two structures are united for a distance of 3 to 4 cm. by means of very carefully and very closely applied interrupted linen sutures (Fig. 90). The attempt to apply a clamp across the esophagus or to a fold of its wall in order to prevent the escape of esophageal contents fails in most instances. The stomach and the esophagus are opened to a corresponding extent and distance from the suture line. By means of closely and carefully applied interrupted linen sutures the anastomosis is completed with a posterior and an anterior Albert

suture and an anterior Lembert suture. If sufficient tissue is available, the
site of suture can be secured by oversewing it with a few additional Lembert
sutures. Finally, the stomach is attached to the margins of the slit in the
diaphragm so that the anastomosis may be relieved of tension as far as
possible.

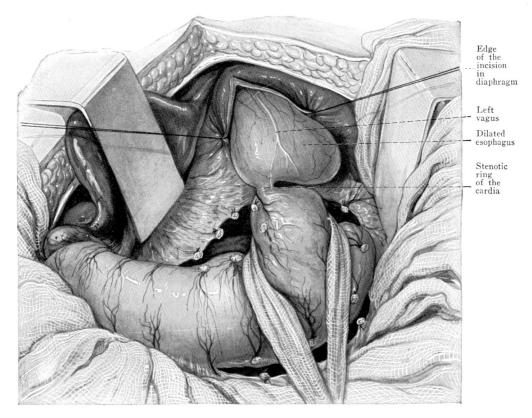

Edge
of the
incision
in
diaphragm

Left
vagus

Dilated
esophagus

Stenotic
ring
of the
cardia

FIG. 89. Esophagogastrostomy. The dilated esophagus has been freed from the incised
diaphragm and drawn downward. The cardia has been mobilized by ligation and division of its
attachments and is being drawn forward by means of a gauze roll.

E. ARTIFICIAL DILATATION OF THE PYLORUS

I. PYLOROPLASTY (FINNEY)

In the treatment of organic pyloric stenosis of adults, pyloroplasty after
the manner of Heinicke-Mikulicz, consisting in the division of all the layers
of the pylorus in the long axis and the transverse suture of the wound, has been
completely displaced, because of the uncertainty of its effect, by gastro-
enterostomy which is certain in its result.

For the same reasons the pyloroplasty of Finney no longer has any great
practical significance. (This opinion is not shared by a great many American
surgeons. I. S. R.) The operation is performed as follows:

At the midpoint of the stenosis a traction suture is applied and made taut,
so that the proximal and distal limbs of the segment approach each other.

Both limbs are then united for a distance of 5 to 6 cm. from the traction suture with interrupted Lembert sutures (Fig. 91). At a distance of ½ cm. from this suture line the proximal and distal limbs are opened, and the incisions are carried through the stenosis and joined into a single incision. In this manner the incision takes the form of a horse-shoe. The two inner walls of this horseshoe which have already been connected by a Lembert suture are now also joined by a three-layer Albert suture. The two outer walls of the

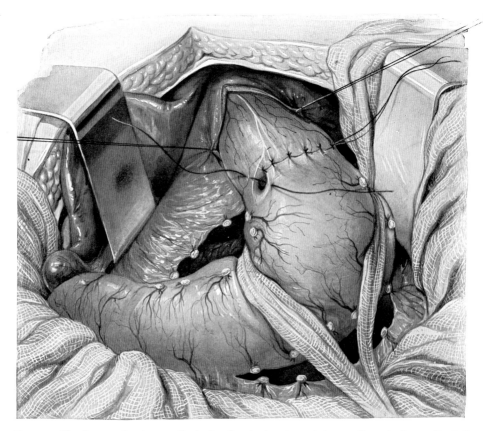

Fig. 90. Esophagogastrostomy. Posterior Lembert sutures between the anterior wall of the dilated esophagus and the anterior wall of the stomach.

horseshoe-shaped incision are then joined by an Albert suture and finally by a Lembert suture. This closes stomach and intestine, and in such a way that the stenosis is replaced by a broad anastomosis between the proximal and the distal limbs. The Finney pyloroplasty is fundamentally a U-shaped gastroduodenostomy.

2. Division of the Pyloric Sphincter from Without (Pyloromyotomy According to Weber-Rammstedt)

The only other plastic operation on the pylorus of practical significance is the extramucosal pyloromyotomy of Weber-Rammstedt in the treatment of pyloric stenosis in infants. This operation is today the most effective, least dangerous and most rapid treatment for this disease and has a mortality of only about 3 per cent.

The infant, whose stomach has been emptied just before the operation by means of a stomach tube, is best anesthetized with a few drops of chloroform, since the anaesthesia can be kept light most of the time and deepened only in a few stages of the operation.

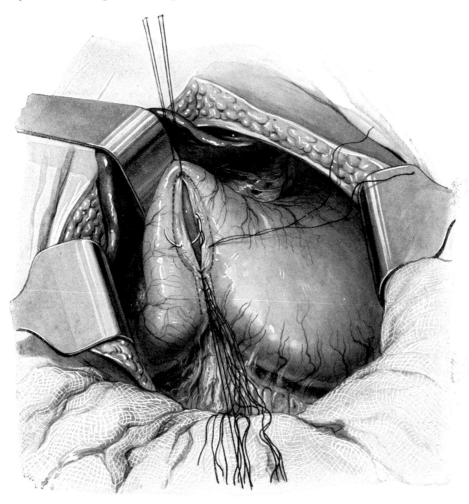

FIG. 91. Pyloroplasty (Finney). The stenosed portion of the pylorus has been drawn forcibly upward by a traction suture. The stomach and duodenum are being joined side-to-side immediately adjacent to the stenosis by means of posterior interrupted Lembert sutures. (The lines along which stomach and duodenum are to be opened after the completion of this suture are indicated in red.)

The abdomen is opened by a small longitudinal incision ½ cm. to the right of the midline and just below the xiphoid process, so that the liver later will protect the sutured wound from buffeting by the abdominal viscera. The right lobe of the liver is displaced upward by means of retractors. The stomach which now comes into view is grasped and followed toward the pylorus until the pyloric tumor is reached. The operator grasps the pyloric tumor from behind between the thumb and index finger of the left hand, which has been covered with a layer of moist gauze to increase the strength of the grip by friction, and makes pressure as if he were trying to pop an almond forward out of its skin (Fig. 92). In this way the anterior wall of the pylorus is put on tension and is made relatively bloodless by pressure. With a small, extremely sharp knife a longitudinal incision is made through the serous coat over the pyloric tumor in a region nearly free of blood vessels, extending from the duodenum to the stomach. The incision is gradually deepened through the muscularis, layer after layer, in the region of the stomach, while the incision gaps widely under the pressure of the fingers grasping the pylorus. Suddenly, with the separation of the divided muscle wall, the silvery outer surface of the mucosa appears at a point in the bottom of the

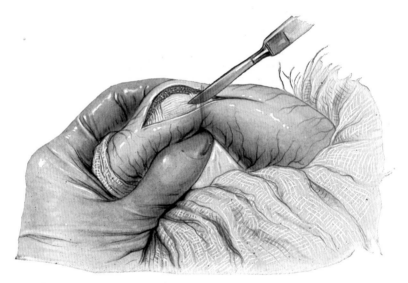

Fig. 92. Pyloroplasty (Weber-Rammstedt) in the infant. The transverse muscle bands of the pyloric tumor are being divided for some distance down to the mucosa. The mucosa appears at the bottom of the wound.

wound. When this layer has been reached at one point, it is not difficult to deepen the incision through the whole of the pyloric circular muscle to the mucosa. With continued pressure of the thumb and finger of the left hand the two muscle walls of the wound are widely separated and the mucosal surface stands out as a broad band. Any injury of the mucosa must be avoided most carefully. Under direct view even the last, most delicate muscle bundle can be divided with the knife toward the cardia as far as the normal gastric wall.

It is at times difficult to carry the incision into normal duodenum without injuring the mucosa. This difficulty is increased by the fact that the mucosa is often prolapsed into the duodenum in the form of a ring-shaped mass by the increased peristalsis of the stomach. This ring of mucosa is injured very easily during the incision. Nevertheless, the division of even the last circular muscle bundle must be accomplished, if the result of the operation is not to be jeopardized by a partial persistence of vomiting. This is best accomplished in this way: after the completion of the incision in the region of the stomach and the pylorus, the two cut surfaces of the muscle toward the duodenum are gently pushed away from the mucosa by means of blunt dissection with the handle of the knife. In this way, while the fingers of the operator's left hand continue uninterruptedly to grasp the pylorus from behind, the mucosa of the beginning of the duodenum is unfolded almost of itself.

If the mucosa is inadvertently opened at one point, a fact which is immediately recognized by the escape of bile-stained, frothy duodenal contents, no attention should be paid to this accident for the time being, but the division of the muscle should be completed. Then, using blood vessel suture instruments, the mucosa and the serosa are separately sutured. The serosal suture should include the superficial layers of the muscle. There must be no further suture of the pylorotomy wound. (The suture line may be reinforced with an omental graft. I. S. R.)

If in the exceptional case there is considerable bleeding from the incision after the grip on the pyloric ring is relaxed, the bleeding points are caught with mosquito hemostats and tied with very fine ligatures.

The stomach is replaced in the abdomen and the abdominal incision is closed with a number of carefully placed sutures. The suture of individual layers is preferable to through-and-through closure. It is important to relieve tension on the abdominal wound and to protect it from contact with urine and feces for ten to fourteen days by a number of strips of adhesive plaster applied across the abdomen from back to back. The postoperative feeding should be controlled by the pediatrician.

Pylorotomy in adults (Payr) has not gained favor, nor has hemipylorosphinctorectomy.

F. ANASTOMOSIS OF THE STOMACH WITH THE INTESTINE (GASTRO-ENTEROSTOMY, GASTROJEJUNOSTOMY, GASTRODUODENOSTOMY)

The anastomosis of the stomach with the small intestine, that is, with the jejunum or the duodenum, makes it possible for the gastric contents to avoid the pylorus in passing from the stomach into the intestine. This operation, conceived by Nikoladoni, and first performed by Wölfler as an anterior antecolic gastro-enterostomy, has since been carried out in numerous variations and in many thousands of cases. It has experienced a very varied evaluation within recent years. The operation must be considered in those cases in which the pyloric antrum, the pylorus, or the duodenum is completely or partially obstructed; in those in which a stenosis is to be expected, or in those in which disease of these parts requires their protection. Gastro-enterostomy is also frequently used to re-establish the continuity of the gastro-intestinal tract after transverse resection of stomach and pylorus. Since emptying of the stomach after a gastro-enterostomy can take place more rapidly and with less difficulty than under normal conditions, the operation has also been advised in ulcer of the body of the stomach.

A number of difficulties may arise from a lateral anastomosis between the stomach and the jejunum. Sometimes immediately after the operation the stomach empties its contents, not into the distal, but into the proximal loop of gut. If the pylorus is patulous, then the gastric contents which are poured through the gastro-enterostomy into the proximal segment of the jejunum return into the stomach, there to repeat the vicious circle. In this way no food, or insufficient food, reaches the efferent small bowel. When this course has become the habitual one the proximal limb, in contrast to the distal, becomes dilated. If the pylorus is not patulous, then the gastric contents may collect in the proximal loop, dilate it and thereby produce a compression of the distal loop, which makes a bad matter worse. In either case, the stomach is overburdened, vomiting occurs, and the body suffers from lack of water and nourishment. (The symptoms of high intestinal obstruction appear and alkalosis is usually present. I. S. R.) Vicious circle can be met by

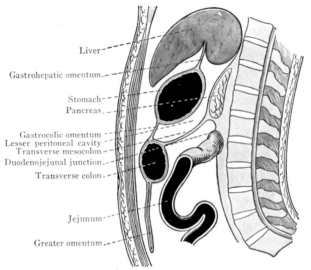

Liver

Gastrohepatic omentum

Stomach
Pancreas

Gastrocolic omentum
Lesser peritoneal cavity
Transverse mesocolon
Duodenojejunal junction
Transverse colon

Jejunum

Greater omentum

FIG. 93. Diagrammatic-sagittal section through the upper abdomen.

anastomosing the proximal and the distal loop of intestine (anastomosis of Braun), below the site of the gastro-enterostomy. (This condition of vicious circle is more apt to be present after anterior gastro-enterostomy or after posterior gastro-enterostomy when a long jejunal loop is used. I. S. R.)

There is the danger that the acid gastric contents will not be well tolerated by the jejunum, intended as it is to receive the alkaline duodenal contents, and that the jejunum will respond to this continued chemical irritation by the formation of a postoperative jejunal ulcer. The intestinal mucosa is apparently more sensitive to the action of the gastric juice the farther it lies below the duodenojejunal junction.

In the development of such a jejunal ulcer other factors are, however, obviously concerned. Chief among these are to be mentioned an ulcer diathesis, primary mechanical damage of the intestinal loop during the operation, as by the pressure of a clamp, or long-continued irritation of the mucosa, as by an unabsorbed suture projecting into the lumen, and the failure to remain on a restricted diet after operation.

The various types of gastro-enterostomy are liable to the dangers mentioned in different degrees. There are certain technical measures, to be mentioned later, which may serve to avoid certain of these untoward events (Fig. 93), but none of them has completely eliminated their occurrence.

In performing a gastrojejunostomy the union between the stomach and a loop of jejunum may be effected either in front of the transverse colon or behind it. In the latter case an opening in the transverse mesocolon must be made. We therefore differentiate between an antecolic and a retrocolic gastro-enterostomy. In either of these procedures we can attach the intestinal loop to the anterior wall of the stomach (anterior gastro-enterostomy) or to the posterior wall (posterior gastro-enterostomy). Theoretically, therefore, there are four types of gastro-enterostomy:

1. Posterior retrocolic gastro-enterostomy (von Hacker, Fig. 94).
2. Anterior retrocolic gastro-enterostomy (Billroth, Fig. 97).
3. Anterior antecolic gastro-enterostomy (Wölfler, Fig. 99) and
4. Posterior antecolic gastro-enterostomy, a procedure which is never used.
5. In addition to these, gastroduodenostomy (Wölfler) is also possible (Fig. 101).

Posterior antecolic gastro-enterostomy has no practical importance, so that its description is unnecessary. I shall also omit a description of the possible variations known as superior and inferior gastro-enterostomy, in which the anastomosis is made to the lesser or to the greater curvature respectively.

In the antecolic anastomoses the intestinal loop, which is fastened by its mesentery to the posterior abdominal wall in the region of the lumbar spine, must be brought in front of the omentum and the transverse colon to the stomach.

In order that the small intestine, the mesentery, the colon and the omentum shall not compress one another, the intestinal loop must be of sufficient length between the duodenojejunal junction and the stomach. This is all the more necessary since the mesentery at the beginning of the jejunum is quite short and only at some distance lower down acquires sufficient length to permit the gut to reach the stomach around the omentum and the transverse colon without tension. The anastomosis is therefore made as a rule at a point in the intestine about 40 to 50 cm. below the duodenojejunal junction. Experience has shown that in the interposition of so long a loop there is considerable danger of a vicious circle. It therefore becomes a matter of fundamental importance in antecolic gastro-enterostomy to make an anastomosis between the proximal and the distal loop (anastomosis of Braun) at the time of the gastro-enterostomy.

In retrocolic anastomoses, especially the posterior retrocolic anastomosis, these difficulties are not present to the same degree. Compression of small intestine and colon can not occur even with a loop on considerable tension. Furthermore, the distance between the posterior wall of the stomach and the duodenojejunal junction is so short that the anastomosis with the intestine can be made a few centimeters below the junction. The danger of a secondary jejunal ulcer is also lessened when this method is used. At the same time the position of the gastro-enterostomy on the posterior wall of the stomach is so favorable for emptying that the flow of gastric contents into the proximal portion of the jejunal loop is practically always prevented. Retrocolic gastro-enterostomy is therefore decidedly superior to the antecolic operation.

I am, however, strongly opposed to making the jejunal loop in the retrocolic gastro-enterostomy too short, as was originally suggested by von Hacker and as is generally advised today. There are three reasons for my attitude. In the first place, it may lessen the freedom of motion of the stomach, which may lead to unpleasant sensations after the ingestion of food. In the second place, with a short hook-up the loop between the duodenojejunal junction and the stomach may be put on such tension that the flow of duodenal contents is at least partially obstructed. This event is particularly to be feared if the jejunal loop must be attached well up toward the cardia and the anastomosis consequently can not be anchored to the slit in the mesocolon, but remains in the lesser peritoneal space together with the attached jejunal loop. Finally, with a very short loop, conditions are so unusually difficult when a secondary operation for jejunal ulcer is necessary that the operation is fraught with considerable danger. I have never seen any harm result from the use of a somewhat longer loop. I make the loop from 15 to 20 cm. long.

The choice between anterior retrocolic gastro-enterostomy and posterior retrocolic gastro-enterostomy is simple. After the necessary opening in the mesocolon we find ourselves in immediate contact with the posterior wall of the stomach. To reach the anterior wall the gastrocolic omentum must be divided. Furthermore, the emptying of the stomach in an anterior gastro-enterostomy is less favorable than in a posterior retrocolic gastro-enterostomy. We therefore prefer posterior retrocolic gastro-enterostomy whenever it is technically possible.

It is obvious that posterior retrocolic gastro-enterostomy is from the view of end-results indisputably the method of choice; the second-best procedure is anterior retrocolic gastro-enterostomy, while anterior antecolic gastro-enterostomy stands third. Posterior antecolic gastro-enterostomy is only of theoretical interest.

The anastomoses between the stomach and the jejunum thus far described are excelled, however, in regard to the restoration of normal physiologic conditions by the anastomosis of the stomach with the duodenum, gastroduodenostomy. The latter anastomosis is possible only when the disease in this region is limited and when the lower part of the stomach and the upper part of the duodenum are sufficiently mobile to permit easy apposition to one another after resection.

The anastomosis between the stomach and jejunum is almost always performed in such a way that the jejunal loop is anastomosed to the stomach side-to-side without interruption of the continuity of the loop. If the line of anastomosis is made transverse to the long axis of the stomach, which is the rule, then the proximal portion of the loop is toward the lesser curvature and the distal portion of the loop toward the greater curvature. If the line of anastomosis is made parallel to the axis of the stomach, which is also permissible, then the proximal portion of the loop is directed toward the cardia and the distal portion toward the pylorus. The direction of a possibly preferred oblique position is obvious. (The observance of these precautions will tend, in a measure, to prevent a vicious circle. I. S. R.)

Only exceptionally, and then only in case of technical necessity, is the jejunal loop transsected before implantation into the stomach, as in the Y-type of anastomosis of Roux. In this procedure the distal limb is implanted end-to-side into the stomach and the proximal limb is joined side-to-side with the distal limb. Aside from its technical difficulties, the Y-type of gastro-enterostomy has been given up primarily because in this anastomosis the limb of intestine connected with the stomach is bathed with undiluted gastric juice as far as the point of lateral anastomosis with the other limb of intestine, conditions under which the danger of development of a secondary peptic ulcer appears to be particularly great.

The stoma of a gastro-enterostomy should always be made sufficiently large so that the stomach contents can freely enter the intestine. The fear that a large stoma might result in excessively rapid emptying of the stomach with consequent symptoms has proved ungrounded. A stoma about 6 cm. long seems to be adequate. Attempts to retard the emptying of the stomach by an intentionally small anastomosis are therefore not only unnecessary, but are to be condemned as extremely questionable because of the difficulty in correctly gauging the degree of subsequent stenosis.

In addition to improvement of the mechanical emptying of the stomach, gastro-enterostomy has been proposed as a means of neutralizing the acid gastric juice with the alkaline intestinal secretions. Since in the usual gastro-enterostomy with a side-to-side apposition of stomach and intestine the entrance of alkaline intestinal contents into the stomach is scant and uncertain, Schmilinsky divides the jejunum and implants the end of the proximal as well as of the distal loop into the stomach. This forces all of the duodenal secretions to be emptied into the stomach, while the food can leave the stomach directly by way of the distal jejunal limb. This procedure has not proved itself, nor has the anastomosis of the gall bladder with the stomach, which has been recommended for the same purpose.

In all anastomoses between the stomach and the intestine the length of intestine to be used in the first line of suture is measured rather scantily in proportion to the length of stomach wall to be used, since the delicate wall of the intestine stretches considerably after being opened, whereas the firm wall of the stomach maintains practically its original length. If this rule is ignored, there may result a disturbing excess of intestinal wall.

1. Posterior Retrocolic Gastro-enterostomy (von Hacker)

After opening the abdominal cavity through a midline or paramedian incision below the ensiform, the surgeon reflects the omentum upward and has an assistant lift the transverse colon vertically so that the mesocolon is put on tension. On the lower surface of the mesocolon and just to the left of the vertebral column the first loop of jejunum comes into view. This loop is pulled forward. It may be recognized even without being seen by the fact that it is fixed at one end.

Its point of passage through the mesocolon has usually a vessel on either side, the middle colic artery and the left colic artery, while the part of the mesocolon enclosed by these two vessels and which therefore lies immediately over the duodenojejunal junction is free of blood vessels. Either the stomach is pressed against this vessel-free portion of the mesocolon by the hand of an assistant or by the right or left hand of the operator introduced above the transverse colon and an incision is then made down to the stomach (Fig. 95), or a free incision is made through this portion of the mesocolon between two forceps and the posterior wall of the stomach is grasped and brought through the opening.

The slit is enlarged in the sagittal plane to a length of 8 cm., any mesenteric vessels crossing the incision being doubly ligated and divided. The stomach wall is pulled through the slit as far as possible, a maneuver which

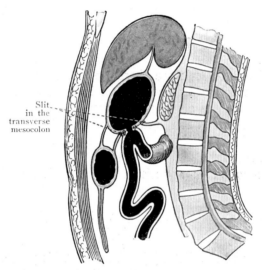

Slit
in the
transverse
mesocolon

FIG. 94. Posterior retrocolic gastrojejunostomy. Diagrammatic. The anastomosis between the posterior wall of the stomach and the highest jejunal loop through a slit in the transverse mesocolon has been sutured to the margins of the slit.

may prove difficult in case of an adherent or a shrunken stomach. The anastomosis should always be made close to the greater curvature and, as a rule, at not too great a distance from the pylorus. If there is a tumor or ulcer in the neighborhood of the pylorus, a point somewhat nearer the fundus is chosen for the anastomosis. (Where it is difficult to deliver the stomach through the opening in the mesocolon I have made a second opening in the gastrocolic omentum and completed the anastomosis in the lesser cavity after the method of Wilkie of Edinburgh. The line of anastomosis is finally sutured to the edges of the slit in the mesocolon. I. S. R.)

The portion of the posterior wall intended for anastomosis with the intestine is grasped in a fold about 8 to 10 cm. long by means of a clamp, and in such a way that the tips of the clamp lie near the lesser curvature while the handle of the clamp crosses the greater curvature. The clamp therefore lies perpendicular or oblique to the long axis of the stomach. Only exceptionally, as for example when in the absence of an electrosurgical knife I fear troublesome bleeding during the opening of the intestine, is a gentle clamp also used in picking up a fold of jejunum for the anastomosis. This clamp, when it is used, is handled with the greatest gentleness, mindful of the danger of injury to the gut, and is removed as soon as possible. The clamp grasps the highest loop of jejunum but at a point sufficiently below the

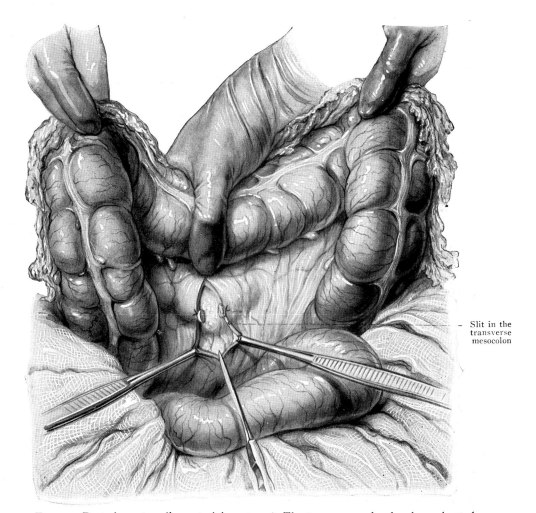

Slit in the transverse mesocolon

FIG. 95.   Posterior retrocolic gastrojejunostomy.   The transverse colon has been elevated. The right hand of the operator forces the stomach down from above against the transverse meso-colon, which has been split in a radial direction after ligation of its vessels, so that the posterior wall of the stomach appears in the opening.

duodenojejunal junction to make the free portion of the proximal limb at least 8 cm. long and to insure against tension. With the tips of the clamp pointing toward the duodenojejunal junction, the clamp grasps a longitudinal fold of the gut wall on the side opposite the attachment of the mesentery and about 10 cm. long. The handle of the clamp lies toward the distal portion of the loop. The gastric clamp and the jejunal clamp are each turned through a 90° angle in such a way that their handles are to the right, their tips to the left and the clamps lie parallel to each other. A gauze roll is placed between the stomach and the intestine.

If an electrosurgical knife is available for opening the gut, the application of a clamp to the jejunum can be dispensed with as a rule. The loop of intestine is then fastened by two traction sutures to the clamped fold of the

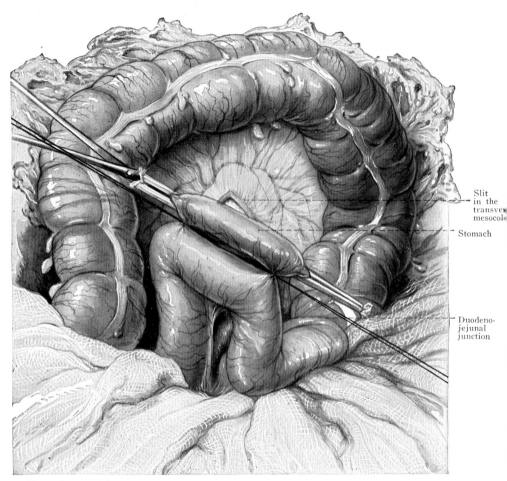

Slit
in the
transver
mesocolo

Stomach

Duodeno-
jejunal
junction

FIG. 96. Posterior retrocolic gastrojejunostomy. A portion of the posterior wall of the stomach has been drawn through the slit in the transverse mesocolon and grasped in the direction from the greater toward the lesser curvature with a gastric clamp. The highest jejunal loop, in a position not too close to the duodenojejunal junction, has been attached to the posterior wall of the stomach by two traction sutures marking the two end points of the posterior Lembert suture line: the proximal limb of the loop lies near the lesser, the distal limb near the greater curvature. The jejunal loop is not clamped.

gastric wall. The free segment between the duodenojejunal juncture and the point of suture must be at least 8 cm. long. The proximal portion is attached toward the lesser curvature, the distal portion toward the greater curvature (Fig. 96). The surrounding field is carefully walled off and a gauze roll is placed between the stomach and intestine.

The posterior interrupted Lembert sutures of silk, linen, or catgut are now applied for a distance of at least 6 cm. between the stomach and the jejunal loop.   The stomach and intestine are opened and their contents aspirated by suction.   A running three-layer catgut suture is now applied, first posteriorly and then anteriorly.   The clamps may now be removed. Finally, the anterior interrupted Lembert sutures are inserted.

After removal of the clamps, if these have been used, the anastomosis lies on the gauze roll beneath it.   With the aid of this gauze roll the site of anastomosis, which after the removal of the clamps tends to slip into the upper abdomen, is pulled through the slit in the mesocolon, and while traction is made, the posterior wall of the stomach in the neighborhood of the anastomosis is sutured to the edges of the slit in the mesocolon with interrupted sutures of catgut.   By this means the anastomosis is fixed permanently in the greater peritoneal cavity and intestinal loops cannot slip through the slit in the mesocolon and thus lead to intestinal obstruction.   After removing the gauze roll, the jejunum is placed in such a way that the distal loop passes to the left so that there will be no kinking of the gut.

The anatomic relations of the anastomosis are as follows (Fig. 94).   The loop coming anteriorly from the duodenojejunal junction passes to the posterior wall of the stomach in a dorsoventral direction and is about 8 cm. long. In the erect posture of the patient it runs an approximately horizontal course, passing along the stomach from the lesser toward the greater curvature.   The distal loop hangs vertically downward, curving away at nearly a right angle from the lower angle of the anastomosis and being thereby expanded in the shape of a funnel.   The contents of the stomach, therefore, at least theoretically, fall by gravity into the distal loop as into an open well.

2. ANTERIOR RETROCOLIC GASTRO-ENTEROSTOMY (BILLROTH)

If the posterior wall of the stomach is so extensively diseased that it can no longer be utilized for the anastomosis or if it cannot be sufficiently delivered, and if the anterior wall is sound and accessible, the anastomosis with the intestine may be made on the anterior surface.   If at the same time the transverse mesocolon is not infiltrated, so that it can be divided without difficulty, retrocolic anastomosis is to be preferred to antecolic since the length of the jejunal loop is not so long.

An opening is made in the gastrocolic omentum corresponding to the point on the anterior wall of the stomach decided upon for the anastomosis. After the surgeon has introduced two fingers of the left hand through this opening into the lesser peritoneal cavity, he turns the transverse colon upward in the manner previously described, forces the two fingers of the left hand from above against the vessel-free portion of the mesocolon over the duodenojejunal junction as seen from below, and divides the mesocolon over the bulge caused by the finger tips.   The two fingers are pushed through the opening and the highest possible loop of jejunum is pulled through the openings in the mesocolon and the gastrocolic omentum to the anterior wall of the stomach (Figs. 97 and 98).

On the anterior wall of the stomach a fold running diagonally downward from left to right is picked up in a clamp near the greater curvature. To this fold the jejunum is attached in such a way that the direction of its peristalsis proceeds from above on the left, downward and to the right (iso-

peristaltic position). The anastomosis between stomach and intestine is
made at such a distance from the duodenojejunal junction that the loop of
jejunum coming from the flexure is about 20 cm. long and therefore has
sufficient play after the anastomosis. The application of a clamp to the
jejunum is to be avoided if possible. An anastomosis 6 cm. long is made
between stomach and jejunum in the usual manner (Fig. 98). After the completion of the anastomosis the proximal limb of the intestinal loop is further
attached to the stomach by a few interrupted sutures (Kappeler suspension) in
order to elevate the proximal limb still more.

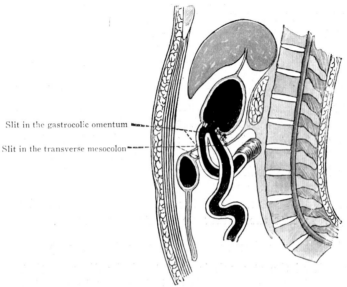

Slit in the gastrocolic omentum

Slit in the transverse mesocolon

FIG. 97. Anterior retrocolic gastrojejunostomy. Diagrammatic. The highest jejunal loop
has been brought through an opening in the transverse mesocolon and in the gastrocolic omentum to the anterior wall of the stomach and anastomosed to the stomach. The intestinal loop
has been sutured to the margins of both openings in the mesenteries.

A vicious circle may develop at times, in spite of the isoperistaltic
anastomosis and the diagonal attachment. It is therefore advisable, though
not absolutely necessary, to make an additional anastomosis between the
proximal and distal loops of the jejunum (entero-enterostomy of Braun).
For this purpose the transverse colon with its mesocolon is pulled upward.
The proximal and the distal loops are placed side by side for a short distance
with or without the aid of a clamp and a small anastomosis 4 to 5 cm. long is
made between them.

The edges of the openings in the mesocolon are fastened with a few
sutures to both of the limbs of the jejunal loop as they pass through, to prevent intestinal loops from being caught in the lesser cavity.

3. ANTERIOR ANTECOLIC GASTRO-ENTEROSTOMY (WÖLFLER)

If disease of the transverse mesocolon prevents making an opening in
the mesocolon for the passage of the highest loop of the jejunum, it becomes
necessary to carry the loop in front of the colon in order to connect it with

the stomach (Fig. 99). Some surgeons prefer the antecolic procedure when an anterior gastro-enterostomy becomes necessary.

The transverse colon is raised and the uppermost loop of jejunum is grasped and followed downward for about 40 cm. This portion is carried in front of the transverse colon and the great omentum and is placed against the anterior wall of the stomach. A fold of stomach in the direction from

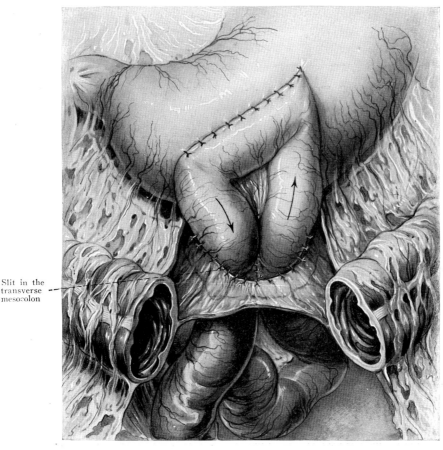

Slit in the
transverse
mesocolon

Fig. 98. Anterior retrocolic gastrojejunostomy. The highest jejunal loop, at a point not too close to the duodenojejunal junction, has been brought through a slit in the transverse meso-colon and through a slit in the gastrocolic omentum to the anterior wall of the stomach and anastomosed to it. The proximal loop will be attached to the anterior stomach wall by a few sutures.

above on the left, downward and to the right, is caught in a clamp near the greater curvature. The jejunal loop is attached to this fold in an isoperistaltic direction and the anastomosis is carried out in the usual manner (Fig. 100). The proximal limb of the jejunal loop is suspended from the stomach by a few interrupted sutures (Kappeler suspension sutures).

In case of a very long and thick omentum I have frequently made an opening through the omentum just below the transverse colon and have carried the jejunal loop through this opening and in front of the colon to the stomach.

It is advisable to provide an entero-enterostomy between the proximal and distal limbs of the loop about a hand's breadth below the gastro-enterostomy.

The **Y-shaped gastro-enterostomy of Roux** was originally a special form of anterior antecolic gastro-enterostomy, but, if it is used at all, it is best applied as a posterior or anterior retrocolic anastomosis. It no longer has any great practical significance, since it is followed more frequently by jejunal ulcer and because the site of anastomosis is more likely to stenose. The operation, therefore, should be considered only when there is a marked lack of jejunal tissue available, as for example, after the removal of a jejunal ulcer. When carried out according to the original technique, the jejunum is divided about 20 cm. below the duodenojejunal junction. The distal loop is carried

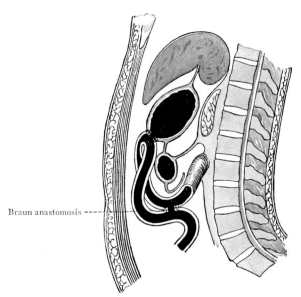

Braun anastomosis ----

Fig. 99. Anterior antecolic gastrojejunostomy with entero-enterostomy. Diagrammatic. A jejunal loop about 50 cm. distant from the duodenojejunal junction has been brought up in front of the transverse colon and anastomosed to the anterior wall of the stomach. The proximal and distal limbs of the anastomosis have been joined by an entero-enterostomy.

upward and forward through a slit in the transverse mesocolon and the gastro-colic omentum to the stomach and is implanted by end-to-side anastomosis into the anterior wall of the stomach near the greater curvature although it may be anastomosed to the posterior surface of the stomach. The edges of the opening through the mesocolon are sutured to the jejunal limb as it passes through. The open end of the limb of jejunum coming from the duodeno-jejunal junction is implanted end-to-side into the distal limb of jejunum at a point 10 cm. below the gastro-enterostomy.

4. GASTRODUODENOSTOMY (WÖLFLER)

If it is possible in avoiding the disease process to bring the pyloric antrum and the upper part of the duodenum side by side for a sufficient distance and without tension, the direct anastomosis of these segments of the gastro-intestinal canal is the operation of choice for short-circuiting the pylorus. In view of the scant mobility of the two structures, the use of clamps must be dispensed with in most cases. The gastric and duodenal walls are first united for a distance of 5 to 6 cm. with a posterior Lembert suture. Both

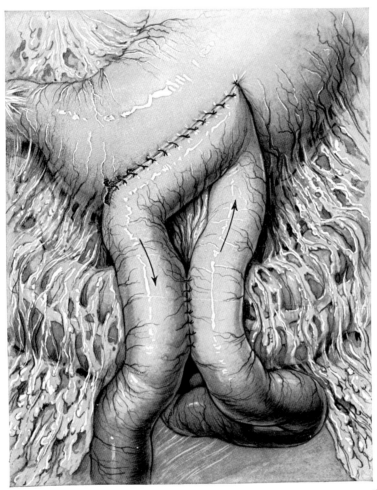

FIG. 100. Anterior antecolic gastrojejunostomy. The jejunal segment at a distance of about 50 cm. from the duodenojejunal junction has been brought up in front of the omentum and the transverse colon and anastomosed to the anterior wall of the stomach in the direction from above on the left to below on the right. The proximal and distal limbs have been anastomosed side-to-side. The proximal loop will be attached to the anterior gastric wall by a few sutures.

lumina are opened and the gastric and intestinal openings are joined in the usual manner by a posterior and an anterior Albert suture and by an anterior Lembert suture (Fig. 101).

Gastroduodenostomy gives excellent results. It largely reproduces the normal anatomic and physiologic conditions and is almost free of the danger of postoperative peptic ulcer. Consequently it should be used more frequently than it has been. Many surgeons however never consider it as a possibility. The operation is simpler than the Finney pyloroplasty which was described on page 111, with which it otherwise has considerable similarity.

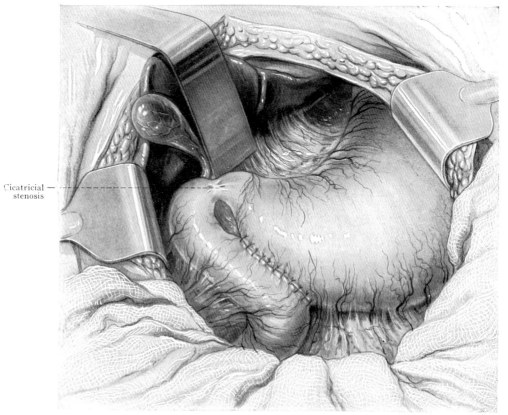

Cicatricial stenosis

FIG. 101. Gastroduodenostomy. The stomach and the duodenum, which can be placed side by side without tension, have been joined by an anastomosis to short-circuit the stenosed pylorus.

5. ABLATION OF A GASTRO-ENTEROSTOMY

Gastro-enterostomies which have been made without sound indications, in the presence of negative gastric or duodenal findings, frequently are the cause of numerous complaints ("gastro-enterostomy disease"), so that the ablation of such an anastomosis often becomes necessary. As a rule this is not particularly difficult if there are no marked adhesions.

After examinations have proved that the pylorus and duodenum are sound and freely patulous, the anastomosis is exposed and completely freed on all sides. The corresponding parts of the gastrocolic omentum and the transverse mesocolon are ligated. The gastric segment of the anastomosis is grasped in a clamp. The anastomosis is then divided, the incision being made at the expense of the stomach rather than the narrow intestine. The two openings so made are closed in the usual way by a two row suture. The division and suture can also be performed to advantage with the Petz suture instrument, which makes clamps unnecessary (Fig. 102).

It is necessary to determine whether the intestine has been seriously narrowed by the suture. If this is the case, then the stricture must be short-circuited by an entero-anastomosis (or the site of the anastomosis may be resected and an end-to-end anastomosis of the jejunum be made. I. S. R.). With a short jejunal loop this may necessitate the mobilization of the lower portion of the duodenum.

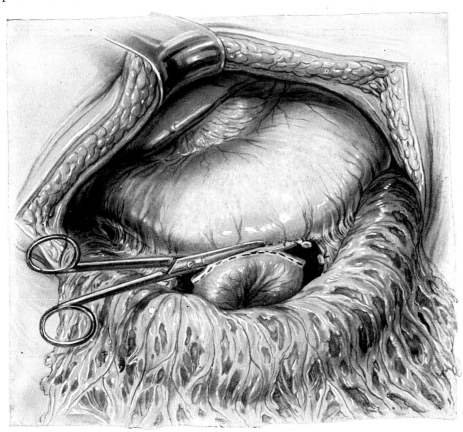

FIG. 102. Ablation of a gastrojejunostomy. The site of the old gastrojejunostomy has been freed sufficiently by ligating and dividing the gastrocolic omentum and the transverse meso-colon so that it can be closed with a double row of clips with the aid of the Petz suture instru-ment. The crushed tissue between the two rows of clips is being divided with the scissors.

Great difficulties frequently result if a marginal or jejunal ulcer has developed at the site of the gastro-enterostomy. The measures to be used under these circumstances are described on page 182.

G. EXCLUSION OF THE PYLORUS AND OF THE DUODENUM

Gastro-enterostomy in itself does not compel the gastric contents to follow the newly made channel; it merely offers this possibility. The contents can continue to use the pylorus and the duodenum. The tendency to use the old channel is particularly marked in those cases in which the pylorus is not at all or only very slightly obstructed, so that the success of the operation is partly vitiated. In such cases the old channel may persist with such obstinacy that the emptying of the stomach continues to take place wholly through the pylorus so that the gastro-enterostomy even closes in the course of time. It is advisable, therefore, when there is no pyloric stenosis of any degree, to constrict or close the pyloric passageway artificially, so that the food is forced through the new stoma.

1. Transsection of the Pyloric Antrum (Unilateral Exclusion of the Pylorus)

Exclusion of the pylorus can be accomplished completely and safely only by dividing the stomach between the gastro-enterostomy and the pylorus —unilateral exclusion of the pylorus as suggested by von Eiselsberg. The assumption that this operation is followed by an unusually high incidence of postoperative jejunal ulcer seems to be unwarranted. But the operation in a restricted sense has largely lost its importance for another reason. If a transverse division of the stomach near the duodenum is to be associated with gastro-enterostomy, it is customary to go farther and to include an extensive resection of the pyloric antrum and, if technically possible, of the pylorus as well, in order to lessen the danger of development of a jejunal ulcer. The extensive removal of the pyloric portion of the stomach, even to beyond the middle of the stomach, serves, by the removal of the pyloric glands, to lessen their influence on most of the fundus glands and consequently to decrease the secretion of hydrochloric acid by the latter, in this way tending to prevent the development of a peptic ulcer. This constitutes a gastric resection of the Billroth II type. (Jejunal ulcer has however been reported even after extensive subtotal gastric resection. I. S. R.)

The technique of pyloric exclusion is simple and corresponds in its details to the procedure of transverse resection of the stomach as described on page 180. The stomach, at a point about 5 cm. above the pylorus, is freed from its attachments on both curvatures with double ligation of vessels so that a zone of stomach about 4 cm. wide is entirely free. The stomach is divided between clamps in the middle of this zone. I do this with the aid of the Petz suture instrument. In so doing, care must be taken that the line of division is not too close to the pylorus. Enough of the stomach is necessary to receive the invaginated end when the infolding sutures are applied, since this tissue cannot be forced through the pyloric ring. The details are given under resection of the stomach. Both the proximal and the distal gastric stumps which have been closed are then invaginated with interrupted Lembert sutures.

Only when this dependable method for transsection of the stomach in its various modifications is for some reason impossible is an attempt made to block the passage of the food through the pylorus by one of the following measures, though they are unsatisfactory and incomplete.

2. Plication of the Pyloric Antrum

The prepyloric portion of the stomach is freed from the gastrocolic omentum and the gastrohepatic omentum for a distance of several centimeters. This portion of the stomach is then plicated with a number of parallel sutures of a Lembert type, taking the first stitch at the lesser curvature and then, after passing transversely across the anterior wall of the stomach, a second stitch just behind the greater curvature. On tying these sutures tightly the anterior wall of the pyloric antrum is folded inward and acts as an internal tampon (Fig. 103).

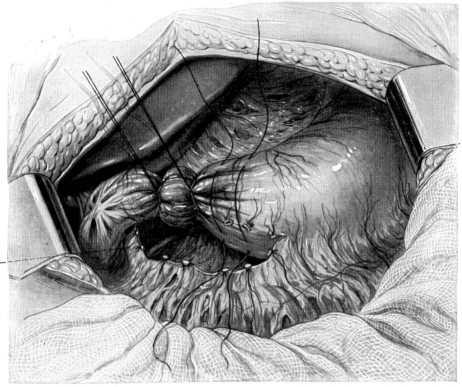

Middle colic artery

FIG. 103. Exclusion of the pylorus by transverse plication of the pyloric antrum after establishing a posterior retrocolic gastrojejunostomy. The latter does not appear in the illustration.

3. Constriction of the Pylorus

A strip of fascia from the anterior rectus sheath or the fascia lata, or the round ligament of the liver, is placed around the prepyloric antrum after this part of the stomach has been completely freed by ligation or blunt separation of the gastrocolic omentum and the gastrohepatic omentum. One end of the fascial strip or the round ligament is provided with a buttonhole through which the other end is passed, drawn tight and sutured to form a tightly constricting ring around the stomach (Fig. 104). The constricting fascial strip can be buried by a few Lembert sutures.

H. EXCISION OF SINGLE PORTIONS OF THE WALL OF THE STOMACH (CZERNY)

Excision of circumscribed areas of the gastric wall is rarely performed today. A double row of infolding sutures leads to a considerable change in

the shape of the stomach in the closure of even small wall defects.   This is
all the more significant since the lesion necessitating operation, usually an old
callous ulcer, usually has already produced a marked change in the shape of
the stomach.   Such changes of shape tend to produce disturbances in the
emptying of the stomach.   Callous ulcers of the lesser curvature are especially
apt to cause distortion of the stomach.   After the excision and suture of such
lesions the cardia and the pylorus are at times brought so close together that
the stomach assumes the shape of a lax bag suspended at these two points.

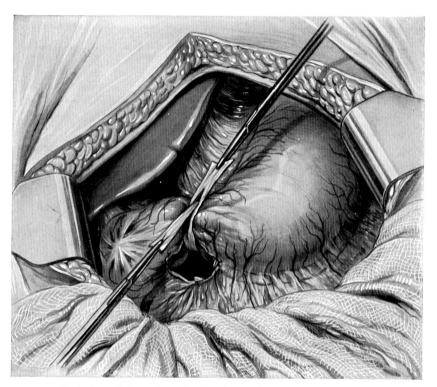

Fig. 104.   Exclusion of the pylorus by ligating the pyloric antrum with a strip of fascia
after establishing a posterior retrocolic gastrojejunostomy.   The latter does not appear in the
illustration.

In case of an ulcer near the pylorus local excision frequently leads to stenosis
so that a gastro-enterostomy is necessary.   The local excision of portions of the
stomach on the lesser curvature and in the neighborhood of the pylorus is
therefore definitely contraindicated unless provision is also made for drainage
of the gastric contents.

The excision of small portions of the anterior or the posterior wall of
the stomach or of an area on the greater curvature is less hazardous, but
here, too, a resection involving the complete cross section of the stomach is
on the whole to be preferred.

If the portion of gastric wall to be excised is adherent to the surrounding
tissues, it must first be completely freed, with or without opening the stomach.
This is done by ligating and dividing tissue strands, by freeing adhesions to

flat surfaces by blunt dissection or by excision with the electrosurgical knife. Visible vessels in the region of the area to be excised are first ligated. Several traction sutures are always applied before the excision is begun to prevent the gastric wall from slipping out of reach. The excision should be carried well into sound tissue, for this increases the chances for a cure of the disease and is most likely to smooth out the cicatricial distortion of the gastric wall usually present in the neighborhood of chronic ulcer. The portion to be excised is isolated with clamps if possible.

The diseased segment of the anterior wall is grasped with a forceps and elevated. An incision, preferably in the form of a pointed oval, is made in the healthy tissue. As soon as the stomach has been opened at one point, it is emptied with an electric suction pump. Bleeding vessels are caught and ligated. After applying the usual traction sutures in the angles, the wound is closed in the long axis by an Albert three-layer catgut suture and by invaginating interrupted Lembert sutures of linen or silk. The local excision of a pathological lesion is performed in a manner similar to the excision of a gastric fistula, as described on page 105, and illustrated in Fig. 87.

Ulcers of the posterior wall of the stomach are frequently adherent to the surrounding structures, most frequently to the pancreas, into which they may at times erode. The procedure of choice for handling such lesions is always gastric resection. If in the exceptional case an excision of the ulcer is to be attempted, the operation is carried out either from in front and through the stomach, or from behind through the lesser peritoneal cavity.

The lesser peritoneal cavity is first exposed through a broad opening in the gastrocolic omentum. If the ulcer is so accessible that it seems possible to operate from behind, it is first advisable to open the stomach with a small incision in the anterior wall, to empty it by suction and to fill it loosely with gauze. Otherwise there is the danger, on opening the stomach from behind, of soiling the lesser cavity with gastric contents. After the stomach has been emptied, the ulcerated portion is excised from behind, if possible in the form of a pointed oval. The opening is closed with a row of three-layer interrupted catgut sutures which, in turn, are buried with interrupted Lembert sutures of silk or linen.

If the exposure through the lesser peritoneal cavity does not appear satisfactory for excising the ulcer, the lesser peritoneal cavity is packed with moist compresses to catch any escaping gastric contents. The anterior wall of the stomach is opened with a transverse incision. The stomach is emptied by suction, and the edges of the wound are retracted with Langenbeck retractors. With the aid of an electric light introduced into the stomach, the location and extent of the ulcer are determined. It will be found advantageous to introduce a hand through the slit in the gastrocolic omentum to raise the posterior wall of the stomach. The excision of the ulcer is then carried out from within the stomach. It is advisable to excise only a small portion at a time, to suture the resultant gap immediately and to pull forward the operative field bit by bit, with the aid of the long ends of the sutures. It is best to place the interrupted catgut sutures which pass through all three layers of the wound edges close together.

After completion of this closing suture, the posterior surface of the stomach with the suture line is brought into the slit in the gastrocolic omentum. This is facilitated by introducing one hand into the opening in the anterior wall of the stomach. The suture line is then buried from without by a row of interrupted Lembert sutures. If it is impossible to apply the second suture row from the outside, one must be satisfied with the Albert suture, applied with particular care from within the stomach.

Appendix: The rare diverticula of the duodenum, which can as a rule be recognized in a roentgenogram, are either amputated flush with the wall of the intestine and the incision closed with a double row of sutures in the usual way, or they are invaginated into the interior of the gut and oversewed.

I. TRANSVERSE RESECTION IN CONTINUITY OF THE STOMACH, OF THE PYLORUS, AND OF THE UPPER DUODENUM

1. CHOICE AND GENERAL TECHNIQUE OF PROCEDURE

The views of individual surgeons concerning the choice and the general technique of procedure in the various diseases of the stomach and duodenum often differ quite materially. Consequently the opinions given here have a decidedly personal slant.

Resection is considered primarily in carcinoma and in ulcer of the stomach. Concerning its indications as opposed to the other operations (excision, gastro-enterostomy and jejunostomy) the following rules apply both in benign gastric ulcer and in carcinoma of the stomach.

Operative Treatment of Gastric Ulcer. The excision of a single circumscribed portion of the stomach (Czerny) is performed only exceptionally today, and then for example in the case of a benign gastric polyp with a narrow peduncle or some similarly local lesion. In all the more extensive lesions which necessitate the removal of larger portions of the gastric wall, resection in continuity is the only procedure which I think should be considered.

In resection with reconstruction of the gastro-intestinal canal in the normal direction (Billroth I, Fig. 125), the pylorus is always removed too, since experience has shown that excision of a segment in the body of the stomach with circular anastomosis of the two portions of the stomach (Payr, Riedel) often leads to stenosis with the formation of an hour-glass stomach. Furthermore, if the pylorus is allowed to remain it may become irritable and produce disturbances in emptying of the stomach.

In the operative treatment of gastric and duodenal ulcer not amenable to conservative measures, resection of the ulcer-bearing portion of the stomach and duodenum is now the operation of choice, although there are still occasional advocates of gastro-enterostomy.

If technically possible, these ulcers of the stomach and duodenum should be removed by resection of both the pylorus and the pyloric antrum. The routine removal of the pyloric antrum to the extent of at least half of the stomach, even in those cases in which the removal of the ulcer does not technically require so extensive a procedure, serves the purpose of diminishing the acid production of the fundus glands by the removal of the pyloric glands which supposedly stimulate them reflexly. This tends to prevent the development of recurrent ulcer in a patient with an ulcer diathesis. (Whether the radical operations will prevent recurrent ulcer is as yet questionable. I. S. R.)

For reconstruction of the gastro-intestinal canal after partial gastrectomy I usually utilize the Billroth II (Fig. 105) method, reserving the Billroth I procedure (Fig. 125) for cases particularly suitable from a technical stand-point. The assumption that the essentially unphysiologic gastric resection and reconstruction by the Billroth II method is frequently followed by post-operative peptic ulcer has been proved incorrect. In fact, jejunal ulcer after resection is observed in less than 1 per cent of cases (Starlinger). The functional results of the Billroth II type of resection after the technique of Krönlein are excellent in my experience.

If an ulcer on the lesser curvature lies so close to the cardia that it cannot be included, or only with difficulty, in a simple transverse resection, I perform a stair-case resection (tube resection) and complete the operation by either the Billroth I (Fig. 133) or the Billroth II (Fig. 135) method.

If an ulcer in the duodenum is situated so far down that an adequate mobilization of the duodenum is difficult, and a dependable closure of the distal duodenal stump after resection is impossible, or if the removal of an ulcer near the pylorus seems to involve too great a risk because of technical difficulties or the poor condition of the patient, the ulcer is left; but it is unilaterally excluded by an extensive resection of the pyloric antrum and, if possible, of the pylorus as well. The operation is completed as in a Billroth II (Fig. 123). (Exclusion resection of Finsterer.) Only when the poor condition of the patient precludes even this palliative resection of the antrum is a posterior retrocolic gastro-enterostomy performed and the ulcer-bearing portion of the stomach isolated as far as possible from the gastro-enterostomy by plicating sutures or by a constricting ring of fascia. (In our experience the plicating sutures are of very little value. I. S. R.)

Unilateral exclusion of the pylorus (von Eiselsberg) with simple transverse division of the stomach between the gastro-enterostomy opening and the pylorus is scarcely to be considered in these cases, since if this is feasible so also is resection of the pyloric antrum which is better and is no more shocking to the patient. The excellent results of palliative resection place the surgeon in the pleasant position that he need not jeopardize the life of the patient in attempting to effect a cure in case of a duodenal ulcer that is difficult to resect.

If the ulcer is high in the fundus, a total resection of the stomach should of course be considered. If this seems impossible, or to entail too great a risk, there are two alternatives, the stomach itself is not interfered with but a temporary jejunostomy is performed (von Eiselsberg, Lameris), or, following the favorable reports of Madlener, the fundus and its ulcer may be left in the body, but an extensive resection of pylorus and pyloric antrum (a two-thirds resection) done, gastro-intestinal continuity being restored by the Billroth II method (Fig. 124).

In case of a completely healed ulcer located at the pylorus which has led to a marked cicatricial stenosis of the pylorus, a posterior retrocolic gastro-enterostomy may be performed without resection. (In many of the above indications for operation pylorectomy followed by a Mayo-Polya anastomosis gives excellent results. In this procedure the jejunum is brought up to the open end of the stomach either ante or retrocolically. I. S. R.)

Operative Treatment of Carcinoma of the Stomach. In carcinoma of the stomach, resection is the only operation which should be considered in the sense of a curative procedure. The reconstruction is accomplished in the form of a Billroth II (Fig. 105) or similar method. Total extirpation of the stomach should also be considered.

The excision of individual parts of the stomach in carcinoma differs from excision in ulcer only in extent. In carcinoma the removal of tissue is carried to the greatest possible limits. This refers not only to the gastric wall itself but to the surrounding tissues as well, particularly the lesser omentum, the gastrocolic omentum and frequently also the transverse mesocolon and the lymph nodes lying in these structures, lymph nodes which must always be suspected of metastatic malignancy. Theoretically, the application of this principle would indicate a total resection of the stomach in every case. Practically, the high mortality of this procedure prevents its routine adoption. In every case, however, we remove as much of the stomach as is possible without too great a risk to the patient. For this reason in itself gastric resection according to the Billroth II method is superior to the Billroth I procedure.

As much as possible of the other structures mentioned must also be removed in every case. Most threatened by malignant metastases are the lymph nodes along the lesser curvature between the layers of the lesser omentum. They are removed by ligating and dividing the vessels of the lesser curvature as close to the cardia as possible and then freeing a band of omental tissue toward the pylorus to the site of the resection; or, what is preferable, by performing a "tube" or "stair-case" resection extending as far as the cardia (Fig. 135). The subpyloric lymph nodes lie along the greater curvature and follow the right gastro-epiploic artery. The retropyloric lymph nodes in the region of the head of the pancreas form the connection between the two groups of lymph nodes previously mentioned. If it is impossible to remove these glands together with the stomach in a single mass, they must be looked for later and removed separately if possible.

If radical operation is no longer indicated, a gastro-enterostomy is performed in the case of all tumors near the pylorus. Whenever possible the posterior retrocolic type of operation is employed and the anastomosis is made as close to the cardia as possible. This is done even when there is as yet no evidence of stenosis. If a gastro-enterostomy above the tumor can no longer be done and if stenosis is present or imminent, a permanent jejunostomy is performed. (When even gastro-enterostomy is no longer possible jejunostomy really has very little to offer. I. S. R.)

Determining the Possibility of a Resection. If resection is planned for ulcer or carcinoma, it must first be determined if the procedure is technically possible, a point frequently not easy to decide. It depends primarily upon the level of the site of the disease and upon the size of the gastroduodenal segment that must be sacrificed in removing the lesion. If the lesion is close to the cardia, only a resection of the whole stomach or of the cardia can be performed. If the lesion only extends fairly high along the lesser curvature, it may at times be possible to remove it by a "tube" resection. If the lesion extends into the duodenum, a 2 to 3 cm. length of duodenum must be available for dependable terminal closure in case of a resection above the orifice of the common bile duct. The question of resection of a pathologic lesion further depends upon the degree to which it is adherent to the surrounding tissues and upon whether these adhesions may be divided without injury to important structures. In benign conditions it is frequently possible to remove such adhesions even though they may be very extensive, as after perforation of the gastric wall. If the ulcer has invaded the anterior abdominal wall, the liver or the pancreas, it may be dealt with in the following manner: The ulcer is excised, preferably with the electrosurgical knife, close to the ring of adhesions. The area which has been excised is closed and covered with a patch of omentum or some other peritoneal reduplication. The most serious complication is the perforation of the ulcer into the transverse colon or mesocolon in the immediate vicinity of the splenic artery. In the former case, if the middle colic artery must be ligated in the removal of the adhesions, it involves a disturbance of nutrition of the transverse colon and necessitates resection of that portion of the colon. This, of course, greatly increases the magnitude of the operation. Injury of the splenic artery must be avoided as far as possible. In an emergency, however, it can be ligated, apparently without serious subsequences as far as the spleen is concerned.

In carcinoma the conditions are often even more unfavorable. Here too, as a rule, it is technically possible to excise the gross lesion when there is invasion at one of the above mentioned points. But in so doing, one can no longer count on a complete excision of the cancerous tissue. Any metastasis that is separated from the primary lesion, as in the liver, in the retroperitoneal glands along the spine, or in the mesenteries of the small or large bowel, precludes radical operation. In such cases, therefore, resection must either be dispensed with, or is performed only as a palliative measure in order to remove a necrotic or bleeding lesion, to relieve stenosis and obstruction, or to remove a cause of pain, but never with the hope of permanent cure or an appreciable lengthening of life. Circumstances are not much more favorable when there are extensive metastases to the regional lymph nodes which can still be grossly removed by the resection.

Whether a diseased gastric segment can be resected or not, depends upon a number of factors. After opening the abdomen, if the lesion is not adherent to the anterior abdominal wall, the transverse colon and stomach are lifted up and examined for adhesions to each other, or the stomach to the liver. The transverse mesocolon is then inspected from below. If the lesion has invaded this structure, it is next determined whether the large mesenteric vessels, particularly the middle colic artery, may be freed, or whether this artery must be sacrificed, necessitating a resection of the colon. An opening is then made between ligatures into the gastrocolic omentum, and the stomach is inspected from behind, especially with regard to possible adhesions to the mesenteric vessels of the transverse colon and to the pancreas. If the lesion extends toward the duodenum, the right lobe of the liver is drawn aside with a broad retractor, the gall bladder and common bile duct are exposed, and the surrounding area closely examined.

The performance of the resection and the reconstruction of the gastro-intestinal canal are carried out either according to the Billroth I method (Fig. 125) or Billroth II (Fig. 105), depending upon the amount of tissue available for the reconstruction of gastro-intestinal continuity. It is a matter of minor importance in which of these two ways the reconstruction of the canal takes place. Of major importance is the extent of the resection.

The Billroth II type of reconstruction is technically easier than the Billroth I type and, if a resection is possible at all, the former can nearly always be performed. The Billroth I method is technically more difficult, is possible only in selected cases, but creates conditions closely approximating the normal. "My heart draws me to the Billroth I, my experience to the Billroth II." Concerning the matter of the ultimate results of the two procedures, the last word has not been said. Jejunal ulcer is rare after the Billroth II type of reconstruction and in my experience no more frequent than after the Billroth I type.

Procedure in the Absence of Pathologic Findings. The surgeon sometimes finds himself in an extremely unpleasant situation, when, after examining the stomach and the duodenum, he does not find the suspected lesion, even after the posterior surface of the stomach has been inspected through an opening in the gastrocolic omentum. To open the stomach or duodenum in such cases in a search for lesions, especially an ulcer not discernible from the outside, does not seem justifiable in my opinion. A simple ulcer, not recognizable from the outside, needs no surgical treatment but belongs to the internist. (With the latter opinion the editor must in part disagree since a posterior duodenal ulcer may at times not be recognizable from an external examination of the duodenum. I. S. R.)

In the absence of positive findings in the stomach and duodenum a careful inspection of the other organs to be considered should be made, notably of the gall bladder, the appendix, the cecum, the kidneys, the flexures of the colon, the sigmoid, finally the small intestine and the pancreas, and in women the pelvic organs. If after a careful search no abnormality of these organs is discovered which might explain the clinical picture, the abdomen should be closed. The surgeon must be extremely careful not to indulge in any operation which is not justified by the findings at exploration. In particular, I wish to warn against a gastro-enterostomy in such a quandary.

If the clinical symptoms in the absence of all positive findings in the abdomen at operation point solely to the stomach so that the assumption of a "gastric neurosis" seems justified, an attempt may be made to ameliorate the trouble by interrupting the nerve supply of the stomach. For this purpose about 10 cc. of 60 per cent alcohol are injected into the lesser omentum, especially in the region of the cardia. If the lesser omentum is too delicate for this purpose, the injection is made subperitoneally along the lesser curvature. A somewhat more formidable procedure is the resection of the lesser omentum which has been recommended for this purpose but which is of very limited value. The structure is divided between ligatures, chiefly in the neighborhood of the cardia in order to interrupt the nerves which reach the stomach in that region. (Either of these procedures is purely empirical and is of limited if any value. I. S. R.)

The General Technique of Gastric Resection. The technical performance of the two types of resection resolves itself into the following individual
steps:

    (a) Mobilization of the segment of stomach or duodenum bearing the
        lesion.
        (1) Division of the corresponding portion of the gastrocolic
            omentum.
        (2) Division of the corresponding portion of the gastrohepatic
            omentum.
        (3) Freeing of the gastric segment from adhesions and accessory
            blood vessels, if necessary.
    (b) Transverse division at both ends of the segment bearing the lesion,
        and reconstruction of the gastro-intestinal canal.
        (1) Resection of the segment and reconstruction of the gastro-
            intestinal tract by gastroduodenostomy (Billroth I)
                (x) by end-to-end anastomosis (Fig. 125), or
                (y) by closure of the distal duodenal limb and an end-
              to-side anastomosis (Fig. 134), or
                (z) by closure of the proximal gastric opening and a side-
              to-end anastomosis (Fig. 127), or
        (2) Resection of the segment, terminal closure of the distal
            duodenal opening and reconstruction of the gastro-intestinal
            passage by gastrojejunostomy (Billroth II),
                (x) by end-to-side anastomosis (Figs. 105 and 116), or
                (y) by closure of the proximal gastric opening and a side-
              to-side anastomosis (Fig. 115), or
                (z) by division of the jejunum, by lateral implantation
              of the proximal jejunal opening into the distal jejunal loop
              and by anastomosis of stomach and jejunum, end-to-end,
              side-to-end (Fig. 117) or end-to-side.

The above-mentioned operative steps almost never follow each other
separately in the order given, but the order varies with the case. At times, a
step which has been started is discontinued for the moment, another step is
undertaken and only after its total or partial performance is the one previously
started carried to completion. No hard and fast rules can be given for the
order of procedure. This is a matter of personal experience and of organization. With the plan of the operation in mind, one usually has no great difficulty in finding the most suitable mode of procedure for the individual case.

    There is no fundamental difference in the course and technique of the
operation, whether a transverse resection is undertaken in the region of the
cardia, the body of the stomach, the pyloric region, or extending into the
duodenum.

    The abdominal incision is, as a rule, closed primarily after a gastric
resection. Drainage and packing are necessitated only by gross offenses
against asepsis, by hemorrhage which cannot be controlled without packing,
by ulcerated surfaces which must be left uncovered in the abdominal cavity
and by large erosions into the pancreas which cannot be adequately covered.

In primary closure of the abdominal wound, the safety of gastro-intestinal sutures is so great that the patient may be given fluids by mouth immediately after operation, a point again to be stressed. (It is our practise to withhold fluids by mouth for several days after all gastric operations and to insert a Jutte tube to drain the gastric segment. There is no doubt that patients so treated do better. The fluid, salt and glucose requirements are met by giving a continuous intravenous drip. I. S. R.)

Because of technical improvements, such as spinal anaesthesia, high-pressure local anaesthesia, the use of the Petz suture instrument, the return to interrupted sutures in the serosal suture, the substitution of the electro-surgical knife, and the abandonment of hopeless radical resections in favor of palliative resection, my operative mortality for gastric resection in gastric and duodenal ulcer and in gastric carcinoma has been materially decreased (in the ulcer group to about 2 per cent).

2. Resection According to the Billroth II Principle (1885). Palliative Resection

I shall first describe gastric resection according to the Billroth II method, and shall consider as the normal procedure the end-to-side anastomosis of the entire gastric opening to the side of the highest jejunal loop (Krönlein) (Fig. 105). This type of gastric resection is also frequently referred to as the Polya-Reichel or Mayo-Polya operation.

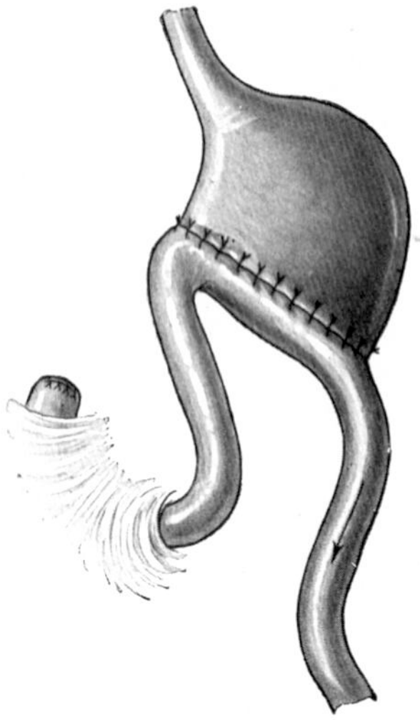

An opening is made through the gastrocolic omentum between ligatures (Fig. 106). A slit is made in the transverse mesocolon parallel to the large vessels. The highest jejunal loop, through the mesentery of which a stout silk suture was passed close to the gut, is drawn forward through both openings, by means of a Korn forceps passed from above and grasping the silk suture. The jejunal segment is fixed by compresses, by a clamp, or by the thread passed through the mesentery.

A forceps is passed behind the stomach through the opening in the gastrocolic omentum and its end is pushed through the extremely delicate gastrohepatic omentum. With the aid of this forceps a rubber tube or a gauze roll is passed around the stomach as a girdle on which the stomach now rides and by which it can be lifted and drawn upward or downward (Fig. 107).

Fig. 105. Gastric resection, Billroth II. Diagrammatic. Anastomosis of the whole cross section of the stomach to the jejunum (Krönlein).

The further procedure may either begin with the division and closure of the duodenum, continue in the direction of the cardia, and conclude with the gastrojejunostomy; or it may begin with the division of the stomach on the cardiac side and the gastrojejunostomy, continue in the direction of the duodenum and conclude with the division and closure of the duodenum. It is advisable to begin the operation in the region of sound tissue where no particular difficulties are present, and to conclude in the region of the diseased portion, because the technical difficulties usually to be encountered in the latter region are lessened by the free movability of the divided end of the segment to be resected.

(a) **The separation of the corresponding segment of the gastro-colic omentum (Fig. 107).** The gastrocolic omentum is made tense by drawing the stomach upward and the transverse colon downward. The gastro-colic omentum is doubly ligated, beginning at the slit made in this omentum. In the case of a benign ulcer this is done close to the stomach, but in car-

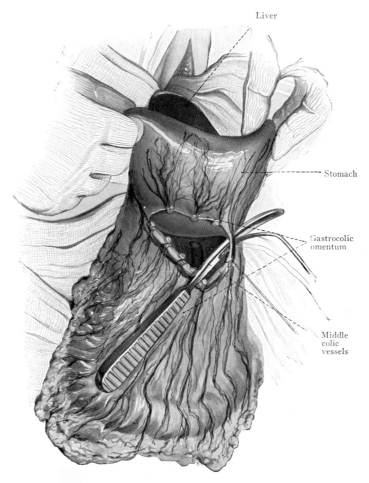

Liver

Stomach

Gastrocolic omentum

Middle colic vessels

Fig. 106. Gastric resection, Billroth II (1). The gastrocolic omentum, which is unusually long, is picked up in segments on an aneurysm needle and divided between ligatures. The transverse mesocolon and the middle colic vessels appear in the opening.

cinoma, especially if glands are demonstrable, the ligation is as close to the colon as possible. It is continued first in the direction of the cardia because, as a rule, no difficulties are encountered here and because the approach to and the inspection of the lesser peritoneal cavity are thus facilitated.

When the separation has proceeded far enough toward the cardia the ligation is continued toward the pylorus. In the region of the antrum the gastrocolic omentum is usually adherent to the mesocolon. The separation of the two, however, is usually accomplished without difficulty, partly by blunt, partly by sharp dissection. Care must be taken to spare the vessels of the mesocolon, especially the middle colic artery. Only when the lesion has invaded the mesocolon is separation by blunt dissection impossible. The diseased portion of the mesocolon must then be excised, and the vessels ligated. As the pylorus is approached, the tissue joining the colon and the pyloric

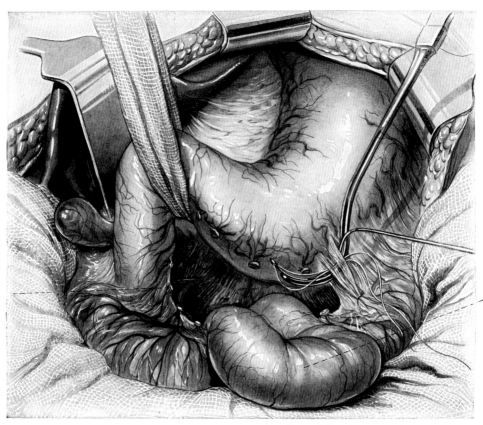

Liga-
tions of
the gas-
trocolic
omen-
tum

Loop
jeju-
num
tende
for t
anas
mosi

FIG. 107. Gastric resection, Billroth II (2). The highest jejunal loop has been pulled up through a slit in the transverse mesocolon and a slit in the gastrocolic omentum. The middle colic artery can be seen through the opening in the gastrocolic omentum. After the ligation and division of a part of the gastrocolic omentum and division of the gastrohepatic omentum, the stomach is elevated by means of a gauze roll (a rubber tube would be preferable). The gastrocolic omentum is divided further in the direction of the fundus between double ligatures.

portion of the stomach becomes thicker and the relations to the middle colic artery are more intimate. This important vessel must therefore be inspected carefully and isolated before tying each ligature. Gradually there become discernible two peritoneal leaflets passing from the hepatic flexure of the colon to the duodenum and to the pylorus, one on the right, the other on the left. The right leaflet contains the right gastro-epiploic artery in addition to numerous veins. This leaflet with its vessels is doubly ligated and divided. The left leaflet leads to the head of the pancreas, and from it numerous short branches of the gastroduodenal artery and numerous veins reach the duodenum. These vessels are small but they must nevertheless be doubly ligated and

divided (Fig. 108). In this manner the duodenum is gradually freed sufficiently from the head of the pancreas.

If it becomes necessary to ligate the middle colic artery because of
inseparable adhesions to the diseased tissue, or if a portion of the transverse
colon after mobilization of the stomach shows circulatory disturbances sufficiently severe to necessitate partial resection further progress is made simpler
by immediately resecting the affected portion of the transverse colon. The

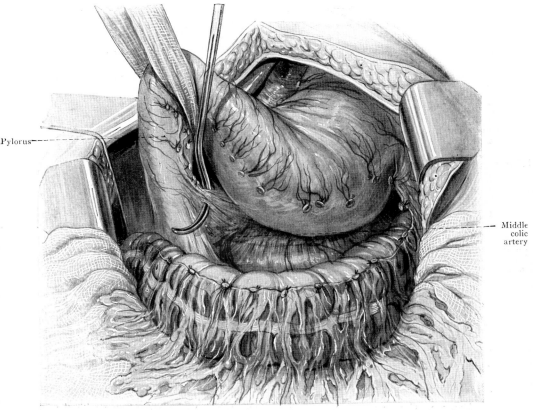

Pylorus

Middle
colic
artery

FIG. 108. Gastric resection, Billroth II (3). The gastrocolic omentum has been sufficiently
divided. The pyloric portion of the stomach is elevated by means of a gauze roll passed around
it. The wall of the duodenum adjacent to the pancreas is freed by dividing between ligatures
the vascular connective tissue strands which join the two organs.

segment of colon is freed from its mesentery, is closed, preferably with the
aid of the Petz suture apparatus, and divided between the two lines of closure
and the two ends of the colon are turned aside to right and left where the
stumps are protected by pads or rubber condoms. The anastomosis of the
ends of the colon follows the completion of the gastric resection as the last
step of the operation.

(b) The separation of the gastrohepatic omentum. In separating
the left side of the duodenum in the region of the lesser peritoneal cavity from
the pancreas in the manner described, the hepatoduodenal omentum which is
continuous with the gastrohepatic omentum is approached. Having arrived at

this point, the stomach is drawn downward and to the left, thus bringing into view the duodenum and the lesser omentum and putting them on tension. Beginning in the middle of the lesser omentum at the point where the rubber tube or gauze roll was pulled through to make traction on the stomach, the delicate tissue is divided between double ligatures. This mobilization of the lesser curvature is carried on toward the duodenum until the region of the previously completed ligations at the upper border of the head of the pancreas

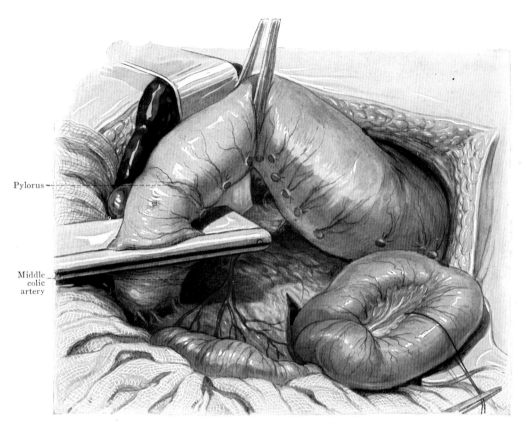

Pylorus

Middle
colic
artery

Fig. 109. Gastric resection, Billroth II (4). Division of the duodenum with the Petz instrument. The pyloric antrum and the upper duodenum have been adequately mobilized. The stomach is elevated by means of a gauze roll. The Petz instrument is applied across the upper duodenum. The loop of jejunum intended for the anastomosis has been pulled through a slit in the transverse mesocolon and provided with a traction suture passed through its mesentery.

are reached. On the duodenal side of the pylorus a number of short vessels are found in the hepatoduodenal omentum which are markedly stretched when traction is made on the duodenum. These vessels enclose the duodenum, as in the limbs of a fork, on its anterior and posterior surfaces. They must be isolated on each side with great care, and then doubly ligated and divided. While traction is made on the stomach and the attached duodenum, first to the right, and then to the left, or upward or downward, the freeing of the duodenum from the pancreas and from the hepatoduodenal omentum gradually proceeds. Any injury to the common bile duct or to the pancreatic duct is of course to be avoided. If there is any danger of injury to the common bile duct, it is better to expose it as fully as possible rather than subject it to the danger of accidental injury.

(c) **Division of the Duodenum.** Division of the duodenum is carried out as soon as the duodenum is sufficiently mobilized on all sides so that sound tissue is available for its division and closure.

The duodenum may be grasped and sutured with the Petz suture instrument (Fig. 109) or it may be divided between clamps. Before the duodenum

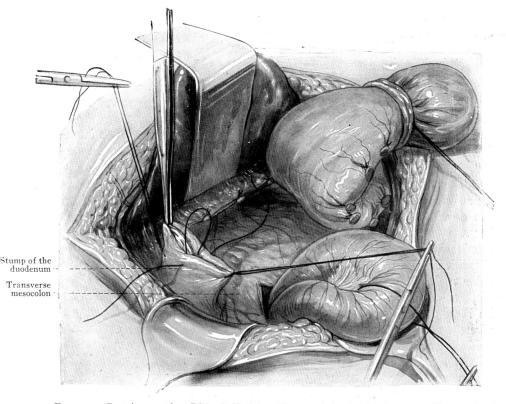

Stump of the duodenum

Transverse mesocolon

FIG. 110. Gastric resection, Billroth II (5). Closure of the duodenal stump. The duodenal transsection which has been closed with Petz clips is infolded by interrupted Lembert sutures. The transsection of the proximal portion of the stomach has had a rubber condom tied over it and has been folded back over the left costal margin. The loop of jejunum intended for the anastomosis has been pulled up through a slit in the transverse mesocolon and has been provided with a traction suture applied through its mesentery.

is divided between the rows of clips after the removal of the apparatus, a continuous sero-muscular purse-string suture distal to the clips is inserted and traction sutures are used to prevent the duodenum from slipping away after division.

After dividing the duodenum between the clips, the cut edge of the distal limb is buried by inverting the stump and making traction on the sero-muscular purse-string suture. Interrupted Lembert sutures may also be used (Fig. 110). Difficulties are at times encountered because often only a little of the duodenal wall is available for suture on the side toward the pancreas. In such a case it is permissible to grasp the pancreas instead of the duodenal wall. The dependability of such an incomplete suture is increased by over-sewing the stump with a piece of omentum or of another fold of peritoneum. When the duodenal stump has been closed, it is dropped and temporarily covered with a gauze pad.

If a Petz instrument is not available, a gentle clamp can be applied to the duodenum if there is enough room. The clamp should be applied as low as possible. The duodenum is then divided on the gastric side of the clamp. If there is too little room, the clamp must be dispensed with. As a result, a good deal of frothy duodenal contents may escape unless adequate suction is provided. The distal duodenal stump is closed with an Albert catgut suture, but applied as an interrupted suture, followed by Lembert interrupted sutures of linen. The duodenum may also be simply ligated and the stump buried with a purse-string suture (Figs. 43 and 44).

Some surgeons prefer to divide and close the duodenum with the aid of the Moynihan or Payr crushing clamp. The technique of this procedure I have previously described and illustrated in Figs. 46 and 47.

Even in patients with ulcer I do not consider it necessary to inspect the interior of the duodenum for ulcers after its transsection. The amount of space available above the bile passages for the terminal closure of the duodenum is so restricted that a still lower resection of the duodenum beyond a newly discovered ulcer is rarely possible. Even when an ulcer is found in the depths of the transsected duodenal stump, it can seldom be resected because of the difficulty of subsequent closure. The discovery of such low duodenal ulcers, not externally visible, is primarily of interest when the Billroth I procedure is contemplated, for if an irremovable ulcer is present a shift to the Billroth II operation might be preferable in order to isolate the ulcer on one side. If the Billroth II procedure is used routinely there need be little fear of overlooking these small ulcers since, as previously stated, ulcers of the non-callous type frequently heal under more conservative or palliative measures and therefore do not require radical removal.

(d) The Division of the Lesser Omentum. The proximal duodenal stump is protected immediately after division with a gauze pad or a condom (Figs. 30 and 110). Stomach and duodenum are pulled forcibly downward so that the attachment of the gastrohepatic omentum to the lesser curvature is stretched. In the region of the cardia the gastrohepatic omentum occurs not as a thin veil, but as a massive semirigid plate, infiltrated with fat, that straddles the lesser curvature on the anterior and posterior surfaces, and whose individual blood vessels and dividing line from the stomach are usually not clearly discernible. If one were to attempt to separate the gastrohepatic omentum from the stomach by blunt dissection under guidance of the eye and with the Kocher grooved director, there would be danger of injuring the gastric wall. The dividing line between stomach and omentum, while not visible, can nevertheless be palpated easily as a rule, by passing the index finger of the left hand behind the omentum and grasping it between the finger and thumb. At this point a small incision is made through the peritoneal covering and the Kocher grooved director is introduced from in front and close to the gastric border against the tip of the index finger; the instrument lifts the omentum with its contained coronary vessels away from the stomach

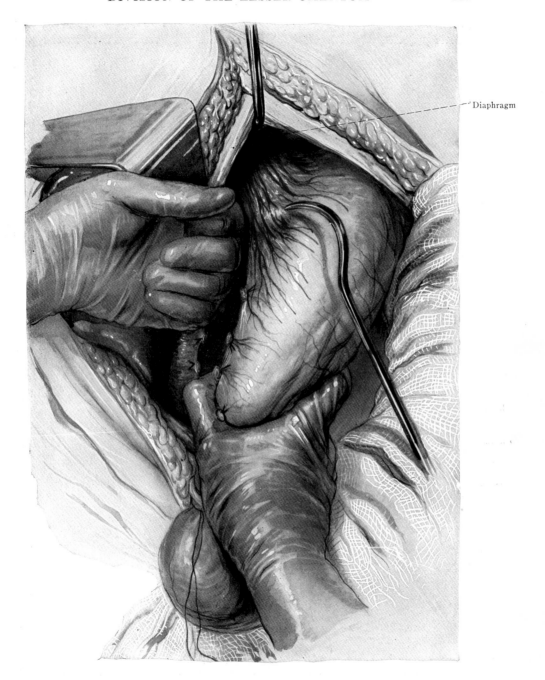

Diaphragm

FIG. 111. Gastric resection, Billroth II (6). Ligation of the gastrohepatic omentum in the region of the cardia. The stomach has been divided transversely at the duodenum and the duodenal stump has been enclosed in a rubber condom. The stomach is now pulled forcibly downward. The border line between the lesser curvature and the gastrohepatic omentum is determined by palpation with the left index finger. The gastrohepatic omentum is picked up on an aneurysm needle directed against the tip of the index finger as close as possible to the esophagus and divided between ligatures.

(Fig. 111). The strand of omentum carried by the grooved director is very carefully doubly ligated. It is advisable to apply two ligatures on the side

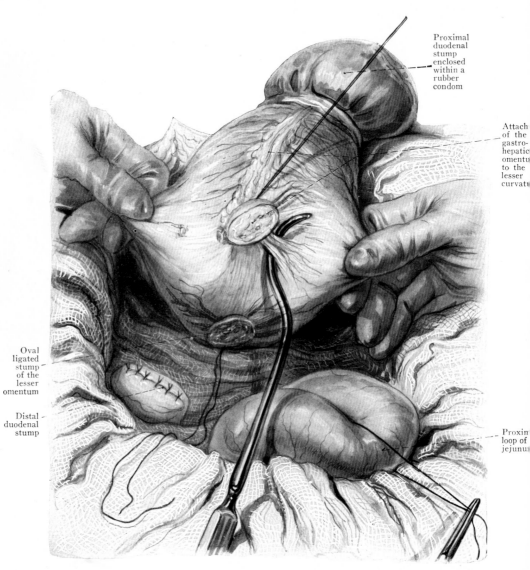

Proximal duodenal stump enclosed within a rubber condom

Attach of the gastro- hepatic omentu to the lesser curvat

Oval ligated stump of the lesser omentum

Distal duodenal stump

Proxin loop of jejunu

FIG. 112. Gastric resection, Billroth II (7). Freeing of the lesser curvature from the gastrohepatic omentum. The stomach has been divided transversely at the duodenum and its free stump covered with a rubber condom. The gastrohepatic omentum has been divided en masse high up, close to the esophagus, between ligatures. The proximal and distal stumps are in view, each provided with a traction suture. The gastric stump has been folded back over the left costal margin. The lesser curvature is exposed and extended by an assistant. The vascular connections of the gastrohepatic omentum, as they run toward the anterior and pos- terior surfaces of the stomach, are picked up with an aneurysm needle and divided between ligatures. The duodenal stump, which has been closed with interrupted Lembert sutures, is in view. The loop of jejunum intended for the anastomosis has been pulled up through a slit in the transverse mesocolon and has been provided with a traction suture passed through its mesentery.

toward the cardia, for the vessels imbedded in the thick tissue have a decided tendency to slip out of the ligature and it may prove very difficult to recapture the freely bleeding retracted vessels. Care must be used in passing the Kocher grooved director so as not to injure the esophagus which at times lies unexpectedly low and to the right.

The most distal ligature of the gastrohepatic omentum on the lesser curvature, in contradistinction to the proximal ligatures, is not cut short but is used as a traction suture, to help in tying off (as far as possible from the lesser curvature) the numerous vessels, branches of the coronary artery, which radiate from this point over the anterior and posterior surfaces of the body of the stomach, and consequently in mobilizing the lesser curvature. They

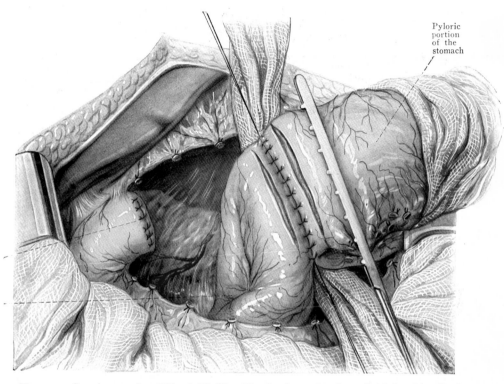

Pyloric
portion
of the
stomach

Distal
uodenal
stump

uodeno-
jejunal
unction

FIG. 113. Gastric resection, Billroth II (8). The duodenum has been divided and its distal stump closed. The pyloric portion of the stomach, wrapped in gauze is reflected over the left costal margin. The highest loop of the jejunum has been attached to the posterior wall of the stomach by posterior Lembert sutures over a gauze roll. The serosa of the stomach and of the jejunal loop has been divided. The stomach has been closed on the pyloric side of the point of opening by means of a heavy clamp. A clamp could not be applied on the fundal side because of lack of room.

stand out clearly on the surface of the stomach if the lesser curvature is pulled up over the left costal margin while the hand of an assistant spreads the stomach transversely (Fig. 112). This retrograde ligation of the gastro-hepatic omentum is continued in the direction of the duodenal stump until the lesser curvature is sufficiently freed. In this procedure the lesser curvature is deprived of its peritoneal covering in a strip several centimeters wide.

The stomach which in this manner has been extensively mobilized is lifted up and turned back over the left costal margin so that its posterior surface may easily be inspected. Here as a rule, the gastrosplenic ligament, a number of adhesions and the vasa brevia arteries remain to be doubly ligated and divided. It is once more determined whether the ligation of the gastrocolic omentum has been carried sufficiently far toward the cardia and any further-needed ligation is performed.

(e) **The Performance of the Gastro-enterostomy.** The stomach is drawn sharply down from beneath the left costal arch and is grasped with a clamp applied as far toward the cardia as possible and from the greater to the lesser curvature. The free tips of the arms of the clamp are tightly tied

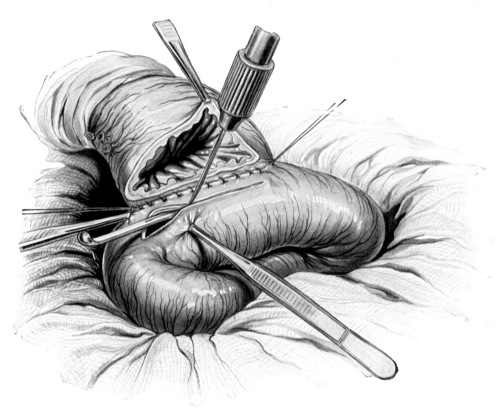

FIG. 114. Gastric resection, Billroth II (9). The stomach and the jejunal loop have been joined by the posterior Lembert suture. The anterior wall of the stomach has been completely divided. The wall of the jejunal loop is being divided with the diathermy knife on an ivory director. The clamp on the portion of the stomach to be removed is not shown in the illustration.

together with a silk thread at the lesser curvature, so that they compress the stomach sufficiently in this region. In case of scantiness of stomach for the anastomosis the application of the clamp may have to be dispensed with. The stomach is then reflected up over the left costal margin (protected by a gauze pad) so that the posterior surface is easily accessible. The highest loop of jejunum which was drawn through the slit in the transverse mesocolon at the beginning of the operation is now applied to the posterior surface of the stomach so that it runs in a downward direction from the lesser toward the greater curvature in an isoperistaltic direction. In so doing, careful measurements are made of the segment between the stomach and the duodenojejunal junction, so that the point of the loop opposed to the lesser curvature is about 10 to 15 cm. from the junction. A gauze roll is placed between the stomach and the loop of gut and the operative field is carefully walled off. The loop is attached to the posterior wall of the stomach with interrupted posterior Lembert sutures, just distal to the gastric clamp (Fig. 113). Difficulties are most likely to be encountered in applying the sutures at the lesser curvature, since a certain amount of tension may scarcely be avoided at this point. Care must be taken to insure that the end traction suture be applied exactly at the lesser curvature and not on the posterior surface of the stomach. It is advisable to apply the sutures at the lesser curvature closely and with particular care, since that portion of the surface of the stomach was denuded of its peritoneal covering to a width of several centimeters during the detachment of the lesser omentum.

After the completion of the posterior Lembert sutures the distal segment of the stomach, which was reflected over the left costal margin is grasped with a clamp from the greater to the lesser curvature, after the band of stomach intervening between this clamp and the clamp previously applied has been milked empty. The stomach and intestine are opened half a centimeter from the Lembert suture (Fig. 114), and the adjacent edge of stomach and intestine are joined with a continuous posterior Albert catgut suture.

The anterior wall of the stomach is now divided, completing the resection of the diseased gastric segment. The two anterior edges of the stomach and intestine are joined by continuous anterior Albert catgut suture and by anterior interrupted Lembert sutures of linen. This completes the anastomosis between the stomach and intestine.

Other Types of Gastric Resection and Reconstruction According to the Billroth II Principle. Billroth originally resected the stomach, closed the gastric cross section and then performed an anterior antecolic or posterior retrocolic gastro-enterostomy (Fig. 115). Von Eiselsberg closed a part of the gastric opening near the lesser curvature and implanted the highest loop of jejunum into the opening remaining at the greater curvature (Fig. 116). Krönlein joined the full length of the gastric transsection to a jejunal loop in an antecolic position, and Reichel, Polya, and Mayo made the same anastomosis in a retrocolic position in the manner I have just described. Finally, one can follow the technique of Roux who transsected the highest loop of jejunum, implanted the distal limb into the remaining portion of the stomach, and the proximal limb into the distal limb end-to-side (Roux Y-shaped gastroenterostomy, Fig. 117). Many of these modifications of gastro-enterostomy after gastric resection no longer have much practical significance.

The von Eiselsberg Method. Some surgeons do not join the intestine to the full width of the gastric transsection but make only a small anastomosis. If this be based on the fear that the stomach will empty too rapidly if the full width of the transsection is used, the premise is fallacious. Any attempt to regulate the gastro-enterostomy by creating a relative stenosis is to be condemned. On the contrary, an anastomosis between stomach and intestine should be made as large as possible and the speed of emptying of the stomach can in the main be ignored. On the other hand, a partial closure of the transsection opening may materially simplify the resection if there is lack of material in the region of the lesser curvature, and can occasionally be recommended for this reason, provided that the residual open-

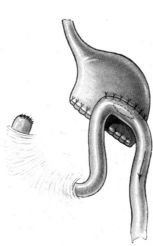

FIG. 115. Gastric resection, Billroth II. Diagrammatic. Closure of the stomach and formation of a gastrojejunostomy. Billroth's original procedure.

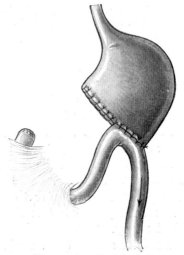

FIG. 116. Gastric resection, Billroth II. Diagrammatic. Partial closure of the stomach, and anastomosis between the remainder of the divided stomach and the jejunum, after von Eiselsberg.

ing is large enough for the unimpeded escape of the gastric contents into the intestine.

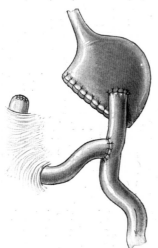

FIG. 117. Gastric resection, Billroth II. Diagrammatic. Closure of the stomach and formation of a Y-shaped gastro-jejunostomy by the method of Roux.

The detailed technique of partial closure of the divided stomach and of the anastomosis of the residual opening with the intestine as practiced in the von Eiselsberg method is described under gastric resection according to the Billroth I on page 163, and illustrated in Figures 128 and 129.

The portion of the gastric transsection adjacent to the lesser curvature is closed by a Czerny double-row suture (Fig. 116), so that a residual opening 3 to 4 cm. long remains near the greater curvature. In order to safe-guard that particularly vulnerable point, where the suture line of the gastric transsection meets the gastro-enterostomy, the proximal loop of jejunum can be fastened over the suture line of the stomach for a short distance for reinforcement. This attachment of the proximal loop at the same time aids the progress of its contents in the manner of a Kappeler suspension suture.

Original Techinque of Billroth. The stomach is closed completely and the loop of intestine is then joined to the stomach by a separate gastro-enterostomy on the posterior or anterior surface of the stomach (original Billroth II, Fig. 115).

Roux Y Anastomosis. In performing a Y-shaped gastro-enterostomy after gastric resection according to the Billroth II (Fig. 117 and 118), the intestine is divided a short distance below the duodenojejunal junction, the proximal loop is implanted into the distal loop and the end of the distal loop is implanted into the stomach end-to-side. The disadvantages of this procedure have already been pointed out. They lie chiefly in the fact that the segment of jejunum between the stomach and the entero-enterostomy receives only pure gastric juice without any admixture of duodenal contents, a condition which predisposes to jejunal ulcer. This procedure is to be considered only in very extensive resections of the stomach, when it becomes difficult to bring a continuous loop of jejunum to the stomach because of the great distance involved, or if the jejunum had to be divided in the resection of a jejunal ulcer. (Even then I question whether some other procedure would not be better. I. S. R.)

(f) **Closure of the Slit in the Transverse Mesocolon.** In every type of gastro-enterostomy after gastric resection according to the Billroth II principle, the site of the anastomosis must if possible finally be sutured into the slit in the transverse mesocolon, so that intestinal loops may not slip through the slit and be caught. If possible, the suturing is to be performed in such a way that the anastomosis comes to lie in the lower abdominal segment. If not, the gut loops are sutured to the slit in the mesocolon. While the transverse colon is lifted high, the gastro-intestinal anastomosis is pulled through the slit in the mesocolon down into the lower abdominal segment. The mesocolon is sutured if possible to the gastric side of the anastomosis by interrupted sutures placed in a circle about the anastomosis (Fig. 118). The anterior wall of the stomach is first sutured to the left edge of the slit in the mesocolon and the posterior surface to the right edge of the slit. If the gastrojejunostomy lies so far toward the cardia that it cannot be drawn completely through the slit in the mesocolon, then the transposition of the anastomosis into the lower abdominal segment must be dispensed with, wholly or in part, and the proximal and distal limbs of the anastomosed loop of jejunum are sutured to the edges of the slit in the mesocolon. Some form of closure of the slit is absolutely necessary if a subsequent obstruction is to be prevented.

The proximal and the distal intestinal loops are examined to make certain that they lie properly in the abdomen. A careful inspection for bleeding is once more made and the abdomen is then closed without drainage.

Resection from the Cardia toward the Duodenum. Instead of proceeding in the manner just described by first completely mobilizing and dividing the duodenum, continuing the mobilization toward the cardia and concluding the operation with the separation of the diseased segment of the stomach from the fundic portion with the anastomosis of the remainder of the stomach to the highest jejunal loop, the order may be reversed. The stomach is first freed and divided in the region of the cardia, the anastomosis is made between the proximal segment of the stomach and the highest jejunal loop, the gastric segment to be resected is freed in the direction of the duodenum and the last stage is the division of the duodenum and the care of the duodenal stump. The procedure in this direction is particularly useful when there are no adhesions and consequently no technical difficulties in the region of the fundus and of the middle of the stomach but when such difficulties are to be expected in the region of the pylorus and duodenum. Aside from the fact that the free mobility of the stomach which has already been divided

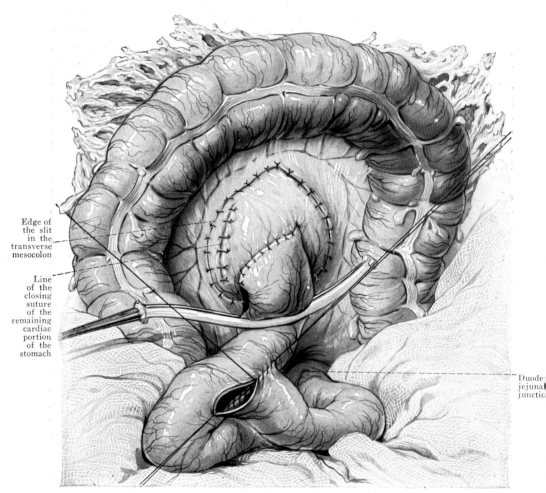

Edge of
the slit
in the
transverse
mesocolon

Line
of the
closing
suture
of the
remaining
cardiac
portion
of the
stomach

Duode-
jejunal
junctic

Fig. 118. Gastric resection, Billroth II, with establishment of a Y-shaped gastrojejunostomy (Roux). After resection of the diseased portion of the stomach and closure of its proximal end and of the duodenal stump, the highest loop of jejunum was divided 20 cm. beyond the duodenojejunal junction. The distal limb of the jejunum was anastomosed to the remainder of the stomach end-to-side and the portion of the stomach used for the anastomosis was sewed into the slit in the transverse mesocolon. The end of the proximal limb of jejunum is implanted into the distal limb end-to-side at a point about 10 cm. distal to the site of the gastrojejunostomy.

near the cardia makes the mobilizing of the pylorus and duodenum easier, this procedure of working toward the pylorus has the additional advantage that, if insuperable difficulties are encountered in the freeing of a lesion in the region of the pylorus, further attempts in this direction can be terminated at any time. The stomach is then divided in the region of the antrum as far as it has been freed and the pyloric end is closed. The total resection is thus converted into a palliative resection with the pylorus remaining as an excluded portion. The procedure in the direction from cardia toward pylorus is therefore to be preferred in the exceptional case presenting serious difficulties in the region of the pylorus and the duodenum, especially if it is impossible to decide at the beginning of the operation whether the lesion can be removed completely.

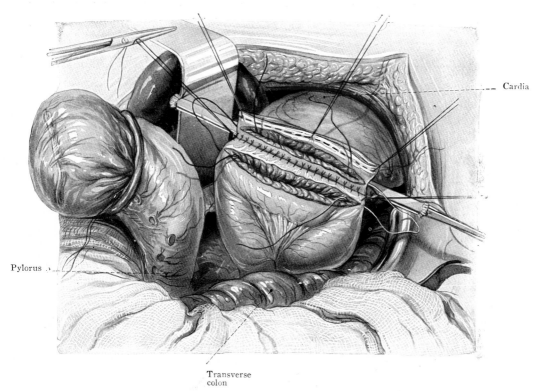

Fig. 119. Gastric resection, Billroth II, in the cardia-duodenal direction (1). The stomach has been divided transversely close to the cardia between two rows of clips inserted by the Petz suture instrument. The distal end of the stomach has been covered with a rubber condom and folded back toward the right. An anastomosis is being established between the highest loop of jejunum, pulled up through a slit in the transverse mesocolon, and the cardia of the stomach, from which leakage is prevented by the clamp. The two structures have been joined by posterior Lembert sutures and have been opened. The end traction sutures of the posterior Albert three-layer suture are being applied.

The operation in this direction proceeds in the main according to the steps already described but in the reverse order, so that only a few sign boards along the road need be mentioned.

After the proximal jejunal loop has been drawn forward through an opening in the transverse mesocolon and in the gastrocolic omentum, a rubber tube is passed behind the stomach through the opening in the gastrocolic omentum and out through an opening made in the gastrohepatic omentum. A forceps is used for this purpose. While the body of the stomach is elevated, the stomach is extensively mobilized, first along the greater curvature and then along the lesser curvature at the point determined on for the transsection.

The stomach is closed and divided at this point and for this purpose I prefer the Petz suture instrument.

The pyloric portion is now covered with a rubber condom and is put aside for the time being. The anastomosis between the proximal end of the stomach and the jejunal loop is completed, either according to the Krönlein-Reichel-Polya principle with utilization of the full width of the transsection, or the gastric opening may be completely closed and a separate gastro-enterostomy

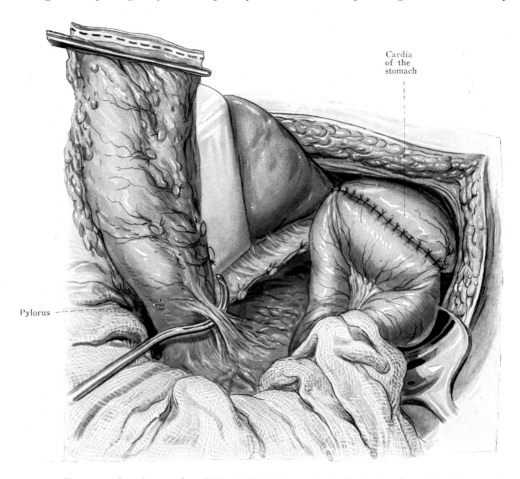

Cardia
of the
stomach

Pylorus

FIG. 120. Gastric resection, Billroth II, in the cardia-duodenal direction (2). The anastomosis between the cardia and the highest loop of jejunum has been completed. The pyloric portion of the stomach and the adjacent duodenum have been freed except for the connections between the duodenum and the head of the pancreas. These connections are being picked up on an aneurysm needle and cut between ligatures.

performed. I prefer the Krönlein procedure (Fig. 119). The cut edge of the stomach, closed with a clamp or Petz clips, is provided with three traction sutures so that the stomach may be reflected upward, exposing its posterior surface. About 1 cm. from the free edge, the proximal jejunal loop is attached to the posterior surface of the gastric stump by interrupted posterior Lembert sutures of silk or linen. The intestine and posterior surface of the stomach are opened ½ cm. from the line of suture (Fig. 119) and their cut edges are united by a continuous posterior Albert three-layer catgut suture which, after division of the anterior wall, is continued as the anterior three-layer suture. The anastomosis is completed by interrupted anterior Lembert sutures.

The pyloric portion of the stomach is picked up and is freed in the usual manner from its attachments on all sides in the direction of the duodenum. Since the stump is only attached at its duodenal portion and can be moved freely in all directions, the mobilization is technically simple. Except for the freeing of the side toward the pancreas, which at times may be particularly difficult, there should be no difficulty (Fig. 120). The mobilization is continued past the diseased portion and beyond the pylorus to the duodenum. The duodenum is closed transversely and divided for which I again use the Petz instrument. The distal stump is invaginated with interrupted Lembert sutures of silk or linen.

At the close of the operation the stomach in the region of the gastroenterostomy is sutured to the slit in the transverse mesocolon.

Special Considerations. If a carcinoma has extensively invaded the tissues around the stomach, there can no longer be any question of a radical operation promising a permanent cure and it is often better to dispense with resection, unless there is only a limited invasion of the tissues. The presence of severe pain, obviously caused by the tumor itself, or the treatment of a necrotic or bleeding lesion justifies the removal of the carcinoma, even when there is no longer any hope of complete extirpation of the carcinoma. In the case of benign ulcer, the involvement of neighboring organs does not contraindicate radical treatment. An ulcer which has invaded the anterior abdominal wall, the liver or the pancreas is either excised in the surrounding healthy tissue with the adhesions closing the perforation remaining attached to the ulcer, thus preserving asepsis, or the lesion is excised at its margins. The latter results on the one hand in an opening in the stomach and on the other in a large necrotic ulcerated surface on the organ affected. The stomach is emptied by suction through the resultant opening and is packed temporarily with a long strip of gauze to prevent the escape of any further gastric contents.

The surface of the organ into which the ulcer has perforated is removed with an electrosurgical loop, or curretted thoroughly with a sharp spoon curette, and then covered with peritoneum. Drainage of the abdominal cavity is not necessary after exposing such an ulcer, since experience has shown that the surface heals excellently if covered with peritoneum.

Almost insuperable difficulties frequently arise in the resection of a duodenal ulcer which has invaded the head of the pancreas, not because an excision of the ulcer is impossible, but because a secure closure of the duodenal stump is hampered by the lack of healthy duodenal wall. The duodenal wall can be freed for only a comparatively short distance because of the nearness to the pylorus of the important structures in the hepatoduodenal ligament. A free edge at least 2 cm. wide is necessary for secure closure of the duodenal stump. It is in this type of case that the removal of a benign ulcer is most frequently found to be impracticable. A palliative resection of the stomach with unilateral exclusion of the duodenum may be substituted with the anticipation of good results from this procedure.

In freeing the stomach, band-like adhesions between the floor of a gastric ulcer and the surrounding structures are picked up on an aneurysm needle, doubly ligated and divided (Fig. 121). They frequently contain fair-sized vessels, so that merely cutting them without previous ligation is never advisable.

Involvement of the Transverse Mesocolon. Invasion of the transverse mesocolon by the lesion is of particular significance because in this

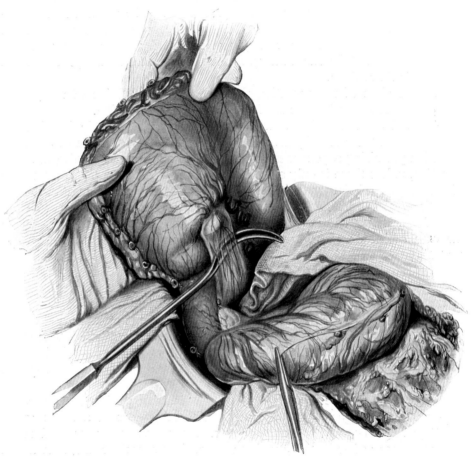

Fig. 121.   Gastric resection. Division of highly vascular band-like adhesions between a partially perforated gastric ulcer and the pancreas.

structure is found the middle colic artery whose ligation results in necrosis of the transverse colon. If it is impossible to preserve the middle colic artery, resection of the transverse colon is inevitable. In case of invasion of this region by carcinoma, the transverse colon and its mesentery are nevertheless the places in which a radical operation, in spite of initial difficulties, offers the greatest hope of success.

If in the course of a gastric resection, the resection of the transverse mesocolon, including the middle colic artery, and the resection of the transverse colon appear to be necessary, the division of the transverse colon is carried out as early as possible, since the approach to the stomach is thereby facilitated. I always use the Petz instrument for the primary closure of the transverse colon (Fig. 122). The two limbs of the colon remaining in the

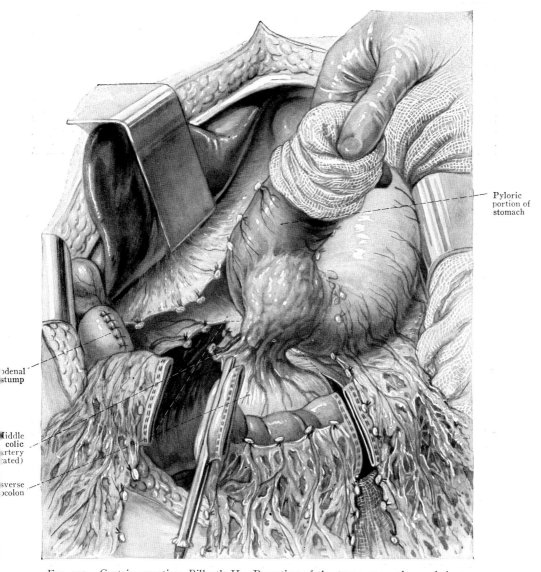

Pyloric
portion of
stomach

odenal
stump

Middle
colic
artery
(ated)

sverse
ocolon

FIG. 122. Gastric resection, Billroth II. Resection of the transverse colon and the transverse mesocolon because of gastric carcinoma which has invaded the mesocolon. The first portion of the duodenum has been divided, the distal duodenal stump has been closed, the proximal stump together with the stomach is being retracted upward and to the left. The transverse colon has been divided at two points with the aid of the Petz suture instrument. The right side of the mesocolon has been divided after ligation of the middle colic artery; the left side has been partly divided, the intended line of division being indicated by the dotted line.

body are for the moment reflected to right and left and are anastomosed at the end of the operation, after their viability has been determined. The lumen is reconstructed as a rule by end-to-end anastomosis, more rarely by lateral anastomosis, and only in case of lack of material by anastomosing the most distal loop of ileum to the descending colon or sigmoid.

The portion of the transverse mesocolon together with the attached portion of the great omentum, is excised in a wedge-shaped piece, with ligation of its vessels, and without separation of any existing connection with the stomach, so that a piece of the colon and of the mesocolon remain attached to the stomach (Fig. 122). At the end of the operation the slit in the transverse mesocolon, through which the gastro-enterostomy is drawn in gastric resections of the Billroth II type, is sutured on the gastric side of the anastomosis.

Palliative Resection of the Stomach (Finsterer, Madlener). The term palliative resection implies a resection in which as large a segment as possible of the prepyloric portion of the stomach (about two thirds of the whole stomach) is removed, including the pylorus if possible, while the ulcer-bearing segment if it is in the duodenum remains. Usually the lesion is a

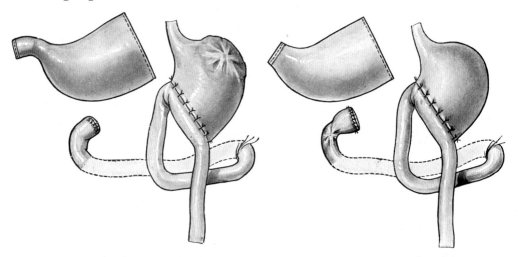

FIG. 123. Palliative resection of the stomach for an irremovable duodenal ulcer (Finsterer). Diagrammatic.

FIG. 124. Palliative resection of the stomach for an irremovable ulcer in the fundus of the stomach (Madlener). Diagrammatic.

benign ulcer. If the ulcer is located in the pyloric region or more especially in the duodenum, the gastric resection and reconstruction are always carried out according to the Billroth II principle because the lesion is thereby short-circuited on one side (Fig. 123). If the lesion is located in the fundus, the resection may be done according to the Billroth II principle (Fig. 124), or it may also be done according to the Billroth I method. The underlying principle of palliative resection is the extensive removal of the pyloric glands, because as I have already stated the production of hydrochloric acid by the fundus glands is supposedly materially diminished by the removal of the pylorus and the pyloric antrum. The permanent diminution of the production of hydrochloric acid is believed to assist in the healing of the ulcer that must be left in the body. In addition an attempt is made to protect mechanically the ulcerated area by diverting the food current from the lesion or by increasing the speed of emptying of the stomach.

When it is impossible to mobilize the pyloric portion of the stomach in the region of an ulcer because of inseparable adhesions with the surroundings, or when the ulcer is located so far down in the duodenum that a dependable closure of the distal duodenal stump no longer seems possible, then a palliative resection is of course indicated (Fig. 123). This operation may be the one originally planned, or it may be decided upon at any time in the course of the resection, that is to say, further mobilization is stopped, the removal of the lesion is dispensed with, the stomach is divided above the ulcer in the region of the duodenum or stomach, the distal opening is closed and the cardiac portion, reduced in size as far as possible, is treated according to the Billroth II principle (Finsterer). Since considerable material is necessary for the invagination of the prepyloric gastric segment if the distal transsection is done at that level, the division of this region must be made at a distance of at least 4 to 5 cm. from the pylorus. Otherwise, one may get into a most uncomfortable situation if it is impossible properly to invaginate the prepyloric stump. To escape this dilemma either the gastric stump may be made smaller and more pliable by excising its mucosa, or the insecurely covered stump may be reinforced with omentum. To conserve material, the application of the Albert suture in the closure of the pyloric segment of the stomach had better be undertaken by hand than with the Petz suture apparatus.

If an ulcer which can no lcnger be removed radically is situated in the cardiac or fundic portion of the stomach, and if it is to be treated by a palliative resection (Madlener), it will be advantageous to carry out the palliative resection in the direction duodenum-cardia with inclusion of the pylorus. The anastomosis between stomach and jejunum is then made distal to the lesion which has been left in the body.

In view of the fact that the purpose of a palliative resection of the stomach is primarily to short-circuit the secreting mucosa of the pyloric antrum, Drüner transsects the stomach, anastomoses the proximal segment with the proximal loop of jejunum and leaves the pyloric segment in the body but removes its mucosa. In closing this pyloric portion which has been denuded of its mucosa, it should be invaginated as far as possible in order to favor the formation of a firm fibrotic pyloric stump.

3. RESECTION OF THE STOMACH ACCORDING TO THE BILLROTH I PRINCIPLE (1881)

The reconstruction of the normal passageway from stomach to duodenum after a gastric resection is contingent upon whether the remaining portion of the stomach and the beginning of the duodenum can be anastomosed without tension. This may often be assured by thrift in the resection and adequate mobilization of the two gastro-intestinal segments.

In the anastomosis between stomach and duodenum there are several possible procedures. The gastric and duodenal openings may be joined end-to-end in their entirety (Haberer, Fig. 125); only a part of the gastric opening may be joined to the duodenal opening (Fig. 126, original Billroth I); the duodenal opening may be implanted into the side of the closed gastric stump by a side-to-end anastomosis (Kocher, Fig. 127), or the gastric opening may be implanted into the side of the duodenum by an end-to-side anastomosis (Haberer, Fig. 134).

If possible the stomach and duodenum are closed by clamps during the anastomosis. Often, however, this may not be possible because of lack of material, at least in the duodenal stump. In such cases one or two sponges attached to a long thread are placed in the lumen of each segment. The sponges are removed just before the completion of the anterior Albert suture.

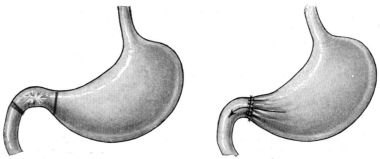

FIG. 125. Gastric resection, Billroth I. Diagrammatic. End-to-end anastomosis of the whole cross section of the stomach to the cross section of the duodenum (Haberer).

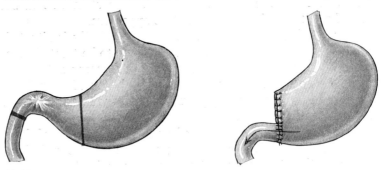

FIG. 126. Gastric resection, Billroth I. Diagrammatic. Partial closure of the gastric cross section, end-to-end anastomosis between the duodenum and the remainder of the gastric cross section (Billroth).

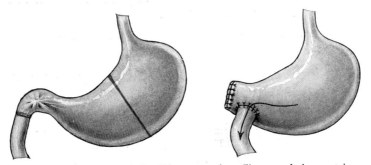

FIG. 127. Gastric resection, Billroth I. Diagrammatic. Closure of the gastric cross section and implantation of the duodenal cross section into the wall of the stomach (Kocher).

The anastomosis between the stomach and the duodenum is most conveniently performed if, after division of the duodenum, the stomach is retracted upward and to the left so that the duodenal opening may be opposed to the intended line of resection on the posterior surface of the stomach (Fig. 128).

The mobilization of the segment of stomach and duodenum to be resected and the division of the duodenum when the operation is to be completed by the Billroth I method are carried out in the same manner already described and illustrated under resection and reconstruction by the Billroth II method. It is therefore unnecessary to describe the technique again at this point.

End-to-end anastomosis between the gastric and duodenal transsection openings (Fig. 125). This procedure presupposes a relative equality in size of the two openings. However, by puckering the stomach, considerable differences in size can be equalized.

After the duodenum has been divided with or without the aid of the Petz instrument, its distal opening is provided with three traction sutures, one each at its upper and lower corners and one joining the midpoints of both sides, and with the aid of these is drawn toward the right. The posterior Lembert sutures may now be placed between the posterior surface of the stomach and the posterior wall of the duodenum at a distance of 1 cm. from the cut edge of the latter. The stomach is opened on its posterior surface at a distance of ½ cm. from the line of suture. The margin of the gastric wound and the posterior margin of the duodenal wound are united by interrupted sutures which pass through serosa, muscularis and mucosa. The anterior wall of the stomach is then divided. Its wound-edge is joined to that of the anterior duodenal wall in the same manner, and over this the anterior Lembert sutures are applied. It is not advisable to protect the suture line by a circular layer of omentum, because shrinking of the omentum may result in stenosis of the lumen.

If it is impossible to anastomose the duodenal opening to the posterior wall of the stomach before the gastric segment to be resected is detached, the stomach is divided and the duodenal and gastric openings are joined end-to-end in the routine manner.

If there is an unusually great disproportion in the size of the gastric and duodenal openings, and if nevertheless an end-to-end anastomosis is preferable, the gastric opening may be made smaller by terminal suture in the neighborhood of the lesser curvature, and the duodenal opening implanted into the residual opening at the greater curvature (original Billroth I, Fig. 126). The procedure is described in the following paragraph.

The duodenum is divided and its distal end provided with three traction sutures as previously described. Its posterior wall is apposed to the posterior wall of the stomach which has been elevated and reflected toward the left. A clamp is applied to the stomach above the intended line of suture. The duodenum is attached to the posterior wall of the stomach with interrupted seromuscular sutures from the greater curvature as far toward the lesser curvature as the duodenal opening permits under slight tension (Fig. 128). After a clamp has been applied to the stomach just below the line of resection, the stomach is completely divided about half a centimeter below the line of suture and the divided portion is removed. The gastric opening is closed from the lesser curvature to the beginning of the attachment of the duodenum with a continuous three-layer suture of catgut and then with interrupted Lembert sutures of linen or silk (Fig. 129). The remainder of the gastric opening is anastomosed to the duodenum in the usual manner. The point at which the angle of the duodenum nearest the lesser curvature meets the line of closure of the stomach is a decidedly weak point in the suture line. Billroth himself called it "calamity corner." This point is reinforced with a triangular sero-muscular suture which grasps the adjacent anterior and posterior walls of the stomach and the wall of the duodenum.

In end-to-side anastomosis (Fig. 134), the duodenum is divided and its distal end is closed and reinforced with a row of Lembert sutures. If possible,

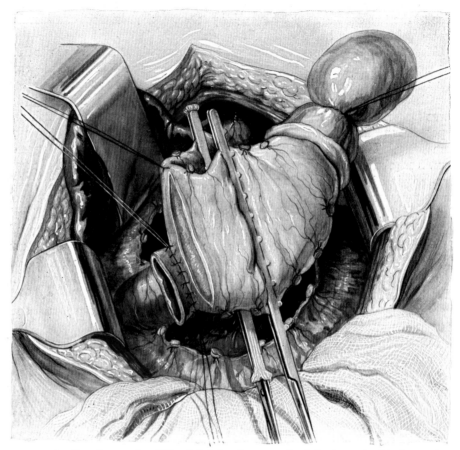

FIG. 128. Gastric resection, Billroth I (1). Anastomosis of the stomach with the duodenum according to the original method of Billroth. After adequate mobilization the gastroduodenal segment has been divided in the region of the upper duodenum; the proximal stump has been inclosed in a rubber condom and reflected upward over the left costal margin. The proximal and distal portions of the stomach have been closed with gastric clamps. The posterior wall of the distal duodenal stump has been joined to the posterior wall of the stomach by means of posterior Lembert sutures, the apposition of the duodenum beginning at the greater curvature and extending about to the middle of the stomach. The serosa of the posterior wall of the stomach has been incised.

division of the stomach is postponed temporarily, and the stomach is elevated and reflected toward the left. The anterior wall of the duodenum is attached by means of Lembert sutures to the posterior wall of the stomach beside the intended line of resection. The subsequent opening of the stomach and duodenum and the completion of the anastomosis follow the customary procedure.

The technique of side-to-end gastroduodenostomy (Fig. 127) is obvious in the light of the preceding discussion. The duodenum and the stomach are divided at the points decided upon for the resection. The gastric opening is closed in the usual manner. The duodenal opening is implanted into the stomach at the side of the gastric stump.

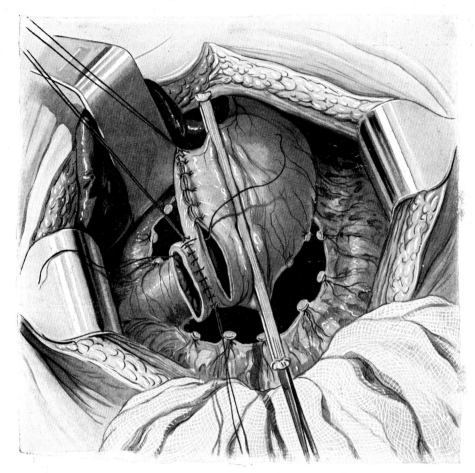

Fig. 129. Gastric resection, Billroth I (2). Anastomosis of stomach and duodenum according to the original method of Billroth. The stomach has been completely divided. The portion of its cross section adjacent to the lesser curvature not required for the anastomosis with the duodenum has been closed with three-layer sutures. The posterior Lembert sutures are in place and the first suture of the posterior three-layer suture row has been applied between the duodenum and the gastric wall.

4. Tube or Staircase Resection of the Stomach

(a) **The Mobilization of Stomach and Duodenum and the Division of the Duodenum.** Tube resection, in which a materially larger portion of the lesser curvature is removed than of the greater, may be performed and then reconstructed according to the Billroth I, as well as according to the Billroth II method. It makes possible the radical removal of a lesion on the lesser curvature close to the cardia without at the same time causing any difficulty through lack of material in anastomosing the remaining portion of the stomach with the jejunum or even with the duodenum. It is applicable when the lesion extends much farther toward the cardia along the lesser curvature than along the greater curvature. On the other hand, I do not consider the prophylactic resection of the lesser curvature indicated in the sense of removing this portion of the stomach because of its tendency to ulceration.

The mobilization of the stomach takes place in the manner previously described, but the blood vessels on the greater curvature are ligated only as far as the point of the intended resection, while the mobilization of the

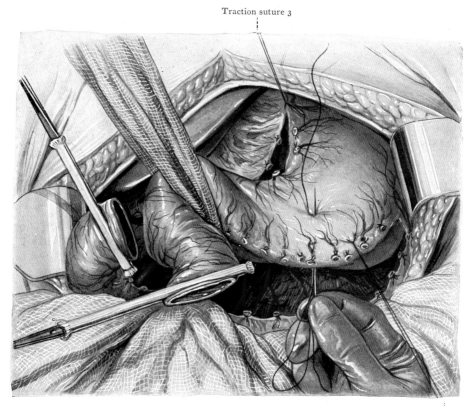

Traction suture 3

Traction suture 1

FIG. 130. Tubular resection of the stomach (1). Application of three traction sutures. The stomach, adequately mobilized, has been divided from the duodenum. The beginning and the end of the intended line of resection are established by traction sutures 1 and 3 at the greater and the lesser curvature. The third important point, the one at which the line of resection deviates at a right angle from the transverse to the long axis, is fixed in the following way: A straight needle carrying a thread is passed through the anterior and posterior walls and back again through both walls and the thread (traction suture 2) tied on the anterior wall.

lesser curvature is carried as far toward the cardia as possible, usually to the right border of the esophagus.

(b) **The Formation of the Gastric Tube.** The duodenum is first divided, preferably after closure with the Petz instrument. If gastro-intestinal continuity is to be re-established by the Billroth I principle in the form of an end-to-end anastomosis, the distal stump of the duodenum is laid aside for the moment. If an end-to-side anastomosis is planned, the distal stump of the duodenum is permanently closed with Lembert sutures.

The point at which the greater curvature is to be divided is provided with a traction suture (traction suture 1). At a point 4 or 5 cm. from this point, in a line toward the lesser curvature and perpendicular to the greater curvature, a suture is passed by means of a long straight needle from in front through the anterior and posterior walls of the stomach and then, at a point close by, is passed from behind forward through posterior and anterior walls of the stomach (Fig. 130) and tied (traction suture 2). This firmly unites the

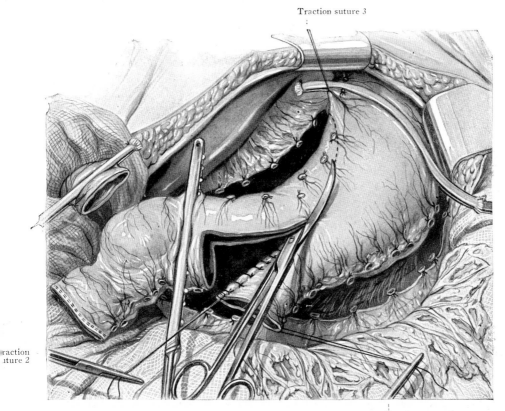

Traction suture 3

Traction suture 2

Traction suture 1

FIG. 131. Tubular resection of the stomach (2). The incision is being carried between the three traction sutures through both walls of the stomach simultaneously by means of a scissors: first from the greater curvature exactly perpendicular to the long axis of the stomach, then toward the cardia a few centimeters, parallel to the greater curvature and then diagonally to the lesser curvature to traction suture 3. The longitudinal incision is closed, bit by bit, by means of three-layer interrupted sutures.

anterior and posterior walls at this point, and fixes the length of the gastric opening which is later to be anastomosed to the intestine. A third traction suture is applied along the lesser curvature as close to the cardia as possible, so that the suture in the form of a Lembert stitch infolds the lesser curvature a little (traction suture 3, Figs. 130 and 131).

In many instances it is not practical to apply a clamp on the proximal side of the line of resection at the lesser curvature, whereas the part of the stomach to the pyloric side is easily clamped off from the line of resection (Fig. 131). It is usually possible, however, to guard against the escape of the contents of the proximal gastric segment. By the repeated application of several clamps the part of the stomach which is being opened and sutured at the moment can be blocked off.

While traction suture 1 (on the greater curvature) and traction suture 2 (which passes through the body of the stomach) are held taut, the anterior and posterior walls of the stomach are divided in a straight line just to the distal side of, and for the same distance as the line joining these traction

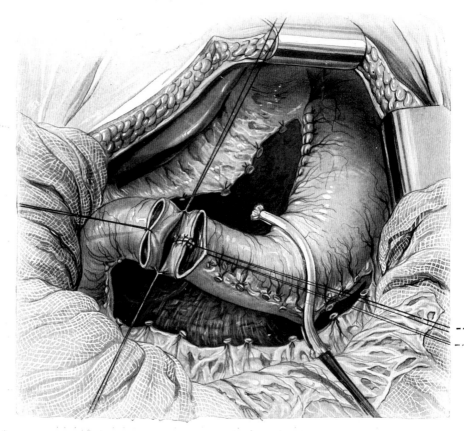

Substitute
traction
suture 2

Traction
suture 1

FIG. 132. Tubular resection of the stomach (3). End-to-end anastomosis of the gastric tube with the duodenum. The resection has been completed. The gastric tube now has the Lembert sutures in place so that a new lesser curvature has been made. The gastric contents are held back with a gastric clamp. The anastomosis with the small intestine is being carried out according to the Billroth I technique. The end sutures of the posterior Lembert suture have been applied, the stomach being rotated on its long axis in such a way that the newly formed lesser curvature comes to lie at the midpoint of the posterior line of the anastomosis.

sutures (Fig. 131). This is done in a single incision. This incision does not reach the lesser curvature but stops about half-way, in the long axis of the stomach. The incision is perpendicular to the greater curvature. The opened stomach is carefully emptied by suction and sponging.

Traction sutures 2 and 3 are now made taut. Both walls of the stomach are then incised a little distal to a line connecting traction sutures 2 and 3. The incision first runs exactly parallel to the greater curvature for a distance of about 4 cm., in order that this segment after being sutured will form a sort of sphincter, and then turns off diagonally, passing proximal to the lesion, toward the lesser curvature which it reaches at a point about 2 cm. to the pyloric side of traction suture 3. The incision from traction suture 2 to traction suture 3 is however not carried out in a single stroke, but is made in a series of small incisions 2 to 4 cm. long, and after each of these small cuts the two divided gastric walls are joined by interrupted three-layer catgut sutures. The gastric lumen is therefore open only temporarily and for a short dis-

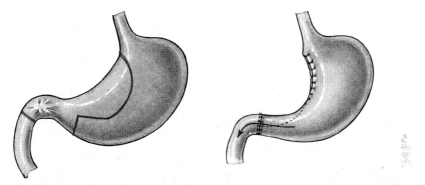

Fig. 133. Tubular resection of the stomach, Billroth I. End-to-end anastomosis of the openings. Diagrammatic.

tance. This opening can usually be shut off easily from the remainder of the stomach by means of clamps. The catgut suture which happens to be nearest the cardia is left long and together with traction suture 3 serves to hold and pull forward the still undivided portion of the stomach.

When the incision reaches the lesser curvature, the piece of stomach to be removed is free. After the closure of this last portion, the whole long line of resection will have been closed dependably with interrupted catgut sutures

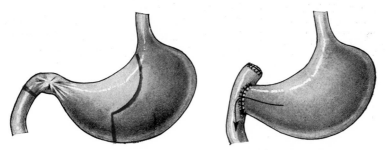

Fig. 134. Tubular resection of the stomach, Billroth I. End-to-side (Haberer) anastomosis of the stomach with the duodenum. Diagrammatic.

which include all three layers of the gastric wall, with the exception of the transverse portion of the incision between traction sutures 1 and 2.

The suture line forming the "new lesser curvature" is buried with interrupted Lembert sutures, during which process traction suture 3 renders valuable service in pulling forward the upper portion of the suture line, while traction suture 2 makes it taut. The last Lembert sutures at the distal end of the resultant gastric tube include as little of the gastric wall as possible so that the resultant nubbin at this point shall be small and cause a minimum of interference during the anastomosis of the transverse gastric opening with the intestine.

This completes the formation of the gastric tube. It possesses a terminal transverse opening about 3 cm. long, to which traction suture 1 is attached at the greater curvature, while the end of the last Lembert suture (substitute traction suture 2) has taken the place of traction suture 2. In most instances the gastric mucosa everts considerably from the small gastric opening. The protruding ring of mucosa may be excised.

(c) **The Anastomosis of the Gastric Tube with the Intestine.** The terminal opening of the gastric tube may be anastomosed either with the duodenum after the Billroth I principle or with the proximal jejunal loop

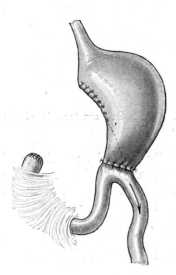

according to one of the Billroth II modifications. Even when the stomach has been divided rather far toward the cardia at the lesser curvature, the new gastric tube tends to be quite long and freely movable, so that one has a free hand in regard to location and type of its anastomosis with the intestine. (The vascular supply of the stomach is remarkably good even after this extensive ligation of the gastric blood vessels. I. S. R.)

Whichever type of anastomosis of the gastric tube with the intestine is selected, in every case the longitudinal gastric suture line, the "new lesser curvature," is joined to the middle of the posterior suture line of the anastomosis by rotating the greater curvature forward 90° from its position (Fig. 136). In the first place, this arrangement facilitates the performance of the suture, because the nubbin at the end of the longitudinal suture can be fitted more easily into the middle of the suture than at one end. In the second place, the new anterior position of the greater curvature of the reduced stomach corresponds to the physiologic position assumed by the stomach in case of marked filling.

FIG. 135. Tubular resection of the stomach, Billroth II. Anastomosis of the entire gastric cross section with the jejunum. Diagrammatic.

(1) Anastomosis of the gastric tube with the duodenum. An end-to-end anastomosis (Figs. 132 and 133) is carried out in the following manner:

The transverse opening of the gastric tube, which already possesses traction sutures at the greater (substitute suture 2) and at the new "lesser" curvature, is supplied with two additional traction sutures, one on each side midway between the other two (Fig. 137a). It now carries four traction sutures. The duodenal opening is provided with additional traction sutures, one at each end and, if necessary, a third midway between which grasps both wound edges. The traction sutures are turned outward and the two viscera are joined to each other by posterior interrupted Lembert sutures at a distance of ½ cm. from the cut edges. The end of the longitudinal gastric suture must be brought to lie in the middle of this suture line as previously stated (Figs. 136, 137a and b).

At this point the connecting Lembert suture grasps both folds of the longitudinal gastric suture and the intestine in a fold parallel to the cut surface
of the stomach (Fig. 137a). Then the posterior suture which includes the
entire thickness of the stomach and duodenum is applied with interrupted
catgut sutures. At the point where the longitudinal gastric suture is encountered, the Albert (three layer) suture is passed through both gastric walls
which form the nubbin at the end of the longitudinal gastric suture (Fig.

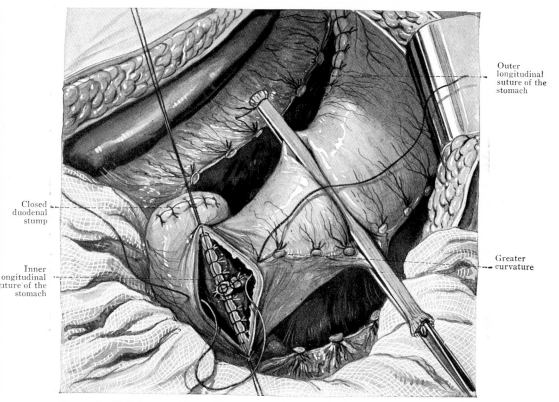

FIG. 136. Tubular resection of the stomach (4). (See Figure 131.) End-to-side anastomosis of the cross section of the gastric tube with the duodenum. The end of the distal limb
of the duodenum has been closed. The cross section of the gastric tube has been attached to
the duodenal stump in such a way that the newly formed lesser curvature lies at the midpoint
of the posterior suture line. The posterior Lembert suture, the opening of the duodenum and
the posterior Albert suture have been carried out in the order named. One suture was so applied
as to include both margins of the longitudinal gastric suture line and the duodenum. The
anterior Albert suture is being started at the midpoint.

137b). The anterior Albert sutures and the anterior Lembert sutures offer
no difficulties.

Anastomosis of the gastric tube with the duodenum end-to-side (Fig.
134). The distal stump of the duodenum which has been closed preferably
with Petz clips is inverted by a row of Lembert sutures. The open end of the
gastric tube, previously provided with 4 traction sutures as above described,
is brought in contact with the distal limb of the duodenum in its long axis in
such a way that the longitudinal suture line of the stomach lies at the midpoint of the posterior line of contact. The two structures are joined in this

position by a posterior row of interrupted Lembert sutures, in which both sides of the longitudinal gastric suture are grasped as above described. The duodenum is opened at a proper distance from this line of suture and in a proper length (Fig. 136) and the anastomosis is then completed in the usual manner.

(2) End-to-Side Anastomosis of the Gastric Tube with the Proximal Loop of Jejunum (Figs. 135, 137a and b). The anastomosis between

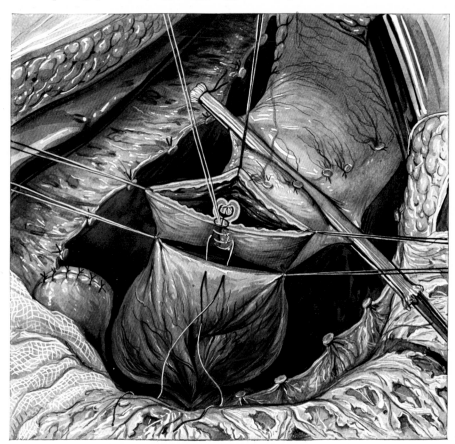

FIG. 137a.   Tubular resection of the stomach (5).   (See Figure 131.)   End-to-side anastomosis of the cross section of the gastric tube with the jejunal loop.   The jejunal loop has been pulled through a slit in the transverse mesocolon into the upper abdomen and apposed to the cross section of the gastric tube in such a way that the newly formed lesser curvature lies at the midpoint of the posterior line of suture.   The two traction sutures at the ends of the posterior Lembert suture line have been applied and the middle one of this line of sutures is just being applied.   It includes both sides of the longitudinal suture line of the stomach and grasps a horizontal fold of the intestinal wall.

the end of the gastric tube and the proximal jejunal loop can be carried out in a similar manner. After the closure of the duodenum, the jejunal loop is brought into the upper abdomen through a slit in the transverse mesocolon (in case this was not done before beginning the gastric resection) and its long axis is approximated to the gastric opening. Here, too, the nubbin on the new lesser curvature is placed at the midpoint of the line of anastomosis. The gastrojejunostomy is then performed in a manner that is quite the same in its details as the gastroduodenostomy just described. Finally, the anastomosis is drawn down into the lower abdomen and the stomach is fastened by a few sutures to the edges of the slit in the mesocolon at the point where it passes through that structure.

Invagination of the Duodenal Stump into the Gastric Tube (Goepel). In an effort to increase the security of the anastomosis of the stomach with the end of the duodenum in a "stair case" or "tube" resection according to the Billroth I principle, Goepel forms a cuff at the new end of the stomach, about 4 cm. long and denuded of mucosa. The duodenum is inserted into this cuff with a broad apposition of surfaces. He proceeds in the following manner.

After extensive mobilizing of the stomach and duodenum, the upper line of division of the stomach is at first carried only through the serosa and

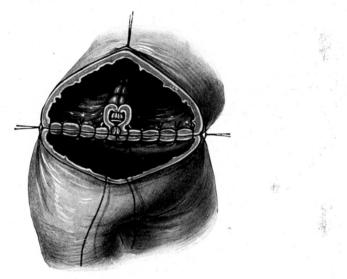

Fig. 137b. Tubular resection of the stomach (6). End-to-side anastomosis of the stomach with the highest jejunal loop. After opening the loop of intestine, the posterior Albert three-layer suture has been applied. The middle suture of this row passes transversely through the ridge of the longitudinal suture line of the stomach.

muscularis. From this point upward the sero-muscular layers are freed from the mucosa for a distance of 4 cm. toward the cardia. Here the mucosa is divided, beginning at the greater curvature and extending toward the lesser curvature for a distance equal to the size of the duodenal stump. The bridge of gastric tissue remaining at the lesser curvature is divided through all its layers diagonally toward the cardia. The pyloric portion of the divided stomach is reflected to the right and the posterior surface of the duodenum which is thereby exposed is sutured to the posterior margin of the sero-muscular incision (Fig. 138). Four centimeters above this suture line the duodenum is divided. All layers of the duodenum are sutured to the cut edge of the gastric mucosa, first in the region of the posterior, then of the anterior wall. Finally the anterior sero-muscular flap is attached by sutures applied at its edges to the anterior wall of the duodenum. The diagonal opening in the stomach extending along the lesser curvature toward the cardia is closed in the usual manner with two rows of sutures.

Since the permanence of a gastro-enterostomy depends primarily on the apposition of broad serous surfaces, it is not to be assumed that the security of the anastomosis is increased by the "cuff" procedure of Goepel. A disadvantage of the procedure is that one of the two apposed surfaces of viscera

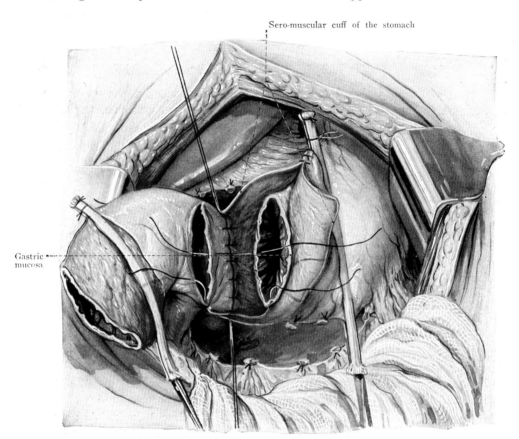

Sero-muscular cuff of the stomach

Gastric mucosa

FIG. 138. "Cuff" procedure (Goepel). A sero-muscular cuff denuded of mucosa has been formed at the distal end of the transsected stomach. The posterior wall of the duodenum has been joined to the posterior margin of this cuff by interrupted sutures. The posterior wall of the duodenum has been incised and the distal margin of the duodenal limb is being joined to the posterior margin of the gastric mucosa by interrupted sutures.

is a fresh wound surface on which complete hemostasis cannot be assured. Therefore hemorrhage can separate the two surfaces which are supposed to adhere to each other, whereas in the apposition of two uninjured serous surfaces their separation by any accumulation of fluid is practically impossible. I do not recommend the "cuff" procedure because I believe it violates fundamental surgical principles.

The late results of "tube" resection, from the standpoint of motor function, are particularly good and are not excelled by those of any other type of resection. The circular muscle of the tube tends to heal so completely that in a few months according to our Roentgen-ray studies it forms a good substitute for the resected pylorus, regulating the escape of the gastric contents by its rhythmic contractions in an excellent manner.

5. RESECTION OF THE CARDIA (RESECTIO CARDIAE, VOELKER) AND RESECTION OF THE WHOLE STOMACH (EXTIRPATIO VENTRICULI TOTALIS, SCHLATTER)

The chief difficulties in extirpation of the whole stomach and in resection of the cardia occur at the same point and consist in establishing a reliable

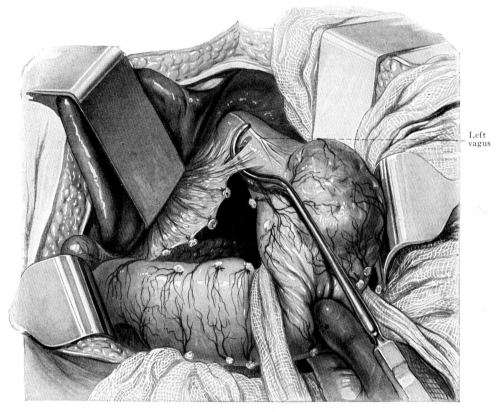

Left vagus

FIG. 139. Total resection of the stomach, freeing of the cardia (1). A gauze roll has been passed around the stomach. The ligation and division of the gastrohepatic omentum proceed in the direction of the esophagus which is gradually freed from the diaphragm. The left vagus nerve is visible through the peritoneum on the anterior surface of the esophagus.

anastomosis between the esophagus and the intestinal segment, difficulties which are occasioned by the inaccessible position of the end of the esophagus and the inferior quality of its wall. A better exposure of the esophagus can sometimes be obtained by the removal of the ensiform process or even by the reflection of the left costal margin. In obese patients with a high-lying diaphragm and protruding intestines it may be practically impossible to perform a satisfactory anastomosis, so that in particularly unfavorable cases the operation should not be attempted. It is of some advantage that the esophagus, as a result of peristaltic action incident to the stenosis at the cardia, or as a result of traction incident to the shrinking of the stomach, is frequently found to extend an appreciable distance into the abdominal cavity and is therefore more easily accessible.

After complete extirpation of the stomach the esophagus is joined to the duodenum or to the proximal jejunal loop. In case the lesion is restricted to the cardia or to the upper half of the stomach, there is no material difference in the technical difficulties, whether one decides upon a resection of the whole stomach or only of the cardia. I base my decision upon whether the remaining

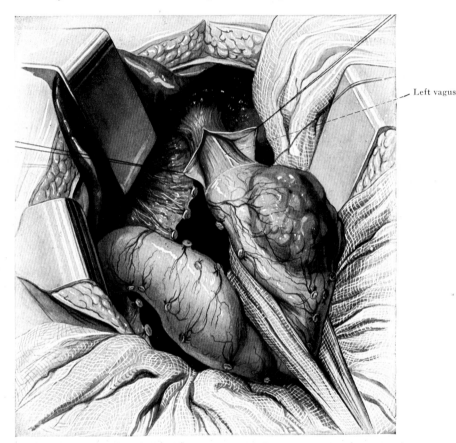

Left vagus

FIG. 140. Total resection of the stomach (2). The stomach which has been adequately freed is being drawn forward by means of a gauze roll passed around it. The serous covering of the diaphragm has been split, picked up by traction sutures and is being dissected free so that the musculature of the esophagus and the left vagus nerve come into view.

pyloric portion of the stomach, or the duodenum, or the proximal jejunal loop can be anastomosed with the esophagus more conveniently. In such cases I have almost always decided in favor of a complete resection of the stomach with an esophagojejunostomy, and I have operated upon a number of cases in this manner with complete success.

After it has been decided that it is technically possible radically to remove the tumor, the midline incision is extended to the left of the ensiform process as far as the costal margin and, under certain circumstances, may be further enlarged by removal of the ensiform, by a transverse incision through the left rectus and by a reflection of the left costal margin. The mobilization of the cardia is the first step, since the whole operation hinges on this point. While the stomach is drawn downward, the gastrohepatic omentum is divided between ligatures at its fan-shaped attachment in the usual way, working closer and closer to the esophagus (Fig. 139). Care is necessary so as not to

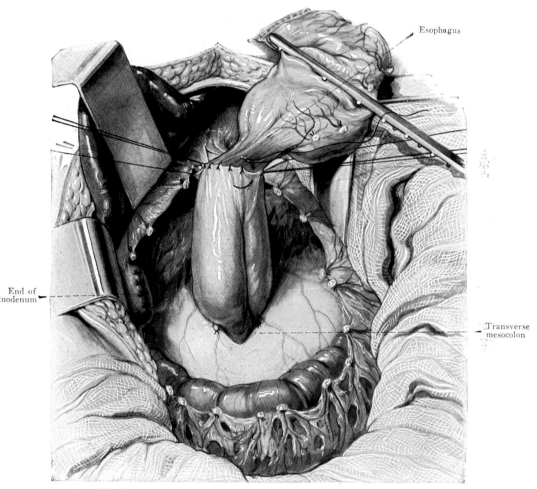

FIG. 141. Total resection of the stomach (3). The duodenum has been divided with the aid of the Petz suture instrument and the distal end closed by Lembert sutures. The stomach is being drawn forcibly upward over the left costal margin. The highest jejunal loop has been brought up through a slit in the transverse mesocolon and is being joined by posterior interrupted Lembert sutures to the posterior wall of the esophagus which has been freed from the diaphragm and drawn forward.

injure the right border of the esophagus by including it in a mass ligature. Its right border is as a rule hard to recognize in the gastrohepatic omentum which becomes thicker and thicker toward the cardia. As a result of the lowered position of the stomach, the esophagus often extends farther down and to the right than is expected. The greater curvature is freed in the same way. Since the fundus of the stomach lies higher than the cardia, the ligation of the vessels must go considerably higher than the level of the esophageal attachment. As soon as the fundus has been completely freed, a great deal more room is available and the stomach together with the esophagus can be pulled down a considerable distance. A rubber tube or a gauze roll is passed around the esophagus or upper portion of the stomach as soon as possible, by which the lower esophagus may conveniently be drawn forward (Fig. 139).

The next step is the freeing of the esophagus from the diaphragmatic foramen and the lowest portion of the posterior mediastinum. An incision in the form of an inverted T is made through the peritoneal covering on the anterior surface of the esophagus and the tips of the two peritoneal flaps are pushed upward with a sponge (Fig. 140). As soon as the proper level is reached, the esophagus can be freed by blunt dissection for a considerable distance from the esophageal foramen and can be pulled downward. By proceeding cautiously it is usually possible to avoid opening the two pleural cavities which extend down this far and have extremely delicate walls. A positive pressure apparatus should be set up ready for use in case the pleura is opened. As the esophagus is drawn down, the vagus nerves appear quite clearly as firm slender cords, the left vagus on the anterior wall and the right vagus on the posterior wall. Unless one is using spinal anaesthesia with local tissue infiltration as routinely employed by me in these cases, they are blocked by an injection of a 1-per cent solution of novocaine and divided, as a result of which the esophagus again moves down an appreciable distance. Although an extensive mobilization of the esophagus is very convenient for the subsequent suture, one must be conservative in this, because an excessively mobilized esophageal stump may easily become necrotic. (This is due to the very poor blood supply which even the normal esophagus possesses. I. S. R.) This invariably leads to a leak in the suture line and to peritonitis. The freed segment of the esophagus must not be longer than 5 cm.

After the esophagus has been mobilized to the extent determined by the lesion and necessary for suture, the mobilization of the stomach is continued toward the pylorus, either to the point in the stomach at which the resection is to be made or on into the duodenum. The division of the stomach or duodenum is conveniently performed with the Petz instrument.

The distal opening, whether in the stomach or the duodenum, is closed by terminal suture. When the esophagus is to be joined to the remaining portion of the stomach, the anastomosis is never made to the terminal opening in the stomach but always to a new lateral opening in the anterior wall of the stomach. Since I routinely perform a resection that extends into the duodenum, I prefer to join the esophagus to the proximal jejunal loop rather than to the duodenum.

If the accessibility of the operative field permits, the diseased segment of the stomach is left attached to the esophagus during the placing of the posterior sutures of the anastomosis between the esophagus and intestine, because it affords an excellent hold to prevent the retraction of the esophagus during suture (Fig. 141). If possible, a curved clamp whose arms are covered with gauze or soft rubber is applied to the esophagus just above the point of anastomosis. This prevents the escape of esophageal contents, and, if the diseased portion of the stomach because of lack of room must be separated from the esophagus before applying the posterior sutures, the clamp at the same time prevents retraction of the esophagus. (The clamp must however not make too much pressure on the esophagus because of the danger of subsequent necrosis. I. S. R.)

The stomach, if it remains attached to the esophagus but has been divided below, is pulled diagonally upward over the left costal margin. This

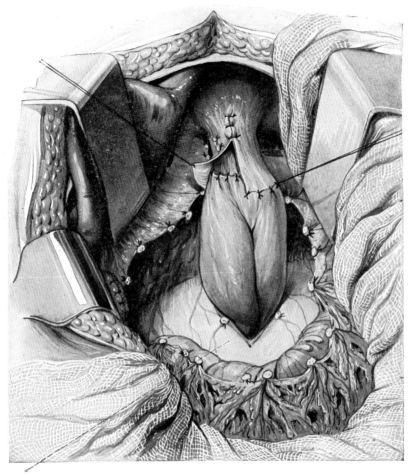

Transverse
mesocolon

FIG. 142. Total resection of the stomach (4). The anastomosis between the esophagus and the jejunal loop has been completed. The flaps of the freed peritoneal covering of the esophagus are being sewed over the esophagojejunostomy to reinforce the suture line.

pulls the posterior wall of the esophagus forward and makes it accessible. The anterior wall of the closed pyloric portion of the stomach, the duodenum or jejunum which can be pulled up farthest through a slit in the transverse mesocolon is placed against the posterior wall of the esophagus and attached to it by interrupted Lembert sutures of linen. These sutures are applied closely and with extreme care (Fig. 141). In order to avoid nutritional disturbances of the esophageal stump, it is advisable to place the sutures through

the esophagus perpendicular, not parallel, to the line of division. The difficulties which are frequently encountered in this suture can at times be lessened by using the "embroidery" stitch described on page 80, and illustrated
in Fig. 66. After the completion of the Lembert suture, the esophagus and
the viscus to be used for the anastomosis are opened at a distance of about 1
cm. from the suture line. The succeeding posterior Albert (three layer)
suture is also applied carefully and closely with interrupted linen sutures.
The anterior wall of the esophagus is now divided, detaching the diseased
gastric segment, and the anastomosis is completed in the usual way with
interrupted anterior Albert and anterior Lembert sutures.

Even if it is technically possible to connect the esophagus directly with
the duodenum, I see no advantage therein, and even in such a case I prefer to
anastomose the esophagus with the proximal loop of jejunum.

I do not concur in the recommendation that in excising the stomach a
portion of it be left attached to the esophagus on the ground that the anastomosis is thereby made easier and more dependable. On the contrary, I have
always had great difficulty in the subsequent anastomosis when I tried this
method.

I must also advise strongly against the use of a Murphy button, since it
is quite impossible in the depth of the wound to get a proper grip for a
dependable joining of the button halves and because the surface of the
esophagus does not possess the peritoneal covering which is indispensable for
a button anastomosis. Nor do other buttons specially devised for resection of
the esophagus seem to have any advantages.

The two peritoneal flaps which were formed from the anterior wall of
the esophagus as above described are sutured together in front of the anastomosis. This forms a peritoneal barrier between the intrathoracic portion
of the esophageal bed and the abdominal cavity (Fig. 142).

In order to relieve the tension on the anastomosis and to keep it immo-
bilized, the viscus which was joined to the esophagus is attached to the diaphragm with a few sutures. The paralysis of the left half of the diaphragm
by phrenic exeresis or better by freezing the nerve, as has been recommended,
is unnecessary. It is however advised in order to relieve any strain on
the anastomosis that a temporary jejunostomy be made so as to feed the
patient through it promptly and freely.

Drainage of the abdominal cavity is not advised, unless the anastomosis
is so insecure that it seems doomed from the start to give way.

6. Transverse Resection of the Stomach (Riedel, Payr). Treatment of Hour-glass Stomach

If a lesion lies in the mid portion of the stomach, while the fundus and
the pyloric portion are normal, it has been suggested that the central diseased
band of stomach be removed and the cardial and pyloric segments reunited by a
circular end-to-end suture. In my experience and according to the opinion of
others, however, this operation almost without exception leads to unsatisfactory anatomic and functional results, because an hour-glass stomach usually
develops in the region of the suture line by shrinkage, scar tissue contraction,
kinking and adhesions, with the resultant disturbances of emptying. I have

therefore eliminated transverse resection from my surgical repertoire.   This
is also true in the treatment of hour-glass stomach as well, a condition in
which transverse resection seems particularly alluring.

The technique of transverse resection is simple and follows clearly defined principles (Fig. 143).   The midgastric girdle to be resected is freed
from its vessels in the region of the greater and lesser curvatures.   The seg-

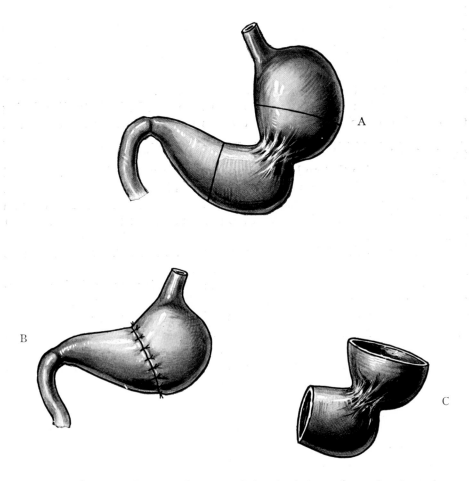

Fig. 143.   Operation for hour-glass stomach by circular resection and end-to-end anastomosis.   Diagrammatic.   (a) Hour-glass stomach before operation.   (b) Residual stomach
after operation.   (c) Resected portion.

ment is squeezed as empty as possible and is then blocked off on both sides
of the constriction by means of clamps.   If room permits, the segment to be
resected is also closed beside the lines of incision by clamps.   The closure of
the area to be resected is made even more simple by the use of the Petz suture
instrument.   In that case the incisions are made between the two rows of
clips, so that each end of the resected gastric girdle and of the remaining parts
of the stomach are closed with rows of clips.

The anastomosis of the remaining gastric segments is most conveniently

performed if the stomach is divided at first only on the pyloric side, while the
cardial portion together with the attached diseased segment is turned upward
over the left costal border. The cut edge of the pyloric segment is provided
with three traction sutures, of which two are applied at the ends and the
third through both wound edges at their midpoint. The posterior wall of the
pyloric portion is attached a centimeter from the cut edge to the posterior
wall of the cardial segment at the level of the intended line of resection by a
posterior row of interrupted Lembert sutures. The posterior wall of the cardial segment is opened at a distance of 1 cm. from the suture line. There
follows a posterior Albert continuous catgut suture. The anterior wall of
the cardial segment is then divided, freeing the diseased middle segment. The
anterior walls of the cardial and pyloric segments are then joined by a continuous Albert and by interrupted Lembert sutures.

If both gastric segments (or only one) were closed with Petz clips during
the resection, the closed margin or margins bearing the clips are excised in
the performance of the anastomosis. Finally, the slit in the gastrocolic omentum is closed.

The suggestion that an hour-glass stomach, a condition in which a normal
fundus is separated from a normal pyloric section by a pathologic constriction,
be treated by a transverse resection has been already dealt with. Nor does an
anastomosis between the fundic and the pyloric segment (gastrogastrostomy)
achieve the desired result of insuring an unhampered emptying of the stomach
in most cases, so that this procedure is also to be advised. Furthermore its
performance is often technically quite difficult.

If the stenosis between the two gastric pouches is very marked, a gastro-
enterostomy using the fundus of the stomach may give a good functional
result. However, it does not remove the lesion underlying the stenosis, which
in most cases is a scarred, indurated ulcer, frequently still in an active state.

By far the best results are obtained by the resection of the diseased segment and also of the pyloric portion of the stomach, including the pylorus.
The reconstruction of gastro-intestinal continuity from the fundus to the
intestine is usually performed according to the Billroth principles. The technique of such a resection in hour-glass stomach entails nothing unusual beyond
that required for gastric resection for other causes. The mobilization of the
stomach in the region of the lesser curvature may be particularly difficult, and
frequently there is only a very small remainder of stomach available for anastomosis to the jejunal loop. Occasionally, therefore, a total resection of the
stomach may be preferable.

7. Treatment of Postoperative Gastrojejunal Ulcer

Postoperative jejunal ulcer is a condition which I believe develops more
frequently after simple gastrojejunostomy than after gastric resection. After
gastric resection it is said to occur with about equal frequency whether the
reconstruction is carried out by the Billroth I or the Billroth II principle.
The unilateral exclusion of the pylorus, in the light of recent studies and contrary to former assumption, does not seem to involve any particular danger of
producing this lesion. In the development of relapsing ulcer a number of
factors are involved. One of the chief causes is obviously the hyperacidity

of the gastric juice, the direct action of which is usually not long withstood by the intestinal mucosa. Therefore the extensive removal of the diseased stomach appears to be the best means of guarding against the later development of an ulcer. (It has been shown however that even after fairly extensive resection of the stomach a high acid concentration may eventually return. I. S. R.)

The lesion, as a rule, steadily progresses, is not amenable to conservative measures, and nearly invariably requires operative treatment. By the time the patient comes under the care of the surgeon the ulcerative process is usually quite extensive, in that it has reached the peritoneal covering of the jejunum, has produced callous changes in the neighborhood, has invaded the stomach and frequently also the colon, and often enough has produced a gastrocolic fistula (Fig. 144). The operator is therefore confronted in most cases by difficult problems of technique and the mortality of the preferable radical operation is high.

The object of the radical operation consists in the removal of the ulcer-bearing segments of the gastrointestinal canal, which in many cases means a resection of the involved segment of the jejunum, of the stomach and often of the transverse colon (Figs. 145, 146 and 147). At the same time, measures must be taken to prevent the recurrence of an ulcer. This, in our opinion, is best effected by an extensive resection of the pyloric portion of the stomach. The operation, which naturally must be suited to the particular conditions met with in each

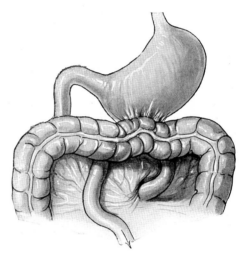

Fig. 144. Peptic (marginal) ulcer of the jejunum, with involvement of stomach and transverse colon. Diagrammatic.

case, is performed according to the following general outline. (The resection of a jejunal ulcer following a gastro-enterostomy will be described as a general type of procedure.)

After opening the abdomen, where difficulties may be encountered because of adhesions, the transverse colon is first inspected in case of a retrocolic anastomosis. If an antecolic anastomosis is present, the gastro-enterostomy is approached first, and the colon examined later. If the colon is involved in the ulcer, and if the ulcer is small, the colon is separated from the ulcer and the opening in the intestinal wall is closed with a double line of sutures. If in the case of a large ulcer this would entail an excessive constriction, the involved portion is adequately freed from its peritoneal attachments and is divided on both sides of the inflammatory lesion, the free ends are reflected to right and left, and the proximal and distal limbs are reunited just before completion of the operation (Fig. 149). The mesocolon is freed from the area of the lesion, or, if this is impossible, this portion of the mesocolon is divided after ligation of the vessels and is left attached to the lesion.

The site of the gastro-enterostomy, if retrocolic, now lies exposed in the slit of the mesocolon (Fig. 149). The distal and proximal jejunal loops are freed to the site of ulceration. It is only rarely possible to excise the ulcer from the jejunal loop in such a way that lateral suture will preserve the continuity of the intestine without producing a marked stenosis (Fig. 146). To let the jejunal ulcer remain in the hope that it may heal spontaneously because it

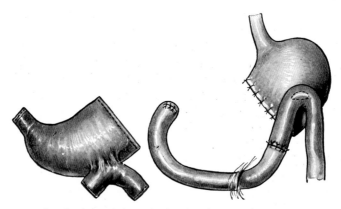

FIG. 145. Operation for jejunal (marginal) ulcer by resection and end-to-end anastomosis of the jejunum, and by extensive resection of the stomach with reconstruction of the gastro-intestinal continuity according to the Billroth II technique.

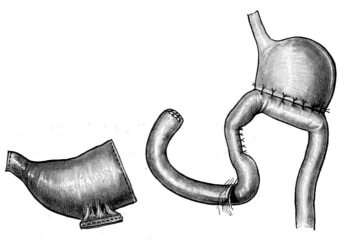

FIG. 146. Operation for jejunal (marginal) ulcer by lateral resection of the diseased jejunal wall, lateral closure of the jejunal opening and extensive resection of the stomach with reconstruction of gastro-intestinal continuity according to a modified Billroth II technique, with implantation of the entire gastric opening into the jejunal wall distal to the site of the former ulcer (Krönlein). Diagrammatic.

will be bathed only in pure duodenal juice after a Billroth II type of stomach resection is illogical and should never be adopted except in case of extreme emergency. In most instances both limbs of jejunum must be divided as close to the ulcer as possible, after ligating and dividing their mesentery (Figs. 145 and 147).

If the continuity of the jejunum was not interrupted during the mobilization, and the resultant opening was closed by lateral suture, then an anasto-

mosis of the Krönlein type is performed between the jejunal loop just beyond
the point of suture and the stomach, with resection of the pyloric portion of
the stomach (Fig. 146). If the two openings resulting from the transsection
of the jejunum can be joined end-to-end or in any other way, this anastomosis
is promptly performed and a gastrojejunostomy is made distal to this point
of suture. Frequently, however, the afferent jejunal loop is too short for this
purpose, usually because of the regrettable but wide-spread practice in gastrojejunostomy of using as short a jejunal loop as possible, so that its immediate
anastomosis to the distal loop offers difficulties which even the mobilization of
the proximal loop beyond the duodenojejunal juncture cannot correct. It is
then necessary to implant the opening of the proximal jejunal loop into the
distal limb end-to-side (Fig. 147).

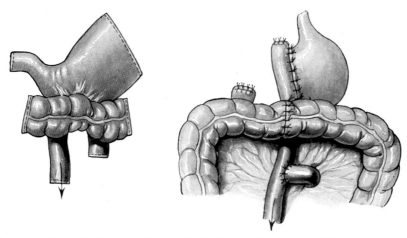

Fig. 147. Operation for jejunal (marginal) ulcer which has invaded the transverse colon
by resection and end-to-end anastomosis of the transverse colon, resection of the jejunum with
closure of its distal end and end-to-side implantation of its proximal end into the distal limb.
Extensive resection of the stomach with reconstruction of gastro-intestinal continuity according
to a modified Billroth II technique, with end-to-side implantation of the entire gastric opening
into the distal jejunal limb (Krönlein). Diagrammatic.

The stomach is freed in the neighborhood of the site of the ulcer or of the
anastomosis with the jejunum, and, insofar as this has not already been done,
the gastrocolic omentum is divided between double ligatures. Since the removal of the pyloric portion of the stomach is desirable in view of the danger
of the recurrence of an ulcer, the mobilization of the stomach is extended to
the lesser curvature and is continued beyond the pylorus to the first portion of
the duodenum (Fig. 148). The duodenum is divided and its distal segment
is closed and buried (Fig. 149), unless in an exceptional case reconstruction
according to the Billroth I principle is to be performed. One can, of course,
begin with the mobilization and division of the duodenum and continue the
mobilization in the direction of the gastro-enterostomy, aided by upward traction on the freed pyloric portion.

The freeing of the stomach is extended in the direction of the fundus
beyond the region of the ulcer as far as the intended point of resection. The
pyloric portion of the stomach, completely mobilized in this manner, is turned
up over the left costal margin.

If the continuity of the proximal jejunal loop was maintained or restored, then a retrocolic anastomosis is made between the fundus segment of the stomach and the proximal jejunal loop, and at a point distal to the former ulcer site, and the mobilized gastric segment is resected. The procedure is either in the form of gastric resection after Krönlein with utilization of the full width of the gastric cross section (Fig. 146), or after von Eiselsberg, using

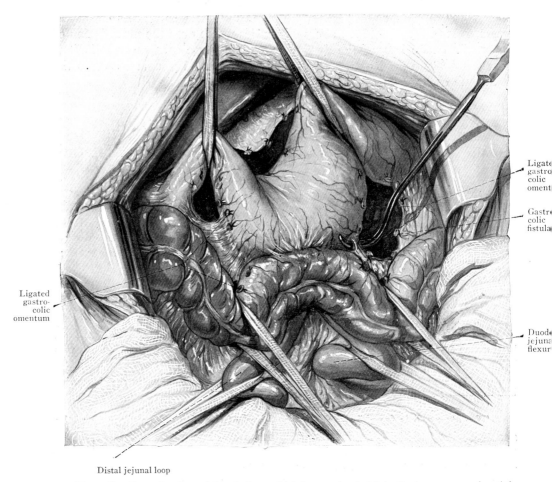

Ligated
gastro-
colic
omentum

Ligate
gastro
colic
oment

Gastr
colic
fistula

Duode
jejuna
flexur

Distal jejunal loop

FIG. 148. Operation for a jejunal ulcer which has perforated into the transverse colon (1). The affected segments of the transverse colon, stomach and jejunum have been mobilized on both sides of the lesion and each surrounded by a gauze roll. The involved portions of the transverse mesocolon are being picked up on an aneurysm needle and cut between ligatures.

the part of the gastric opening at the greater curvature after closure of the rest of the opening, or according to the original Billroth procedure with complete closure of the gastric transsection and a subsequent gastro-enterostomy at another point (Fig. 145). If after the jejunal resection the proximal jejunal limb was implanted into the distal limb, the unattached jejunal limb is anastomosed to the stomach, end-to-end or side-to-side (Fig. 147).

If the transverse colon was divided, its proximal and distal limbs are reunited end-to-end (Fig. 147) or side-to-side at the close of the operation.

The edge of the slit in the transverse mesocolon is sutured to the stomach around the new anastomosis. The abdomen is then closed without drainage.

If a resection appears to be impossible or too dangerous, the ulcer must be permitted to remain. In every instance, as in the case of primary gastric ulcer, one can make use of a temporary jejunostomy. If an irremovable secondary ulcer is located in the duodenum after a gastric resection and reconstruction according to the Billroth I method, a palliative resection of the stomach with gastrojejunostomy or infrapapillary gastroduodenostomy may be performed.

Case 1. Example of radical operation for jejunal ulcer with resection of the stomach, resection of the jejunum with a Roux Y-shaped anastomosis according to the Billroth II principle and resection of the transverse colon with end-to-end anastomosis.

H. P. I. A man of 40, in whom a posterior retrocolic gastro-enterostomy had been performed 3 years previously because of a prepyloric ulcer on the lesser curvature, suffered a return of symptoms 2 years later. Within the last few weeks particles of food appeared undigested in the stool a few minutes after they had been eaten. Fluoroscopy after an opaque meal disclosed a tender niche in the upper jejunum and the passage of gastric contents into the transverse colon, while after a barium enema the material passed from the transverse colon into the stomach.

Diagnosis: jejunal ulcer and gastrocolic fistula.

Operation. A midline incision was made above the umbilicus in the region of the old scar. Because of numerous adhesions it was at first impossible to enter the free peritoneal cavity. While the left side of the abdominal wall was forcibly elevated, the exposed layer of adhesions was partly separated by dissection from the abdominal wall and partly divided in small sections between ligatures. In this way the free peritoneal cavity was finally reached far to the side. With continued retraction of the left anterior abdominal wall, the surgeon passed the index finger around the midline adhesions, in which the omentum was extensively involved, and divided them between a series of ligatures. In this way there was gradually effected a complete separation of the anterior abdominal wall from the intestinal mass beneath. The same procedure was followed on the right side where the firm adhesions between the abdominal wall and the surface of the liver greatly impeded the exposure. The surface of the liver was torn in several places, resulting in troublesome bleeding and necessitating temporary packing and in several instances suture of the torn liver.

The exposed conglomerate tumor consisted of the stomach, the transverse colon, several jejunal loops and the greater omentum. The freeing of the transverse colon was undertaken first, the adhesions being picked up in small sections on an aneurysm needle and divided after double ligation. The transverse colon was followed on both sides to the point where it seemed inseparably adherent to the tumor mass. A rubber tube was then passed around the colon on each side by means of a forceps. By gentle traction on these tubes the colon with the attached conglomerate tumor was lifted up (Fig. 148). At these two points the transverse colon was divided with the aid of the Petz suture instrument. A piece of the transverse colon about 6 cm. long remained attached to the mass (Fig. 149). The other two free ends of the transverse colon were covered with condoms and reflected lateralward.

Attention was then directed to the stomach. After completing the ligation and division of the gastrocolic omentum, the gastrohepatic omentum was likewise divided. The stomach could now be freed on the cardial and pyloric sides of the mass and a rubber tube was passed around it on each side (Fig. 148).

By making gentle traction, first on the proximal, then on the distal colonic stump, the transverse mesocolon could be separated from the main tumor, with the formation of a considerable gap but with preservation of the middle colic vessels (Fig. 149).

With the aid of the rubber tube tractors, the stomach was mobilized in the direction of the pylorus along the lesser and greater curvatures as far as the upper part of the duodenum. The duodenum was divided with the help of the Petz suture instrument. The distal limb was closed with an infolding Lembert suture and dropped (Fig. 149).

While traction was made on the stomach by its free pyloric end and by the rubber tube passed around it to the cardial side of the adhesions, the gastro-enterostomy site was freed more and more from the surrounding adhesions. Several intestinal loops had to be dissected out of the mass before it was possible to find the jejunal loop attached to the stomach by the gastro-enterostomy and to separate its adhesions to the transverse mesocolon to the extent that the proximal and distal limbs of the gastro-enterostomy could be individually identified. Each was then surrounded with a rubber tube passed through the mesentery (Fig. 149). While working toward the tumor mass, at times from the stomach, at other times from the jejunum, the distal jejunal loop tore in the region of the ulcer. The division of the loop was completed with the electrosurgical knife and its end closed with an intestinal forceps.

By raising the stomach forcibly, the proximal loop leading from the duodenojejunal junction to the stomach was put on tension. It was unfortunately very short. It was therefore divided as close as possible to the stomach by means of the electrosurgical knife. There was not sufficient room to apply a clamp. The escape of bile-stained froth was prevented by the temporary insertion of a gauze tampon provided with a long thread.

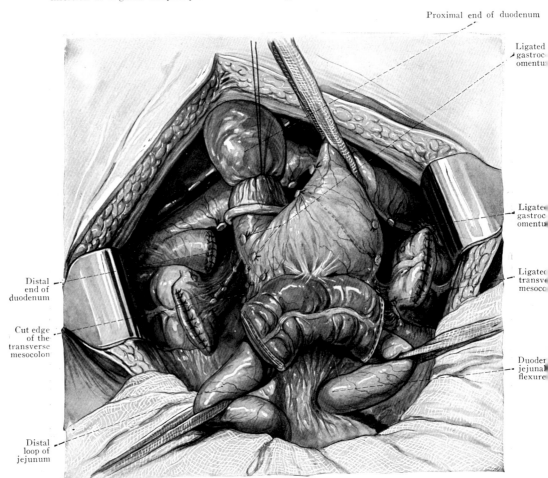

FIG. 149. Operation for a jejunal ulcer which has perforated into the transverse colon (2). The transverse colon with the corresponding portion of the mesocolon has been divided on both sides of the diseased portion with the aid of the Petz suture instrument, and the ends of the colon have been closed by Lembert sutures, since the continuity of the colon is to be restored by side-to-side anastomosis. The duodenum has been divided and its distal limb closed by Lembert sutures, since the reconstruction of gastro-intestinal continuity is to be by the Billroth II method. The proximal duodenal end has been covered with a rubber condom. The stomach has been surrounded by a gauze roll proximal to the diseased portion and is being pulled forward. The faintly dotted line indicates the intended line of gastric resection.

The divided opening of the distal loop of jejunum was closed. The stomach was turned up over the left costal margin, and the distal jejunal loop brought up and placed against the posterior surface of the stomach in the direction from the lesser to the greater curvature. The jejunal loop was then anastomosed to the stomach side-to-side in a line transverse to the long axis of the stomach. In the course of the anastomosis the stomach was divided and the pyloric portion together with the old gastro-enterostomy site excised (Fig. 147). Only a part of the body and the fundus of the stomach remained.

The opening of the proximal jejunal loop coming from the duodenojejunal junction was implanted into the side of the distal jejunal loop 15 cm. below the gastrojejunostomy. This anastomosis was extremely difficult because of the shortness of the proximal jejunal loop, in spite of the fact that the afferent limb of the duodenum had been separated for some distance from the posterior abdominal wall.

Finally, the two ends of the transverse colon were joined end-to-end, after making sure that the blood supply to them had not been affected. The slit in the transverse mesocolon was closed to the point where the jejunal loop coming from the stomach passed through and the edge of the slit was sutured in a circle around it (Fig. 147).

The abdominal incision was then closed without drainage.

J. RESECTION OF THE DESCENDING PORTION OF THE DUODENUM

Resection of the descending portion of the duodenum must be considered if a malignant process arises within it or if such a process beginning in the pancreas involves the common bile duct or the papilla of Vater, also in primary carcinoma of the papilla of Vater, where resection of the papilla alone is no longer feasible. The dangers of this extremely difficult and prognostically highly dubious procedure lie in its long duration, the laborious technique and the vascularity of the operative field; in the increased tendency to bleeding due to the jaundice and the reduced general resistance; in the difficulty and the uncertainty of establishing a passageway for the pancreatic juice and the bile and in the lack of reliability of the sutures which come in contact with the secretion of the opened pancreas and which are dependent for their holding qualities upon the inadequate peritoneal covering of the duodenum. The operation has thus far been performed successfully in only a single case by Kausch.

In only exceptional instances will the diagnosis of the disease be known preoperatively in such detail that the resection of the duodenum can be decided upon in advance. In the great majority of instances the abdomen is opened with a diagnosis of tumor or gall-stone obstruction of the papilla of Vater and the resection of the duodenum is not decided upon until after inspection of the lesion.

The first step of the operation is the proper exposure of the operative field. The abdomen is opened by a midline incision extending down from the ensiform process and enlarged transversely if necessary or else by one of the incisions commonly used in operations on the biliary system. In view of the magnitude and duration of the operation, spinal anaesthesia is much to be preferred. The transverse colon is displaced downward, and the hepatic flexure, if it blocks the approach to the duodenum, is freed and displaced downward and toward the midline.

Since the nature and the extent of the lesion can rarely if ever be determined from the exterior, the duodenum is opened in the manner described under transduodenal choledochotomy and is inspected from within (Fig. 150). If the resection of the duodenum is decided upon, the gut is closed again and the operation is continued with clean instruments.

The second step is the performance of a gastro-enterostomy, preferably a posterior retrocolic gastrojejunostomy.

The **third step** begins with the division of the afferent portion of the intestinal tract. The mobilization required for this purpose had better be

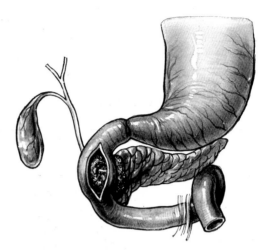

FIG. 150. Carcinoma of the papilla of Vater, with involvement of the adjacent portions of the duodenum and pancreas (1). The duodenum has been opened on its anterior aspect by a longitudinal incision in order to determine the extent of the tumor. Diagrammatic.

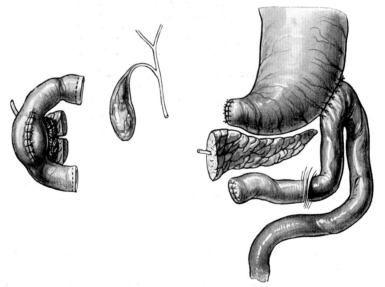

FIG. 151. Resection of the descending portion of the duodenum for carcinoma of the papilla of Vater (2). Diagrammatic. The opening in the duodenum was closed and a retrocolic posterior gastrojejunostomy established. The stomach was transsected in its prepyloric portion and the proximal end closed blind. The distal portion of the stomach, the first portion and the descending portion of the duodenum were freed from their attachments, the common bile duct and the pancreatic duct divided and the diseased portion of the pancreas removed. The duodenum was then divided in the region of its distal transverse portion. The pyloric portion of the stomach, and the proximal two-thirds of the duodenum together with the attached diseased portion of the pancreas were then removed. The resected mass is on the left.

started in the region of the stomach rather than of the duodenum because after the division it is easier and safer to close the proximal opening if it is

in the stomach than in the duodenum. Furthermore, it is easier to handle
the segment of duodenum to be resected if a piece of stomach is attached to it.
It is advisable, therefore, to make the division in the region of the prepyloric
portion of the stomach. Otherwise, the duodenum may be divided just distal
to the pylorus. The Petz suture instrument will be found of great advantage
in the required resections. The opening on the proximal side of the transsection is permanently closed with a further row of interrupted Lembert sutures
(Fig. 151).

The fourth step includes the actual resection of the lesion. The distal
stump of intestine (pyloric antrum or first portion of duodenum), which is
closed with Petz clips, is gradually freed in a downward direction from its

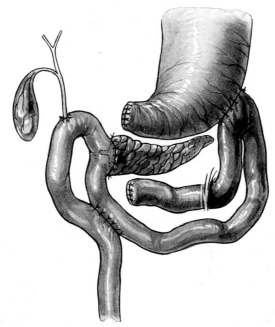

FIG. 152. Resection of the descending portion of the duodenum (3). Diagrammatic. The
cut surface of the pancreas has been implanted into a lateral opening of the proximal jejunal
loop and the stump of the common bile duct into an opening at another point in the same
jejunal loop. The proximal and distal limbs of this loop have been joined by a side-to-side
anastomosis.

connections. All strands of tissue which are put on stretch are picked up in
small segments on an aneurysm needle and cut between ligatures. The diseased portion of the pancreas is excised with the electrosurgical knife in the
manner described under the surgery of the pancreas on page 540. The external wound in the pancreas must be as small as possible. In cutting the
pancreatic tissue the small accessory pancreatic ducts in the upper part of
the organ will be divided. If they are recognized they should be ligated
singly. The main excretory duct should be exposed separately, caught with
a traction suture or temporarily closed with a clamp.

On the right side of the duodenum the common bile duct is dissected
free from the hepatoduodenal ligament, divided and also caught with a traction suture or a clamp. As soon as the duodenum has been freed into normal

tissue it is divided distal to the lesion. Here again, if the distal limb of the duodenum is to be closed blind, the Petz suture instrument should be used if possible. This completes the resection of the lesion (Fig. 151).

Two tasks remain to be performed—the establishment of a passageway for the bile into the digestive tract and a similar passageway for the pancreatic secretion. These tasks may be carried out in one of several ways.

Fifth step. If the biliary tract from the liver to the gall bladder is open, it is simplest to do a cholecystogastrostomy (Fig. 153). The anastomosis can however be made between the gall bladder and the distal limb of the duodenum or a loop of jejunum (Fig. 154).

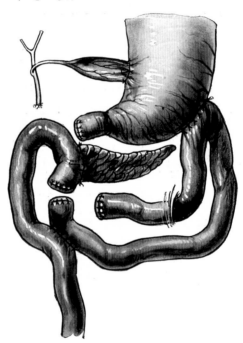

Fig. 153. Resection of the descending portion of the duodenum (4). In this illustration the duodenum is divided in its first portion, instead of in the pyloric portion of the stomach. Diagrammatic. The cut surface of the pancreas has been implanted into a lateral opening in the proximal jejunal loop. The proximal and distal limbs of the jejunal loop have been joined by a side-to-side anastomosis. The limb of jejunum leading from the anastomosis to the pancreas has been divided and both ends closed. The stump of the common bile duct has been closed and a cholecystogastrostomy performed.

If the gall bladder is not suitable for making such an anastomosis, the end of the divided common bile duct is anastomosed to any point of the intestine, as a rule most conveniently to the distal limb of the duodenum or to a loop of jejunum pulled up for the purpose (Fig. 152). In doing this, a temporary prosthesis as described under surgery of the biliary tract may be useful.

Sixth step. It is more difficult to establish a passageway into the intestine for the pancreatic secretion. It is probably never possible to use the pancreatic duct as an isolated structure for anastomosis. Furthermore, the presence of the large wound surface of the pancreas resulting from the resection demands that the whole cross section of the pancreas be joined to the intestine. Occasionally the open end of the distal limb of the duodenum will prove suitable for this purpose. The pancreatic wound surface is inserted into the intestinal opening or is at least covered by the opening, and the two structures are united as firmly as possible with interrupted sutures and the suture reinforced with omentum. If the end of the duodenal stump is not suitable for the purpose, a loop of jejunum is brought close, and the open end of the pancreas is joined to the open intestine (Fig. 154) or to a lateral opening (Fig. 153) in its distal limb after division and implantation of the proximal end into the distal limb; or the pancreas is joined to a lateral opening in a jejunal loop whose continuity has been preserved (Fig. 152). In the latter

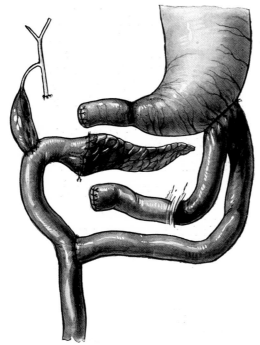

FIG. 154. Resection of the descending portion of the duodenum (5). Diagrammatic. The proximal jejunal loop has been divided. The proximal end has been implanted end-to-side into the distal limb at a point about 50 cm. below the point of division. The cut surface of the pancreas has been implanted into the distal end and the fundus of the gall bladder has been anastomosed to this limb a short distance beyond this point. The stump of the common bile duct has been closed.

instance it is advisable to perform an entero-enterostomy between the bases of the limbs of the loop.

All uncertain suture lines are secured by placing omentum over them. In spite of this, the lack of security of individual sutures and the injury of the pancreas will nearly always necessitate packing and drainage of the abdominal cavity.

K. TREATMENT OF PERFORATED GASTRIC AND DUODENAL ULCERS. TREATMENT OF VOLVULUS OF THE STOMACH

Treatment of Perforated Gastric and Duodenal Ulcers. The treatment of perforated peptic ulcer really belongs in the chapter on the treatment of general suppurative peritonitis. The technique of the operative procedure presents so many peculiarities, however, that it is pertinent to describe it separately under the stomach and duodenum, and to refer the reader to the above mentioned chapter for the general measures.

When the abdomen is opened, the presence in the upper abdomen of air, food particles or turbid sour-smelling fluid makes certain the diagnosis of perforated ulcer and frequently leads promptly to the site of the lesion. The perforated ulcer is usually situated in the anterior wall of the stomach or duodenum near the lesser curvature and close to the pylorus. The perforation, gastric or duodenal, is therefore usually easy to find on lifting the edge of the liver and pulling the stomach downward. In every case it is first sought for in this region and in this manner. If the ulcer is not promptly found there or on the rest of the easily accessible anterior wall of the stomach or in the upper part of the duodenum, then it can only be on the posterior wall. A knowledge of this position of the perforation is important, since the attendant peritonitis may be limited wholly to the lesser peritoneal cavity, so that on opening the abdomen one fails to find any evidence of soiling of the greater cavity.

To inspect the posterior wall of the stomach the gastrocolic omentum is divided. The presence of food particles in the lesser peritoneal cavity confirms the suspected diagnosis. By passing the hand behind the stomach through the slit in the gastrocolic omentum, the stomach is examined bimanually. Suspicious points on the posterior wall are brought into view by means of retractors and specula and by rotation of the walls of the stomach.

As soon as the ulcer is found the further escape of food is prevented by placing a finger tip over the opening. The opening may then be temporarily plugged with a piece of gauze.

The much debated question as to whether a perforated ulcer should merely be oversewed or whether it should be removed by resection, I decide on the following grounds: An acute peritonitis after perforation is a condition which immediately threatens life and in which the simplest procedure should be employed as a rule. In such instances I resort to simple suture and reinforcement of the ulcer site. Of course, in a particularly favorable case an exception is justifiable, or in a particularly unfavorable case in which the perforation cannot be closed by suture an exception must be made. My opinion is strengthened by the fact that, on changing from resection to suture and gastro-enterostomy, the mortality in the Tübingen Clinic fell materially. Besides, simple oversewing is recommended by experience, in that many perforated ulcers apparently heal completely after this simple operation, provided that unrestricted emptying of the stomach is assured at the same time by a gastro-enterostomy.

The closure of the perforation is carried out with Lembert sutures. Difficulties, however, may be met with because of the friability and the edematous infiltration of the surrounding tissue. Nevertheless, it is usually successful if the sutures include sufficient tissue (Fig. 155). A stenosis of the channel is possible in this procedure but the gastro-enterostomy provides for this. If the closure with Lembert sutures seems insecure, the suture line may be reinforced by a bit of omentum or other peritoneal reduplication.

If a dependable closure cannot be effected in this way, three alternatives remain:

(a) Resection of the ulcerated gastric segment.

(b) An adjacent peritoneum-covered viscus may be sutured over the opening.

It is usually possible to suture a piece of omentum into the opening or to stretch a bit of omentum over the ulcer. At times the perforation may be closed by suturing its edges to the under surface of the liver or to the anterior

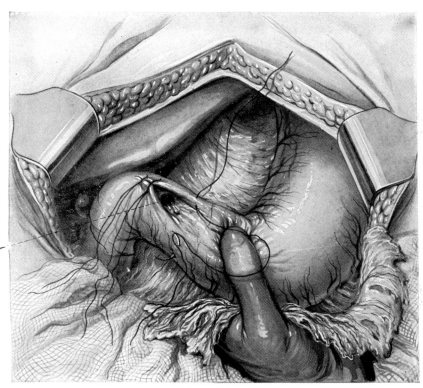

Point of perforation

FIG. 155. Oversewing a perforated gastric ulcer on the lesser curvature in the region of the pyloric antrum. The point of perforation of the ulcer is being closed by wide Lembert sutures.

abdominal wall. In an emergency, an excised piece of omentum may be used.

(c) A tightly fitting drainage tube is inserted into the opening. Its tip, inside the stomach and pointing toward the duodenum, is surrounded on all sides by omentum and is led to the surface of the body (Fig. 156). This omental cuff (Newmann) is fastened by suture to the stomach on one side, and to the parietal peritoneum on the other.

The drainage tube is clamped off for short periods after a few days and is removed in 10 to 12 days. The opening then closes rapidly of itself.

If the perforation cannot be dealt with in one of the ways described, or if further destruction of the gastric wall is anticipated, as after the recent action of a caustic, then the threatened segment of the abdominal cavity is drained and walled off with packing, and a jejunostomy is performed to side-track the stomach and place it at rest.

If, as is the rule, the ulcer is located near the pylorus then oversewing it usually leads to stenosis of the pylorus or increases an existing stenosis. In such instances an immediate gastrojejunostomy is obligatory; and in every

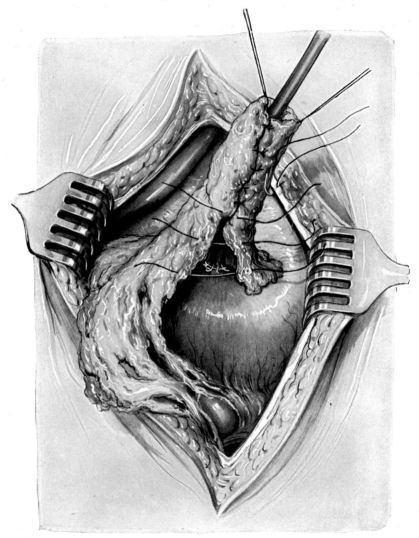

FIG. 156. Treatment of a perforated gastric ulcer on the lesser curvature by drainage and a cuff of omentum. A drainage tube is inserted into the perforation and surrounded by a cuff of omentum which is attached by sutures to the stomach and the adjacent portion of the abdominal wound.

other case I believe it is advisable. In addition, one may obstruct the access of food to the ulcer by means of one of the measures for excluding the pylorus, for example, by transverse plicating sutures.

The gastro-enterostomy is placed at some distance from the ulcer so that in case of continuance of the disease the possibility of a subsequent extensive resection of the diseased gastric segment remains.

After the usual cleansing of the abdominal cavity by sponging and aspiration, the abdomen is closed without drainage. (In perforations of more than 8 hours duration I prefer to drain. The drainage tube should not lie adjacent to the line of suture however. I. S. R.)

THE TREATMENT OF VOLVULUS OF THE STOMACH

Volvulus of the stomach is frequently mistaken for a perforated ulcer because of the previous history, and in view of the stormy upper-abdominal manifestations which consist of the symptoms of a high ileus and peritonitis. A midline incision is made above the umbilicus. It should be large enough to permit full orientation of the anatomic conditions. The stomach is found rolled on its long or its transverse axis into a sausage-shaped tumor. In extreme cases the transverse colon may be involved in the twisting and may be forced against the diaphragm behind the stomach and beneath the left costal margin. The untangling of the gastro-intestinal mass may be very difficult, or, in case of adhesions, quite impossible.

After a successful untwisting and replacement, if the general condition of the patient permits, a search should be made for the lesion underlying the volvulus. This, for example, may be a pyloric stenosis, a tumor (usually benign), a diaphragmatic hernia or a wandering spleen. The underlying cause should be removed if possible, but this must frequently be deferred for a second operation in view of the condition of the patient. In case of simple volvulous without recognizable cause, the stomach is anchored as well as possible to prevent a recurrence. This is best accomplished by attachment to the anterior abdominal wall according to the procedure of Rovsing, described under the treatment of gastroptosis on page 198.

If the volvulus cannot be untwisted, there is nothing else to do but isolate the stomach from the rest of the abdominal cavity with packing and establish a jejunostomy for feeding the patient. A total resection of the stomach, although theoretically applicable for the cure of this condition, cannot be considered because of the poor condition of the patient.

L. TREATMENT OF GASTROPTOSIS

In many instances gastroptosis is simply a result of some other lesion. The treatment then is the removal of the underlying cause. In other cases, gastroptosis is only part of a general visceroptosis. In the latter cases no relief of the complaints caused by the general enteroptosis is brought about by an elevation of the stomach, even if this is permanently successful. Only rarely is the gastroptosis a simple clinical entity. The tendency is more and more away from the operative treatment of this condition. It is justified only in extremely rare and exceptional cases, if at all. The frequently reported successes of such operations are to be accepted with caution, since gastroptotic complaints are so often of a neurotic character.

Recently resection of the stomach has occasionally been recommended for the treatment of a true gastroptosis (Martin). The results of this measure can not be called uniformly successful and involve a serious and mutilating operation, of which I gravely doubt the wisdom.

A few writers insist on gastro-enterostomy for those cases associated with a dilatation of the stomach, even when there is no mechanical obstruction at the pylorus. The good results which are alleged frequently to be observed are usually to be explained by the short-circuiting of a spastic irritable sphincter and by a more rapid emptying of the stomach. In other similar cases the complaints are increased by the gastro-enterostomy, so that this procedure cannot be advised in the absence of stenosis at the pylorus.

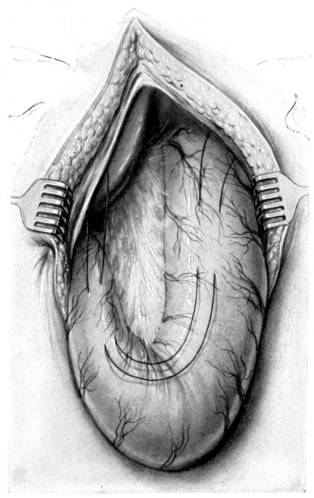

Fig. 157. Attachment of the stomach to the anterior abdominal wall for the relief of gastroptosis (Rovsing). The sutures are passed through the abdominal wall and the anterior wall of the stomach in such a way that they will elevate the stomach when they are tied after the closure of the abdominal incision.

Two types of specific procedure are available for the treatment of true gastroptosis:

1. Attachment of the Stomach to the Anterior Abdominal Wall (Rovsing-Klapp)

Through a midline abdominal incision above the umbilicus, Rovsing applies three heavy linen or silk sutures in a transverse direction in such a way that each suture passes through all layers of both abdominal wound edges including the skin, and between grasps the anterior surface of the stomach in two Lembert sero-muscular folds (Fig. 157). The uppermost suture

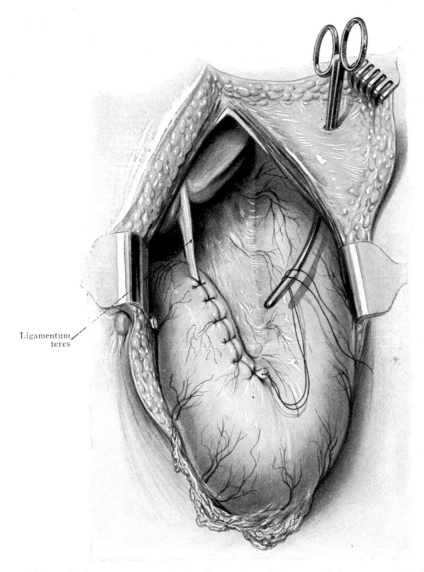

Ligamentum
teres

FIG. 158. Gastropexy (Perthes). Suspension of the stomach by means of the ligamentum teres for the relief of gastroptosis. The ligamentum teres has been separated from the umbilicus and attached to the lesser curvature of the stomach by means of a Witzel canal. The free end of the ligament through which a suture has been passed is pulled through the left anterior abdominal wall just above the lower costal arch by means of a forceps where it is fastened under tension at the point of exit so that the lesser curvature of the stomach will be elevated and put on tension.

lies 1 cm. below the lesser curvature, the lowest, 3 cm. above the greater curvature and the third, half way between the other two. The peritoneum of the abdominal wall and that of the anterior wall of the stomach are scarified over an appropriate area to promote adhesions. The surfaces may also be painted with tincture of iodine for this purpose. After closure of the abdominal wound in the usual manner, the three sutures are tied over a gauze roll and are not removed for three weeks.

2. SUSPENSION OF THE STOMACH BY THE GASTROHEPATIC OMENTUM (BIER, BEYA) AND BY THE LIGAMENTUM TERES (PERTHES)

The gastrohepatic omentum is transfixed in its full width from cardia to pylorus by four silk or linen sutures parallel to each other and perpendicular to the lesser curvature. Each suture picks up three folds, each about 1 cm. wide, one fold close to the liver, one in the middle and one at the lesser curvature. By tying all these sutures at the same time, the gastrohepatic omentum is plicated like a curtain, lifting the stomach toward the portal fissure. The difficulty of the procedure lies in the fact that the gastrohepatic omentum is often so poorly developed that the sutures have only a very weak hold on it and on the portal fissure.

In Perthes' operation the ligamentum teres is divided at the umbilicus, dissected free as far as the portal notch and used for the suspension of the stomach. Perthes originally advised making a tunnel under the peritoneum of the lesser curvature by blunt dissection to receive the round ligament. This procedure is not without danger and occasionally leads to perforation of the stomach with resultant peritonitis. It is therefore preferable to fasten the ligament to the anterior surface of the stomach along the lesser curvature by means of a Witzel canal from the region of the pylorus toward the cardia (Fig. 158), as recommended by Vogel. The free end of the ligament, to which a silk suture is tied, is drawn out through a slit made in the abdominal wall at the outer border of the left rectus and as close to the costal margin as possible. The ligament is fastened under tension to the anterior rectus sheath and the excess removed.

CHAPTER IV

OPERATIONS ON THE SMALL INTESTINE AND THE LARGE INTESTINE

A. GENERAL CONSIDERATIONS OF THE ANATOMY OF AND ORIENTATION IN THE LOWER ABDOMEN. INCISIONS FOR INTESTINAL OPERATIONS

The lower abdomen, in which lie the small and the large intestine, is divided from the upper abdomen by the transverse mesocolon, horizontally attached to the posterior abdominal wall at the level of the second lumbar vertebra, and by the transverse colon. The great omentum attached to the transverse colon hangs like an apron over the small intestine. In order to make the lower abdomen and its contents, especially the small bowel, accessible, the transverse colon and the great omentum must be reflected upward.

It cannot be too much emphasized that the search for and the exposure of a particular portion of the intestine are greatly simplified by placing the patient in such a position that the abdominal segment in question forms the highest point of the abdomen. In this position the remainder of the small intestine gravitates out of the field of operation and affords free access to the lesion. Additional help is afforded by a lordotic position of the patient, best procured and adjusted by the use of a pneumatic rubber cushion in the manner previously described. Even with these aids the orientation in the lower abdomen may become extremely difficult as a result of the great motility of protruding intestines, especially when the patient strains or when the gut is distended. Therefore an anaesthetic which completely relaxes the abdominal wall is one of the most important prerequisites for orientation and for the exposure of a particular intestinal segment. Spinal anaesthesia is ideal for these purposes. Bulging loops of intestine may be held back with the hand or with broad flat retractors after being protected with moist compresses.

The amount of abdominal fat and, above all, the amount of contents in the intestines are of decided significance in working in the abdomen. The differentiation between small and large intestine is easy. Only in case of extremely distended and hypertrophic intestinal loops could any difficulty arise in this differentiation.

The large bowel is recognizable less by its size, in case of stenosis the small bowel may be greatly dilated, than by its taeniae, its sacculations or haustrations and its epiploic appendages. The transverse colon is distinguished by the attached omentum, the ascending and descending colon by the lack of a mesentery, the rectum by its attachment behind the promontory of the sacrum and by its disappearance into the pelvis.

The small intestine, which is attached throughout to a long mesentery, is

easily accessible in all its parts. Its mesentery is attached to the posterior
abdominal wall in a line running from the second lumbar vertebra to the right
sacro-iliac joint. It contains the branches of the superior mesenteric artery
(Fig. 159) which arises from the aorta in the upper abdomen (Fig. 73), passes
behind the pancreas and in front of the lower horizontal limb of the duodenum
into the lower abdomen, enters the root of the mesentery, and supplies the

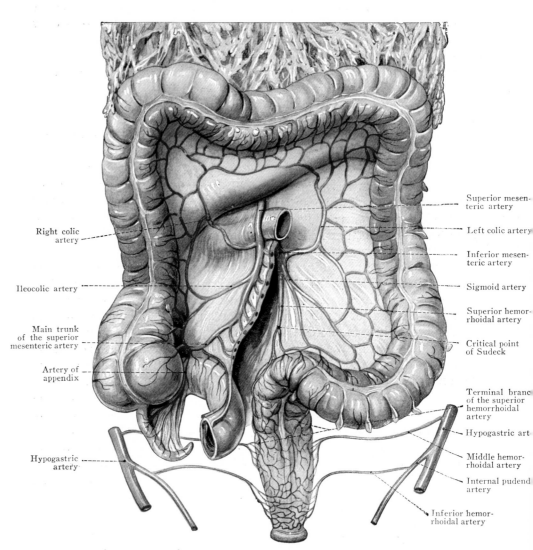

Right colic
artery

Ileocolic artery

Main trunk
of the superior
mesenteric artery

Artery of
appendix

Hypogastric
artery

Superior mesen-
teric artery

Left colic artery

Inferior mesen-
teric artery

Sigmoid artery

Superior hemor-
rhoidal artery

Critical point
of Sudeck

Terminal branc
of the superior
hemorrhoidal
artery

Hypogastric art

Middle hemor-
rhoidal artery

Internal pudend
artery

Inferior hemor-
rhoidal artery

FIG. 159.   The arterial supply of the intestine.

whole small intestine, the ascending colon and, through its highest branch, the
middle colic artery, the major part of the transverse colon. With the superior
mesenteric artery and its branches run the veins of the same names, which
finally go to form the portal vein.

The small intestine is freely movable on its mesentery, so that the mesentery is accessible on both sides. The mesentery is not attached to the intestine

in a narrow line but grips it as in the limbs of a fork, a point of importance in separating the mesentery from the intestine. (This must also be kept in mind in end-to-end anastomosis of the small intestine since this area is not peritonealized. I. S. R.)

The transverse colon and the sigmoid are the only parts of the large bowel with a mesentery. The ascending colon and the descending colon are as a rule attached to the posterior abdominal wall by a broad surface and are therefore only slightly movable. The blood vessels approach the ascending and descending colon and the sigmoid from the median side in accordance with the developmental shifts of these organs (Fig. 210). The large bowel receives only a few vessels from the lateral side, and these are of no significance in its nutrition.

The blood supply of the appendix is by vessels coursing in the meso-appendix, and arising from the superior mesenteric vessels. The meso-appendix may be absent or nearly obliterated by preceding inflammation.

It makes a great difference in the matter of searching for particular organs in the abdomen whether the intestines are comparatively empty or excessively full. If the intestines are not overfull, the inspection of the abdominal contents is simple and the delivery into the incision of even deeply seated lesions is in most cases easily possible without removing large portions of the small bowel from the abdominal cavity. I presuppose a relatively empty intestine in the following procedures.

There is no sure mark of identification of the level of a loop of small intestine picked up at random. Nor is it possible to tell at a glance which is the proximal and which the distal end of an intestinal loop. To determine this, there is nothing else to do but follow the intestine in one direction until either the duodenojejunal junction or the ileocecal valve is reached. While tracing the bowel in this way, it is necessary that the loop which is the point of departure be held fast by an assistant or marked by a clamp, the direction also being noted, so that, in case the search was made in the wrong direction, it will not be necessary to follow the whole length of intestine back again, but the search can be continued in the other direction from the original loop. In examining the intestines only a short loop should be delivered at a time. The operator lets this loop glide between the fingers of both hands and replaces on one side as much bowel as he withdraws on the other, in doing which he must have the aid of an assistant. In this way, only a short section of intestine is outside of the abdominal incision at a time.

The duodenojejunal junction and the proximal jejunal loop can easily be found if the surgeon passes his hand along the under surface of the stretched transverse mesocolon just to the left of the spine and picks up the intestinal loop which emerges at this point. This loop can be brought into view in most cases without difficulty. It is recognizable by the fact that it can be delivered only in one direction.

The cecum, the appendix and with it the end of the ileum and the beginning of the ascending colon, if not discovered at a glance, are found by displacing the small bowel to the left as far as possible and picking up that part of the intestine which lies farthest down to the right. If this fails, then the small bowel must be followed as far as the cecum, or the ascending colon be used as a guide, downward.

The hepatic flexure of the colon is reached by following the ascending colon upward or the transverse colon to the right. The descending colon and the sigmoid are made accessible by displacing the small intestine to the right. By following the descending colon upward, one reaches the splenic flexure, to which the transverse colon also leads to the left. Following the sigmoid downward leads to the rectum.

In order to inspect the pelvic organs, the anterior wall of the rectum, the bladder and the internal female genitalia, it is convenient to use the Trendelenburg position, so that the small intestine gravitates upward out of the field of vision. To bring the female genital organs into the operative wound, the uterus is grasped with a uterine forceps and drawn forward. The adnexa on each side are then easy to find. In doing this, one often sees the ureter, with its characteristic worm-like contractions, glistening through the posterior layer of the peritoneum in the region of the sacro-iliac joint (Figs. 278, 279, 343 and 344). Here, too, can be seen and palpated the common iliac artery, crossed in front by the ureter, and its bifurcation into the external and internal iliac arteries.

The kidneys can be palpated in the retroperitoneal space to the right and left beside the spine and, depending on their position, above or below the transverse mesocolon.

The aorta to the left of the spine is easily recognizable by its pulsations. In the corresponding position on the right lies the vena cava, which is not palpable and only stands out when stasis is produced by raising the head and lowering the pelvis or by applying pressure on the cardiac side.

Thus it is possible in most cases to find individual organs which before operation are suspected of being diseased, surely, quickly and with little manipulation, and in cases of doubtful diagnosis any or all of the abdominal organs may be subjected to a systematic inspection by bringing them into view or palpating them with the hand. The points of particular importance in orientation are the duodenojejunal junction, the ileocecal valve, the transverse colon with its hepatic and splenic flexures and the sigmoid.

It is much more difficult to become oriented in the abdomen when the intestines are excessively distended, as occurs particularly in cases of ileus. The technique of procedure under these circumstances is described in detail in the section on the treatment of mechanical ileus.

B. THE OPENING AND SINGLE-STAGE ARTIFICIAL EVACUATION OF THE INTESTINE (ENTEROTOMY)

1. THE OPENING OF THE INTESTINE

It is only rarely that the intestine is opened for the inspection of or operations on the interior of the bowel. In the great majority of cases, if we exclude division of the bowel and lateral anastomosis, this is done for the removal of a foreign body, as for example, an object that has been swallowed, a gall stone or a clump of ascaris worms. The intestine may be opened temporarily to evacuate its contents in the presence of a mechanical or paralytic ileus. The technique of enterotomy is in the main the same as in gastrotomy, as described on page 92, and illustrated in Figures 76 and 77.

The intestinal loop to be opened is delivered from the abdominal wound if possible and the surrounding field is walled off with wet sponges. After milking the loop as nearly empty as possible, the site of the intended opening is closed off from the rest of the intestine by means of a clamp applied to a longitudinal fold of the gut or by two clamps applied transversely, one on each side (Fig. 160).

The incision for opening a loop of gut is made in the long axis because in this direction it may be extended if necessary. The wall opposite the mesenteric attachment is selected because the fewest blood vessels lie here. In the colon the incision is made in the middle of a taenia.

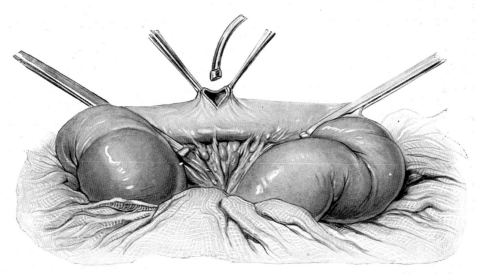

Fig. 160. Enterotomy in a distended loop of gut. To prevent the escape of intestinal contents the intestinal loop to be opened has been milked empty and closed on each side with a light clamp. The enterotomy is held with two forceps and the intestinal contents removed by suction. (An incision in the long axis of the gut is preferable.)

The electrosurgical knife should preferably be used for dividing the wall of the gut, but a scalpel is also used. When the removal of a palpable foreign body is concerned, the part is carefully walled off with gauze compresses and the body is squeezed against the intestinal wall and the stretched wall is incised down on the foreign body. The foreign body is then removed, either as a whole, for example, a gall stone (Fig. 261), or in its component parts, for example, a clump of ascaris worms (Fig. 262), through the smallest possible opening.

If the gut wall is to be divided for a considerable distance the line of incision is at first carried only through the serosa. At one point of this serosal incision the outer surface of the mucosa is picked up with two toothed forceps and is incised at the top of the raised fold. Through this small opening the intestinal contents are aspirated while the edges of the wound are elevated by means of the two forceps to prevent overflow (Fig. 160). Using a grooved director as a guard, the incision is completed to the desired extent by means of an electrosurgical knife or a scissors (Fig. 114). Bleeding vessels are caught and ligated in the usual way. The cut edges of the intestinal wound are held apart with traction sutures or Kocher forceps and the intended operation in the interior of the intestine is performed.

Operative wounds of the intestine should usually be sutured in such a way that the corresponding points of the wound edges are reunited. Longitudinal incisions should therefore be sutured in the long axis. In transverse incisions the same procedure may also be followed, as a rule. An obstructive narrowing of the lumen is usually not produced thereby, so that the old rule to cut in the long axis and to suture transversely seems unnecessary. Only in case of loss of tissue of the intestinal wall or in case of a previously existing stenosis is the transverse suture of a longitudinal incision indicated. If, after closure of an intestinal opening, there is any doubt as to the adequate patency of a narrowed lumen, the area should be short-circuited. This is usually done by a side-to-side anastomosis of the proximal and distal loops.

The closure of the intestinal opening follows the usual technique with an Albert three-layer catgut suture and interrupted Lembert sutures with silk or linen. The three-layer suture may be carried out as a continuous or an interrupted suture. The serosal suture is always an interrupted one. Any excessive bulging of the mucosa at the wound edges must first be trimmed off.

A very small opening in the intestine, such as is made for the removal of a slender object like a lead pencil, may also be closed with a purse-string suture. The first purse-string suture must be secured and buried by a second purse-string or by a few Lembert sutures (Figs. 42, 43 and 44).

2. The Artificial Evacuation of the Small Intestine

In evacuating an isolated segment of distended intestine, the chief concern is to prevent soiling of the surrounding field with intestinal contents. The field must therefore be carefully walled off with moist sponges. The intestine is milked as empty as possible. The further access of intestinal contents from neighboring loops to the site of the intended opening is blocked by two intestinal clamps applied across the bowel. The isolated loop may then be aspirated by means of a cannula or large-bore needle with a syringe or suction pump. In most cases, however, the gut can be incised without previous aspiration and without soiling of the surrounding field, by cutting between two Allis forceps with which the wall is elevated. The gas-bubble escapes first, while the fluid contents are removed by aspiration (Fig. 160).

The operative evacuation of the whole intestine of its excessive accumulation of contents in case of ileus is not an independent operation but is undertaken in the course of an operation directed against the cause of the ileus. The emptying of the bowel not only serves the purpose of facilitating inspection and accessibility during the operation, the subsequent reposition of the intestines and the closure of the abdominal wound, but also effects the collapse of the overdistended gut whose circulation has been impaired thereby and gives its musculature a chance to recover. It also protects the body from the absorption of toxins which may have accumulated in the gut, even though peristalsis is not immediately resumed. The single complete artificial evacuation gives the intestine a chance for rest and recovery and there is no harm if the next evacuation by the natural route does not occur until several days later. These advantages are achieved, however, only if the evacuation of the whole intestine is practically complete.

The complete evacuation of the whole intestine cannot be secured through a simple puncture or by the mere opening of an intestinal loop, even though the gut is milked by stroking or if a catheter or stomach tube is inserted for some distance. It is possible only by the insertion of a straight Moynihan glass tube attached to a suction apparatus. This must be done gently. My suction apparatus for emptying the intestine has recently been modified by using an electrically driven suction pump and, as proposed by my assistant, Stör, by the presence of a side-valve in the handle of the aspirating tube, through the opening of which the suction at the tip may be reduced or stopped entirely. This prevents the aspiration of the intestinal wall, as frequently occurred in the past.

The evacuation of the intestine with the aid of an electrically driven suction apparatus may be done as follows: Precautions are taken to separate clearly the clean operative field of the primary operation and the infected secondary operative field of the intestinal evacuation. This is done by stretching a sterile sheet perpendicularly over the abdomen in the long axis of the body. The operator and the second assistant with the opened loop of gut and the handle of the aspirating tube are on the one side, and the first assistant with the bulk of the intestines and the tip of the aspirating tube in the interior of the gut on the clean side.

The surgeon stands on the right side of the patient. In case of ileus of the large bowel the lowest loop of the small intestine, in case of a small bowel ileus the intestinal loop just above the obstruction is sought and delivered to an extent of about 30 cm. The surroundings are carefully walled off with moist gauze compresses. A laparotomy sheet is spread tent-like, as above described, in such a way that the first assistant standing at the left of the patient is completely separated from the operator and from the second assistant standing at the side of the operator. This barrier is low enough that one can look over it from one side to the other.

The exposed loop of ileum is milked empty and a length of about 30 cm. is clamped off above and below with intestinal clamps. A piece of narrow rubber tubing is passed through a small slit in the mesentery quite close to the gut. If necessary, the loop is first emptied by aspiration with a cannula and suction pump. The gut is then opened with a small longitudinal incision 6 cm. distal to the rubber tube. Every drop of exuding intestinal contents is immediately caught. The straight Moynihan intestinal tube is quickly inserted in the direction of the proximal clamp. As soon as the tube has passed the point where the rubber tubing pierces the mesentery the tubing is pulled together tightly over the intestine and the glass tube within, forming an air- and water-tight closure around the latter, and is held with a hemostat or ligature. The proximal intestinal clamp is then removed and suction is started.

The glass tube is slowly advanced in the intestine in the direction of the duodenojejunal junction (Fig. 161). The operator makes use of the lateral safety valve in the handle in such a way that suction is maintained but without sucking the gut wall into the opening of the tube. While advancing the tube, the operator, looking over the tent-like cover, watches the progress of the tip of the tube in the intestine and by appropriately moving the other end of the tube gives it the proper direction. The first assistant, working in the clean field, assists him by threading the intestine, loop for loop, over the slowly

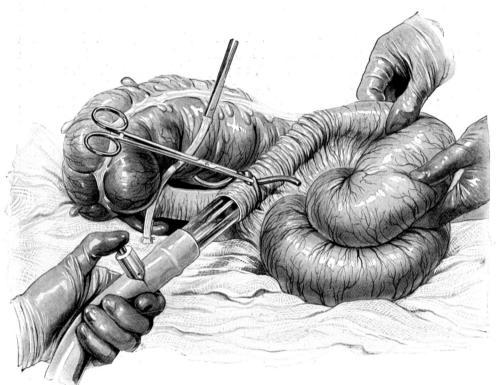

Fig. 161. Evacuation of the entire small intestine in intestinal obstruction by suction. The ileum is clamped just proximal to the ileocecal valve. A short distance above this point a straight glass tube was introduced into the gut through a small opening and tied securely in place by means of a rubber tube passed through an opening in the mesentery. The glass tube was pushed along as far as the duodenojejunal junction, threading the whole small bowel on the tube. The suction exerted by an electric suction pump is regulated by means of a by-pass safety valve.

advancing tube, by guiding the top of the tube, and by avoiding all undue traction on the gut.

In this manner the tip of the tube progresses slowly, picking up the whole small bowel, until it arrives at the duodenojejunal junction. By carefully regulated suction the gut is in this way emptied of nearly all of its fluid and gaseous contents. After reaching the duodenojejunal junction the glass tube is withdrawn somewhat more rapidly than it was introduced, while the suction is continued, aspirating the last of the intestinal contents. When the tip of the glass tube has been brought back to the opening in the gut wall, the glass tube is removed.

The opening in the side of the intestine is closed in the usual way with a two-tier suture. The rubber tubing is withdrawn from the slit in the mesentery and the distal intestinal clamp is removed.

In case of ileus of the large bowel it is usually not necessary to extend the aspiration downward into the large bowel. It is also rather difficult to pass the straight glass tube through the ileocecal junction and through the remaining flexures of the large bowel. If the patency of the large bowel to the anus is re-established, the relatively short colon usually empties itself promptly and thoroughly through a rectal tube which we use routinely in every abdominal operation.

If individual segments of the large bowel are unusually distended, they are preferably punctured with an aspirating needle and emptied by suction or milking. Asepsis is more easily maintained when this is done because the contents of the large bowel usually consist of firm or thick mushy material and gas, and not of fluid, and the gas can be evacuated as a rule without the escape of the rest of the contents. The gas-filled large bowel can usually be emptied for a considerable distance by milking after puncture at a single point because its various segments, in contrast to the small intestine, form fairly uniform connecting sacs. However this procedure is rarely necessary.

3. Intestinal Tapping Through the Abdominal Wall—Percutaneous Puncture

If in desperate cases of ileus the peristaltic power of the overdistended intestine can no longer evacuate its contents over long stretches of gut through the natural or an artificial anus or through an intestinal fistula, multiple punctures of the gut with a fine needle may bring about a resumption of activity of the gut. This measure is theoretically fraught with the danger of an infection of the peritoneal cavity by the seepage of intestinal contents into it through the opening in the intestine made by the needle and the procedure would therefore seem questionable at first glance. Experience has shown, however, that this danger is very slight since the puncture wound in the gut, if made with a sufficiently fine needle, closes at once, so that no further contents escape from the emptied and collapsed gut. Nevertheless, in view of the danger of the procedure, it should be used only in desperate cases. That it may be life-saving in such cases is beyond doubt in my opinion, which is based on numerous experiences.

It is usually possible by inspection and palpation to determine the position of a few especially distended loops in the swollen abdomen of the patient. These points are marked with a colored solution. As a rule 5 or 6 such points are selected. The region is painted with a tannin-alcohol solution and the point of puncture is anesthetized by skin infiltration with novocaine. A hollow needle, 5 cm. long and 0.6 mm. in diameter, of the type used for the injection of local anesthetics, is thrust perpendicularly through the abdominal wall into the gut. One can feel clearly when the needle point has overcome the resistance of the abdominal wall and lies within the gas-filled intestinal loop. The needle is left in place and the same procedure is undertaken with another needle at the second of the indicated puncture points. This is continued until all the points have been punctured (Fig. 162).

The needles are left in place for some time, sometimes as long as half an hour, while the intestinal gases in favorable cases escape through the needles and the abdomen slowly collapses with an attendant improvement in the general condition of the patient. It is possible to hear and see the escape of the gas by applying a drop of fluid to the free end of the needle. Or it may be recognized by the movements of a bit of cotton or the flame of a burning match held in front of the needle opening. Occasionally the needles show a pendulum motion as a sign of the resumption of peristalsis. A needle from which no further gas has escaped for some time is withdrawn.

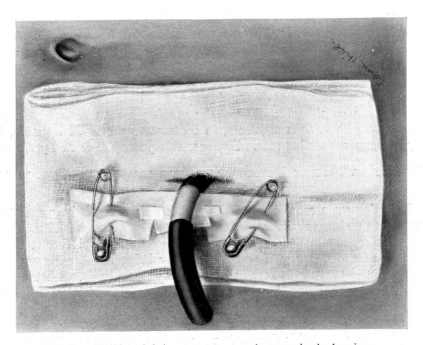

Fig. 162. Method of fixing enterostomy tube to patient's dressing.

Percutaneous puncture of the intestines may be repeated a number of times. (It is a procedure which should be used however only as a last resort. I have never used this method but it violates basic surgical principles. I. S. R.)

C. ESTABLISHMENT OF AN INTESTINAL FISTULA (ENTEROSTOMY)

An enterostomy is performed either for the purpose of introducing nourishment into the intestine or to permit the evacuation of the intestinal contents. For nutritive purposes, the enterostomy is placed in as high an intestinal loop as possible, preferably in the upper jejunum, while a fistula for the evacuation of feces is placed in as low a loop as possible, preferably the terminal ileum or the large bowel. An enterostomy may be temporary or permanent. Enterostomy openings which have fulfilled their purpose must be closed.

The chief difficulty in the establishment of an intestinal fistula lies in preventing the invasion of the abdominal cavity by bacteria from the gut and from the outside. It is essential, therefore, that the canal joining the gut with the exterior be absolutely tight. This is effected by the direct union of the visceral peritoneum of the intestinal loop with the parietal peritoneum of the abdominal wall around the fistula. (I have not found this necessary in small bowel enterostomies. After the tube, preferably a soft rubber catheter, has been fixed in the intestine I pass the tube through the greater omentum and attach this with several interrupted sutures around the enterostomy. When the tube is removed the opening rapidly closes without leakage into the free cavity. I. S. R.)

1. Establishment of a Nutritive Fistula (Jejunostomy)

Feeding through a jejunostomy becomes necessary when the stomach can not be used for the purpose, or is to be short-circuited for its own protection. This is the case in carcinoma of the stomach which interferes with nutrition or will soon so interfere, and which can no longer be resected and in which a gastro-enterostomy is no longer possible. In the treatment of benign gastric ulcer, jejunostomy for feeding purposes may be used if resection of the diseased gastric segment is impossible and the position of the ulcer near the cardia makes the success of a gastro-enterostomy unlikely. I can testify on the basis of numerous observations to the good effect of such a temporary jejunostomy through which the patient is fed entirely for several months while the stomach is short-circuited and placed at rest. If it is desired to begin prompt feeding of a greatly undernourished patient after a gastric operation of unusual magnitude, perhaps with sutures not wholly secure, as for example in case of a total gastric resection, a prophylactic jejunostomy is an excellent measure to add to the major operation. Finally, jejunostomy is to be preferred over gastrostomy in those cases in which esophageal disease, especially cicatricial stenosis, necessitates fistula feeding, but in which the stomach itself is to be used later for an esophagoplasty and should therefore not have its shape and mobility unfavorably altered.

As high a loop of intestine as possible should be selected to secure complete digestion and utilization of the food. The jejunostomy however is placed at least 50 cm. below the duodenojejunal junction to prevent backflow of the food toward the duodenum and the stomach.

If jejunostomy is performed in connection with another abdominal operation or in the course of an exploratory laparotomy, the major operation is completed first and the jejunostomy is carried out as the last step of the procedure. If the jejunostomy is an independent operation, the abdomen is opened with a median longitudinal incision which begins a few centimeters above the umbilicus and ends a few centimeters below the umbilicus. The total length of the incision is about 8 cm. and depends in the individual case on the accessibility of the proximal jejunal loop. A lateral rectus incision beginning just below the left costal margin may also be used. The operation can be performed under local anesthesia.

After the abdomen is opened the transverse colon is lifted and pushed upward toward the stomach, putting the transverse mesocolon on stretch. The right hand of the surgeon or an intestinal forceps is slipped along the under surface of the mesocolon just to the left of the spine and the proximal jejunal loop is caught. This can be recognized by its origin from the duodeno-jejunal junction and the fact that it can be drawn forward in only one direction. At a distance of about 50 cm. from this fixed point a section of gut is milked empty for a length of 12 cm. and clamped off. On the side opposite the mesenteric attachment a rubber tube is inserted into the jejunum in the manner of a Witzel fistula as described below, the short end of the tube being directed toward the ileocecal junction. If the jejunostomy is to be permanent, a tube with an outer diameter of 7 mm. and a caliber of 4 mm. is used. If the jejunostomy is to be temporary these dimensions are 4 mm. and 2.7 mm. respectively. The tube should be exactly 50 cm. long so that at any time from

Loop of jejunum

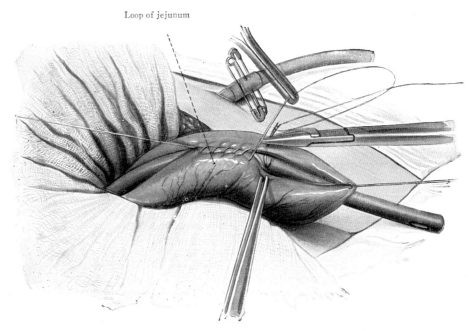

Fig. 163. Jejunostomy (1). A rubber tube, its short end directed distally, is attached to the surface of the gut opposite the mesenteric attachment by the formation of a Witzel canal. The long end of the tube is carried to the exterior through a stab wound in the abdominal wall.

the outside the length of the tube inside the fistula can be determined. The technique of the formation of a Witzel canal in the jejunum corresponds to the procedure described under gastrostomy.

The tube with its short end pointing downstream is fastened to the intestinal wall opposite the mesenteric attachment for a distance of 5 to 6 cm. by throwing up two lateral sero-muscular folds of the intestinal wall around the tube (Fig. 163). The lower end of the tube which is eventually to lie within the intestine should extend below these folds for a distance of 8 to 10 cm. It is important in attaching the tube that one is not mistaken in the direction of the intestinal tract, lest the end of the tube be directed toward the stomach. The two ends of the serosal tunnel are formed first by means of two traction sutures. The intervening portion is formed either by interrupted sutures or by a running suture. In forming the canal the intestinal wall must be used sparingly, just enough to fit snugly around the rubber tube but without narrowing the intestinal lumen too much.

The distal end of the tube is bent back and the wall is picked up close to the point of exit of the tube in two Lembert folds with sutures the ends of which are not yet tied. Between these two Lembert folds and the point of exit of the tube a small incision is made in the gut. The edges of the incision are immediately caught with three small Kocher hemostats or Allis forceps. While these hold the wound open, the free end of the tube is inserted through it with a dissecting forceps (Fig. 164). The last-placed double Lembert sutures are at once drawn taut and tied, which closes and buries the opening in the intestine and the point of entrance of the tube. A few additional sutures secure the closure of the opening. Care must be taken that the free end of

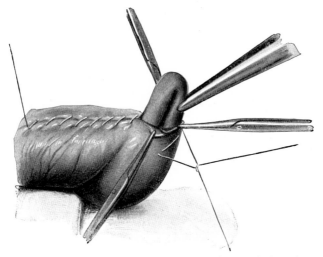

FIG. 164. Jejunostomy (2). The distal end of the tube attached to the surface of the gut is introduced into the gut at the end of the Witzel canal, while the opening of the gut is held open with three hemostats. The first Lembert suture closing the opening in the gut has been applied but will not be tied until after the insertion of the tube into the intestine.

the tube is not bent backward after its introduction into the intestine. It is advisable at this point to inject some fluid through the tube to make sure of its proper placement.

The Witzel canal in the dimensions here advised does not block the intestinal lumen, so that the bile, the other digestive juices and small amounts of food have sufficient room to pass. It is, however, always necessary to test the lumen of the gut as to its adequate patency. Should there be any doubt as to its patency, an entero-enterostomy 4 cm. long is made around the site of the fistula between the proximal and distal loops. (If the jejunostomy has been made properly this should not be necessary. I. S. R.)

A long silk thread is knotted firmly around the tube at the proximal point of exit from the Witzel canal. Each end of the thread is passed from within outward through one each of the two folds of the wall bordering the point of exit of the tube.

If the tube was not carried through a special opening in the abdominal wall at the beginning of the operation, it must next be decided whether the tube is to be carried out through the laparotomy wound or through a special opening.

Since the presence of the tube in the laparotomy wound endangers asepsis, it is better to make a special opening. The free end of the tube is provided with a spear-head bent at a right angle. To this the two ends of the long silk thread previously tied around the tube are fastened by means of a second thread. The left side of the abdominal wound is forcibly elevated with a retractor so that the surgeon standing on the right can see the inner side of the adjacent abdominal wall (Fig. 82). The spear-head is forced through the abdominal wall from within outward at a point a little to the lateral

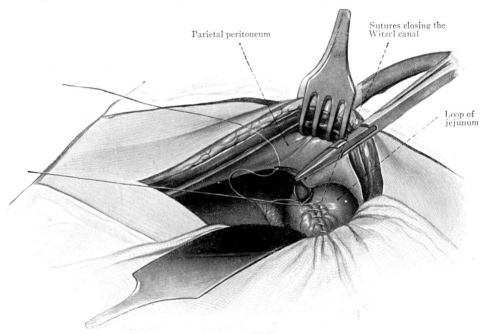

Parietal peritoneum

Sutures closing the
Witzel canal

Loop of
jejunum

FIG. 165. Jejunostomy (3). The tube inserted into the gut has been drawn through a stab wound in the abdominal wall. The visceral peritoneum and the parietal peritoneum are being sutured together at the point of exit of the tube.

side of the lateral border of the left rectus and just below the costal margin. The tube with the two ends of the long silk thread attached to it is pulled through the abdominal wall until the intestinal wall lies tightly against the abdominal wall. One end of the silk thread, which is now on the outside of the abdomen, is mounted on a straight needle and passed through the skin edge of the fistula opening from within outward, and the two ends then are tied together on the skin surface. This pulls the upper end of the Witzel canal against the parietal peritoneum.

Instead of drawing the silk thread, which is attached to the tube and the gut at the end of the Witzel canal, through the abdominal wall to the body surface, it may be mounted on a curved needle and, while the left edge of the abdominal wound is forcibly elevated, passed through the parietal peritoneum just beside the point of exit of the tube and tied (Fig. 165). This also brings visceral and parietal peritoneum into close union. It is also advisable to apply a few such auxiliary sutures in the first type of procedure.

If the tube is to be brought out through the laparotomy wound itself, the two ends of the long thread are passed through the parietal peritoneum from within outward at the lower angle of the abdominal incision, one end on each side of the wound. Here they are tied, so that the end of the Witzel canal is pulled against the parietal peritoneum at the lower angle of the wound (Fig. 166). A second suture can be passed in a similar manner on the other side of the tube through the intestinal wall and the peritoneum. The abdominal incision is closed in the usual way up to the point of exit of the tube. The tube is again fastened to the skin by a separate suture and attached to the body in the manner described in Vol. I, page 287.

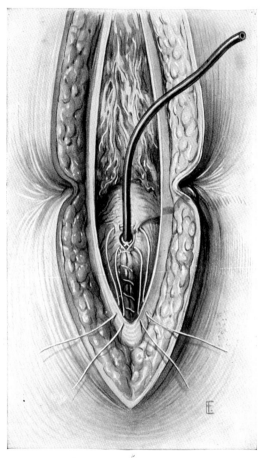

If the tube should slip out of the fistula prematurely, or if it is removed purposely at the end of 2 to 3 weeks, its reintroduction must be attempted only with the greatest care. If it cannot be reintroduced easily, a new jejunostomy must be established by means of a second laparotomy.

If the fistula does not enclose the tube snugly, a smaller tube is inserted for a few days, which is followed by a rapid narrowing of the fistula. The skin around the fistulous opening must always be carefully dressed and covered with zinc oxide ointment.

The administration of food and fluids through the jejunos-

FIG. 166. Jejunostomy (4). The tube, one end of which has been inserted into the gut, may be carried out of the abdominal cavity at the lower end of the midline abdominal incision. The visceral peritoneum is being attached to the parietal peritoneum with two sutures.

tomy is begun at once in a patient operated upon under local anaesthesia; in case of general anaesthesia, as soon as the patient has regained consciousness and the post-anaesthetic vomiting is over. In general, the patient may be given 500 to 1000 cc. of fluid and an equal number of calories on the day of operation. On the following day, the fluid and caloric intake through the tube is raised to 1000 to 2000. This will depend, however, on the subjective feelings of the patient which are the most important and deciding guide as to quantity, frequency and concentration of feedings. Fluids and nourishment may at first be given to the patient gradually, drop by drop, by attaching an irrigator and a Martin drop-bulb (Vol. I, Fig. 242) to the jejunostomy tube. Patients usually soon tolerate larger quantities, the food being injected very slowly with a 50 cc. syringe. One or two syringefuls are given at each feeding. An increase of the individual feeding usually gives the patient a sensation of pressure in the abdomen. The material must be warmed carefully to 40° C. I use a specially made glass syringe whose tip is larger than the caliber of the tube (Fig. 167). The syringe can also be used to inject semi-fluid food and finely-chopped meat.

Under ordinary conditions the patient receives sufficient fluid and nourishment through the jejunostomy to meet his needs completely, so that oral feeding can be dispensed with.

It is well known that patients may be kept indefinitely in an excellent state of nutrition and strength by jejunostomy feeding alone. While experienced jejunostomy patients can plan their own diet in time, it is necessary to feed patients freshly operated upon according to strict rules. For this purpose the following mixture has proved most satisfactory.

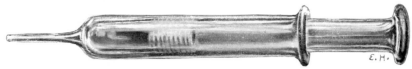

FIG. 167. Glass syringe for introducing material through the jejunostomy tube.

Jejunostomy Feeding Mixture. A feeding mixture sufficient for 24 hours is prepared in the following manner:

1750 cc. whole milk	= 1225 cal.	(100 cc. = 70 cal.)
50 g. barley meal	= 200 "	(100 g. = 400 ")
50 g. glucose	= 200 "	(100 g. = 400 ")
200 cc. cream + 5 g. table salt	= 400 "	(100 cc. = 200 ")

This mixture = 2025 calories.

After cooking, the quantity is brought up to 2 liters with water. On cooling, 5 cc. of lactic acid are added with constant stirring. The mixture is cooled and kept in the refrigerator. The amount needed for each feeding is warmed just before it is used to 40° C. and is passed through a fine strainer.

One cubic centimeter of the mixture contains about one calorie. In exclusive jejunostomy feeding the patient as a rule should receive 2 liters of the mixture, which equals about 2000 calories, in 24 hours. Morawitz and Hennig give 40 calories per kilo, or 2800 calories for a 70 kilo patient. A somewhat smaller amount meets the subjective desire for fluid and nourishment. Not more than 100 cc., 2 syringefuls, are usually given at a feeding. The injection of 100 cc. should take from 3 to 5 minutes. Each feeding is followed by the injection of a little luke-warm water to cleanse the tube.

If the patient complains of pain, pressure sensations or discomfort during the injection of the feeding mixture, the mixture is diluted with water and the quantity of the feeding is reduced. In exceptional cases one may resort temporarily to 5 per cent glucose solution or physiologic salt solution, or jejunal feeding may have to be stopped completely for a time. The subjective sensations of the patient are the best guide to the amount and frequency of the feedings and should always be considered. If digestive disturbances (diarrhoea) arise, barley water or rice water should be used, to which may be added the usual medicaments (paregoric, bismuth, chalk or tincture of kino). I have never observed the flow of the nutriment material toward the stomach if the lumen of the gut toward the ileocecal region is patent.

2. ESTABLISHMENT OF A FECAL FISTULA (FISTULA STERCORALIS)

(A) GENERAL CONSIDERATIONS

An external fistula for the evacuation of the gaseous, fluid and solid contents of the intestine may be established for a limited time or it may be established permanently.

In making a temporary fistula it is necessary to consider its eventual closure at the time the fistula is established. This requires that only a lateral opening be made for the escape of the fecal matter while the natural channel is preserved so that the intestinal contents can reach the distal portion of the bowel. For a permanent fecal fistula, a lateral opening should rarely be used and only when the patient is so weak that he can no longer be subjected to the more formidable operation for a permanent artificial anus.

On the other hand, a permanent opening for the evacuation of the intestinal contents is usually made in such a way that all of the fecal matter must pass through the artificial channel. Such a terminal opening is called an artificial anus (anus praeternaturalis).

The establishment of a lateral fecal fistula is done as a preliminary operation before attacking a lesion of the intestine, especially when the lesion causes a stenosis. This makes it possible to evacuate the intestinal contents before the main operation for the removal of the lesion, to "detoxify" the patient and to empty the intestine thoroughly before attacking the major lesion. Such a fistula is allowed to remain for some time after the major operation in order to relieve the operative site of any tension. The advantages of such postoperative relief can be so great that a lateral intestinal fistula is often established at the end of intestinal operations of unusual magnitude, especially when the security of the intestinal sutures at the site of the main operation seems doubtful.

In acute mechanical ileus without circulatory changes in the intestine a fecal fistula is established if the mechanical obstruction cannot be removed at the time, or if a short-circuiting operation in the form of an entero-enterostomy between the proximal and distal intestinal loops cannot be performed. (I frequently provide a fistula after an operation for acute intestinal obstruction when the proximal portion of the bowel is distended with fluid even though the obstruction has been relieved. I. S. R.) In paralytic ileus an intestinal fistula in the small bowel should be considered when peristalsis is not reestablished after the main operation directed against the peritonitis and when there is reason to assume that only individual segments of intestine are paralysed and the relatively normal segments do not have the strength to force the intestinal contents through the paralysed segments, or that the intestinal paralysis is caused by the overdistention of a restricted part of the intestine and will disappear if these loops are sufficiently evacuated. For these reasons an ileostomy is also recommended as a prophylactic measure at the end of an operation for peritonitis where paralytic ileus is feared (Heidenhain).

A lateral fecal fistula may be established at any point in the intestinal canal. To obtain the maximum absorption from ingested contents, a site is selected as low as possible in the intestinal canal, contingent of course on the site of the lesion. The order of preference is therefore, sigmoidostomy, colostomy, cecostomy and ileostomy.

In the individual case the choice of location depends upon the site of the lesion. Since a water-tight closure of the fistulous canal from the abdominal cavity is a fundamental prerequisite, only those parts of the intestinal canal are considered for the establishing of fistulae which because of their mobility can be brought without difficulty to the anterior or lateral abdominal wall. These are the sigmoid, the transverse colon, the cecum and all parts of the small intestine. The ascending and the descending colon cannot be used for a lateral fecal fistula. If there is a localized lesion, if its position can be accurately determined and if an operative attack on the lesion is to be made later, the site of the subsequent laparotomy incision is considered in selecting the location of the fistula, so that the cleanliness of the later operative site will be safeguarded. For example, if the lesion is to be attacked through a midline incision, the cecum is to be preferred to the transverse colon as the site of the fistula, even though the lesion is in the sigmoid.

In most instances the site of an obstruction in the large bowel can be established by a barium enema. However if, in the case of ileus, an accurate localization of the lesion is impossible at the moment, and if it does not seem advantageous to localize it and determine its character by an extensive laparotomy, the fistula should be made in a loop of intestine whose excessive distention shows that it is proximal to the obstruction. The abdomen should then be opened over the point where peristaltic waves stand out most clearly, or where, in case of paralytic ileus, the most markedly distended loops are situated as determined by the X-ray and the fistula is made in the first greatly distended loop which presents itself. If there is absolutely no indication of the exact site of a possible obstruction, and if an exploratory laparotomy does not seem expedient, the abdomen is opened in the right hypogastrium, and the distended cecum or, if it be empty, the first distended loop of intestine which can be reached is used.

For a sigmoidostomy, the abdomen is opened by a lateral rectus incision below the umbilicus or by a gridiron incision on the left side. For a colostomy in the region of the transverse colon, a midline longitudinal incision just above the umbilicus is used. For a cecostomy, one employs a lateral rectus incision below the umbilicus or a gridiron incision on the right side. For an ileostomy, an incision is made directly over the most distended part of the lower abdomen.

(B) THE ESTABLISHMENT OF A FECAL FISTULA WITH FORMATION OF A SEROUS CANAL (WITZEL)

The tube used in forming the fistula is usually brought to the surface through the laparotomy wound. It is often better from the standpoint of technique however, in order to maintain asepsis in the main laparotomy wound, to lead the tube out through an opening immediately overlying the segment of gut used for the fistula. To pass the tube through a separate opening in the abdominal wall, the spear-head which was described and illustrated on page 101 under jejunostomy and gastrostomy, may be used to advantage. The operation can be performed under local anaesthesia.

The technique for establishing a lateral fecal fistula in the small bowel differs in no fundamental respect from the technique for a nutritive fistula. The Witzel canal is preferable for a temporary fecal fistula because it can be depended upon to prevent leakage. The free end of the rubber tube within the gut is however pointed upstream, if the direction of the loop of gut can be determined. Only in a cecostomy is the tube end directed downstream, since the head of the cecum is more mobile than the remainder of it and can therefore be fastened more easily to the anterior abdominal wall for the exit of the tube. (In a temporary fistula of the cecum I prefer to pass the tube through the stump of the excised appendix. I. S. R.)

In acute ileus, especially acute paralytic ileus, there may be difficulty in delivering an intestinal loop in the presence of the marked overdistention of the gut which frequently exists. In these cases the wall tears easily and the loops, because of their huge size, can only be brought through a small laparotomy wound with difficulty. Further difficulties which may arise are that the loop intended for the site of the fistula cannot be milked empty because of the excessive amount of its contents as well as that of the neighboring intestinal segments. The marked tension of the intestinal wall often does not permit the folding necessary for the Witzel canal. The needles pass all the way through the wall which may be as thin as paper. The sutures cut out with the slightest tension. In such cases the loop is delivered as carefully as possible and, without any regard to its contents, is closed at both ends by a spring clamp. The isolated segment, after careful walling off of the surroundings, is punctured with a medium-sized trocar and cannula with a diameter of 3 to 5 mm. to which is attached an electric suction pump (Fig. 168), or with a large-bore needle on a large syringe, and is emptied of its contents. When the loop has been collapsed and relieved of tension, the Witzel canal can usually be constructed around the tube without further difficulty. The puncture opening is used as the portal of entry for the tube or else is included within the Witzel canal.

The gaseous and fluid contents of the small bowel will as a rule pass through a fairly small tube without difficulty. However a tube of fair size should be selected, in view of the fact that solid food particles may occasionally be present. Because of the inspissation of the feces in the large bowel, a fairly large rubber tube must be used here, not less than 3.5 to 4 mm. in bore and 7 mm. in external diameter. Even such a tube will transmit only gas, fluid and possibly mushy material, but not inspissated feces. Although the evacuation of gas and fluid in acute ileus of the large bowel may temporarily result in a material and adequate relief, it is not permanently adequate, so that in case of an unrelieved obstruction in the large bowel it will eventually be necessary to enlarge the fistula.

Such an enlargement of a Witzel fistula can be carried out as follows: After several days, when the parietal and visceral peritoneum are firmly adherent in the region of the fistula, the Witzel canal is stretched by inserting glass or rubber tubes of increasing size. The edge of the tract may have to be nicked with a knife. This procedure is however not always successful, covers a long period of time, and is not without danger, in view of the chance

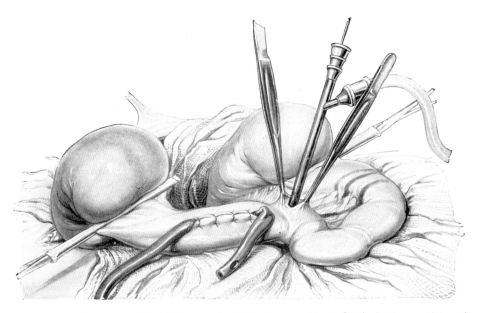

FIG. 168. Ileostomy. Establishment of a Witzel type of fecal fistula in the small bowel. A fairly heavy rubber tube is attached by means of a Witzel canal to the surface of the gut which was first milked empty and clamped on each side. The gut is punctured at the proximal end of the canal and is emptied by suction. After the removal of the trocar and cannula the short end of the rubber tube is introduced into the gut through this opening and buried with Lembert sutures.

of opening the free peritoneal cavity. It is better to make the opening large enough at the start, in which case the formation of a Witzel canal is usually dispensed with.

(c) THE ESTABLISHMENT OF A DIRECT FECAL FISTULA

The surface of the gut is sutured in a circle to an opening in the abdominal wall and the communication of the gut lumen with the exterior is made directly or by means of a wide glass or rubber tube. Before opening the bowel an absolutely tight closure against the general abdominal cavity must be provided for. For this purpose, the surface of the loop to be opened, in an area two to three centimeters in diameter and opposite the mesenteric attachment, is sutured to the parietal peritoneum of the wound edge with a sero-muscular suture (Fig. 169). If the loop is greatly distended, it may at times be impossible to avoid piercing its wall with the needle. Intestinal contents which may escape through the stitch wounds must be sponged off at once and the site reinforced. The head of the cecum, because of its great mobility, is especially well fitted for the establishment of such a lateral fistula.

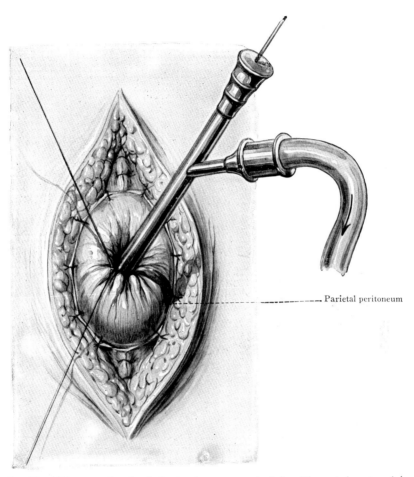

Parietal peritoneum

FIG. 169. Establishment of a fecal fistula (enterostomy) (1). The gut is sutured in a circle to the opening in the parietal peritoneum. It is punctured with a trocar through the midpoint of a purse-string suture applied to the gut wall and is emptied by suction. The purse-string suture is pulled taut as soon as the trocar is inserted to prevent the escape of intestinal contents.

The circular suture of the intestinal loop to the parietal peritoneum is facilitated and the adhesion of gut to abdominal wall is hastened, if, in the abdominal wound, the free edge of the parietal peritoneum is first attached by suture to the edge of the skin and the loop is then sutured to the parietal peritoneum lining the abdominal wound.

It is best to wait several days, if possible, before opening an intestinal loop sutured to the wound in this manner, until the parietal and visceral peritoneum are tightly adherent and the wound is covered with granulation tissue. This greatly lessens the danger of infection of the abdominal cavity and of the wound. In the meantime, the exposed loop may be aspirated repeatedly, effecting a certain amount of deflation and relief, but without flooding the wound with intestinal contents. The final opening is made with the electrosurgical knife.

However, in most cases of acute intestinal obstruction the bowel must be opened at once. The following measures will protect the operative wound from excessive soiling by the intestinal contents at the time the opening is made and for the next few days: In the center of the exposed loop, which has been carefully walled off from the general abdominal cavity, a purse-string

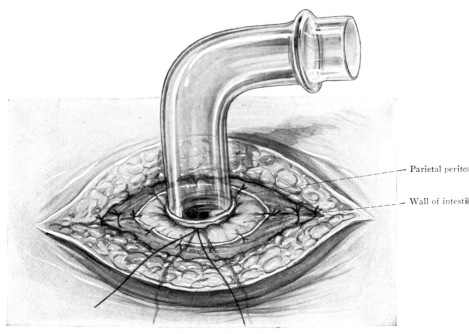

Parietal perito
Wall of intesti

Fig. 170. Enterostomy (2). After the gut is evacuated by suction, a glass tube is tied into the opening by means of the purse-string suture.

suture is applied in a circle about one centimeter in diameter, the ends being looped but not tied. The gut wall is picked up in the center of the purse-string with two tissue forceps. A trocar and cannula, not too small, and provided with a lateral exit with rubber tube attached, is plunged through the intestinal wall between the forceps (Fig. 169). At the moment the tip of the trocar enters the gut, an assistant tightens the thread of the purse-string around it, but without knotting the ends. The obturator is withdrawn and the intestinal contents are evacuated.

When the gut is sufficiently emptied so that no more contents flow out of the cannula, it is replaced by a firm-walled rubber tube or by a Paul-Mixter glass tube (Fig. 170). After the removal of the cannula from the gut, the edges of the opening are caught with three Allis forceps, raised and spread, reopening the purse-string, the ends of which have been only looped together. The tube is inserted into the opening and is fastened by knotting the purse-string. The rubber or glass tube is anchored to the abdominal wall so that it will not exert any traction on the intestinal wall. Such a closure remains tight for 5 days or longer. If it begins to leak, it may again be secured for a few days by adding a second purse-string around the first.

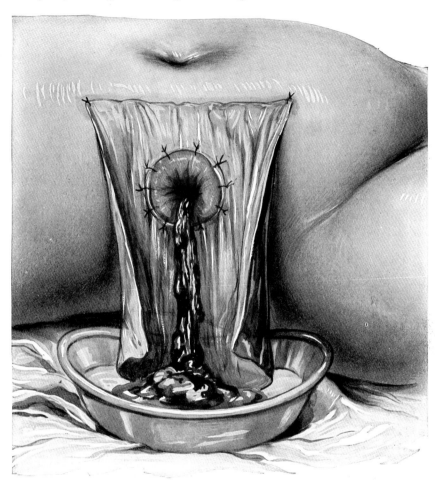

FIG. 171. Fecal fistula apron (Hartert) (3). A rectangular piece of rubber dam is attached to the skin and a circular opening in the material sutured to the muco-cutaneous junction of the fecal fistula.

In order to prevent soiling of the surrounding field by a fecal fistula, Hartert covers the skin in the immediate neighborhood of the fistula with a thick layer of zinc oxide ointment and then glues a rectangular piece of some impervious material over the fistulous opening, cuts a round hole in the material directly over the fistulous opening and sutures the edge of the hole to the edge of the intestinal opening (Fig. 171). The two upper corners of the rectangle can be fastened to the skin by sutures. The lower border of the rectangle is gathered together and placed into a basin for the collection of the fecal matter. Such an apron can be made with Billroth batiste and mastisol, or preferably with Ultraplast and Ultrasol which is made by Schack and Pearson, in Hamburg.

If an intestinal fistula is to be permanent, the edge of the mucosa of the intestine is sutured all around to the skin edge, forming a lipped fistula (Fig. 172).

If a fecal fistula shows a tendency to premature narrowing or closure, this may usually be prevented by bouginage or by the insertion of glass or rubber tubes. Otherwise the opening is enlarged by a radial incision and the new wound edges of skin and mucosa are sutured together.

An excessive bulging of the mucosa of an intestinal fistula is only rarely observed and can be removed by trimming with the electrosurgical knife. In case of frank prolapse, the measures described on page 362 under the treatment of prolapse of the natural anus are employed.

The skin around an intestinal fistula, as far as it comes in contact with intestinal contents, is cleansed daily and is covered with a thick layer of zinc oxide ointment.

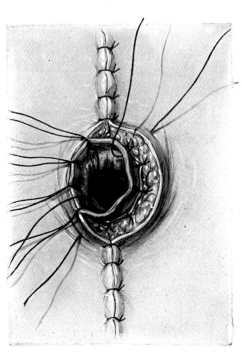

FIG. 172. Enterostomy (4). Establishment of a lipped fistula. Several days later, after the removal of the glass tube the mucosa of the intestinal opening is sutured on all sides to the margin of the skin.

(D) APPENDICOSTOMY AND CECOSTOMY

Appendicostomy. The establishment of a fistula leading into the cecum may be carried out by using the appendix. Since the caliber of the appendix is quite small, a fistula made in this way is less suitable for the evacuation of solid fecal matter than for the evacuation of gases and for the irrigation of a chronically inflamed colon. The narrowness and the length of a fistulous canal formed by the appendix insure a fairly certain closure of the structure around a catheter inserted into it, so that the patient is scarcely bothered by the undesired escape of gas and feces.

The appendix is sought for and mobilized through a lateral rectus or a gridiron incision, made as small as possible as described on page 299. The appendix is partly freed from its mesentery and is sufficiently mobilized that its tip can be drawn out of the abdominal wound. Trophic disturbances of the appendix, the result of too extensive ligation of its mesentery, are to be avoided because of the danger of peritonitis. A long forceps is introduced into the abdomen and is pressed forward from within against the abdominal wall near the right groin. An incision is made from the outside down on the forceps and its tip is forced outward from within, making a small opening. A second forceps, inserted into the jaws of the first, is pulled into the abdomen, grasps the appendix by its tip and pulls the appendix out through the opening. A few sutures fasten the appendix to the skin (Fig. 173). The laparotomy wound is closed. After a week the appendix is cut off flush with the skin. The mucosa is sutured to the skin, forming a lipped fistula.

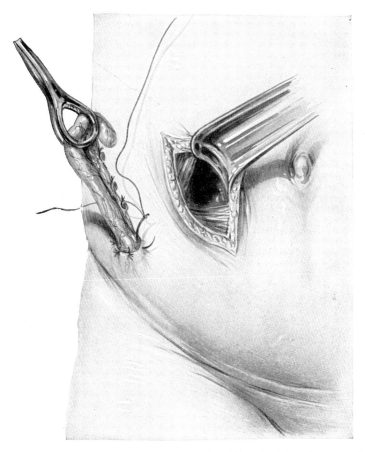

Fig. 173. Appendicostomy. Through a lateral gridiron incision the appendix is found and partly freed from its mesentery. The appendix is then pulled out through a small opening in the abdominal wall and sutured on all sides to the margin of the skin.

A Nelaton catheter can now be passed at any time through the stump of the appendix and through it accumulated gases can escape and irrigations be performed.

If the appendix is brought out through a gridiron incision, it can easily be pulled out as far as its funnel-shaped junction with the cecum, and sutured to the parietal peritoneum at this point. By amputating the appendix at this level, the diameter of the fistula is enlarged.

Cecostomy. In the further development of this procedure, the appendix can be used as an excellent handle for the establishment of a cecal fistula

(Figs. 174 and 175). The cecum is pulled out by the appendix for a short distance through a gridiron incision. It is sutured to the wound edge in a larger circle, and a portion of the cecum is later excised so that the opening will permit the insertion and anchoring of a fair-sized tube. Before suturing the cecum to the wound edge, the abdominal wound may be lined throughout with peritoneum by suturing the edge of the parietal peritoneum to the skin.

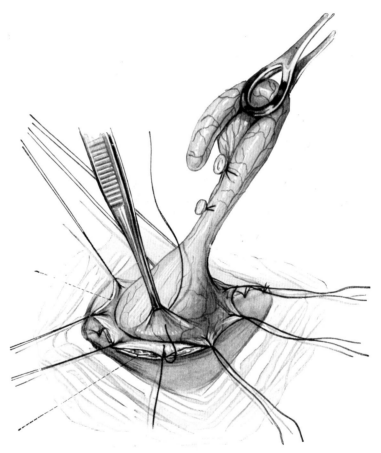

Fig. 174. Cecostomy. The cecum is reached through a lateral gridiron incision and is delivered by traction on the appendix which has been freed of its mesentery. The parietal peritoneum in the region of the abdominal wound is sutured to the skin edge on all sides. The dome of the cecum is attached to the edge of the wound by means of the same sutures.

This facilitates the attachment of the cecum and hastens the formation of adhesions. The circular suture of cecum and parietal peritoneum can be further secured by tying a slender gauze roll (cigarette wick) along the line of suture. Cecostomy makes possible a free evacuation of feces. (It has been the experience in our clinic that a cecostomy is never as satisfactory as a sigmoidostomy. The procedure outlined is satisfactory for a permanent cecostomy. If the obstructing lesion is in the lower sigmoid I prefer a sigmoid colostomy so that a large portion of the colon does not remain between the

artificial anus and the obstructing lesion. In a temporary cecostomy I place
a Paul's tube in the cecum with a double purse-string suture or when it is
used both for the relief of colonic distention and for the administration of
fluids I insert a Nelaton catheter through the stump of the amputated appendix. A larger tube is threaded over the catheter and pushed down to the point
where the purse-string sutures hold the catheter into the cecum. The cecum

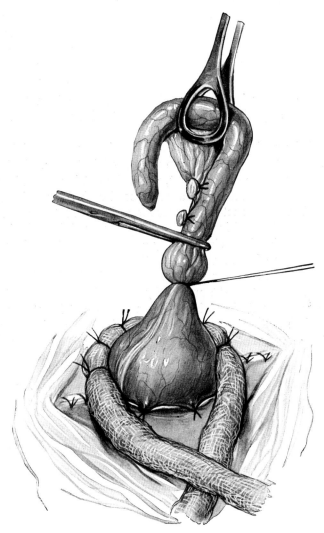

Fig. 175. Cecostomy. With the same sutures by which the cecum was attached to the
edges of the abdominal incision, a cigarette tampon is fastened in a circle around the cecum.
The appendix has been ligated and will be amputated.

is not sutured to the parietal peritoneum. The catheter may be used for the
relief of distention and for the introduction of normal saline solution at a very
advantageous point. When the catheter is withdrawn leakage of intestinal
contents rarely occurs and if it does the larger drainage tube takes care of
this. The method was described a few years ago by Wilson. I. S. R.)

D. ESTABLISHMENT OF AN ARTIFICIAL ANUS (ANUS PRAETERNATURALIS)

The functional difference between a fecal fistula and an artificial anus lies in the fact that a fecal fistula merely forms a lateral escape-valve and the intestinal contents can still pass into the distal portion of the intestine as before. With an artificial anus, on the other hand, all of the fecal matter must escape through this passage and its entrance into the distal segment of the gut is prevented. The anatomic difference lies in the fact that in the establishment of an artificial anus the continuity of the gut is interrupted and the open end at least of the proximal loop, frequently of both loops, is implanted into an opening in the abdominal wall, while in a temporary fecal fistula only a lateral opening is made into an intestine the continuity of which is preserved.

In view of the radical nature of this procedure, an artificial anus is used only as a permanent measure in the majority of instances. It is used after the extirpation of a whole gut segment, when the gut is removed as far as the anus, or the bowel can no longer be anastomosed with the proximal limb, as in case of amputation of the rectum, or resection of both rectum and sigmoid. It is also used in short-circuiting an incurably diseased intestinal segment, if this segment cannot be short-circuited by an entero-anastomosis, as in case of inoperable carcinoma of the lower colon, the rectum and the sigmoid. From these considerations it becomes evident that the indication for the establishment of a permanent artificial anus rarely occurs in the small intestine. (In certain cases of advanced ulcerative colitis a permanent ileostomy is indicated however. I. S. R.) Moreover, such a measure is to be avoided for the reason that sufficient fluid may not be absorbed after the short-circuiting of the entire large bowel. As a rule, therefore, a permanent artificial anus is established only in the large bowel.

An artificial anus is established as a temporary measure only when, after an intestinal resection, the normal intestinal passage cannot be primarily reestablished. In such a case, the procedure takes the form of a double-barreled anus if at all possible, with a view to its subsequent closure.

The division of the intestine necessary for the complete exclusion of the distal segment is either performed at one operation, or the gut may retain its continuity for the time being and be eventrated and subsequently divided. Subsequent division is to be preferred in view of the lessened danger of infection. In primary division of the bowel for the formation of an artificial anus, only the proximal loop needs to be brought to the surface; the distal loop may be closed and dropped. In secondary division, the full diameter of the continuous loop of gut, that is, both its proximal and distal limbs, must be fixed outside the abdominal wall.

1. Establishment of an Artificial Anus in an Eventrated Continuous Loop of Intestine

The eventration of a continuous loop of the large bowel is possible only in its mobile segments or in segments which can be sufficiently mobilized without endangering their nutrition. This restricts the procedure to those portions of the bowel which have a free mesentery, the transverse colon and the sigmoid. Difficulties are encountered even at the hepatic and splenic flexures. Eventration is impossible in the region of the ascending and descending colon. The establishment of an artificial anus in the large bowel as the sole operative procedure is theoretically, therefore, performed only in the transverse colon and in the sigmoid.

(A) ESTABLISHMENT OF AN ARTIFICIAL ANUS IN A LONG EVENTRATED LOOP

The technique of establishing an artificial anus with preservation of the continuity of the bowel is essentially the same in all regions. It is only necessary to describe the most frequently used type of artificial anus as performed in the sigmoid on a long eventrated loop as an example of the procedures generally used.

The abdomen is opened by a left lateral rectus incision below the umbilicus or by a gridiron incision close to the left anterior superior iliac spine. If the gridiron incision does not provide sufficient room to bring out the intestinal loop, it is enlarged by lateral incisions. Rigid aponeuroses or muscle bundles which would constrict the bowel as it passes through are radially incised. The nearer the anal opening is to the groin, the less it will annoy the patient.

The sigmoid flexure may usually be picked up easily close to the left ilium after the abdomen is opened and be delivered without difficulty. At times, however, adhesions on the left side of the mesosigmoid must be cut; this is made easier by making strong traction on the sigmoid loop. Only rarely is the mesosigmoid so short that it is difficult to draw the apex of the flexure out of the wound. The loop is so placed that the proximal limb is at the upper angle of the wound and the distal limb at the lower angle. It must be remembered that the position in which the loop happens to be found in the abdomen tells nothing of its direction. In each case the direction of the course of the loop must be determined by following the limbs to the rectum and the descending colon. The confusion of the proximal and the distal limbs and the consequent closure and dropping of the proximal loop has repeatedly proved disastrous.

The mesosigmoid is pierced at its widest point close to the gut by a forceps. With the aid of the forceps, a rubber tube or a strip of gauze is pulled through the opening. This opening is further enlarged by tying off and dividing bit by bit a strip of the mesentery close to its attachment to the gut for a distance of 3 to 4 cm. In view of the fork-like attachment of the mesentery, the ligatures are placed alternately on the right and left sides of the mesentery. As soon as the slit in the mesentery is large enough, a second rubber tube or a second strip of gauze is passed through it.

The abdominal wound may be prepared to receive the sigmoid loop by suturing the edge of the parietal peritoneum in a circle to the edge of the skin. This measure, which is intended to effect an organic closure of the abdominal cavity and a protection for the wound in the abdominal wall against the later escape of feces, is however unnecessary and seems particularly superfluous if the gut is not to be opened for several days.

The central portion of the abdominal wound is now sutured together through the slit in the mesentery (Fig. 176). The freed loop of the sigmoid lies over the suture line, while the limbs of the loop enter the abdominal cavity at the angles of the wound. During the suturing, the loop of gut is elevated and drawn to the right by means of the rubber tubes or strips of gauze beneath it. The midportion of the right edge of the wound is grasped from the left with two Kocher forceps which were passed through the slit in the mesentery and is pulled through the slit into contact with the left edge. Two or three sutures can now be passed with ease through the right and left edges of the wound and tied beneath the loop of intestine. All the layers of the abdominal

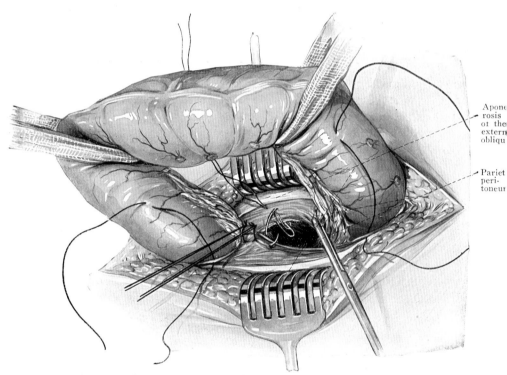

Apone
rosis
ot the
extern
obliqu

Pariet
peri-
toneur

FIG. 176. Artificial anus. The dome of the sigmoid loop is freed from its mesentery for a distance of about 6 cm. and elevated by two gauze loops. Beneath the gut the two edges of the abdominal wound are sutured together so that the loop of intestine lies on the abdominal wall. On each side there has been inserted, but not yet tied, one of the sutures which will fasten the limbs of sigmoid to the parietal peritoneum as they pass through the abdominal wall.

wall except the skin may be included in each suture, or the sutures may be placed in separate layers, usually peritoneum and the deeper layers in the first tier of sutures and the superficial layers in the second.

If the abdominal incision is so long that the two limbs on reentering the abdomen are too widely separated, the upper angle of the wound is closed as far as desired before beginning the suture through the mesenteric slit. As a rule, however, the original wound is too small so that the limbs of the loop are encroached upon, with resultant interference with the passage of feces and with the nutrition of the gut. The incision must then be lengthened before its central portion is sutured. The distance between the two limbs of the loop as they pass through the abdominal wall should be about 3 cm.

Traction on the rubber tube or the strip of gauze is relaxed, permitting the limbs of gut to be replaced as far as possible in the abdomen. They are then securely sutured in a circle to the parietal peritoneum at the point where they pass through the abdominal wall. This completes the closure of the abdominal cavity. Finally the edges of the skin are sutured through the mesenteric slit and beneath the eventrated loop of gut (Fig. 177), and are attached to the limbs of the loop with a few sutures. When the dressing is applied, a layer of gauze is placed beneath the loop so that the intestine does not lie directly on the skin.

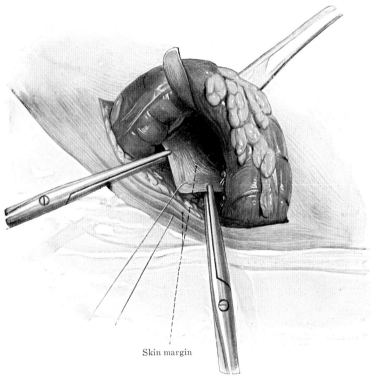

Skin margin

FIG. 177. Artificial anus. The skin wound is sutured beneath the eventrated loop of sigmoid.

If there is no need for haste in opening the artificial anus, the patient is given opiates to splint the bowel. During the next few days the intestine may be relieved of accumulated gases by aspirating the eventrated loop with a medium-sized needle. At times one can observe the passage of intestinal contents through the eventrated loop to be evacuated through the normal channels. When it becomes necessary in a day or in a few days, a small incision for the escape of gases is made at the apex of the intestinal loop for which incision I use the electrosurgical knife (Fig. 178). A few days later, the anterior wall of the loop is divided longitudinally. The complete division of the bowel and the amputation of the eventrated loop at the level of the skin should be delayed until the end of two weeks, since the segments, when deprived of their contents, often show a tendency for some time to slip back into the abdominal cavity.

If it is necessary to open the bowel sooner, it may be done either immediately at the end of the operation or on the following day by dividing the anterior wall.

The establishment, just described, of an artificial anus with a long eventrated loop in which the proximal and distal limbs are separated by a narrow bridge of abdominal wall as they reach the exterior has the following advantages over an artificial anus with a short eventrated loop (to be described in the next section) in which both limbs lie in a common opening: The eventrated loop cannot slip back into the abdomen under any circumstances, and later, it

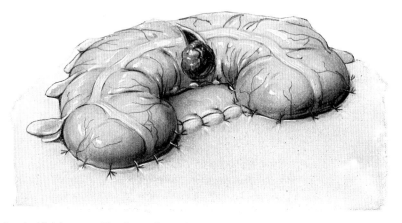

Fig. 178. Artificial anus. The loop of gut lies on the closed abdominal wall. The sigmoid is opened 24 to 48 hours later for the evacuation of feces.

is possible to carry out separate treatment of the distal loop with irrigations, etc., without involving the proximal loop.

The skin, instead of being closed beneath the eventrated loop of colon at the end of the operation, may be sutured over it, so that the segment of colon lies subcutaneous for some distance. Later the loop is divided only at the distal angle of the wound and the open ends of the proximal and distal limbs are sutured to the edge of the skin wound. After healing has taken place it is then possible to compress the subcutaneous limb of gut leading to the artificial anus by means of a pressure pad, and in this way to exert a regulating influence on the evacuation of the feces. If this type of formation of the artificial anus is decided upon in advance, it is better to make the skin incision in the form of a flap so that the pressure pad will not lie directly on the cutaneous scar.

(B) ESTABLISHMENT OF AN ARTIFICIAL ANUS IN A SHORT EVENTRATED LOOP

Somewhat simpler is the establishment of an artificial anus according to the original procedure of Maydl. After the abdomen has been opened, the sigmoid loop is found and mobilized and a rubber tube or a gauze strip is passed beneath it in the manner just described. The proximal and distal limbs are sutured together side to side for a distance of a few centimeters, the sutures being placed so that they do not include the mesosigmoid. The abdominal incision, if it be too large, is closed at one end until the two limbs of gut can just comfortably pass through side by side. The ∩-shaped loop of intestine is replaced in the abdomen as far as the level of the rubber tube or gauze which supports it, and is sutured in its circumference to the parietal

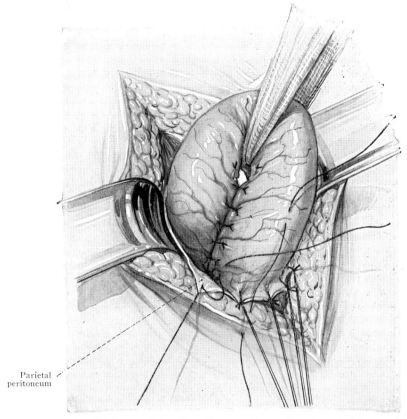

Parietal
peritoneum

FIG. 179. Artificial anus (Maydl). The two limbs of an intestinal loop, which has been elevated on a gauze roll, are sutured together for some distance, avoiding their mesenteric attachments. The serous surface of the two limbs of gut is sutured to the parietal peritoneum in such a way that the dome of the intestinal loop remains outside of the abdominal wall. One of the sutures with which the loop will be attached on all sides to the skin has been inserted but not tied.

peritoneum (Fig. 179). The skin may be attached to it with a few sutures. The rubber tube or gauze strip lying beneath the loop of gut is attached to the skin by one suture on each side.

In a corresponding manner an artificial anus may be established after the eventration procedure at other points in the bowel, especially in the transverse colon. The greater omentum is first separated from the eventrated loop so as not to lie outside of the wound. It is at times necessary to resect the gastrocolic omentum for a short distance in order to obtain sufficient mobility.

If evacuation through an artificial anus is insufficient at first, a catheter, a rectal tube, or a stomach tube is passed into the proximal loop and an enema is given. Obstructing hard fecal masses can be removed with a gall stone spoon or with the exploring finger. In case of doubt the patency of the proximal loop at its point of exit through the abdominal wall must be determined by inserting a gloved finger.

(c) ESTABLISHMENT OF A DOUBLE-BARRELLED ARTIFICIAL ANUS

If it is intended to close an artificial anus at a later time, this subsequent closure is provided for at the establishment of the artificial anus by suturing the proximal and distal limbs of the gut to each other for a distance of 8 to 10 cm. like the double barrel of a shotgun. The line of suture is kept as far away from the line of the attachment of the mesentery as possible (Figs. 234 and 235). If the mesentery is avoided, there is no danger of severe bleeding when the septum dividing the two lumina is subsequently crushed. The doubled portion of bowel is replaced within the abdominal cavity as far as the point where the rubber tube passes through the mesentery and the projecting dome of the loop is sutured to the edges of the abdominal wound which is made small for the purpose. After the subsequent opening and amputation of the projecting dome of the loop, the proximal and distal limbs lie in direct contact for a considerable distance inside the abdominal cavity, and the septum which separates them can be crushed without danger of injuring either loop of intestine. The technique of closure is described and illustrated on page 253.

Almost the same type of procedure is used in the two-stage intestinal resection, in which the diseased loop is eventrated before it is opened. The technique of this procedure, which includes in a single operation the formation of a special type of artificial anus and intestinal resection of a special type, differs from the procedure just described simply in that the eventrated segment consists not of a small normal dome, but of a large loop which is the site of the lesion. For details, see intestinal resection, page 286.

2. ESTABLISHMENT OF AN ARTIFICIAL ANUS WITH TRANSSECTION OF THE INTESTINE

The second method of establishing an artificial anus consists in the eventration of the end of the proximal loop of the gut which has been divided at a given point. The formation of such an artificial anus may be an independent operation or it may be the temporary or final step of an intestinal resection. The description given here is of the establishment of such an artificial anus as an independent operation. It should be considered when the distal segment of the gut is not suitable or is inaccessible for an entero-enterostomy.

The establishment of an artificial anus at the end of an intestinal segment can be carried out at any point in the intestine. It is even possible in the region of the ascending and the descending colon, since these portions of the intestine may as a rule be mobilized sufficiently without danger to their nutrition to permit bringing the end of the divided bowel through the anterior abdominal wall.

After the division of the gut, the distal segment is closed and buried, in the manner described on page 59.

It is also advisable to close temporarily the opening of the proximal segment intended for the artificial anus after the division. This is done to prevent contamination of the operative field with intestinal contents during the operation and to make possible the opening of the artificial anus at any desired time after the conclusion of the operation. For this reason, the bowel is best divided with the aid of the Petz suture instrument which closes both ends of the bowel with a single manipulation. The clip suture line on each end of the bowel is inverted by interrupted Lembert sutures of linen. The threads on the proximal end are left long to facilitate its handling.

The proximal loop of gut is brought to the surface through the main laparotomy wound or through a special opening. In the first instance the abdominal incision is partly closed until the intestine can just pass through it. If the length of the proximal segment permits, its end should not be flush with the skin but should project beyond it for several centimeters. This will guard against the bowel slipping back and will permit a tube to be tied into the gut to evacuate the feces.

The peritoneum of the eventrated intestinal end is sutured in its whole circumference to the parietal peritoneum at the level of its exit. The parietal peritoneum of the abdominal wound may first be sutured to the edge of the skin. After the complete closure of the remainder of the abdominal wound up to the point of exit of the gut, the skin edges are sutured to the intestine.

If a separate opening is to be used, as when the abdomen was opened through a midline incision which is not suitable for an artificial anus, the operation is carried through the stage of division of the intestine and the care of the ends of the segments in the manner described. Next, if an artificial anus is to be made in the sigmoid, a 4-cm. skin incision is made above and parallel to Poupart's ligament on the left side. The aponeurosis of the external oblique is split by a crucial incision and the muscles are separated by blunt dissection down to the peritoneum. The position of the incision is selected in such a way that the proximal loop can easily be drawn out at this point.

The left side of the main laparotomy wound is lifted up with forceps. The peritoneum of the small wound is pushed forward by a Korn forceps which was introduced through the major incision and the peritoneum is opened by a cruciform incision. The edge of the peritoneum may be sutured to the skin edge; if so, the ends of the sutures are left long. The bridge of abdominal wall between the two abdominal incisions is forcibly elevated by means of a Langenbeck retractor introduced from the large into the small wound. By means of a forceps introduced through the small wound, the long ends of the sutures at the end of the proximal segment are grasped (Fig. 180) and the loop of bowel is drawn out through the small wound. After it has been determined that the eventrated loop has not been twisted on its axis, it is sutured to the edges of the small abdominal wound in such a way that its end projects several centimeters beyond the skin. The long ends of the peritoneum-skin suture are used for this purpose. The main laparotomy wound is then closed.

If the opening of the loop to be used for the artificial anus cannot be delayed, this is now carried out and a glass or rubber tube is inserted into the

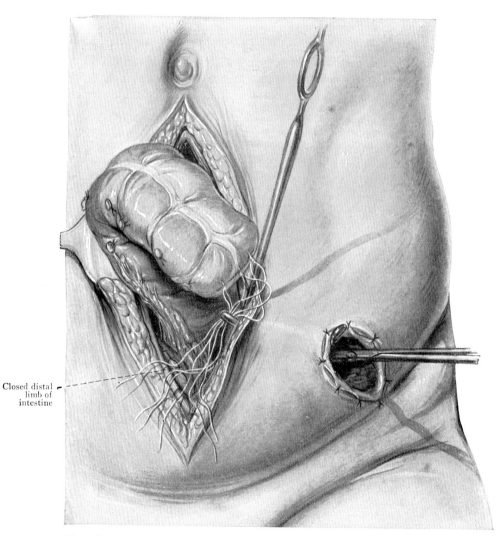

Closed distal
limb of
intestine

Fig. 180. Terminal artificial anus. The sigmoid is picked up through a midline incision and divided. The distal limb is closed and dropped. The proximal limb is also closed and mobilized by ligation and division of its mesentery. In the left inguinal region a second small abdominal incision is made and the parietal peritoneum sutured to the skin margin. By means of a forceps introduced through the small abdominal incision the proximal limb is pulled out through this incision to the margins of which it is sutured. It is subsequently opened.

opening (Fig. 170). A ligature tied around the free cuff of intestine above the skin level effects a tight closure around the tube. A drainage system to receive the intestinal contents is attached to the tube. This protects the operative wound for a number of days against soiling with intestinal contents. If the tube is not used the opening of the loop should be deferred for several days if possible, but in the meantime there may be repeated aspirations of it.

Subsequently the protruding part of the intestinal loop is amputated at the level of the skin with the cautery or preferably the electrosurgical knife. Within a very short time a very efficient lipped fistula has formed.

From the preceding considerations it will be seen that the establishment of an artificial anus of the terminal type may be carried out without the performance of an intestinal resection. For example, the most frequent type of artificial anus, the sigmoid anus, in case of inoperable carcinoma of the rectum, may be established as a single-barrelled anus instead of the double-barrelled form as previously described. The loop intended for the formation of the artificial anus may be brought through the original abdominal wound or through a separate opening.

In case of inoperable carcinoma of the rectum, I personally prefer the double-barrelled anus, because the single-barrelled anus robs the patient of the advantage of irrigation of the short-circulated segment. Furthermore, obstruction of the closed loop leading to the carcinoma may occur and may lead to rupture of the blind sac. Finally, the double-barrelled anus leaves open all the possibilities for the later radical treatment of the rectal lesion if this becomes feasible.

3. Operative Measures for the Regulation of Fecal Evacuation from an Artificial anus

The subjective feeling of well-being, the capacity for work, and the fitness for society of an individual with an artificial anus depend largely upon his ability to control defecation and flatus and on whether the disturbance of the patient by soiling and by offensive odors can be avoided.

The most important aid consists in the regulation of the diet and the wearing of a suitable closure or storage appliance. The individual application and testing of such appliances is a routine duty of the surgeon and should be considered scarcely of less importance than the operation of forming the artificial anus.

The appliances are fastened to the body after the manner of a hernial truss. Tightness of closure is effected either by means of a ring, often provided with a rubber cushion, which is pressed tightly against the skin around the artificial anus by means of an adjustable spring or elastic bands or by means of a sausage-shaped projection which can be inserted into the gut. The fecal reservoir consists of a flattened metal container or of a rubber bag.

In my own patients the most satisfactory appliance for nearly two decades has been a simple metal shell which is pressed against the skin by elastic bands or by a gentle spring and is fastened to the body by a belt (Fig. 181). This well-tried apparatus, which has been patented in various forms and thereby unduly increased in price, is easy to clean and all its parts can be boiled.

Recently, the metal shell has been made detachable without removal of the bandage, which is a great advantage to the patient.

The efforts to attain by operative measures a voluntary control over an artificial anus have not as yet produced a completely satisfactory solution of this problem. I therefore use such measures only in very exceptional cases, and only when a permanent cure of the underlying disease is possible. Most of the plastic procedures employ only the proximal loop and they require considerable length and mobility of this loop. These prerequisites are most

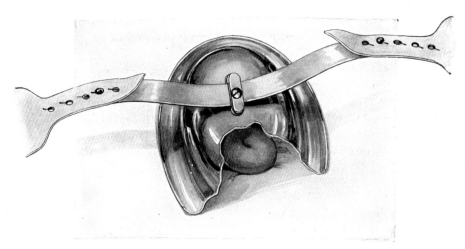

Fig. 181. Metal cover for a colostomy. A belt holds it in place and it is pressed firmly against the abdominal wall by means of a spring. It can easily be removed, cleansed and boiled. Instead of a spring an elastic rubber belt may be used which is fastened directly to the metal cup.

frequently met with in practice after a combined resection of the rectum for rectal carcinoma with establishment of an artificial abdominal anus.

(A) ARTIFICIAL STENOSIS OF THE ARTIFICIAL ANUS

Procedures involving a relative stenosis of the artificial anus or of the proximal loop are obviously inadequate and untrustworthy. A stenosis means a permanent obstruction, not a regulated alternation between opening and closing of the passageway. When the evacuation of the dammed-up contents finally begins, it continues for a long time as a rule. An attempt to produce such a stenosis is made by twisting the end of the gut through 180 to 360° (Gersuny) at the time of suturing it to the abdominal wall. This gives the end of the gut a spiral course. In this group belongs the longitudinal plication of the end of the gut by a number of gathering sutures transversely applied just above the artificial anus (Schmieden); also the narrowing of the gut opening by a subcutaneous Thiersch wire ring placed around the anus or by a fascial ring.

(B) THE FORMATION OF A CANAL OF MUSCLE

The hope of voluntarily controlling the anus by leading the gut through a canal of muscle is based on an erroneous physiological concept. No one can keep a striated muscle in a continuously contracted state for fifteen minutes much less for hours at a time and relax it only for the few moments of a desired bowel evacuation. The conveniently situated rectus muscle is usually chosen for this operation. From the original midline or lateral incision the lateral or the medial border of the rectus muscle is exposed. A Korn forceps is forced transversely through the muscle, dividing its fibre bundles either into a medial and a lateral or into an anterior and a posterior half. The skin is incised over the tip of the forceps pressed against it and the resultant canal is stretched by opening the jaws of the forceps. A second Korn forceps is inserted into the jaws of the first, and is drawn into the abdomen and this is used to draw the adequately mobilized gut through the tunnel in the muscle. The edge of the gut is sutured to the skin edge of the tunnel. The original laparotomy wound is closed without drainage.

The sartorius muscle has been used in the same way by drawing the end of the gut through the muscle, or by dividing the muscle below and folding it upward, or by transmitting its power by means of a transplanted fascial loop.

In establishing a sacral artificial anus after amputation of the rectum, the end of the gut can be led through the gluteus maximus muscle, split by blunt dissection, and then opened on the surface as a "gluteal" anus in the upper region of the right or the left buttock.

(C) SUBCUTANEOUS DISPLACEMENT OF THE PROXIMAL LOOP

The proposal of Frank to lead the bowel for some distance between the surface of the abdominal muscles and the skin falls in that group of promising procedures which would close the end of the gut by mechanical pressure voluntarily exerted. At the end of the description of the establishment of an artificial anus with a long loop on page 232 attention was called to the fact that in this procedure the terminal gut can be placed subcutaneously for some distance and can be compressed from without by a pressure pad to regulate the evacuation of the feces.

In the Frank procedure, the end of the bowel is pulled out of the wound for a distance of about 10 cm. and is sutured firmly to the edges of the wound, with the exception of the skin. The remainder of the laparotomy wound is closed. The skin is undermined in the subcutaneous fat by a tunnel the length of the available segment and in a transverse or a downward direction (Fig. 182). The skin is incised at the end of the tunnel. The bowel is drawn through the subcutaneous tunnel and the small skin opening and is sutured to the edge of the latter. Later the subcutaneous segment can be compressed against the muscles of the abdominal wall by a pressure pad, producing a certain degree of closure of the intestine.

(D) UNDERMINING THE PROXIMAL LOOP WITH A SKIN TUBE

The only really dependable procedures for voluntary regulation of an artificial anus are those of Kurtzahn, and of Haecker, who form a tube of skin under the terminal portion of the gut. This makes it possible to compress the end of the gut with a spring, a clamp, or a rubber tube sufficiently to prevent the escape of feces or even of gas. It is easily understood that carrying these measures to excess could lead to a pressure ulcer of the skin, and this has been my experience in several otherwise successful cases.

In the procedure of Kurtzahn the skin tube is placed in the immediate neighborhood of the opening of the anus, while the procedure of Haecker has the great advantage that it involves the proximal loop at some distance from the artificial anus and is therefore independent of the position of the latter.

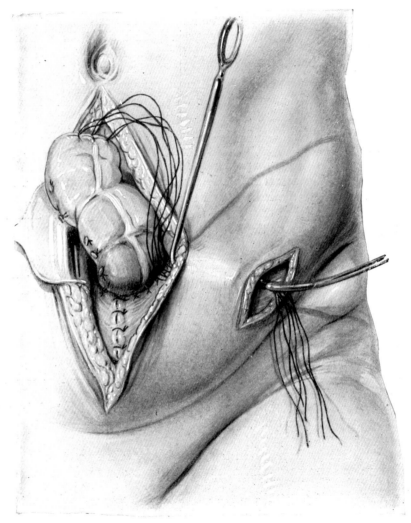

FIG. 182. Colostomy with a controllable artificial anus. The gut is divided and both ends invaginated and sutured. The distal end is dropped back. The proximal (mobilized) end is brought out through the midline incision which is then closed except for the skin. A skin incision is made in the left inguinal region and connected with the midline incision by a subcutaneous tunnel through which the proximal limb of gut is drawn to the surface by means of a forceps and the ends of the sutures which were left long for this purpose.

The Procedure of Kurtzahn is carried out as follows:—The terminal bowel is well mobilized and is brought out of the abdomen through a separate transverse slit in the abdominal wall for a distance of 8 to 10 cm. and is sutured to the edge of the slit at the point where it passes through (Fig. 183). The intestinal segment is then laid flat on the skin in the direction of the intended anal opening, which is usually downward. The line of contact between the transversely cut end of the segment and the skin forms one side of a rectangular skin flap; the skin is incised in this line. The intestinal segment having been folded up out of the way, the two short sides of the skin flap are outlined by two parallel incisions beginning at the two ends of the first incision and carried upward toward and half way to the ends of the opening through which the gut leaves the abdomen. The base of the skin flap formed by these three incisions therefore lies parallel to and about 4 cm. below the

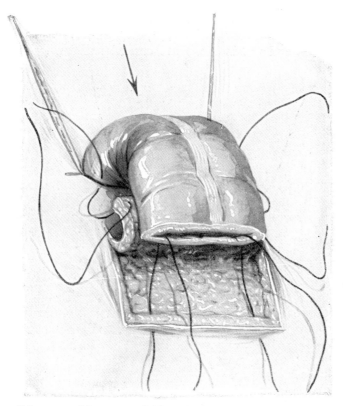

FIG. 183. Colostomy with a controllable artificial anus. The sigmoid has been transsected, the distal end closed and dropped back. The proximal end has been mobilized for a considerable distance and drawn to the surface through a small incision in the abdominal wall. A rectangular skin flap has been outlined by incision on three sides and is being converted into a skin tunnel by suturing its free margin to the skin margin at the point of exit of the sigmoid. The lower cut edge of the sigmoid is being sutured to the transverse margin of the skin wound. On the other side of the point of exit of the bowel a tongue-shaped skin flap is being outlined in such a way that when it is displaced it will cover the sigmoid in the direction of its long axis.

point of exit of the gut from the skin. The skin flap is now dissected up to its base and its long free edge is sutured to the skin edge of the lower border of the wound through which the gut emerges from the abdomen. The flap is thus converted into a skin tube with the epithelial surface on the inside (Fig. 183). The intestinal segment is now placed over the skin tube and over the fresh wound surface from which the skin flap was just freed, and the under surface of the end of the segment is sutured to the transverse skin edge of the fresh wound surface. The posterior surface of the bowel therefore lies on the anterior abdominal wall and on the skin tube and completely covers the wound surface which resulted from the plastic procedure. The lateral margins of the segment may be attached by a few additional sutures to the edges of the wound.

The problem now is to cover the anterior surface of the bowel with skin. This may be done with the aid of a Thiersch graft. Since such a graft has little resistance, it is advisable to use a pedunculated skin flap (Fig. 183). A tongue-shaped skin flap is formed whose narrow free side is the upper free wound edge where the gut leaves the abdomen. The two lateral incisions begin at the two ends of this edge and are carried upward, in the opposite direction from the present course of the gut, diverging slightly as they proceed. This flap is freed and the incisions are carried sufficiently high to permit

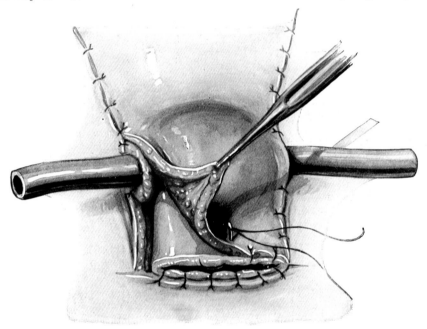

Fig. 184. Colostomy with a controllable artificial anus. A rubber tube has been passed through the skin tunnel. The lower cut edge of the bowel has been sutured to the transverse margin of the skin wound. The tongue-shaped skin flap has been placed over the sigmoid and its edges are being sutured on all sides to the edges of the wound resulting from the freeing of the rectangular flap which went to form the skin tube.

pulling the tongue-shaped flap down over the gut and suturing the free border of the tip to the anterior edge of the intestinal opening (Fig. 184). In tense abdominal walls with scant skin, difficulties may arise because of a lack of material.

The same possibility of mechanically compressing the terminal segment leading to an artificial anus is achieved by surrounding the terminal portion of the artificial anus with skin so that it looks very much like a penis. In addition to continence, patients claim for such an anus that they can grasp the intestinal tube and evacuate the feces in a stream, without soiling the skin. At the same time the difficulties incident to cleansing and caring for a cutaneous tunnel are done away with.

For the formation of a trunk-like tube end, the intestinal segment at the

first operation has a tube of skin placed beneath it and a skin flap in front of
it in the manner just described. At a second operation the segment is dissected away from the abdominal surface in such a way that the abdominal skin

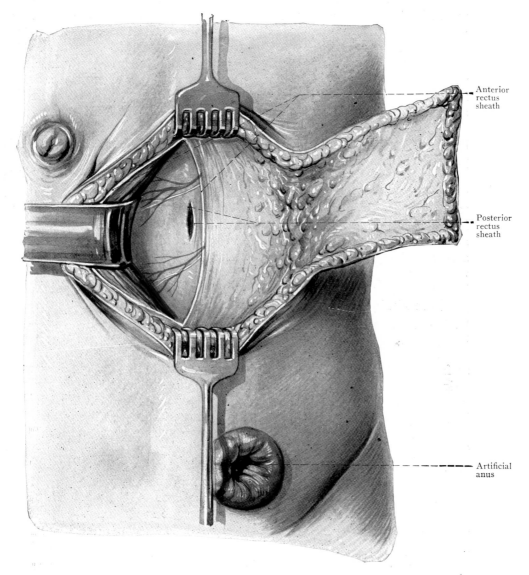

Anterior
rectus
sheath

Posterior
rectus
sheath

Artificial
anus

FIG. 185. Colostomy with a controllable artificial anus according to the method of Haecker
(1). In the region of the sigmoid a rectangular skin flap has been dissected free, with its
pedicle on the side and with its midpoint over the lateral edge of the rectus muscle. The
anterior rectus sheath has been opened in the long axis of the body and the rectus retracted
toward the midline. The abdominal cavity will be opened along the line of incision of the
posterior rectus sheath.

flap remains attached to the anterior surface of the gut and the skin tube to
its posterior surface. The tube skin is now cut open parallel to the line of its
original base and is unrolled. The wound surface so freed is used to clothe
the posterior surface of the gut and the fresh cut edge is united to the margin

of the opening of the gut. The raw wound resulting on the surface of the abdomen from the separation of the gut segment is covered by a Thiersch graft.

Procedure of Haecker. A prerequisite for this procedure is that a segment of gut proximal to the artificial anus can be mobilized sufficiently so that it can be eventrated for a short distance in the form of a closed loop. The sigmoid is best suited for the purpose, the transverse colon next best. The ascending and the descending colon as a rule cannot be sufficiently mobilized without causing trophic disturbances. Roentgen-ray studies yield valuable information as to the suitability of the sigmoid and the transverse colon and as to the location of the most favorable incision to deliver them.

I shall describe the formation of a controlling mechanism in the sigmoid because it is most frequently carried out in this region. The technique of this procedure in the transverse colon will then be obvious.

At a point which according to the roentgenogram seems most suitable and which is as far as possible from an existing artificial abdominal anus, a rectangular skin flap with a lateral pedicle is formed. The middle of the flap is about in a line with the lateral border of the left rectus. The flap measures about 5 cm. in the long axis of the body and about 7 cm. in the transverse axis of the body. The flap is dissected free to the lateral side and the abdominal cavity is opened in the region of the rectangular cutaneous defect by a lateral rectus incision (Fig. 185). The sigmoid is delivered. At the point of its greatest mobility, the mesosigmoid is pierced close to the gut and enough of the mesentery is ligated and cut so that a thumb can easily be passed through the opening.

The rectangular flap of skin is sutured to form a tube with the epithelial surface on the inside. This tube is drawn through the slit in the mesosigmoid (Fig. 186) and its free end is sutured to the corresponding edge of the rectangular skin wound so that the sigmoid lies over the skin tube. The sigmoid is sutured, as far as is possible, to the parietal peritoneum at the point where it passes through the peritoneal wound, and the abdominal wound, in case it is too large, is made smaller. One must take care that the limbs of the sigmoid are not compressed as they pass through the abdominal wall.

After mobilizing the skin at the upper and, if necessary, the lower angle of the wound, the skin is sutured over the skin tube in such a way that both openings of the skin tube drawn beneath the gut are freely accessible from the outside (Fig. 187). If the neighboring skin fails to cover the wound, a plastic is necessary.

The skin tube must be carefully taken care of. After three weeks the use of closing appliances may be begun. A hairpin-like device, one arm of which is covered with a rubber tube and inserted into the tube, is particularly suitable. Since the skin forming the tube is not sensitive while the patient usually has a strong desire for complete continence, there is often a tendency to use too much pressure with the closing device, with consequent damage to the skin tube.

The procedure just described can be carried out at the same time as the formation of an artificial anus, or it can be performed as an independent operation. Of particular value is the fact that it can also be used in case of a sacral artificial anus. The closer the controlling mechanism is to the artificial anus, the better does it regulate the evacuation of feces.

The controlling device of Haecker can be used not only at a distance from the artificial anus but also in its immediate neighborhood.

Mucosal Prolapse. If the mucosa of the artificial anus tends to prolapse in the course of time, it may be freshened by multiple nicks with the electro-

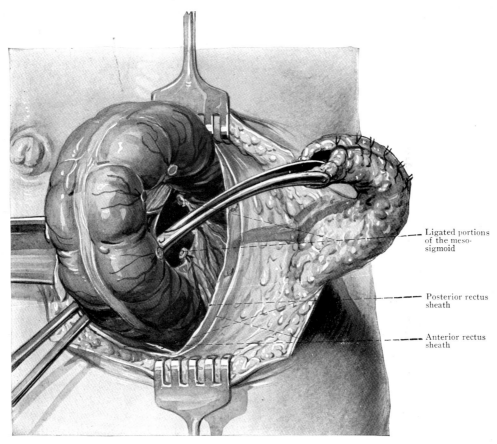

Ligated portions of the meso- sigmoid

Posterior rectus sheath

Anterior rectus sheath

FIG. 186.   Colostomy with a controllable artificial anus according to the method of Haecker (2).   The abdominal cavity has been opened.   The sigmoid is delivered and the mesosigmoid separated from it for a very small area.   The rectangular skin flap has been sutured to form a tube with the epithelium on the inside.   A forceps which has been passed through the opening in the mesosigmoid is pulling the tip of the skin flap beneath the sigmoid and through the opening in the mesosigmoid.

surgical knife with a resulting formation of scar tissue and shrinkage. If the prolapse is excessive, the proximal end sometimes being gradually projected by peristalsis as much as a whole meter, the measures described on page 372 under the treatment of prolapse of the rectum are necessary.

Before beginning any procedure the prolapse must present to its full extent. This is brought about, in addition to active straining by the patient, by repeated traction on the inside of the gut with Kocher forceps.

Stenosis of an Artificial Anus. Troublesome stenosis of the anal open-ing can frequently be met successfully by blunt dilatation. Otherwise, the anus is split by an adequate radial incision in the direction in which the gut seems most extensively attached to the abdominal wall as determined by digital examination. The cut edges of skin and mucosa are united to form a lipped fistula. After healing, further stenosis must be prevented by furnishing the

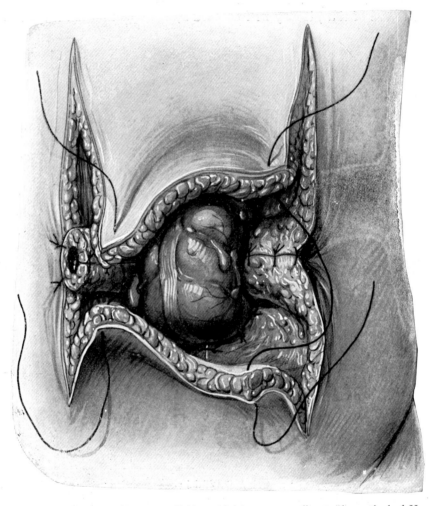

FIG. 187. Colostomy with a controllable artificial anus according to the method of Haecker (3). The skin tube has been pulled beneath the bowel and its tip has been fastened by a few sutures to the corresponding edge of the skin. The upper and the lower skin margins bordering the rectangular skin defect have been dissected free from the underlying tissue and the two skin flaps so formed are being sutured to each other as they overlie the bowel.

patient with a bulbous dilator with a handle or a Hegar sound which he inserts into the opening from time to time.

E. CLOSURE OF AN INTESTINAL FISTULA AND OF AN ARTIFICIAL ANUS

The closure of an intestinal fistula or an artificial anus by local measures restricted to the region of the external opening will be successful only if the intestinal contents can pass without obstruction from the proximal to the distal limb of intestine and can be evacuated freely through the terminal gut. If these conditions are not present the free passage of the feces must be established either before closing the fistula or at the time of its closure. The measures for the reconstruction of the intestinal canal in the region of the fistula consist either in a resection of the stenosed fistula-bearing gut segment, in an entero-enterostomy between the proximal and distal loops or in the crushing of a common wall separating the two limbs. The first two procedures presuppose that it is possible to expose the proximal and the distal limbs of the gut for a sufficient distance. If this mobilization fails because of extensive adhesions, the closure of the fistula may become impossible, which in case of a high fistula draining the major part of the intestinal contents may lead to death from loss of fluid and food.

The presence and the size of the passage between the proximal and the distal limbs of a fistula must be determined before operation by functional testing, by barium Roentgen-ray studies and, if possible, by exploring with the palpating finger or a sound.

1. Closure of a Tubular Fistula of the Intestine

Those fistulae which were established with the formation of a serosal canal, according to Witzel or Kader, usually close of themselves when the tube is withdrawn. It is only necessary in the first few days, when a little of the intestinal contents seeps out at times, to treat the skin around the fistula carefully with applications of zinc oxide ointment and to draw the edges of the fistula together with strips of adhesive plaster. Protruding granulations are first removed with a scissors or an electrosurgical knife. Also those fistulae which in the absence of a special serosal canal reach the surface through a long granulating passageway frequently close spontaneously with this simple palliative treatment.

If the fistula does not close under this conservative treatment, the closure must be effected by operation. Particularly stubborn in this regard are those fecal fistulae which arise spontaneously, as after an appendectomy, in abdominal drainage for suppurative peritonitis, at times from the pressure of a drain, in gangrene of the intestine, in inflammatory lesion of the intestinal wall or after traumatic or operative injury of the intestine. The closer such fistulae are to the stomach, the more resistant they are to conservative measures and the more difficult it is to keep the skin around the fistulous opening in good condition. Particularly difficult in this regard are duodenal fistulae. Their treatment is described separately on page 106.

The operative removal of a tubular fistula consists in the isolation of the whole fistulous canal from the skin to its entrance into the gut, its separation from the skin and the gut and the closure of the resultant defects in the skin, abdominal wall and intestine (Fig. 188).

The fistulous tract can be more easily followed if it is filled with an indigo carmine or methylene blue solution. During the operation the introduction of a probe facilitates the finding of the tract. It is, however, not difficult as a rule to trace the fistulous canal because it is clearly differentiated from the surrounding tissue by its firmness and fibrous structure.

An elliptical incision with pointed ends is made in the skin around the fistula and this skin area is dissected free at its borders. The margins of the opening are sutured together to prevent soiling of the operative field by the escape of intestinal contents (Fig. 87). The ends of the elliptical incision are prolonged to permit free dissection of the tract and of the separate layers of the abdominal wall. First one side then the other of the skin oval is dissected free, using sharp hooks as retractors, until the uppermost layer of the abdominal wall beneath the skin is exposed into sound tissue. This layer is

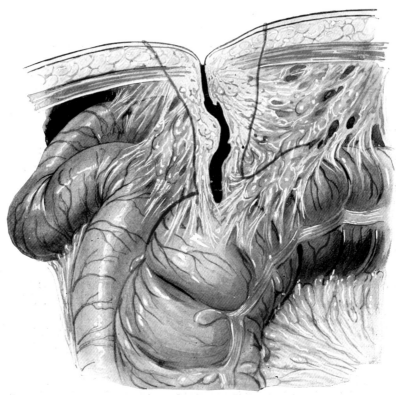

FIG. 188. Closure of a fecal fistula. The fistulous opening is dissected free on all sides, corresponding to the red lines. The individual layers of the abdominal wall are dissected free and the tract is followed downward, with freeing of the viscera encountered, until its entrance into the gut is reached and the adjacent surface of the bowel exposed.

then divided in an elliptical form by deepening the original incision and its edges are again freed into the region of normal tissue. The excision and dissection of the individual layers are continued until the peritoneum is reached.

The careful dissection of the individual layers of the abdominal wall in the manner described serves the purpose of removing the incisional hernia which is associated with the fistula in most cases. It also prevents the later development of such a hernia after the operation for closure of the fistula.

When the peritoneum has been reached, the fistulous tract and the portions of the abdominal wall attached to it are grasped with a Museux forceps and elevated. This lifts the peritoneum in a cone and as a rule brings into view a portion of the parietal peritoneum to which no intestine is attached. At this point the peritoneum is incised. There now comes into view a mass of tissue which may consist of intestine, omentum, parietal peritoneum and other viscera situated in the vicinity. The fistulous tract enters this mass. The parietal peritoneum is excised in a circle around this conglomerate tumor and adhesions and cords of omentum are doubly ligated and divided (Fig. 189). Finally the fistulous tract and the mass of tissue around it may be

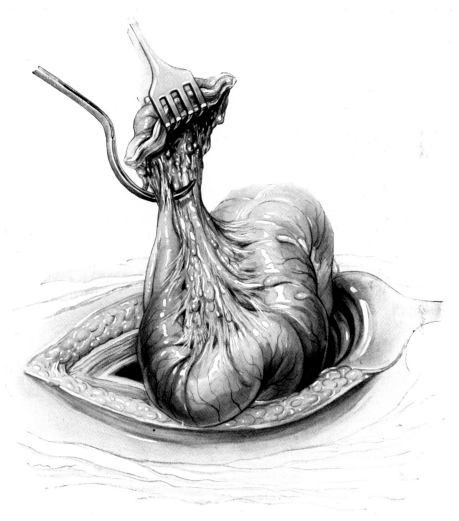

FIG. 189. Closure of a fecal fistula. The fistulous tract is now free and is being held with a Museux forceps. The attached viscera will be dissected free, the adhesions being picked up on an aneurysm needle and divided between ligatures until the point of entrance of the fistula into the gut and the adjacent gut surface are exposed.

lifted out of the abdominal wound. After the surrounding field is carefully covered with gauze pads, the fistulous tract is dissected out of the adherent mass of tissue to the point of its entrance into the intestine. When this has been reached, the tract is tied off and amputated, and the site of ligation is carefully covered by interrupted Lembert sutures of silk or linen.

An examination must now be made to see whether the intestine has become stenosed in the region of the fistulous opening. If there is the slightest question on this point, the stenosis must be obviated, either (and usually) by an entero-enterostomy between the proximal and the distal loops, or more rarely by a resection of the diseased segment and an anastomosis of the proximal and distal loops. A resection of the intestinal segment bearing the fistula is indicated ab initio if the intestine is involved in extensive adhesions, the freeing of which is impossible or offers great difficulties, whereas the loops proximal and distal to it can easily be found and exposed. The abdominal wound is carefully closed by tier suture. Drainage is not, as a rule, necessary.

2. Closure of a Lipped Fistula of the Intestine

A lipped fistula, that is, one in which there exists a direct union between the skin and the intestinal mucosa, whether at a single point or in its full

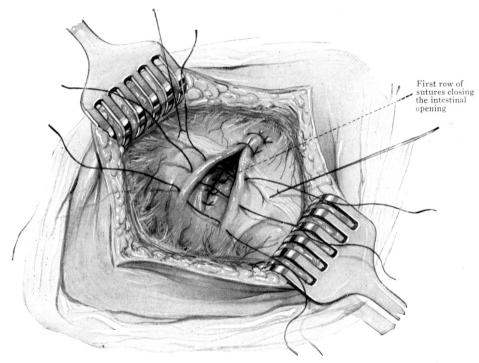

First row of sutures closing the intestinal opening

Fig. 190. Closure of a lipped fistula of the intestine by freshening and suturing the margins. An elliptical incision has been made in the skin close around the fistulous opening, and the opening closed by suture after infolding the skin edge. The surface of the bowel has been freed from its surroundings without opening the abdominal cavity. The first row of sutures closing the fistula is being infolded by Lembert sutures.

circumference, will never heal without operation. In a lipped fistula the intestine is usually in direct contact with the abdominal wall without an intervening canal. It is therefore not absolutely necessary to open the general abdominal cavity to reach the surface of the intestine.

An elliptical incision with pointed ends is made around the fistula in such a way that a border of skin 1 to 2 millimeters wide remains attached to the fistula. The incision is enlarged if necessary by incisions continued at its ends. The incision is carried down through the individual layers of the abdominal wall in the manner described until the full extent of the surface of the intestine is reached. The opening of the fistula is closed by interrupted silk sutures in the direction in which its edges can be brought together most easily, usually transversely. The border of skin surrounding the opening is folded inward and the sutures are applied to the margins of the skin where they can be pulled taut without cutting through. This suture line is buried by a Lembert suture (Fig. 190). If the intestine is not sufficiently mobile for the performance of this suture, it is freed a little more from the surrounding tissue. This is possible in most instances without opening the general abdominal cavity, since the adhesions in the region of such a fistula as a rule cover a considerable area. If the abdominal cavity happens to be opened at one point, the opening is closed with a few sutures before suturing the abdominal wall, even though the double-row suture of the fistula is dependable.

After the closure of the intestinal orifice by the double suture, the wound in the abdominal wall is closed. If possible, the individual layers are sutured separately, which at some points may require further dissection. If tier suture is rendered difficult by a lack of material, the abdominal wall may be drawn together with wire tension sutures including the skin. They are left in place for from 10 to 12 days.

Even though primary union does not take place and a little pus or even fecal matter exudes in the next few days, the wound tends to heal completely in most cases after some time.

If the external opening of a lateral intestinal fistula is very large, its closure by simple suture in the manner described may fail. In such cases the measures for the closure of an artificial anus are applied as described in the following section.

3. Closure of an Artificial Anus

The closure of an artificial anus consists in the anastomosis of the proximal to the distal segment of intestine and in the closure of the orifice of the artificial anus.

The anastomosis of the proximal to the distal segment of intestine. Since in the case of an artificial anus all of the feces are evacuated through the terminal opening of the proximal segment and since the proximal segment has no communication with the distal segment, the first task in the closure of an artificial anus is to reestablish a free communication between the proximal and distal limbs of the intestine.

In case of a double-barrelled artificial anus, the passageway may be reconstructed without a laparotomy by gradually crushing the common wall between the two limbs.

If, however, instead of a double-barrelled artificial anus, there are proximal and distal limbs which open on the surface side by side but without an extended lateral attachment to each other, or if their openings reach the surface of the abdomen at two separated points, or if the distal end was closed and not brought to the surface at all, a special operation involving laparotomy is necessary to reestablish communication between the proximal and the distal segments.

The abdomen is opened either by an incision which encircles the artificial anus or by an incision at another site, usually in the midline. An incision encircling the artificial anus is particularly indicated in the single-stage resec-

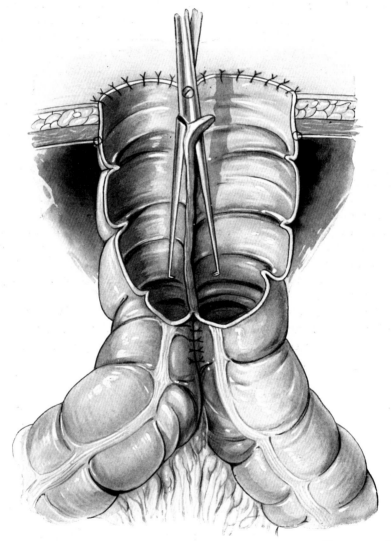

Fig. 191. Crushing the septum of the double-barrelled artificial anus. The septum is being grasped and crushed between the limbs of the forceps.

tion of the artificial anus or when the proximal and the distal loops open side by side. This procedure has the advantage of avoiding a weakening of the abdominal wall by a second incision.

The opening of the abdomen at a new site has the advantage that there is no immediate soiling of the operative field or of the general abdominal cavity by fecal matter from the artificial anus. This plan is advisable if the resection of the loops involved in the artificial anus is to be dispensed with, if the resection is to be performed in two stages, if the proximal and distal loops reach the surface at separate points, or if the distal loop lies closed within the abdominal cavity.

The closure of the orifice of the artificial anus may be effected by suture of the orifice or by resection of the intestinal loop bearing the anus.

Closure of the anal orifice by suture. After a free communication between the proximal and the distal loop has been re-established, thereby short-circuiting the artificial anus and converting it functionally into a lateral fistula, the closure of the anal orifice may be effected by freshening and suturing its edges in the manner just described. This leaves a blind segment of gut within the abdomen between the artificial anus and the anastomosis. Such blind sacs short-circuited out of the direct channel may very occasionally give rise to fecal accumulations and consequently to symptoms.

Resection of the gut segment bearing the artificial anus. The resection of the intestinal segment bearing the artificial anus creates conditions which functionally most nearly approach the normal. This procedure is therefore to be preferred. It is, however, the most extensive.

The two procedures, the establishment of a new intestinal passageway and the ablation of the artificial anus, can be carried out at a single sitting or in two stages. This depends on the condition of the patient and on the difficulties encountered. If both procedures are carried out at a single operation it is immaterial in which order this is done.

In practice there are three main procedures for the closure of the various types of artificial anus:

Closure of a double-barrelled artificial anus.

Closure by means of an abdominal incision excising the artificial anus.

Closure by means of an abdominal incision at a distance from the artificial anus.

(A) CLOSURE OF A DOUBLE-BARRELLED ARTIFICIAL ANUS

The crushing of the septum of a double-barrelled anus for the purpose of reestablishing the natural fecal channel is carried out in the following manner:

The exact position of the proximal and the distal loops, the form and extent of the septum and the extent of firm adhesion of the two loops are determined by inserting the gloved fingers. A large Billroth clamp, toothed at its tip, is introduced as far as possible, one limb into the proximal, the other limb into the distal segment, so that the septum comes to lie between the jaws of the clamp (Fig. 191). The clamp is then tightly closed, crushing the septum. Since the crushing of the septum is usually quite painful for the patient, the septum is infiltrated with 1 per cent novocaine solution before applying the clamp. The clamp is left in place until it drops off. This occurs in a few days, after necrosis of the clamped tissue.

The result of the first crushing of the septum is determined by digital exploration of the artificial anus. In most cases the crushing must be repeated one or more times in the same manner until the septum between the proximal and the distal limbs is sufficiently divided and a broad communication exists between the two limbs.

If adequate crushing of the septal spur is impossible because of its breadth, the angle formed by the two limbs of gut may occasionally be smoothed out by the insertion of a stout rubber tube over a long period of time. One half of the tube lies in one limb of the gut, the other half in the other limb (Fig. 192). The pressure exerted by the drainage tube at times brings about a gradual flattening of the septal spur. In order that the tube shall not be carried along by peristalsis and so be lost, a stout silk thread is tied around the middle of the tube and is led out of the artificial anus. It later serves for the removal of the tube. The tube may remain in

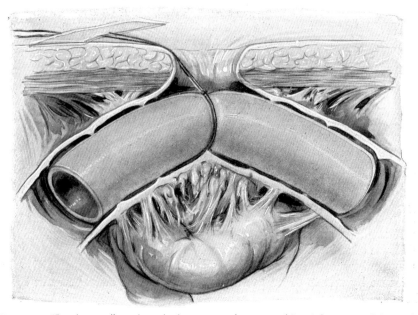

FIG. 192. "Ironing out" an intestinal septum. A stout rubber tube, secured by a thread, has been inserted into both limbs of a double-barrelled artificial anus, flattening out the septum and conducting the intestinal contents from the proximal to the distal limb.

place for a number of days since the intestinal contents can pass through its lumen. The treatment must be continued over weeks.

Only after the septal spur has been sufficiently flattened out, should the closure of the artificial anus be undertaken. This is done in the manner already described for the closure of a lipped intestinal fistula.

(B) CLOSURE OF AN ARTIFICIAL ANUS BY MEANS OF AN ABDOMINAL INCISION EXCISING THE ANAL ORIFICE

If the resection of the loop bearing the artificial anus is to be carried out at the same operation, the abdomen may be opened by an incision carried around the anal orifice (Fig. 193). The openings of both intestinal segments are included in a single incision which leaves a narrow border of skin around them. The segments are packed for a short distance with vioform gauze and are then closed by sutures which invert the skin edge of the wound. By careful dissection of the successive abdominal layers the incision is gradually carried down on all sides to the peritoneum which, in turn, is opened by a circular incision. If the incision around the artificial anus is too small for the dissection of the separate layers of the abdominal wall and for the inspection of the abdominal cavity, it is elongated at one or both ends.

After the peritoneum has been opened, the two intestinal segments are followed and freed to a point where sound tissue is available for their division and anastomosis.

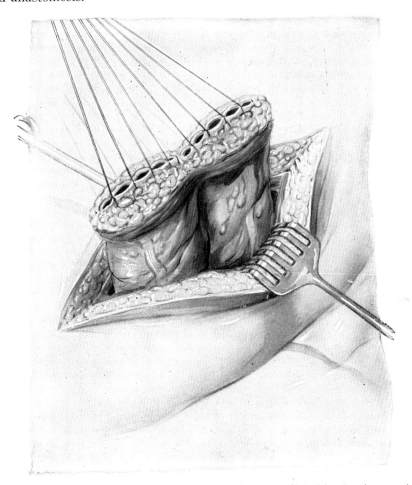

Fig. 193. Excision of an artificial anus (1). An elliptical incision has been made around the anal opening and the individual layers of the abdominal wall have been dissected free. The artificial anus was closed by suture before the peritoneum was opened. The two limbs forming the artificial anus have been freed and are held up by some of the suture ends left long for the purpose.

A side-to-side anastomosis may first be made between the proximal and the distal intestinal limbs, the redundant ends resected and the remaining stumps closed (Fig. 194); or the proximal and distal loops may first be divided, which removes the ends bearing the artificial anus, and the proximal and distal intestinal segments then anastomosed by one of the various possible methods.

The abdominal wound is closed in layers. Drainage is usually unnecessary.

(C) CLOSURE OF AN ARTIFICIAL ANUS BY MEANS OF AN ABDOMINAL INCISION
AT A DISTANCE FROM THE ARTIFICIAL ANUS

The end of the loop forming the artificial anus, and also the distal loop
if it is open to the exterior, are tightly packed with vioform gauze to a depth

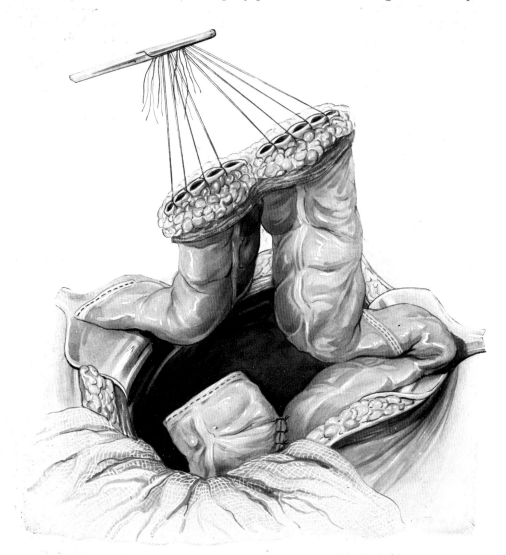

Fig. 194. Excision of an artificial anus (2). A lateral anastomosis has been made between
the proximal and the distal limbs of the bowel. Both limbs have been sutured across with the
Petz suture instrument and one limb has been divided.

of about 10 cm. The abdomen is then opened at another site, usually in the
midline. The side of the abdominal wound nearest the artificial anus is elevated and the loops of gut forming the artificial anus are sought for. They
can be recognized by their attachment to the abdominal wall and by their
distension with the vioform gauze. In case of doubt an assistant may introduce a finger into the artificial anus, which the operator can then feel from

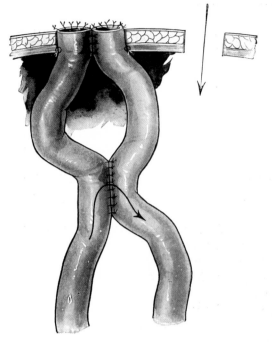

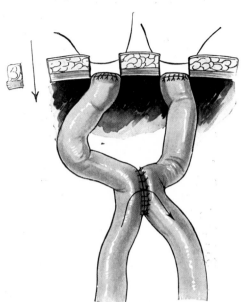

FIG. 195. Short-circuiting an artificial anus at a distance from the artificial anus. Establishment of an anastomosis between the proximal and the distal limb. Diagrammatic.

FIG. 196. Short-circuiting an artificial anus and closure of the anal orifices. Establishment of an anastomosis between the proximal and the distal limb. Closure of the artificial anus from without. Diagrammatic.

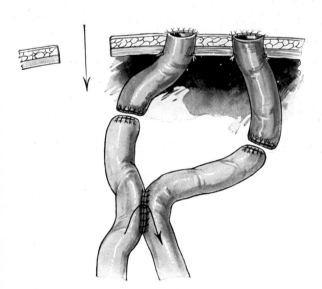

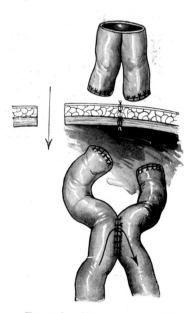

FIG. 197. Closure of an artificial anus at a distance from the anal openings. Establishment of an anastomosis between the proximal and the distal limb and transsection of both limbs. The short-circuited segments remain in the body. Diagrammatic.

FIG. 198. Closure of an artificial anus at a distance from the anal openings. Establishment of an anastomosis between the proximal and the distal limb, transsection and removal of the segments leading to the artificial anus. This is the procedure of preference. Diagrammatic.

within the abdomen. If the distal intestinal loop does not enter into the formation of the artificial anus, but lies closed within the abdominal cavity, it must be looked for separately.

The best plan is first to make an anastomosis between the proximal and the distal loops (Fig. 195). The anastomosis is made as close as possible to the artificial anus to avoid short-circuiting unnecessarily long intestinal segments. Only if the two loops cannot be placed side by side easily should a location at a greater distance from the artificial anus be chosen. A side-to-side anastomosis is usually made.

After the completion of the anastomosis there are three possibilities for further procedure. The choice depends upon the condition of the patient and the difficulties encountered.

The first possibility is to do nothing further than the anastomosis for the time being and to close the abdomen (Fig. 196). The artificial anus is thus converted into a fecal fistula. The escape of feces from the artificial opening is limited as far as possible by drawing the edges of the opening together with strips of adhesive plaster.

If this measure does not suffice, the anal opening, which has been short-circuited out of the normal fecal channel by the anastomosis, can subsequently be closed from without in the manner described for the closure of an intestinal fistula. An incision is carried around the anal orifice, the intestine is closed by suture and buried and the abdominal wall is closed over it by tier suture (Fig. 196).

If closure from without is not successful, it is possible at a later operation to resect the short-circuited loop between the anastomosis and the anal orifice. This is done by making an incision around the anal orifice, by opening the abdomen and resecting and closing both limbs of gut, as described in the preceding chapter.

The second possibility is to divide the proximal loop, at the time of the anastomosis, between the site of the anastomosis and the anal orifice (Fig. 197). If the distal loop is also involved in the artificial anus, it is divided in the same manner. The four resultant openings are closed by terminal suture.

Of course the intestinal loops can be divided first and the proximal and distal limbs anastomosed, while the limbs leading to the skin are closed and oversewed. The state of affairs so established is more favorable than the procedure first described in that the artificial anus is now permanently excluded from the fecal channel. It is less favorable in that the discharge of mucus formed in the excluded gut segment takes place permanently through the orifice of the old artificial anus. This, however, does not greatly inconvenience the patient. It may be done away with by the resection of the short-circuited and divided loops, together with the excision of the artificial anal orifice.

The third possibility, and the best, but at the same time the most radical procedure is that at the first operation the anastomosis of the two intestinal limbs is followed immediately by the resection from within the abdominal cavity of the intestinal loops attached to the artificial anus (Fig. 198). The loops attached to the artificial anus are mobilized within the abdomen by

dividing their mesenteries and adhesions bit by bit between ligatures. Finally
the two loops remain attached only to the abdominal wall in the region of
the artificial anus. While the corresponding side of the laparotomy wound
is forcibly lifted with a Meseux forceps or a sharp hooked retractor, the loops
are put on stretch, dissected free and removed (Fig. 199). The resultant open-

Anastomosis between the proximal and the distal limbs of the intestine

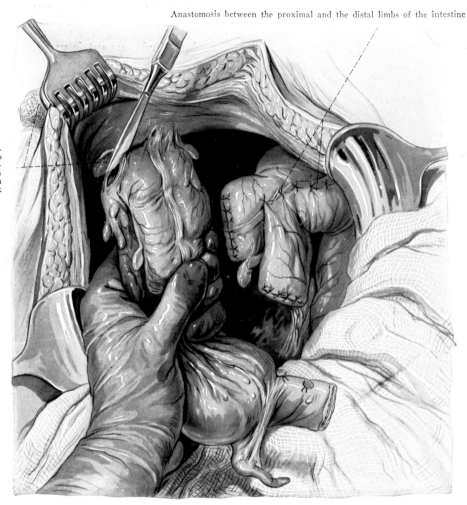

ize in-
ed into
 artifi-
l anus
from
without

FIG. 199. Closure of an artificial anus at the hepatic flexure of the colon. The abdominal
cavity has been opened in the midline. The proximal loop (ileum) and the distal loop (transverse colon) have been divided, the two ends remaining in the body closed and laterally anastomosed. The bowel leading to the artificial anus has been freed from its mesentery and its
other attachments. It remains attached only to the abdominal wall in the region of the artificial
anus. While firm traction is made on the bowel, it is freed at this point by sharp dissection, in
doing which the gauze which was inserted into the artificial anus from without before beginning
the operation is exposed.

ing in the abdominal wall is closed temporarily by a compress introduced from
within the abdomen and pulled out through the opening. The main laparotomy
wound is closed and a dressing applied.

Here, too, one can first sever the intestinal loops from the artificial anus
and then carry out the anastomosis and resection.

The compress in the opening of the former artificial anus is removed from without. Any intestinal mucosa remaining in the opening is trimmed away. The separate layers of the abdominal wall are dissected free and freshened and the wound is closed by tier suture.

F. SHORT-CIRCUITING AND RESECTION OF AN INTESTINAL SEGMENT

The indication for the extirpation of an intestinal segment is present in every intestinal lesion, the existence or further development of which is incompatible with life or health and which can not be successfully treated in another way. Among chronic conditions, carcinoma of the intestine is by far the most common indication for this type of operation, but tuberculosis and other severe chronic ulcerative diseases in which perforation or stenosis has occurred or can occur are also to be considered. Among acute conditions, gangrene of the intestine, as seen for example in mesenteric embolism or thrombosis, is the most common indication. There are also other conditions involving nutritional disturbances, such as occur in strangulation and volvulus. Here must also be included acute injuries of the gut which cannot be taken care of by suture, or in which suture involves the danger of stenosis. Short-circuiting or resection of the obstructing segment may also become necessary in stenoses which are not dangerous at the moment, as in a scar-tissue stricture, or in functionally deranged sections of the intestine, as a chronically costive colon. The short-circuiting of a segment of intestine is indicated if resection, though preferable, is impossible or too dangerous, or if leaving the segment in the body does not constitute a danger for the time being or in the future.

A large number of procedures are at our disposal for short-circuiting and for removing a diseased intestinal segment. Which of these possibilities is to be applied in a given case depends upon the particular conditions of that case. Occasionally a number of procedures are applicable, any one of which may be successful. The individual surgeon must then give preference to that procedure in which he is most skilled and with which he has experienced the best results. In general, the following plan of attack is advisable.

In the individual case a choice between short-circuiting and resection must first be made. In benign lesions involving no danger of subsequent peritonitis, short-circuiting operations are often more suitable than resection or equally as good. Every short-circuiting procedure which preserves the normal channel for the evacuation of the feces is to be preferred to the short-circuiting of a loop by establishing an artificial anus. On the other hand, resection should be performed in malignant lesions or in those involving present or future danger of perforation. Resection is applicable, of course, only when it is technically possible. If resection is technically impossible, the only alternatives are short-circuiting by entero-enterostomy, by an artificial anus or by an intestinal fistula, or else an abandonment of all operative procedure.

If resection has been decided upon, the next question is whether resection of the intestinal loop at a single operation is possible and advantageous, or whether a two-stage resection is necessary or preferable.

Two-stage resection is preferable if the patient's condition is unfavorable, or in case of marked fecal accumulation, or in those instances where the bowel wall over a considerable area is not in good condition. In cases with fecal accumulation, the possibility of thoroughly emptying the gut with a suction apparatus, such as I have described, has increased the scope of indications for resection. In case of the large bowel, a few surgeons prefer a two-stage resection as the routine operation, provided that the eventration procedure can be carried out. This, however, does not seem necessary. (Resection is not indicated in the presence of an acute obstruction. I. S. R.)

If a two-stage resection is decided upon, the next question is whether the diseased loop must be removed at once or whether it may still remain attached to the body, and especially, whether it may still remain in the interior of the abdomen.

If in a two-stage resection the diseased loop must be removed from the abdominal cavity at once, it is eventrated if possible. If eventration is impossible, the loop is resected in the first stage and at least the proximal gut is led out of the abdomen to form an artificial anus.

If in a two-stage resection the diseased loop may be left attached temporarily, it is eventrated if possible. Here, too, the mobility of the diseased loop is the deciding factor.

If in a two-stage resection eventration is impossible, and if the loop is to remain for the time being, an anastomosis is made between the proximal and distal limbs and the diseased loop is permitted to remain within the abdomen. In such cases, if the condition of the patient permits, the first operation should be carried so far that as little as possible remains to be done at the second operation. If possible, therefore, the proximal or even both limbs are divided. In the latter case, the short-circuited loop must possess or must be supplied with an external fistula.

The various types of short-circuiting of a loop of intestine may constitute an independent operation or may be the first or the last step in a single-stage, or a two-stage intestinal resection.

In short-circuiting, the intestinal contents are directed by means of a by-pass more or less completely away from an intestinal segment in otherwise undisturbed communication with the body. There are, in general, three types of short-circuiting, bilateral short-circuiting by lateral anastomosis, unilateral short-circuiting, and complete short-circuiting.

1. Bilateral Short-circuiting of a Loop of Intestine by a Lateral Anastomosis of Its Two Limbs

In short-circuiting by lateral anastomosis between the proximal and the distal loops (Figs. 200 and 201), the intestinal contents are given the opportunity to pass from the proximal to the distal limb without traversing the diseased loop. The use of the new passageway is however not made obligatory. The functional conditions are therefore similar to those in gastro-enterostomy without exclusion of the pylorus. Experience shows that the by-pass is used extensively only when there is a stenosis in the region of the diseased intestinal loop which materially obstructs the passage. Even then clinical disturbances may occasionally arise because of distension of the proximal segment. These are usually the more marked, the longer the segment of intestine between the anastomosis and the stenosed point. It is advisable, therefore, to place the anastomosis as close to the lesion as possible.

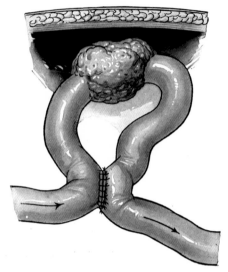

Fig. 200. Short-circuiting of an intestinal loop which is the site of a neoplasm by anastomosing the proximal and the distal loop. Diagrammatic.

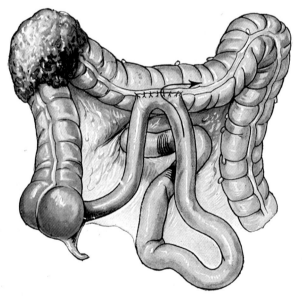

Fig. 201. Side-to-side anastomosis of the lower ileum with the transverse colon because of a carcinoma of the hepatic flexure. Diagrammatic. Stasis phenomena may arise in the ascending colon if the carcinomatous segment is obstructed and the ileocecal valve is not patulous in a retrograde direction.

The accumulation of intestinal contents may be a source of danger if the drainage of a short-circuited segment of intestine is obstructed on both sides. So, for example, in case of a stenotic lesion of the colon with a lateral anastomosis between the ileum and the colon distal to the lesion, there can develop an overdistension of the segment of colon between the lesion and the ileocecal valve if the diseased point in the bowel becomes completely obstructed and if the ileocecal value is not patulous in a retrograde direction (Fig. 201).

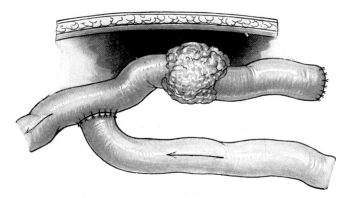

Fig. 202.   Short-circuiting of an intestinal loop.   Diagrammatic.

2. Unilateral Short-circuiting of a Loop of Intestine

Unilateral short-circuiting (Figs. 202 and 203) is performed by dividing the proximal loop, closing the distal opening and anastomosing the proximal opening end-to-side or side-to-side to the distal loop at a point beyond the

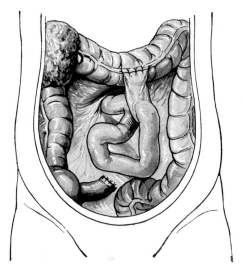

Fig. 203.   Short-circuiting of the cecum and ascending colon by transsection of the terminal loop of ileum, closure of its distal end and end-to-side implantation of the proximal end into the transverse colon, in a carcinoma of the hepatic flexure.   Diagrammatic.   If the carcinoma obstructs the bowel completely there is danger of overdistension of the ascending colon.

site of the lesion.   In this type of short-circuiting the intestinal contents are prevented from passing through the diseased loop, but may reach it by back-flow.   Experience shows that the latter event is of frequent occurrence, so that in this type of operation trouble may also arise.   Therefore when this type is used the short-circuited segment should be as short as possible.

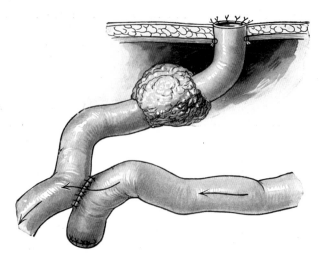

FIG. 204. Short-circuiting of an intestinal loop with establishment of a fistula on one side of the short-circuited loop. Diagrammatic.

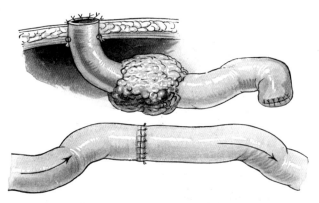

FIG. 205. Complete short-circuiting of an intestinal loop with formation of a fistula on one side of the short-circuited loop. Diagrammatic.

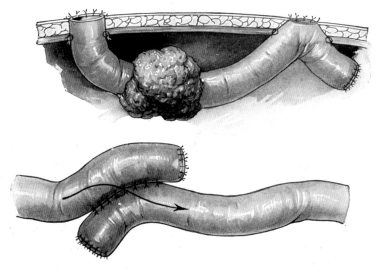

FIG. 206. Complete short-circuiting of a diseased intestinal loop with formation of a fistula on each side of the short-circuited loop. Diagrammatic.

A prerequisite for short-circuiting in this simple manner is that the type of lesion does not and will not block the emptying of the blind sac of the short-circuited loop. Otherwise, an overdistension of this part of the bowel by secreted mucus will arise.

If there are any doubts on this point, the portion of the unilaterally short-circuited loop proximal to the lesion must be provided with an external fistula (Fig. 204).

3. Complete Short-circuiting of a Loop of Intestine

Only by complete short-circuiting is the site of the lesion guarded against all contact with the intestinal contents (Figs. 205, 206 and 207). Complete short-circuiting consists in division of both the proximal and the distal limbs. The intestinal channel is reformed by anastomosing the proximal to the distal segment.

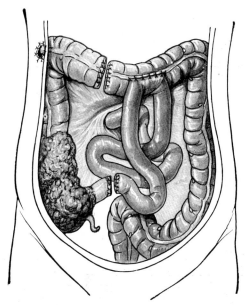

Fig. 207. Complete short-circuiting of the cecum, the ascending colon and half of the transverse colon because of ileocecal tuberculosis. The short-circuited bowel has been provided with an external fistula at the hepatic flexure to insure its emptying. Diagrammatic.

The short-circuited loop must be provided with a free communication with the exterior, since the accumulation of mucous secretion or the products of the lesion can produce a filling, an overdistension, and even a rupture of the blind loop. The communication with the exterior is effected by suturing one (Fig. 205) or both ends (Fig. 206) of the short-circuited loop into the abdominal wound, either using the open ends of the loop or making a lateral fistula after blind closure of the ends. Communication of the short-circuited loop with the exterior by a single opening is permissible only if a stenosis of the loop does not exist or can not arise to prevent the flow of intestinal mucus from the far end of the loop to the end which has the opening. Such an impassable stenosis in an antiperistaltic direction is formed, for example, by the ileocecal valve.

The establishment of an external fistula at each end of the short-circuited loop (Fig. 206) has the advantage that the diseased intestine may be irrigated.

In many cases, intestinal short-circuiting in one of the forms described is only the first step of a multiple-stage intestinal resection that has been carried up to the point of the actual resection. The resection of a loop of intestine can therefore be performed at any time after the loop has been short-circuited.

4. General Considerations Concerning the Resection of a Loop of Intestine

Large, almost unlimited, segments of the intestine can be removed without material damage to the body economy. The question, how much of the approximately 5 meters of small intestine and of the 1.5 meters of large bowel can be removed, had better be put:—how much intestine must be preserved to avoid any recognizable harm to continued existence? On the basis of experience, the only answer is that as much intestine must remain as can possibly be saved, and as much intestine can be removed as absolutely must be removed. In an extreme emergency the patient can get on with a few meters.

Intestinal resection consists of (1) **the actual resection**, which includes the division of the mesentery and the division of both ends of the intestinal segment, and (2) **the reestablishment of the intestinal channel**, which includes the final care of the divided ends resulting from the resection.

The resection of the intestine and the reestablishment of the normal channel may be carried out in a single operation:—**One-stage Intestinal Resection**; or, these two measures may be carried out at two or more operations:— **Two-stage or Multiple-stage Intestinal Resection.** In the latter case, the resection can be undertaken at the first operation, and the intestinal channel reestablished at the second; or the new channel be formed at the first operation, while the resection of the diseased loop is undertaken at the second. If the diseased loop is left in the body at the first operation, it may either be eventrated or it may be allowed to remain within the abdominal cavity. Based on these possibilities, there are the following methods of practical procedure:

(a) Primary resection of the diseased loop; primary reestablishment of intestinal continuity.

(b) Primary resection of the diseased loop; secondary reestablishment of intestinal continuity.

(c) Primary establishment of a new intestinal channel; secondary resection of the diseased loop.

(d) Primary establishment of a new intestinal channel and primary eventration of the diseased loop; secondary resection of the eventrated loop.

Since a single-stage intestinal resection "cures" the patient at a single stroke, as it were, it is the ideal procedure and should be the aim in all cases. If, however, the condition of the patient does not permit combining the various phases of the operation in a single procedure, as for instance is usually the case in acute ileus, or if there is some doubt on the basis of asepsis about the primary opening of the intestinal lumen in an otherwise normal abdominal cavity, the resection must be carried out in multiple stages. A few surgeons consider the normal flora of the large bowel to be so highly infectious that they make it a rule to resect even the fairly empty large bowel in two stages, with primary eventration of the diseased loop. I personally do not share this fear, so that I do not avoid a single-stage resection of the large bowel but I routinely perform it in the absence of contraindications.

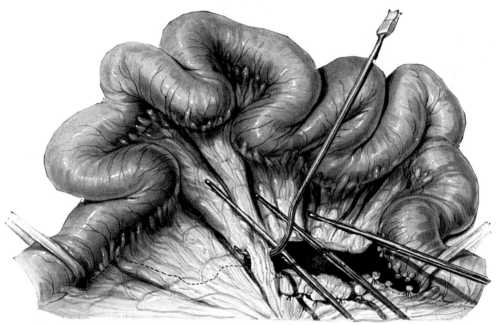

Fig. 208. Resection of a large segment of small intestine: division of the mesentery. At the two points of intended transsection of the gut a linen tape has been passed through the mesentery around the gut. On the right the mesentery has been tied off in small segments close to the gut and has been divided between ligatures. The line of division then deviates toward the root of the mesentery, the ligations including somewhat broader segments. In view of the danger of the ligatures slipping off, the mesentery is always divided at some distance on the intestinal side of the ligatures, so that the ligatures pass through closed circular openings in the mesentery. The mesentery remaining attached to the gut is grasped with large clamps before being divided.

The removal of a segment of intestine usually begins with the detachment of the mesentery, the "mobilization" of the loop.

The Mobilization of an Intestinal Loop with a Free Mesentery. If the intestinal loop possesses a free mesentery (which is everywhere the case with the exception of the duodenum, the ascending and the descending colon and the rectum) the mesentery is tied off between ligatures en masse and is divided, step by step.

The two points at which the intestine is to be divided are first secured. At each of these two points the mesentery is pierced close to the gut with a Deschamp needle or a Korn forceps and a stout silk thread, or better, a piece of tape or a thin rubber tube is pulled through the opening (Fig. 208). The line of division of the bridge of mesentery between these two tractors is as follows:—at each end the line of division runs close to the gut for about 4 cm. and then describes a curve toward the root of the mesentery, the middle of the curve coming closest to the origin of the root of the mesentery near the spine.

A proper division of the intestine and the management of the resultant openings by terminal closure with lateral anastomosis or end-to-end anastomosis require that the gut be freed completely from its mesentery for several centimeters. In the case of the large bowel the epiploic appendages must also be removed from this zone. However, in the loops which are to remain in the body, the length of the intestinal segment robbed of its mesenteric blood supply must not be too great, lest disturbances in nutrition arise. Such nutritional disturbances can be recognized during the operation by a bluish-red discoloration of the gut and by the absence of pulsation of the vessels on its surface. If such signs appear, and they must be looked for with particular care in every case, the end must be shortened as far as the normal tissue before suturing.

The reason for the curved line of division of the mesentery as above described (Fig. 208) is based upon the fact that in extensive resections the distance which must be ligated is materially shorter than if the mesentery were divided close to the bowel along the line of its attachment. In view of the fan-shaped form of the mesentery, the path from one loop of gut to another is shorter the closer it lies to the root of the mesentery. In the case of malignant and other lesions which have invaded the mesentery, the curve of the line of resection toward the root of the mesentery has the additional advantage of a wider removal of the threatened or invaded zone.

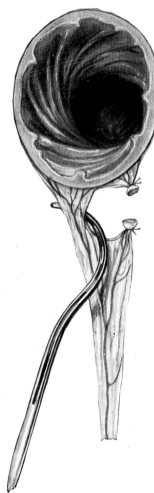

FIG. 209. Ligation of the mesentery at its attachment to the bowel. The mesentery which fans out as it joins the bowel is picked up on both sides, ligated and cut close to the gut so that the ligated stumps remaining attached to the bowel shall be as small as possible.

The division of the mesentery is performed in steps, after double ligation with silk passed with the aid of an aneurysm needle (Fig. 208). If there is sufficient room, the control of bleeding on the side of the segment of gut to be removed may be effected by the application of hemostats. Frequently, however, the mass of attached hemostats obstructs the view and impedes further work on the gut, so that the time saved by applying hemostats instead of ligatures is counterbalanced by the obstruction of view and interference with the progress of the operation.

In the region of the line of division of the intestine the ligation of the mesentery is carried out in very small portions at a time, with regard to subsequent closure or end-to-end anastomosis. Because of the fork-shaped form of the mesenteric attachment to the gut, the ligatures here are applied alternately on one side, then the other (Fig. 209). When ligating close to the gut, particular care must be exercised in the case of the large bowel that the ligature does not include a diverticulum, since a perforative peritonitis can result if the ligature subsequently cuts through.

As the line of division of the mesentery becomes farther from the gut, the individual ligations should be very carefully placed. The vessels in the loose tissue of the mesentery have a decided tendency to retract, especially in the obese, which may lead to dangerous and even fatal bleeding. Therefore, the individual ligations should not exceed a certain breadth, the ligatures must be tied slowly and tightly, and in cutting the mesentery a long nubbin of tissue is left on the side of the mesentery which remains in the body.

In spite of these precautionary measures, the slipping-off of ligatures is not always prevented with certainty in the case of an unusually fat or extremely edematous mesentery. In such cases the surgeon can avoid difficulty by dividing the mesentery peripheral to the holes in the mesentery resulting from the passage of the ligatures, so that the ligatures after the completion of the resection do not lie at the ends of separate tips of mesentery but in a chain of closed circles out of which they cannot slip. This is done as follows (Fig. 208):—A segment of the mesentery is transfixed with an aneurysm needle carrying the ligature, and the ligature is tied. The attached but considerably broader segment of the mesentery peripheral to the ligation is tightly clamped across with a Kocher clamp. The mesentery is cut with a scissors between the clamp and the ligature, but not to the full width of the ligated portion and without opening the gaps in the mesentery through which the ligature passes. The succeeding ligatures are applied in the same manner until the whole sector of mesentery has been divided.

By the continued ligation and division of its individual segments, the whole stretch of mesentery between the two tractors passed around the gut is finally divided in its full extent. In so doing, it is often advisable, after the division has been carried from one end as far as the middle, to begin at the other end and work back to the middle.

At the end of every intestinal resection the gap in the mesentery resulting from the removal of a portion of the mesentery must be closed by suture to prevent intestinal loops from slipping through and possibly becoming strangulated (Figs. 64 and 65). During the suture of the mesentery the vessels must be carefully avoided.

The Mobilization of the Ascending and the Descending Colon. In the region of the ascending and the descending colon, where a free mesentery is not present, the colon lies with its posterior surface against an expanse of the posterior abdominal wall. The separation of the gut from its vascular connections in these areas is somewhat different.

During fetal life the afore-mentioned parts of the colon originally had a free mesentery attached medially, which after the rotation of the bowel became adherent to the posterior abdominal wall. Consequently, the blood vessels

reach these parts of the colon from its medial side, with only a few unimportant vessels from the lateral side. The mobilization of the gut must therefore
be carried out from the lateral toward the medial side. The peritoneum is first
incised on the outer side of the colon along the line of reflection of the peritoneum from the posterior abdominal wall to the gut (Figs. 210 and 211).
By pulling on the gut, the peritoneum on its outer side is made tense and can
usually be divided with a few passes of the knife. Only an occasional vessel
must be caught and tied (Fig. 211). As soon as the medial side of the gut is
reached, the vessels approach the gut in a broad, highly vascular layer of
connective tissue. This connective-tissue layer is carefully divided close to
the gut between double ligatures (Fig. 212). In so doing, care must be taken
of the ureter which runs retroperitoneally on the posterior surface of the

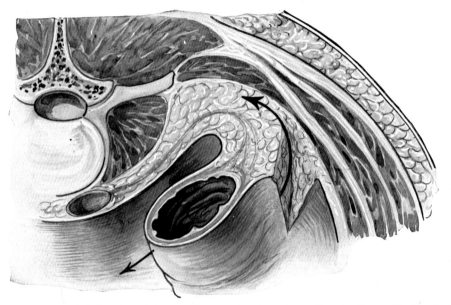

FIG. 210. Chief direction of the vascular supply of the descending (and ascending) colon.
Separation undertaken from without inward in the direction of the large arrow does not injure
the vessels as they approach the bowel from within outward. Diagrammatic.

peritoneal reflection to the medial side of the ascending and the descending
colon and which can easily be picked up while detaching the peritoneum from
the posterior abdominal wall. In its upper portion the ureter lies quite close
to the colon or even just beneath it. In its lower segment it lies some distance
to the medial side of the colon, crossing over and in front of the internal iliac
artery.

Division of the Intestine. The technique of transsection of the intestine
has been described in Chapter II. The management of the openings resulting
from the resection depends upon the manner in which the intestinal channel
is to be reconstructed, whether end-to-end, side-to-side, end-to-side or side-to-
end, and whether the anastomosis is to be made at the point of division or at a
distance from this point in one or both segments, or whether there is to be no
anastomosis at all, while one or both loops are brought to the surface.

In the small intestine, there is usually a free choice of the location and the method of anastomosis. All of its segments, with the exception of the duodenojejunal junction and the ileocecal junction, are extremely mobile and can be displaced quite a distance. Being covered on all sides with peritoneum, they can readily be closed by terminal suture and can be used for every type of anastomosis. The large bowel, on the other hand, often gives trouble in this regard. It is only slightly mobile, and in the region of the

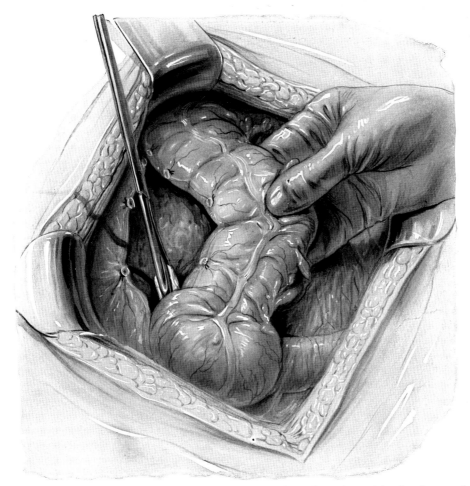

FIG. 211. Mobilization of the cecum and the ascending colon. An incision has been made in the peritoneal fold at the outer side of the colon which is freed toward the midline by blunt dissection. In so doing, only a few small vessels must be ligated.

ascending and the descending colon is only partially covered with peritoneum, and chiefly on its anterior surface.

Since the dependability of the closure of a transsection opening of the intestine depends largely upon its peritoneal covering, many surgeons have misgivings as to the terminal closure of the ascending and the descending colon with their posterior surface devoid of peritoneum. In case the position of a lesion would lead to division in the region of these sections of the bowel the operator often prefers to extend the resection to the next portion of the gut which is completely clothed with peritoneum: the ileum, the transverse colon or the sigmoid. I do not consider such misgivings justified. In my opinion the open end of a gut only partly covered with peritoneum may be closed quite dependably.

Nevertheless, it may become necessary in the course of a resection to leave behind individual segments of the gut as blind ends or to remove them by carrying the resection beyond the point required by the lesion. It is never permissible to leave in the abdomen an intestinal segment which has been closed at both ends. The mucus which is constantly secreted will in time

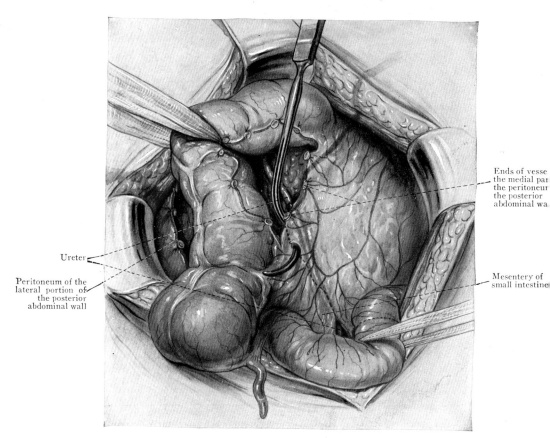

Ends of vesse
the medial par
the peritoneur
the posterior
abdominal wa.

Ureter

Peritoneum of the
lateral portion of
the posterior
abdominal wall

Mesentery of
small intestine

FIG. 212. Resection of the cecum and the ascending colon. The colon has largely been freed from its attachments. Tapes are passed around the bowel at the intended points of division. The mesentery of the ileum remains still to be ligated. The ureter can be seen beneath the peritoneum.

distend a closed loop and may lead eventually to its rupture. Every short-circuited segment of gut must therefore remain in connection with the rest of the intestinal canal or must be brought into communication with the intestinal canal or with the exterior so that it can constantly empty itself. In this connection, the rules laid down in the preceding sections for the short-circuiting of a loop of intestine are to be followed.

5. SINGLE-STAGE INTESTINAL RESECTION. (PRIMARY RESECTION AND PRIMARY REESTABLISHMENT OF INTESTINAL CONTINUITY.)

After the diseased loop has been removed by dividing its mesentery and both its ends, the proximal and the distal segments are immediately anastomosed end-to-end, side-to-side, side-to-end, or end-to-side, whichever happens to be most suitable (Fig. 213).

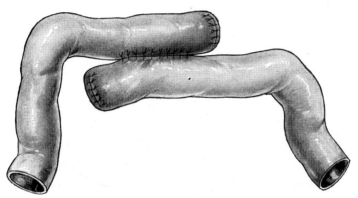

FIG. 213. Completed one stage intestinal resection and anastomosis. The proximal and distal loops have been anastomosed side-to-side near their ends. Diagrammatic.

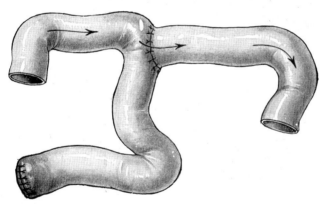

FIG. 214. Completed one stage intestinal resection and anastomosis. The end of the proximal loop could not be joined to the end of the distal loop. Diagrammatic.

If the two cut ends of the intestine cannot be brought together for an end-to-end anastomosis of the proximal and distal loops, the anastomosis may also be performed at another point in the course of the proximal loop (Fig. 214), or of the distal loop (Fig. 215) or of both (Fig. 216). The end which does not take part in the anastomosis is closed, and is thereby short-circuited on one side. It is obvious that the short-circuited segment should be as short as possible. The loop, short-circuited on one side, must be able to drain into the intestinal channel or to the exterior in accordance with the previous discussion. In this regard, the ileocecal valve cannot be considered patent in a retrograde direction (Fig. 217).

Case 1. Example of a single-stage intestinal resection for the cure of ileocecal tuberculosis
(Fig. 218). The terminal ileum and the lower half of the ascending colon were resected during
an inactive stage of the disease. The proximal loop of ileum and the distal limb of the ascending

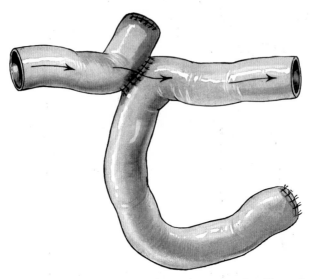

FIG. 215. Completed one stage intestinal resection and anastomosis. The end of the distal loop
could not be joined to the end of the proximal loop. Diagrammatic.

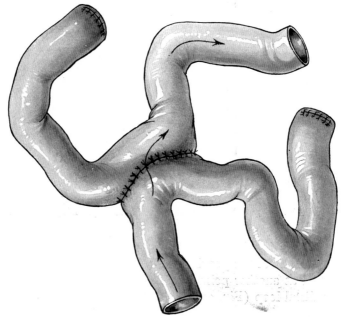

FIG. 216. Completed one stage intestinal resection and anastomosis. The ends of the proximal and distal loops could not be used in the anastomosis. Diagrammatic.

colon could not be brought together. Both gut ends were therefore closed blind and the ileum
was anastomosed side-to-side to the transverse colon.

Case 2. Example of a single-stage intestinal resection, sacrificing a normal ileocecal valve
(Fig. 219). The removal of a carcinoma of the hepatic flexure coming to operation without

signs of obstruction would of itself require the resection of a segment extending from the middle of the ascending colon to the middle of the transverse colon. It would have been impossible to bring together the two resultant open ends, and the reestablishment of the intestinal channel would have required the anastomosis of the terminal ileum to the distal limb of the transverse

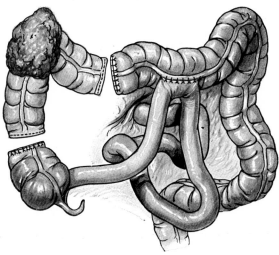

FIG. 217. Improper short-circuiting of the cecum in case of a primary resection for carcinoma of the hepatic flexure. Diagrammatic. There is no assurance that the ileocecal valve is patulous in a retrograde direction, so that the short-circuited cecum may become over-distended.

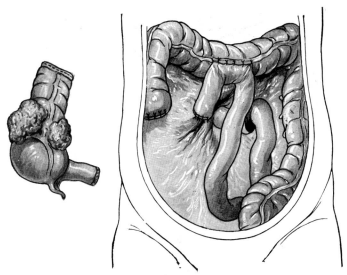

FIG. 218. Example of a one stage intestinal resection. Diagrammatic. Resection of termi-nal ileum and cecum, blind closure of both openings, reestablishment of intestinal continuity by side-to-side anastomosis of the lower ileum with the transverse colon.

colon. This would have left the short-circuited cecum in communication with the rest of the gut only by way of the ileocecal valve. Since the retrograde patency of this valve is uncertain, this procedure would not have been satisfactory. The resection was therefore extended from the ascending colon beyond the ascending colon and the cecum to the lowest loop of ileum. After a blind closure of the proximal ileum and of the distal loop of the transverse colon, these two intestinal segments were anastomosed side-to-side.

In a single-stage intestinal resection the fresh suture line between the proximal and distal loops is immediately subjected under ordinary circumstances to a full functional load by the intestinal contents. The proximal intestine can get rid of its contents only by the use of the full length of the

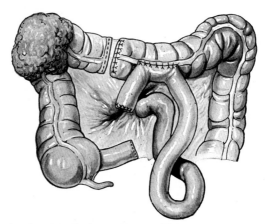

Fig. 219. Example of an intestinal resection sacrificing a normal ileocecal valve. Diagrammatic. Although it would have been possible to divide the colon between the lesion and the cecum and thereby preserve the latter, the cecum and the ileocecal valve were removed because it could not be assured that the valve would be patulous in a retrograde direction.

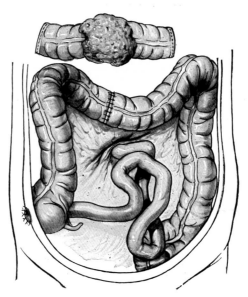

Fig. 220. Example of a one stage intestinal resection with simultaneous establishment of a protective fecal fistula. Diagrammatic. After the resection of the diseased segment of the transverse colon and the end-to-end anastomosis of the colon, a cecal fistula has been made to protect the suture line of the colon.

distal intestinal canal. In case of a difficult intestinal suture or of excessive accumulation of intestinal contents, the need therefore arises to relieve the intestinal suture and to make the work of evacuation easier for the gut. This may be accomplished by establishing a safety-valve near and proximal to the anastomosis in the shape of an intestinal fistula or an artificial anus. Such a relief opening can be made some time before the intestinal resection, at a separate preliminary operation. The fistula is allowed to remain for some time after the main operation. Or the fistula may be established at the time of the main operation. The intestinal resection as such is nevertheless carried out at a single sitting. It is simply a matter of custom and terminology whether this type of intestinal resection with preliminary establishment of an intestinal fistula is to be designated as "single-stage" or "two-stage" operation.

Case 3. Example of a single-stage intestinal resection with simultaneous establishment of an intestinal fistula (Fig. 220). In a case of carcinoma of the transverse colon the middle segment of the transverse colon had to be resected. The openings of the transverse colon were anastomosed end-to-end. The small intestine was greatly distended so that it seemed that the intestinal suture would be subjected to marked tension. To relieve the intestinal suture line, a fecal fistula was established in the cecum. Three weeks after the operation the fistula was closed.

6. MULTIPLE-STAGE INTESTINAL RESECTION

The dividing of an intestinal resection into two or more separate operations may be necessary for any of the following reasons: The condition of the patient does not permit the major procedure of a single-stage resection. The resection of the diseased intestine or the anastomosis between the proximal and distal loops appears to be unusually difficult. The excessive filling of the intestine makes advisable the immediate external evacuation of the obstructed fecal masses in the proximal loop, with short-circuiting of the distal gut. The increased infectiousness of the intestinal contents makes an extensive procedure in the abdominal cavity undesirable after opening the intestine. Such contra-indications to a single-stage resection are particularly frequent in acute intestinal obstruction, and not rare in chronic obstruction. In general, the two-stage procedure is only rarely used in the small intestine, while in the large bowel it is the procedure of choice for some operations.

A two-stage intestinal resection may be carried out in one of three ways:

(A) PRIMARY SHORT-CIRCUITING AND SECONDARY RESECTION OF A LOOP OF INTESTINE

The short-circuiting of the diseased loop at the first operation follows one of the methods already described for intestinal short-circuiting by the formation of a new fecal channel. The loop to be resected remains in connection with the body and in the interior of the abdomen. At the second operation the loop is resected. The diseased gut may be left within the abdomen at the first operation only if the disease process neither at the moment nor in the immediate future entails any danger of infection for the peritoneal cavity. It is therefore not permissible to permit it to remain in infections, marked nutritional disturbances or possible perforation of the diseased gut.

The short-circuiting of a diseased loop which is to be resected is carried out most simply at the first operation by a side-to-side anastomosis of the proximal and distal loops (Fig. 200). If it is technically difficult or impossible to bring the proximal and distal loops together for a sufficient distance to perform a side-to-side anastomosis, the diseased loop may also be short-circuited by dividing the distal loop, closing the proximal end of the transsection and implanting the distal end into the proximal loop. Or, the proximal loop is divided, the distal end of the transsection is closed and the proximal end is implanted into the distal loop (Figs. 202 and 221). The blind closure of one end of a short-circuited diseased loop presupposes that the site of the lesion is passable for fluids arising in the lesion (mucus, pus, blood and gases). Therefore, if the gut is not patulous at the site of the lesion, as for example in case of a carcinoma completely obstructing the lumen, the segment short-circuited on one side must be brought into communication with the exterior. This is accomplished either by a lateral fistula or by suturing the divided end into the abdominal wound (Fig. 204).

At the second operation the short-circuited diseased loop is removed by dividing the attached mesentery, transsecting the proximal and distal loops and closing the ends remaining in the body. If one of the two loops was already divided at the first operation, there remains only the transsection of the proximal loop or of the distal loop between the anastomosis and the diseased segment. In order to simplify the second operation the division of one limb of the diseased loop is frequently undertaken at the first operation.

It is possible at the first sitting of a two-stage intestinal resection to divide and anastomose the proximal and the distal limbs (Fig. 204), the resection of the diseased loop being deferred to the second operation as being too great a tax on the patient. In that case the completely short-circuited loop must have a communication for drainage to the exterior. This is done, for example, by suturing the end of one of the limbs of the segment into the abdominal wound or by making a lateral fistula. At the second operation only the resection of the isolated diseased loop remains to be performed.

Case 4. Example of a two-stage intestinal resection with primary unilateral short-circuiting of a tuberculous ileocecal region and secondary resection of the diseased intestine. A woman of 35 had had gradually increasing signs of partial intestinal obstruction, which according to the Roentgen-ray study was due to stenosis of the intestine in the region of the ileocecal valve. A vague mass was palpable in this region. Nevertheless the bowel could be emptied easily with enemata and laxatives. The patient was in a very weakened condition. Tubercle bacilli were present in the stool. A diagnosis of ileocecal tuberculosis was made.

The patient was anesthetized with spinal anesthesia, placed in the Trendelenburg position and tipped well to the left. The abdomen was opened through a right lateral rectus incision. Tuberculosis of the ileocecal region was found involving 15 cm. of the terminal ileum and the adjacent portion of the mesentery and the proximal third of the ascending colon. In view of the patient's poor condition, a single-stage resection seemed inadvisable. Eventration was out of the question because of the firm adherence of the mass to the posterior abdominal wall. It even seemed doubtful whether the patient would recover sufficiently that a major resection might ever be risked.

A short-circuiting anastomosis was therefore performed (Fig. 221). At a point 30 cm. above the cecum, that is, 15 cm. proximal to the beginning of the lesion, the ileum was freed from its mesentery for a distance of 4 cm. by multiple ligation and division of the mesentery. The operative field was carefully walled off. In the middle of this freed segment the gut was transsected with the aid of the Petz suture instrument. Both ends were invaginated with Lambert sutures.

The transverse colon, easy to recognize by the greater omentum attached to it, was drawn down and delivered. The ileum was anastomosed side-to-side to the transverse colon at a point in the ileum 10 cm. above the site of its closed end. In the anastomosis, a taenia of the colon was used for the first suture line. The abdomen was closed without drainage (Fig. 221).

The patient made an excellent postoperative recovery in the course of the next few weeks and had regular bowel movements. Occasionally there were loose mucous stools in which tubercle bacilli could be demonstrated. A month later the radical removal of the diseased segment was decided upon. The patient, under spinal anesthesia, was placed in the Trendelenburg position and tipped to the left. The abdomen was opened through the scar. The cecum and ascending colon were exposed, pulled forward and followed to just below the hepatic flexure where the gut seemed to be healthy. Beginning in sound tissue, an incision was made on the lateral side of the ascending colon through the line of reflection of the peritoneum from the posterior abdominal wall of the colon. Drawn sharply to the left, the normal portion of the colon could easily be freed from the posterior abdominal wall. Only a few vessels were encountered and these were doubly ligated and cut. On the medial side of the colon, however, was the attachment of the thick mesenteric plate, richly supplied with blood vessels. This was ligated in sections and divided close to the colon.

In this way the normal part of the ascending colon was freed from its connections on all sides. A rubber tube was placed beneath it. At its distal end the freeing of the ascending colon was continued by ligation and sharp and blunt dissection beyond the hepatic flexure as far as the anastomosis between the transverse colon and the lowest loop of ileum. Ten centimeters proximal to this point the colon was divided with the aid of the Petz suture instrument. The distal end was invaginated with Lembert sutures and dropped, while the proximal end was covered with a condom.

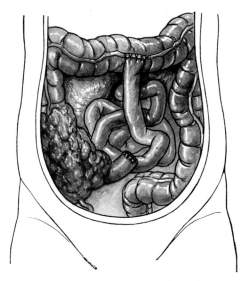

Fig. 221. Example of a two-stage intestinal resection with primary shortcircuiting and secondary resection of the diseased loop, at the end of the first operation. Diagrammatic. Because of tuberculosis of the ileocecal region, the terminal ileum has been divided, its distal end closed and its proximal end joined end-to-side to the transverse colon.

Traction was made on the proximal end, and the colon was easily freed as far as the ileocecal junction. At this point difficulties arose because of a large mass of tuberculous glands in the angle of the mesentery between the ileum and the ascending colon, the mass being tightly adherent to the posterior abdominal wall. Since it was impossible to tell at a glance to what extent the ureter and the iliac vessels were involved in this mass, these structures were looked for on the posterior abdominal wall above this point. By pulling the colon and the cecum vertically and to the left, while the vessels and the ureter were pushed against the posterior abdominal wall with dissecting forceps, it gradually became possible by blunt dissection to separate the mass and the intestine from the posterior abdominal wall and from the ureter and vessels. In so doing, the dissection was carried on constantly from the lateral toward the medial side. A triangular tuberculous mass in the mesentery extending toward the spine caused particular difficulty. Finally it, too, was freed without injury to the main trunk of the superior mesenteric artery passing close to its tip. The mesentery of the lowest loop of ileum was divided between ligatures. Since the ileum had been divided at the first operation, the whole diseased portion of gut, including also the appendix, was now free and was removed from the abdomen (Fig. 222).

The large raw surface, whose floor was formed by the iliopsoas muscle with the large vessels and the ureter, was once more carefully inspected for bleeding points and was covered as far as possible by suturing the adjacent edges of the peritoneum. This was successful except for an area the size of a silver dollar, which was covered by drawing the right tube over it. The abdomen was closed without drainage.

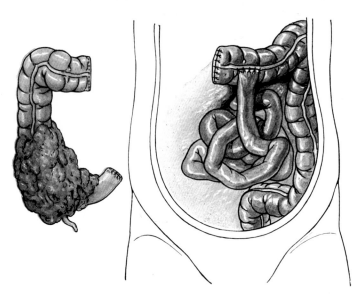

Fig. 222. Continuation of conditions of the preceding illustration, at the end of the second operation. Diagrammatic. The transverse colon has been divided proximal to the end-to-side anastomosis and the distal end closed blind. The short-circuited bowel with the lesion has been resected.

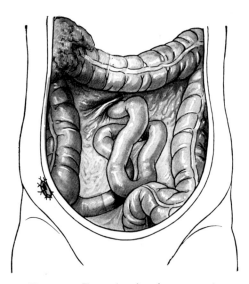

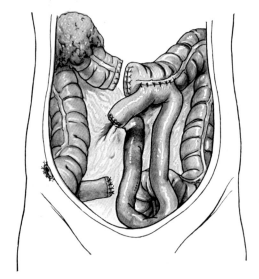

Fig. 223. Example of a three-stage intestinal resection, at the end of the first operation. Diagrammatic. A cecal fistula has been established because of a carcinoma of the hepatic flexure coming under treatment in a state of acute obstruction.

Fig. 224. Continuation of the preceding illustration, at the end of the second operation. Diagrammatic. A side-to-side anastomosis has been established between the terminal loop of ileum and the transverse colon, the proximal and distal limbs of the diseased loop have been transsected and the intestinal openings closed blind. The completely short-circuited segment is drained externally by the cecal fistula.

Case 5. Example of a three-stage intestinal resection. (Primary establishment of fecal fistula, secondary, complete short-circuiting of the diseased loop, tertiary resection.) A patient with a carcinoma of the hepatic flexure was admitted in acute ileus and in such a poor condition that the only feasible procedure was the establishment of a cecal fistula to relieve the obstruction (Fig. 223).

After the patient had sufficiently recovered three weeks later, the abdomen was opened through a midline incision below the umbilicus. A single-stage resection of the diseased intestine was decided upon. The ileum was divided 10 cm. above the ileocecal valve and the transverse colon at its midpoint. The four transsection openings were carefully closed by suture. The proximal loop of the ileum was anastomosed side-to-side to the distal limb of the transverse colon. In the meantime the condition of the patient had grown so much worse that an early termination of the operation appeared desirable. The short-circuited segment which had a communica-

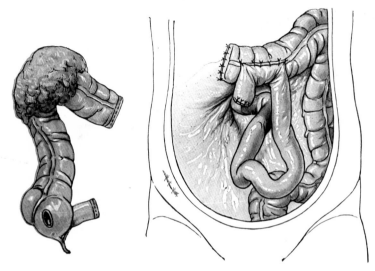

Fɪɢ. 225. Continuation of the preceding illustration, at the end of the third operation. Diagrammatic. The segment which was completely short-circuited at the preceding operation has been removed.

tion with the exterior through the cecal fistula made at the first operation, (the patency of the carcinomatous portion of the hepatic flexure had been ascertained during the operation), was therefore left in the abdomen (Fig. 224). The laparotomy wound was closed without drainage.

After 3 weeks the short-circuited carcinomatous segment was removed through a right rectus incision (Fig. 225).

(B) PRIMARY RESECTION OF AN INTESTINAL LOOP WITH ESTABLISHMENT OF AN ARTIFICIAL ANUS; SECONDARY REESTABLISHMENT OF INTESTINAL CONTINUITY AND CLOSURE OF THE ARTIFICIAL ANUS

An intestinal resection of this type may be done if a single-stage resection is not feasible for any of the reasons previously given; if the nature of the lesion nevertheless demands the immediate removal of the diseased loop and if the over-distension of the proximal gut makes the free and adequate evacuation of the intestinal contents through an artificial anus desirable. Such conditions are occasionally found, as for example, in an operation for strangulated hernia with a gangrenous loop of intestine.

At the first operation the diseased intestinal segment is resected and at the same time the evacuation of the feces from the proximal loop is provided for by making an artificial anus. This can be performed in the following ways. Both the proximal and the distal limbs are brought to the surface. If both limbs can be led through the abdominal wall at the same point, they are placed side by side and, for the later reestablishment of the intestinal channel, a double-barrelled type of anus is constructed if possible (Figs. 226 and 230). If the two limbs of gut cannot be brought together, they can be brought to the surface at two separate points (Fig. 227). It is permissible, however, in such a case to bring only the proximal limb to the surface, the distal limb being closed blind and left in the abdomen (Fig. 228). It is preferable, although more difficult in the presence of distended gut, to attach the proximal loop

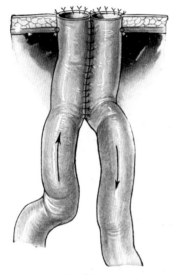

FIG. 226. Two-stage intestinal resection, at the end of the first operation. Diagrammatic. The diseased loop has been resected, the proximal and distal limbs have been brought to the surface in the form of a double-barrelled artificial anus.

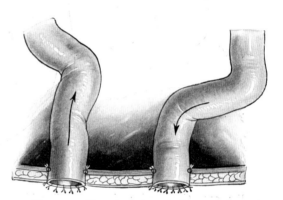

FIG. 227. Two-stage intestinal resection, at the end of the first operation. Diagrammatic. The diseased loop has been resected, the proximal and the distal limbs have been brought to the surface separately.

side-to-side to the distal loop which has been carried to the exterior (Fig. 229), because this simplifies the second operation, the reestablishment of the intestinal channel.

The second operation consists in the reestablishment of the intestinal channel and closure of the artificial anus. The procedures applicable in this operation have already been discussed.

Case 6. Example of a two-stage intestinal resection with primary resection, formation of an artificial anus and secondary closure of the artificial anus. In an operation for strangulated inguinal hernia a knotted mass of gangrenous ileum was found in a phlegmonous hernial sac. The gangrenous intestinal loops were resected. In view of the poor general condition of the patient, the severe infection in the hernial sac and in the abdominal cavity and the marked distension of the whole gut, a primary anastomosis of the proximal with the distal loop was not done. Both ileal loops were brought out through the enlarged hernial orifice, attached to the parietal peritoneum and walled off against the general peritoneal cavity with vioform gauze, the open ends of the loops pointing outward. A large drainage tube was tied into the proximal loop and connected by a rubber tube to a collecting receptacle.

Three weeks later, the proximal and distal loops were picked up through a midline incision, the two limbs anastomosed side-to-side, and divided between the anastomosis and the artificial anus. The blind ends of the proximal and distal loops were securely closed. The intestinal segments attached to the hernial orifice were then resected.

Case 7. Example of a three-stage intestinal resection in a case of gangrene of the transverse colon, with primary resection and establishment of a terminal artificial anus in the proximal loop and terminal closure of the distal loop; with secondary entero-enterostomy between the ascending colon and the sigmoid, and with tertiary closure of the artificial anus. A man of 50 with a cardiac lesion was suddenly taken ill with severe abdominal pain localized in the region of the umbilicus and with the general symptoms of peritonitis. A tentative diagnosis of a perforated gastric ulcer was made and the abdomen was opened through a median incision under spinal anaesthesia, ten hours after the onset of illness. A 20 cm. section of the transverse colon was found to be bluish black. After delivering the transverse colon into the wound so as to inspect the transverse meso-colon from below, there was discovered an occlusion of the middle colic artery.

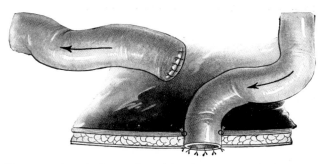

Fig. 228. Two-stage intestinal resection with primary removal of the diseased loop, at the end of the first operation. Diagrammatic. The diseased loop has been removed, the proximal loop has been brought to the surface as an artificial anus, the distal loop has been closed blind and dropped.

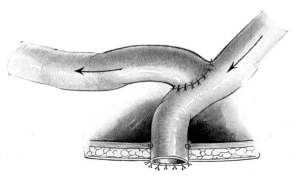

Fig. 229. Two-stage intestinal resection with primary removal of the diseased loop, at the end of the first operation. Diagrammatic. The diseased loop has been removed, the proximal limb has been brought to the surface as an artificial anus, the distal limb has been anastomosed to the proximal limb by end-to-side anastomosis.

It was of course necessary to resect the gangrenous segment of gut immediately, since eventration of the loop was impossible because of a short transverse mesocolon. Experience has shown that such vascular occlusions frequently tend to extend in a short time, so that the resection of the entire transverse colon was decided upon. Direct anastomosis of the two ends of the colon was impossible because of the great distance between them.

With a blunt forceps, cotton tapes were passed through the transverse mesocolon close to the gut, one each at the hepatic and splenic flexures. The gut was pulled out and put on tension by means of these two tractors, while the stomach and the remaining intestines were replaced in the abdominal cavity. The operative field was carefully packed off. First the gastrocolic omentum and then the transverse mesocolon were picked up in small segments on an aneurysm needle, doubly ligated and divided. In so doing, the line of division ran close to the colon for a distance of about 4 cm. at each end, then curved toward the spine, in order to remove the thrombosed vessels of the mesocolon as completely as possible. In a similar manner the greater omentum was divided bit by bit on the right and the left. In the region of the splenic flexure, at the starting point of the mobilization of the colon, the epiploic appendages were carefully ligated and cut away, so that the gut was entirely free for a distance of about 5 cm. At this point the colon was divided with the aid of the Petz suture instrument, the line of division passing between the two rows of clips. The proximal end was covered with a rubber condom and the distal end was closed and buried by a second row of invaginating Lembert sutures (Fig. 231).

Since the patient's general condition was not very good, an early termination of the operation was advisable. It did not appear feasible, therefore, to anastomose the proximal and distal segments of the gut at this time, especially since there were already present the signs of a beginning peritonitis.

An incision 5 cm. long was therefore made in the right hypochondrium just at the point where the transverse colon, still attached at the hepatic flexure, could be led to the exterior with ease. After the skin and the external oblique muscle had been incised, the deeper muscle layers were separated by blunt dissection. Retraction was obtained with two hooked retractors, resulting in a round hole, 3 to 4 cm. in diameter, in the bottom of which the peritoneum appeared. While the

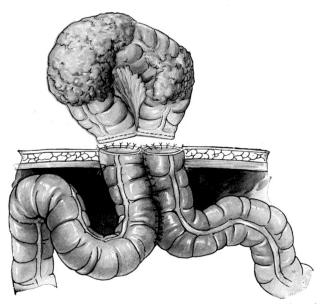

FIG. 230. Two-stage resection of the colon with eventration and double-barreled arrangement of the proximal and distal limbs. Diagrammatic.

right side of the midline laparotomy wound was held high, a forceps was introduced through the median incision and pushed forward through the wound in the right hypochondrium, so that the parietal peritoneum presented in a tent-like projection. The peritoneum was opened by a crucial incision and the four tips were sutured to the skin.

The right abdominal wall was further elevated and a Langenbeck retractor was inserted from the outside into the small abdominal wound in the right hypochondrium. With a forceps introduced through the smaller opening, the operator grasped the end of the transverse colon, which had been closed with Petz clips and covered with a condom, and pulled it out through the opening until there was no more slack in the loop of transverse colon leading to the hepatic flexure.

The median laparotomy wound was closed without drainage.

The transverse colon was sutured all around to the parietal peritoneum at the place where the gut passed through the small abdominal incision. The skin was also sutured to the colon. The eventrated transverse colon was amputated 5 cm. above the surface of the skin with an electro-surgical knife. A Paul-Mixter glass tube was inserted into the proximal limb of the gut and tied securely. The glass tube was provided with a rubber drainage tube which was carried to a receptacle (Fig. 231).

After three weeks the patient had recovered sufficiently so that the continuity of the intestinal channel could be reestablished at a second operation. For this purpose the abdomen was again

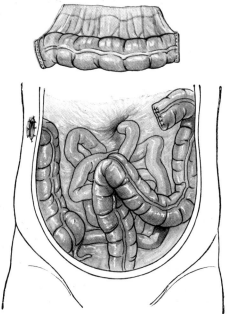

Fig. 231. Example of a three-stage intestinal resection, at the end of the first operation. Diagrammatic. The transverse colon has been resected. The ascending colon has been brought to the surface as an artificial anus. The distal end of the transverse colon is closed.

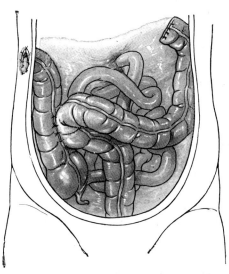

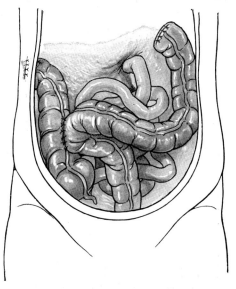

Fig. 232. Continuation of conditions of the preceding illustration, at the end of the second operation. A side-to-side anastomosis has been established between the ascending colon and the sigmoid.

Fig. 233. Continuation of conditions of the preceding illustration, at the end of the third operation. The artificial anus, which was shortcircuited on one side by the preceding operation has been closed.

opened through a midline incision. The freely movable dome of the sigmoid loop was anastomosed, side-to-side with the cecum (Fig. 232).

In the period which followed, the anastomosis between the cecum and the sigmoid functioned satisfactorily. The artificial anus in the right hypochondrium was then closed at a third operation. Under local anaesthesia the tissue around the artificial anus was freshened, leaving a narrow edge of skin attached to the anal opening. The individual layers of the abdominal wall were dissected free to the parietal peritoneum without opening the peritoneal cavity, the opening in the colon was closed and the abdominal wall repaired by tier suture (Fig. 233).

(c) INTESTINAL RESECTION AFTER AN EVENTRATION PROCEDURE

The eventration procedure owes its development to the desire to avoid all contamination of the general abdominal cavity by the escape of intestinal contents. The diseased loop of intestine is eventrated in a closed state at the first operation and is later resected outside the abdomen at a second opera-

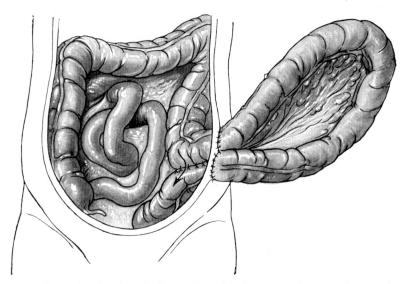

FIG. 234. Example of an intestinal resection with the eventration procedure, at the end of the first operation. Diagrammatic. The diseased sigmoid has been eventrated and sutured to the abdominal wall, the proximal and distal limbs have been sutured side to side for some distance with the purpose of forming a double-barreled artificial anus.

tion after the abdominal wound has healed and the peritoneal cavity has been completely sealed. The subsequent anastomosis of the proximal and distal limbs and the closure of the artificial anus resulting from the resection can also be carried out without opening the abdominal cavity by utilizing a "double-barreled" apposition of the proximal and distal limbs. In this way the whole operation actually becomes an "aseptic intestinal resection" from the standpoint of the abdominal cavity. Furthermore, since eventration is a simple, short operation, and since the resection dwindles to a harmless extraperitoneal procedure, the measure is particularly indicated in patients with low powers of resistance and in case of highly infective intestinal contents. The accumulated intestinal contents can be evacuated on the day after, or even on the same day of the eventration by aspiration of the intestinal loop or by burning a small hole into it with the cautery.

The eventration procedure is dependent upon a considerable mobility of the loop to be resected as possessed particularly by the small intestine, the transverse colon, the cecum and the sigmoid.

The secondary operations consist in the resection of the eventrated loop and in the closure of the resultant artificial anus. (It should however be con-

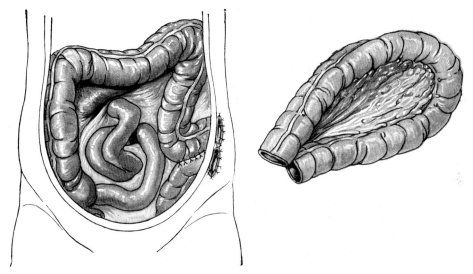

FIG. 235. Continuation of conditions of the preceding illustration, at the end of the second operation. The eventrated loop has been amputated and the double-barrelled artificial anus formed.

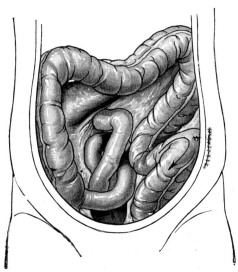

FIG. 236. Conditions at the end of the third operation. Diagrammatic. The double-barrelled artificial anus has been closed and intestinal continuity reestablished.

sidered that such multiple procedures prolong convalescence, and leave the patient with a weaker abdominal wall. Although they should be used in specially selected cases they should not be used as routine measures. I. S. R.)

The first operation is carried out as follows. The mesentery is punc-

tured at the midpoint of the diseased intestinal segment. A strip of gauze is
pulled through the opening. The diseased intestinal segment is lifted with the
aid of the gauze strip. The connections with the surroundings are sufficiently
freed so that the loop to be resected can be drawn wholly out of the wound and
so that its proximal and distal limbs can be placed side by side for a distance
of 8 to 10 cm. (Fig. 234). For this distance they are sutured together, side
by side, avoiding their mesenteries. The double-barrelled structure so formed
is replaced in the abdomen and at the level of its emergence from the abdomen
is carefully sutured to the parietal peritoneum.

In most cases the main laparotomy wound, made smaller to fit, is used
to bring the loop of intestine to the surface. If, however, the laparotomy

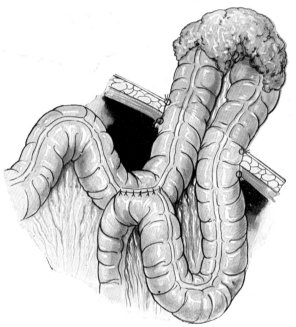

Fig. 237. Example of an intestinal resection after eventration, with primary anastomosis
within the abdominal cavity between the proximal and the distal loop, at the end of the first
operation. Diagrammatic. The diseased loop has been eventrated and sutured to the abdominal
wall. At some distance from the abdominal wall an anastomosis has been made between the
proximal and the distal loop.

wound is located at some distance from the diseased segment, it is better to
make a new incision immediately over the loop and to eventrate the loop
through the new opening which is made just large enough for the purpose. The
skin is attached by sutures to the gut loops at the point of their emergence.

If it seems necessary to open the bowel, the proximal loop of the eventrated segment is aspirated at once or on the following day, or it may be
opened by making a small hole in the gut. Otherwise, the opening of the
bowel and the attendant contamination of the operative field can be delayed
for several days while the eventrated loop is emptied by repeated aspiration.

Up to this point the operation proceeds in almost the same manner as the
formation of a double-barrelled artificial anus, described on page 234, except
that in the former the diseased intestine is eventrated to a large extent, whereas

in the latter only sufficient intestine is eventrated for the transsection of the loop.

Second Operation.   Not until about one to two weeks later is the eventrated loop with its mesentery amputated at the skin level with a cautery (Fig. 235).   Since the cutting of the mesentery is painful for the patient, the mesentery is infiltrated with a local anaesthetic solution before the amputation. The mesentery is ligated en masse and divided in the usual manner, and any spurting vessels are caught and tied.

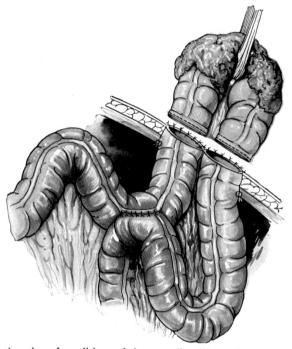

FIG. 238.   Continuation of conditions of the preceding illustration, at the end of the second operation.   The diseased eventrated loop has been amputated.   The proximal and distal loops, which have been shortcircuited on one side by an anastomosis, open to the exterior.

Later the double-barrelled artificial anus resulting from the amputation is closed by crushing the septum and suturing in the manner described in detail on page 253 (Fig. 236).

Case 8.   Example of intestinal resection after use of the method of eventration in a case of volvulus of the sigmoid flexure.   A patient, who had had several attacks of volvulus of the sigmoid due to megacolon, came to operation during a free interval.   After opening the abdominal cavity through a midline incision below the umbilicus, it was decided to resect the excessively dilated and lengthened sigmoid loop.   Because of the presence of a large number of hard fecal masses in the distended proximal loop, a one-stage resection did not seem proper and a two-stage resection, with eventration of the gut segment to be removed, was decided upon.   The bases of the sigmoid loop were sutured together side-by-side for a distance of 10 cm.   The sigmoid loop itself was eventrated through the laparotomy wound which was closed around it (Fig. 234).

After several days a small opening was made with a cautery into the proximal limb of the eventrated sigmoid, permitting the escape of gas.   A few days later, the opening was enlarged, so that solid fecal masses could then be evacuated.   After two weeks the mesentery was ligated and the sigmoid loop was resected at the level of the skin (Fig. 235).

After a few days more, the crushing of the septum was begun.   Two weeks later the artificial anus was closed by freshening and suture (Fig. 236).

It is at times impossible to mobilize the diseased loops of gut sufficiently to place the proximal and distal limbs side by side for a sufficient distance to form a double-barrelled artificial anus. On the contrary, it may barely be possible to bring sound portions of the proximal and distal limbs through the abdominal wound. Nevertheless, it is not necessary in such a case to give up

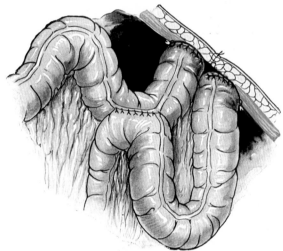

FIG. 239. Continuation of conditions of the preceding illustration, at the end of the third operation. The external openings of the proximal and distal limbs have been closed.

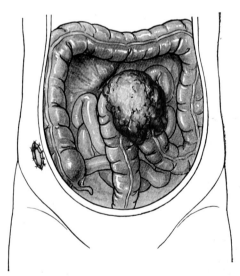

FIG. 240. Example of a five-stage intestinal resection, at the end of the first operation(1). Diagrammatic. A cecal fistula has been established.

the idea of an eventration procedure. One merely loses the opportunity to anastomose the gut openings resulting from the amputation of the eventrated loop and to close the artificial anus without performing a second laparotomy.

A second laparotomy may be avoided also in such unfavorable cases if at the first operation the proximal and distal segments of the gut are anastomosed with each other at a distance from the site of the eventration (Fig. 237).   In that case, since the proximal and distal gut segments were anastomosed at the first operation, it will suffice, after amputating the eventrated loop (Fig. 238), to freshen the edges of the fistula and to close the intestinal openings by suture (Fig. 239).

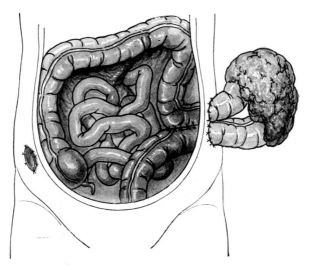

FIG. 241.   Conditions at the end of the second operation.   The diseased loop of colon has been eventrated and sutured to the abdominal wall.

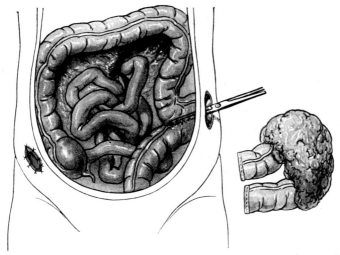

FIG. 242.   Condition at the end of the third operation.   The eventrated loop has been resected.

Case 9.   Example of a multiple-stage intestinal resection after eventration and with primary establishment of an entero-anastomosis.   A patient in acute ileus was found at operation to have a complete obstruction of the sigmoid flexure by a carcinoma.   Primary resection of the diseased loop was fraught with too great danger because of the great distension of the proximal loop.   On the other hand, the patient's general condition was so good that we did not seem justified in limiting the operation simply to the establishment of an artificial anus.   It was impossible, however, to bring together the limbs of the diseased loop for a sufficient length for the formation of a double-barrelled artificial anus.   An anastomosis was therefore made between the proximal and distal loops at some distance from the carcinoma. At the same time the carcinomatous loop was eventrated through a separate abdominal incision on the left side (Fig. 237).

Ten days later the eventrated loop was amputated (Fig. 238).

After another two weeks the double intestinal fistula was closed (Fig. 239).

Case 10. Example of a five-stage intestinal resection in a case of carcinoma of the sigmoid flexure: (1) Establishment of a cecal fistula, (2) eventration of the diseased loop, (3) resection of the eventrated diseased loop, (4) closure of the sigmoid artificial anus, (5) closure of the cecal fistula. A 60-year old patient with a stenosing carcinoma of the sigmoid flexure developed signs of ileus.

First operation. Under local anaesthesia a cecal fistula was established through a gridiron incision in the right iliac fossa. The cecum adjacent to the appendix was delivered and sutured to the parietal peritoneum which was attached to the skin and after a few days the cecum was opened (Fig. 240).

Second operation. After thorough evacuation of the gut by means of irrigation, the abdomen was opened under spinal anaesthesia through a left lateral rectus incision, with the patient in the Trendelenburg position and tipped toward the right. A scirrhous carcinoma in the upper portion

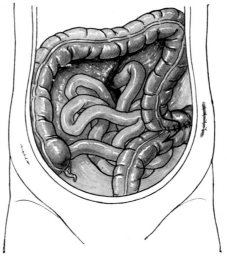

FIG. 243.   Conditions after the fourth (removal of spur) and at the end of the fifth operation. The sigmoidal artificial anus and the cecal fistula have been closed.

of the sigmoid flexure was found. A single-stage resection seemed inadvisable in view of the lowered resistance of the patient and the infectious nature of the contents of the large bowel. A two-stage resection with the aid of an eventration procedure was therefore decided upon.

The mesosigmoid was pierced at its most mobile point close to the gut and a rubber tube was pulled through this puncture hole, by the aid of which the sigmoid loop could easily be delivered. The sound proximal and distal limbs of the diseased loop were sutured together side by side for a distance of 12 cm., the mesentery being carefully avoided. This double-barrelled section of intestine was then replaced in the abdomen to the point where sound gut and sound mesentery still projected from the abdominal wound. The double limbs of the sigmoid were carefully sutured to the parietal peritoneum at their point of emergence from the abdomen and the abdominal wound was closed up to the emerging limbs of sigmoid (Fig. 241).

The cecal fistula remained open and through it the evacuations were obtained during the succeeding days.

Third operation. After 10 days the eventrated loop was amputated under local anaesthesia at the level of the skin, after ligation of the mesentery (Fig. 242).

Fourth operation. A week later, the crushing of the septum was begun. In ten days it had proceeded far enough that the artificial anus could be freed by a circular incision and closed by suture without opening the abdominal cavity.

Fifth operation. Two weeks later the cecal fistula was closed from without in a similar manner (Fig. 243).

(D) INTESTINAL RESECTION AFTER AN INVAGINATION PROCEDURE

The desire for an "aseptic" intestinal resection, that is, an intestinal resection and immediate reestablishment of intestinal continuity without primarily opening the intestinal lumen and without the interior of the gut coming in contact with the abdominal cavity, has led to no generally useful procedure in resections of the intestine in continuity. Only at the beginning and the end of the gastro-intestinal canal, where it is possible by means of instruments introduced through the natural openings to work toward an intra-abdominal procedure, have efforts in this direction gained a foothold in the form of an invagination procedure, as in the resection of the esophagus and the cardia and in the resection of the sigmoid and the rectum. The avoidance of a primary opening of the intestine appears to be particularly important in the region of the terminal bowel, in view of the increased danger of infection from this area. Invagination-resection of the large bowel is rarely used in favorably situated tumors of the sigmoid, but it is occasionally used in the treatment of congenital megacolon. I will therefore describe it under the treatment of the latter condition (invagination procedure of Grekow). In Hirschsprung's disease, conditions are especially favorable for this purpose in that the length and diameter of the diseased bowel permit a considerable mobility and a certain waste of material.

The abdomen is opened through a midline incision. The diseased segments of the large bowel are completely freed in the manner already described. A Babcock probe or a ring probe (described and illustrated later in the description of the combined procedure for amputation of the rectum on page 450) is introduced through the anus into the bowel by an assistant not engaged in the abdominal operation. The operator grasps the tip of the probe, as it lies in the interior of the intestine, within the abdomen and guides it upward within the sigmoid as far as the midpoint of the gut segment which has been freed from its mesentery. At this point the gut and the probe within it are tied together by a stout silk thread just below the tip of the sound (Fig. 244). If a ring probe is used, the thread is passed through intestinal wall-ring-intestinal wall with a needle and is tied tightly around intestine and probe on both sides just below the ring.

The assistant working at the anus now slowly withdraws the stem of the probe, pulling the segment of intestine above the point of ligation into the distal portion of the gut. The operator watches and guides this invagination from within the abdomen. The invagination is continued until the externally visible wall of the receiving segment and the wall of the invaginated segment show no nutritional disturbances. At the margin of the invagination the surfaces of the two gut segments are sutured together in their full circumference by closely-placed interrupted Lembert sutures (Fig. 245). It is advisable to apply these sutures in a double row by applying one row just before the invagination is completed and a second after its completion.

The abdomen is closed without drainage. The patient is turned over and the reduplicated intestine which hangs out of the anus is amputated in layers. In so doing, the cross-sections of the two gut segments which are to remain in the body are joined by a row of interrupted three-layer sutures (Fig. 246).

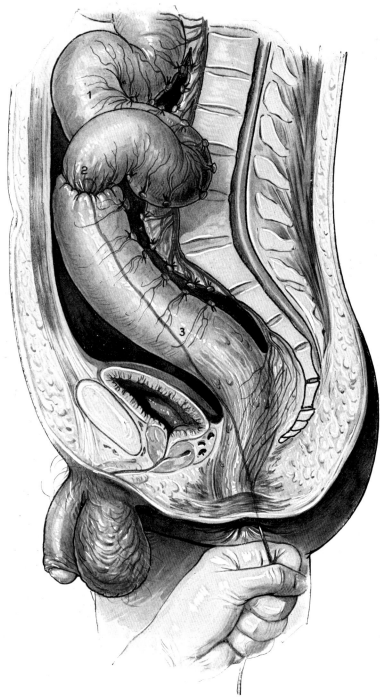

Fig. 244. Invagination-resection of the large bowel (1). Diagrammatic. The segment of colon to be resected has been freed of its mesentery. The midpoint of the mobilized segment has been tied to a probe introduced through the anus and the gut is being invaginated and drawn out of the anus by traction on the probe.

If the mesentery was removed to the proper extent, the main part of the reduplicated intestine lying within the rectum becomes necrotic in a few days and is sloughed off (Fig. 247). This results in conditions which largely correspond to the normal.

The chief difficulty of the invagination procedure lies in properly judging how far the intestine can and must be deprived of its blood supply. "Too

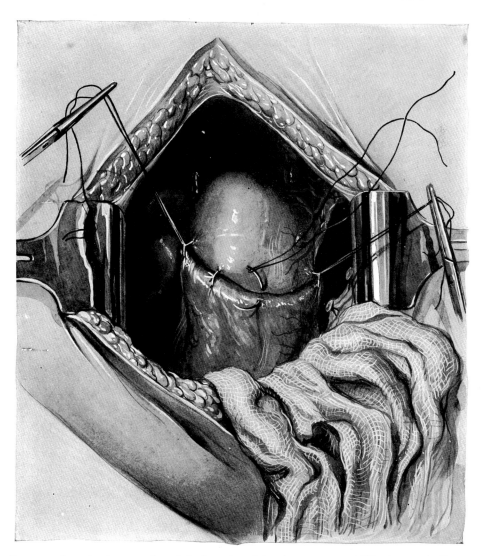

Fig. 245. Invagination-resection of the large bowel for the treatment of Hirschsprung's disease. The wall of the invaginated bowel is being sutured to the wall of the receiving segment.

much" gives rise to nutritional changes of the gut wall lying free within the abdominal cavity and leads to peritonitis. "Too little" prevents the invaginated gut from becoming necrotic to the extent desired. It is best to sever too few vessels at first and to undertake the invagination in stages. The cutting of vessels and the invagination are then continued until the gut has

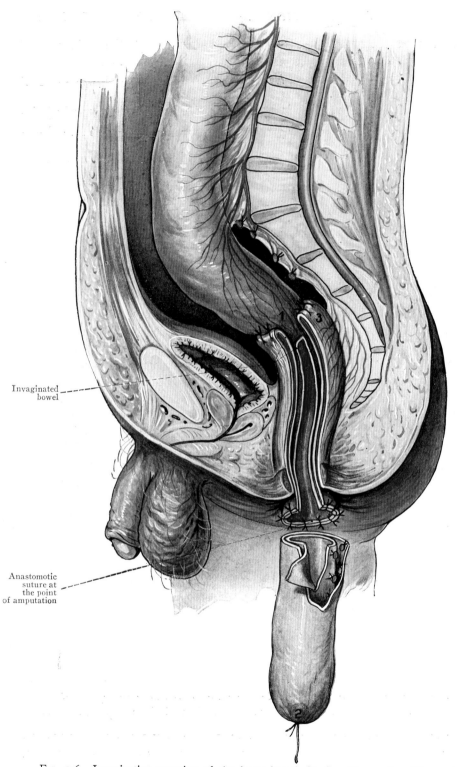

Invaginated
bowel

Anastomotic
suture at
the point
of amputation

FIG. 246. Invagination-resection of the large bowel (2. See Fig. 244). Diagrammatic.
The bowel has been pulled out through the anus. At the point of invagination the surface of
the invaginated bowel has been sutured in a circle to the surface of the receiving segment. The
two segments after being pulled out through the anus are amputated at the level of the anus
and their ends joined by suture.

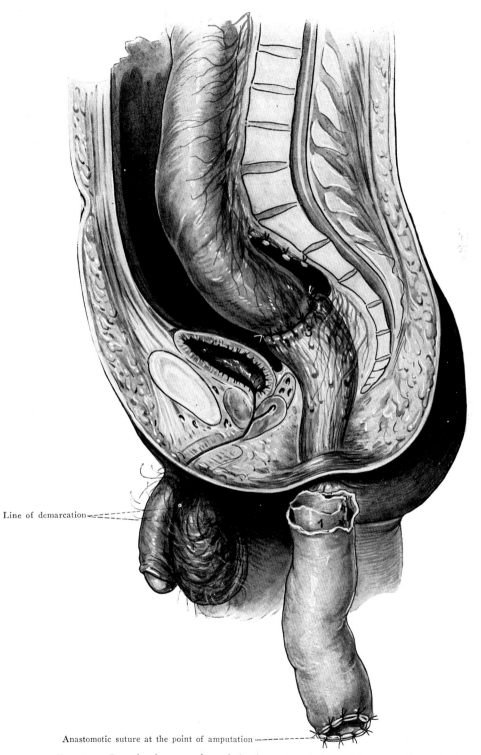

Line of demarcation

Anastomotic suture at the point of amputation

FIG. 247. Invagination-resection of the large bowel (3). Diagrammatic. The two segments which were freed of their mesentery and invaginated have become necrotic, sloughed off and been discharged through the anus.

been sufficiently shortened and no fair-sized vessel enters the intussusceptum. (On the whole this procedure has little to commend it. It is fraught with the danger of sepsis and intestinal obstruction and the desired end can usually be attained by a method which is better from the standpoint of initial technic and end-result. I. S. R.)

7. Appendectomy and Excision of Meckel's Diverticulum

(A) Indications

Inflammatory disease of the appendix can come to operation in the most widely different stages and the same is largely true of inflammation of Meckel's diverticulum. It is generally recognized today that in acute appendicitis, when the inflammation is still limited to the appendix itself and no pathologic-anatomic complications have yet arisen, the appendix should be removed at once, and without regard to whether the case is a mild or a severe one. In this regard no distinction should be made between adults and children. In children the diagnosis is often difficult to make, and consequently operation is more often delayed, to the detriment of the patient.

As to further indications there is, however, no unanimity of opinion. Some surgeons demand an immediate radical operation in even the most advanced stages of the disease. Most surgeons, however, adopt a selective policy when the extension of the inflammation to the surroundings is extensive. In general, immediate operation may be delayed if the general and local manifestations of inflammation have subsided. In the presence of acute manifestations of inflammation, when the peritonitis is not widely diffused, or when an abscess is demonstrable, immediate operation is indicated. In the latter instance this may often be restricted to the mere opening of the abscess.

Frequently, therefore, those patients who were not operated upon because of the subsidence of the first acute manifestations of inflammation, or who were treated simply by the opening and draining of an appendiceal abscess, retain their appendix for the time being. It is true, however, that in the latter case the necrosed appendix may be discharged through the drainage tract, so that it cannot be found at a subsequent operation. Experience has shown that an appendix which has once been the site of severe inflammation shows a decided tendency to repeated similar attacks because of the residual pathologic-anatomic changes. It is therefore not only justified but becomes a matter of duty to remove a suspicious appendix "in a free interval" by an operation that may be designated as almost without danger. Between the subsidence of an acute attack and an interval operation a period of 1 to 3 months should elapse, provided that a new acute attack does not demand an earlier operation. (I do not believe that an interval of 3 months is necessary or even desirable. I. S. R.)

Then there are patients who have constant or very frequently recurring pains in the appendiceal region, and without any single severe attack to help in the diagnosis. Such cases of so-called chronic appendicitis frequently should be operated on if no more definite diagnosis can be established. (In these cases the most astute clinician will frequently make mistakes. The end-results of operation in such cases are frequently unsatisfactory. Each patient should be very carefully studied before being subjected to appendectomy and at the time of operation an exploratory laparotomy should be made. I. S. R.)

(B) THE TECHNIQUE OF APPENDECTOMY

Appendectomy should be performed in the Trendelenburg and semi-left-lateral position, because in this position gravity removes the small intestine from the operative field. This position also holds for an operation in the acute stage, for there need be no fear that an infectious exudate will gravitate into the normal parts of the abdominal cavity.

Two incisions come into consideration for the routine exposure of the appendix and its surroundings, the lateral gridiron incision (page 25) and the lateral rectus incision (page 16). The gridiron incision does less damage and is therefore preferred when the diagnosis is certain. The lateral rectus incision can be extended up or down more conveniently, so that in cases with a doubtful diagnosis it is easier to inspect and operate upon more distant organs, for instance, the gall bladder or the female internal genitalia. This incision is therefore better suited for doubtful cases. (In cases with evident suppuration I prefer by all means the gridiron incision. It provides a direct approach, while when the rectus incision is used it is frequently necessary to break through protective barriers to get to the suppurative focus. Thus the infection is spread in the free cavity. I. S. R.)

It cannot be too much emphasized in acute cases to make the incision large to begin with and to enlarge it in the manner previously described just as soon as the primary incision proves to be too small. Visibility and a free approach to the operative field are important in view of the serious technical difficulties so often encountered in the acute inflammatory stage.

On the contrary, the conditions in an interval operation are often quite simple. The abdominal walls in a gridiron incision can easily be retracted. The incision can be enlarged at any time without difficulty. It is therefore permissible in an interval operation to keep the size of the incision within reasonable limits, without at the same time going to the senseless extreme of "button-hole" incisions.

Although most surgeons prefer general anaesthesia, spinal anaesthesia is excellently suited for the operation. The operation can also be performed easily under local anaesthesia, provided that there are no extensive adhesions which may necessitate prolonged search, or separation of the adhesions and undue traction on the intestines. In acute cases one had therefore better dispense with local anaesthesia, and if one meets the above mentioned difficulties in a case begun under local anaesthesia, one should promptly decide to induce general anaesthesia.

When the peritoneum is opened in acute cases, a more or less turbid exudate escapes as a rule. As soon as this has been aspirated, the abdominal cavity must be walled off systematically and with particular care in acutely inflamed cases, provided that the appendix does not promptly present itself. The edges of the wound are lifted with retractors. As soon as the cecum comes into view it is caught, so as not to be packed away with the small intestine. A long sponge forceps carries a moist gauze roll strip toward the ileum and glides along the posterior abdominal wall toward the midline, pushing before it any free loops of small bowel. These strips of gauze are introduced into the abdomen with the same gentle wiping motion until a gauze wall has been erected on the inner side of the appendiceal region, blocking off the general peritoneal cavity and the bulging loops of small intestine. It may be necessary to form a second gauze wall up toward the liver. It must fit snugly against the first gauze wall and should be carried far out into the flank. A third gauze barrier is placed below, blocking off the true pelvis. In this manner the operative field is guarded in two-thirds of its circumference by a ring of gauze which holds back the small bowel, is prepared to prevent leakage into the free cavity and at the same time acts as an absorbent.

In an interval appendectomy the walling off of the abdominal cavity may be omitted or carried out less thoroughly if no loops of small intestine get into the way and if an abscess can be ruled out with certainty, as is the case for example when the free appendix promptly comes into view or can be palpated.

The appendix often pops up of itself or after the first few orienting manipulations. It is grasped as close to the tip as possible with a special forceps and is drawn out of the wound. In other cases the appendix is hard to find because its position is quite variable. It may lie free in the abdominal cavity between the loops of the small bowel. It may be matted in a conglomerate tumor, commonly overlaid by, or enclosed in omentum. It may be tightly adherent to the anterior, lateral or posterior abdominal wall. It may hang far down into the pelvis. Together with the cecum, it may lie high up in the region of the liver. It may be in the left side of the abdominal cavity attached by its tip to the sigmoid. It may be tucked behind the cecum and the ascending colon so that the colon pins it to the posterior abdominal wall, wholly extraperitoneal.

If the surgeon has difficulty in locating the appendix, the search must be conducted according to a strict routine in the following manner: First look for the cecum. It must be remembered that not every segment of large bowel encountered in the right iliac fossa is necessarily the cecum or the ascending colon. At times the sigmoid flexure or the transverse colon strays into this region. On attempting to deliver the lower pole of the supposed cecum, the sigmoid becomes taut in the direction of the pelvis. The transverse colon is recognizable by the dependent free omentum. On the other hand, the cecum may always be recognized by the point of emptying of the small bowel. Segments of the large bowel which have proved not to be cecum or ascending colon are packed off as was the small intestine.

In case of a high-lying cecum whose lower pole can be above the level of the umbilicus, the cecum will of course not be found in the right iliac fossa. In such cases the search must be continued upward toward the liver. This occurs when there has been faulty rotation or descent of the cecum.

When the cecum has been brought into the wound, the taenia on its anterior surface is followed downward over the head of the cecum. It leads to the base of the appendix. If the anterior taenia cannot be followed, the ileocecal junction is looked for on the medial side. The appendix is usually to be found in the lower angle between the cecum and the ileum. Occasionally the appendix is more easily felt than seen when the cecum is put on stretch. The crooked right index finger is slipped down behind the cecum in the angle between the cecum and the ileum and an attempt made to palpate the vermi-form structure. (Occasionally a fetal funnel-shaped cecum is present and the appendix appears to be the stem of the funnel, or it may at times be attached to the lateral side of the cecum. I. S. R.)

If the appendix is fixed by old or recent inflammatory adhesions, it is freed partly by blunt, partly by sharp dissection. The skilful exposure of the operative field with variously shaped retractors and spatulae is of the greatest value in working down into the depths of the wound. In the case of recent

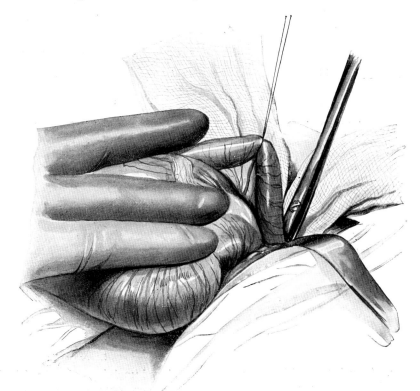

FIG. 248. Appendectomy. The appendix, which is hard to free, is being freed and delivered by means of a ligature around its midportion.

inflammatory adhesions, the freeing is often performed most safely by blunt separation with the index finger. Every cord of tissue that becomes taut is picked up on an aneurysm needle and is cut only after double ligation or after it has been doubly clamped with hemostats. Tearing roughly through such adhesions often results in troublesome bleeding which is difficult to control in the depths of the wound. If the separation has been skilfully done it finally becomes possible in most cases to crook the index finger around the appendix and deliver it into the wound.

If this is not possible the appendix is first freed at some easily accessible point. A stout silk thread is passed beneath it and is tied tightly around it (Fig. 248). By this thread the appendix is gently pulled forward and freed from its connections for a short distance. As soon as the appendix has been freed on all sides a bit farther, another "climbing ligature" is applied and the appendix is drawn out a little farther. In this way one works ahead, centimeter by centimeter, until the tip is reached and freed.

If the appendix is retroperitoneal, the cecum must be mobilized and turned upward and to the left. The cecum is put on stretch and the peritoneum is incised on the lateral side at its line of reflection from the cecum to the posterior abdominal wall. Under continued traction, the cecum and the ascending colon are freed by blunt dissection and are turned upward and to the left, so that their bed, their posterior surface and the appendix located in the retrocecal connective tissue come into view. Very long appendices may extend as high as the liver. The ascending colon must then be freed for a considerable distance before the appendix can be safely removed.

All these measures must be carried out with the greatest care in the case of a turgid appendix filled with pus, in order to avoid rupture of the appendix

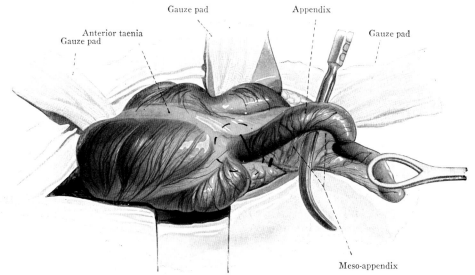

Fig. 249. Appendectomy. The cecum and appendix have been delivered and the abdominal cavity walled off with gauze. The meso-appendix is being picked up in segments, doubly ligated and divided.

and the spread of its infectious contents. In spite of every precaution, the escape of the purulent contents cannot always be prevented, because of a perforation that is present before the operation, or because the necrotic wall tears as the appendix is being delivered. In such cases the material which escapes is aspirated and sponged away as completely as possible. A fecolith that may have been extruded is carefully removed. An enveloping covering of omentum is resected without being unfolded.

A stump of the appendix remaining in the depths of the wound is grasped with a forceps and, if at all possible, is freed and removed. Leaving such a portion of the appendix in the wound is permissible only in case of extreme necessity, and then only if the cylinder of mucosa was separated and pulled out of the serosa like a sword out of its scabbard.

As soon as the acutely inflamed appendix has been freed from its bed, the bed is packed with a strip of gauze which protects it from soiling during the remainder of the operation, controls oozing, and absorbs inflammatory exudate. The appendix is picked up by its tip.

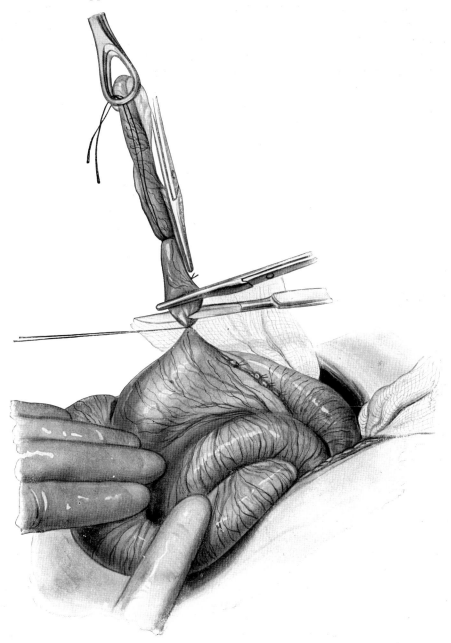

FIG. 250. Appendectomy. The appendix, freed of its mesentery, has been ligated at its base and clamped off peripheral to the ligature. The appendix is being divided close to the ligature with a knife.

When the appendix has been found and exposed, it is spread out and freed of its mesentery and the vessels therein. A free mesentery is unfolded by pulling up the appendix by its tip; the mesentery is ligated en masse and divided (Fig. 249). In so doing, several centimeters at a time are picked up on an aneurysm needle, doubly ligated and cut. This is continued until the appendix is freed to its base. The last segment of the appendix is often without a mesentery and is held close to the wall of the cecum by a common peritoneal covering The appendix must then be dissected free from the cecum until its perpendicular entrance into the cecum is clearly seen.

The amputation of the appendix and the care of its stump have led to the proposal of many measures whose number is in inverse proportion to the im-

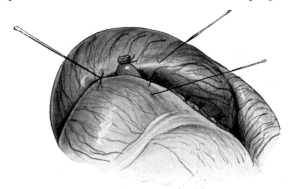

Fig. 251. Appendectomy. The stump of the amputated appendix is buried by means of interrupted Lembert sutures.

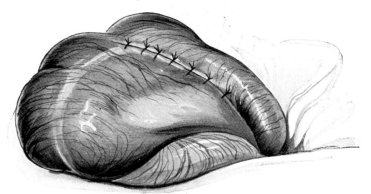

Fig. 252. Appendectomy. The stump of the appendix and the first part of its bed have been buried by Lembert sutures.

portance of the problem. The simpler the procedure, the better. The appendix, without any preliminary crushing, is ligated tightly with a silk thread close to its entrance into the cecum (Fig. 250). It is grasped with a hemostat 0.5 cm. peripheral to the ligature and is divided between these two points with a knife. A few Lembert sutures are used to bury the stump (Fig. 251). If the appendix had been situated along the wall of the cecum, the series of Lembert sutures can be continued to close the appendiceal bed (Fig. 252). Some surgeons prefer to bury the stump with a purse-string suture (Figs. 42 and 43), others with a cross-stitch suture (Figs. 44 and 45). Care must always be taken not to produce a stenosis of the ileocecal orifice by the sutures.

In case of a markedly infiltrated cecum that is fixed in the bottom of the wound, it may be impossible to ligate the appendix in the usual way and to bury its stump by suture.   Sometimes it is possible to grasp the appendix at its base with a curved renal pedicle clamp, cut off the appendix and ligate the stump on the cecal side of the clamp.   If the threads cut through when the Lembert suture is attempted it may be necessary to forego the burial of the stump.   If this occurs I prefer to drain the area.   This is best accomplished

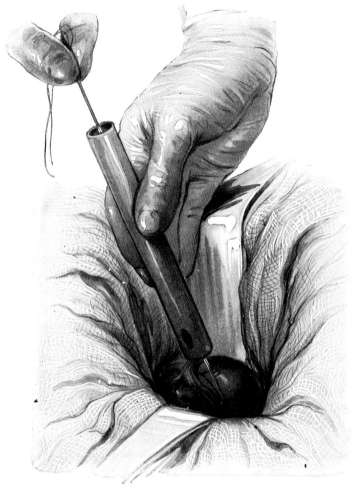

Fig. 253. Focal drainage of the appendiceal stump in case its closure is insecure.   The drainage tube is directed with certainty to the desired point by means of the ends of one of the inverting ligatures which are left long for the purpose.

by threading the drainage tube over the thread ligating the stump (focal drainage) (Fig. 253).

The principles underlying primary abdominal closure, or drainage, or packing after appendectomy are the same as those described on page 334, under the treatment of general peritonitis.   Primary closure is the rule, drainage and packing must be based on particular conditions.   If the appendix has been completely removed, if no necrotic purulent parts of it remain in the abdomen, if hemostasis has been complete and the stump securely taken care of, then the wound is closed without drainage. I do this often even in cases of severe suppurative peritonitis. If, however, necrotic parts remain in the abdomen, if the closure of the appendiceal stump is not secure, if there is deep bleeding, if a tip of the appendix could not be completely removed, if fecal material escaped from a perforation, drainage should be instituted. This is, however, rarely the case. A drain is led to the surface from the center of the suppurative focus and the free abdominal cavity is walled off from the drain-

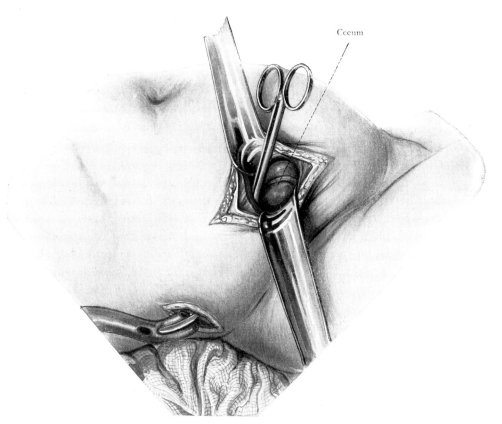

Cœcum

Fig. 254. Drainage of the appendiceal region into the loin. A forceps has been passed from the anterior laparotomy wound toward the loin and then to the exterior through a counter incision through the abdominal wall. The forceps grasps the tip of a drainage tube to carry it to the appendiceal region.

age tract and the site of the infection by vioform gauze packing. A bleeding point is packed with vioform gauze if it cannot be successfully ligated. (I very rarely use gauze packing unless this is protected by a surrounding wall of rubber dam. Intestinal obstruction occurs too frequently after the use of rubber drainage tubes and is I believe even more frequent after gauze drainage. When a bleeding point cannot be safely ligated I catch it with a hemostat and close the wound around this, removing the hemostat in from 48 to 96 hours. I. S. R.)

Since the mechanical conditions for drainage after appendectomy are unfavorable through an anterior laparotomy wound, it would at times seem advisable to bring the drainage out through the right loin space. This method of drainage has become much less frequent as drainage in general has become less frequent. To drain through the loin space, a forceps is pushed firmly against the posterior abdominal wall from within. An incision is made down on the point of the forceps which is then forced through (Fig. 254). A stout drainage tube is grasped in the jaws of the forceps and the tip of the tube is pulled into the appendiceal bed while the other end comes out through the posterior opening. The anterior laparotomy wound is closed completely.

The treatment of generalized suppurative peritonitis arising from the appendix and of appendiceal and secondary abscess is described on pages 329 and 339.

For the treatment of cecum mobile which is occasionally interpreted as chronic appendicitis see the section on chronic constipation, page 324.

(The policies in regard to drainage which Professor Kirschner has laid down in the preceding paragraphs may leave the reader with an erroneous idea in regard to drainage. The dictum enunciated some years ago, "when in doubt drain" is still a good one.

The thin turbid fluid so often encountered in early acute appendicitis is filled with phagocytic cells and is indeed often protective rather than harmful. There is no necessity to drain such a case. On the other hand where definite suppuration and necrosis exist I believe drainage for a few days is indicated. The drainage tubes should be so placed as not to cross loops of intestine. When placed in the pelvis they should lie along the postero-lateral wall of the pelvis. I frequently place a rubber coffer-dam around the drainage tubes so as to prevent a loop of ileum becoming attached to them. I. S. R.)

(c) EXCISION OF MECKEL'S DIVERTICULUM

Acute appendicitis and acute Meckel's diverticulitis belong together, not only because of the similarity of the clinical pictures, leading frequently to confusion of the diagnosis, but also because of the similarity of the treatment and the operative technique for the removal of the structure underlying the disease.

Meckel's diverticulum is a congenital remnant of the vitello-intestinal duct which projects from the small bowel when present, at a distance of 30 to 150 cm. from the ileocecal valve. It may exist as a completely patent duct from the region of the umbilicus to the intestine; it may exist as a solid cord, it may be a mucosa-lined blind sac opening at the umbilicus or into the intestine or it may lie as a closed cyst within the abdomen.

A blind sac attached to the small bowel most frequently leads to surgical interference. It may be slender like an appendix or it may be a broad out-pouching of the intestinal lumen (Fig. 255). Frequently there is a narrowing of the gut lumen in the region of the mouth of the diverticulum, congenital in origin (Fig. 256) or due to inflammation or to kinking.

The treatment of acute inflammation and of perforation of Meckel's diverticulum follows the same rules as does the treatment of acute appendicitis. It consists in most instances in the removal of the diseased diverticulum. After the diverticulum has been exposed, vascular connections are doubly ligated and divided. If it is slender, it is ligated like an appendix. If it has a broad base, it is cut off in the direction of the long axis of the intestine (Fig.

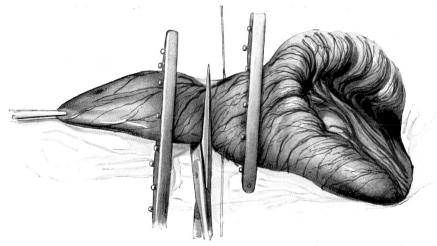

Fig. 255. Amputation of Meckel's diverticulum. The diverticulum has been closed on both sides with clamps and its base provided with two traction sutures.

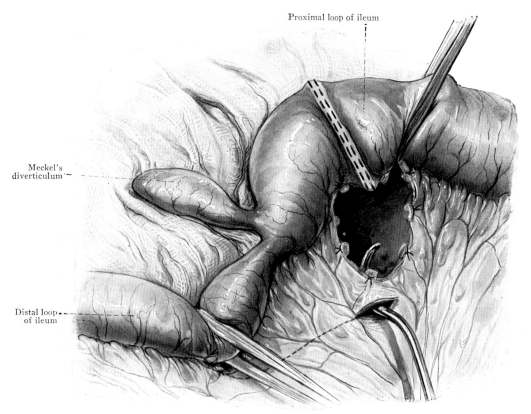

Proximal loop of ileum

Meckel's diverticulum

Distal loop of ileum

Fig. 256. Removal of Meckel's diverticulum by resection of the involved segment of small intestine. Tapes have been passed, at the intended points of resection, around the segment of ileum to which the diverticulum is attached and which is stenosed distal to the latter. The intervening mesentery is picked up in segments on an aneurysm needle and divided between ligatures. The intended line of division of the remainder of the mesentery is indicated by the dotted line. The proximal loop of intestine has been closed at the transsection point by means of the Petz suture instrument. The distal transsection site is indicated by the dotted line.

255) and the wound is closed by a double suture. Great care must be taken in this to avoid any narrowing of the lumen of the small intestine. If a stenosis is unavoidable, or if one already exists before the amputation of the diverticulum (Fig. 256), it must be short-circuited by an entero-enterostomy. Occasionally the simplest thing to do is to resect the segment in which the diverticulum is located (Fig. 256) and reestablish the intestinal channel by an entero-enterostomy.

If the diverticulum is in communication with the umbilicus in the form of a mucosa-lined tube or a fibrous cord, this condition may lead to strangulation or volvulus of intestinal loops. These conditions are treated surgically in the usual manner, the umbilical-intestinal communication being removed at the same time.

The peripheral remnant of the vitello-intestinal duct may show itself as a moist rosette of mucous membrane at the umbilicus. This should not be treated by cauterization, which is a dangerous procedure. All of the mucous membrane should be carefully removed. This is quite easy if there is only a small everted bit of mucosa. At times, however, in following the mucosal tube one may get into a deep funnel which is difficult to remove. This is best accomplished by an excision of the umbilicus, in which the cosmetic plastic procedure described under the operation for umbilical hernia is to be followed.

G. TREATMENT OF MECHANICAL INTESTINAL OBSTRUCTION (MECHANICAL ILEUS)

1. General Considerations

Orientation in the abdominal cavity usually offers no material difficulties when the intestines are empty. In the presence of ileus, however, especially of acute ileus, it can be extremely difficult, since the distended intestinal loops may impede or almost make impossible the access to and the view of individual portions of the abdominal cavity. Even the differentiation between small and large intestine is not always simple in an overdistended bowel.

The surgeon's first problem is to ascertain the nature and the site of the obstruction. Without this knowledge it is impossible to carry out suitable therapy directed against underlying causes and one is limited to symptomatic measures. It is of vital importance, in view of the type of operative procedure, to determine whether in a given case one is dealing with an obstructive ileus, in which drainage of the intestinal contents meets the vital indications, or whether there exists strangulation, which if unrelieved will result in suppurative peritonitis, even though the intestinal obstruction is relieved by the drainage of the intestine proximal to the site of the obstruction.

It is obvious that all applicable measures of examination must be employed to answer this cardinal question. If the question can not be answered before operation, its investigation at the beginning of the operation may be omitted only in exceptional instances, and then only if the condition of the patient no longer warrants exploration, and the risk of subsequent peritonitis attached to the establishment of an intestinal fistula seems less than that of exhausting the patient by actual visualization of the etiologic factor. In such desperate cases and in those favorable ones in which strangulation can be ruled out, an intestinal fistula is established proximal and as close as possible to the obstructed loop. In those cases in which the cause of the obstruction is not clear this should be determined at the operating table if the patient's condition permits of it, since the danger of subsequent peritonitis is very great.

Even with a patient in good condition, every operation for acute ileus is dangerous and should therefore be made as limited and as simple as possible.

My own experience has been that patients with intestinal obstruction are least affected by spinal anaesthesia. This form of anaesthesia is therefore to be preferred, unless only an intestinal fistula or an artificial anus is to be established, in which case local anaesthesia is adequate. (The only contraindication to spinal anaesthesia is the late stages of intestinal obstruction when circulatory collapse is present. I. S. R.)

The establishment of an accurate localizing diagnosis by operation may, however, by no means be insisted upon in all cases. If no definite information on this point could be obtained before the operation, the abdomen is opened by a midline incision below the umbilicus, and the incision is enlarged as needed. If, on the other hand, the site of obstruction is known, the abdomen is opened directly over it, if possible. In this connection one should remember the old rule that in a patient with a hernia, who also has obstruction, it should always be assumed that the hernia stands in an etiologic relation to the ileus. The neighborhood of the hernial orifice should therefore always be the point of operative attack.

It is often possible to locate the obstruction by palpating the abdominal cavity with a hand introduced through the midline incision (Fig. 257). The right hand is inserted into the laparotomy wound and is passed gently along the anterior abdominal wall in the direction of the cecum, which it attempts to grasp and deliver. If the cecum and ascending colon are not distended, no further attention need be paid to the large bowel, since the obstruction must be in the small intestine. If the cecum is distended, or if this is uncertain, the hand is passed down to the right inguinal canal and the right femoral canal, then back over the cecum along the ascending colon to the hepatic flexure, along the transverse colon to the splenic flexure, then down along the descending colon to the sigmoid, from there to the left inguinal canal and the left femoral canal. The rectum and the true pelvis are palpated. The hand then glides upward over the promontory of the sacrum and, as it is withdrawn, palpates the small intestine for any resistance. If this examination is fruitless, we can exclude with reasonable certainty all lesions of the intestine involving femoral, inguinal, umbilical and epigastric hernia, or hernia of the wall of the true pelvis, or involving the large bowel. There remains only a careful inspection of the small bowel. If a loop of collapsed small bowel is encountered this is followed to the point of obstruction. If in the course of this blind search the hand encounters a pathologic lesion, it is often possible to determine by palpation not only the site but also the nature of the lesion and the necessary therapeutic procedure. At times the diseased segment can be drawn out of the wound, inspected and then subjected to the necessary treatment.

In some instances the blind search with the hand may fail to ascertain the lesion. An attempt must then be made to make the lesion visible by systematic inspection of the gut. If collapsed loops are encountered near the distended portions, the surgeon knows that the stenosis is proximal to the empty loops.

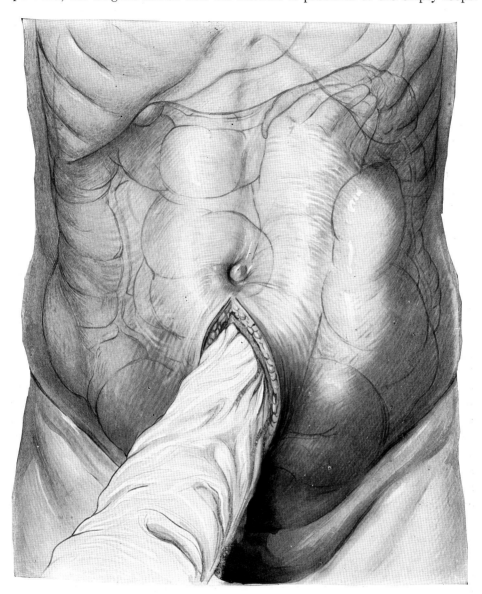

Fig. 257. "Blind" search of the abdominal cavity, in a case of intestinal obstruction, by inserting the hand through a small abdominal incision.

In cases of chronic ileus, the marked hypertrophy of the loops proximal to the stenosis often leads quickly to the obstruction. If, for example, an empty cecum or an empty loop of small bowel is found, it is known that the obstruction must be in the small bowel. If a distended transverse colon and an empty sigmoid are found, the obstruction must lie between these two segments. In most cases the lesion can be found by following the gut first in one direction and then, if this fails, in the other. In doing this, only a short loop of gut is to be drawn out at a time and immediately replaced in the manner described on page 203, for the inspection of the empty intestine.

If this attempt also fails to attain the objective promptly, and if the condition of the patient is good enough to permit further exploration the whole small bowel should be delivered from the wound without delay. The shock which might be produced by this is usually more than made up for by the shortening of the operation.

The intestines must be handled with the greatest care during their delivery, since an overdistended gut and its mesentery tear easily. The tearing, drying and cooling of the intestinal loops are to be prevented as far as possible by supporting and covering the distended intestines with compresses wrung out of warm saline solution.

Orientation and the whole further operative procedure are extraordinarily facilitated as soon as the overdistended small bowel is thoroughly emptied. This is accomplished in the manner described in Section D, 2, b, page 207, by emptying completely the whole of the distended small bowel by means of my evacuation apparatus. The hard struggle is followed suddenly by quiet, by visibility and accessibility. An early evacuation is all the more to be advised in such difficult cases because the emptying of the gut materially facilitates the replacement of the bowel and the closure of the abdominal wound. It lessens the danger of injury to the intestine. It detoxifies the body and saves it the task of the natural evacuation of the bowel for days.

If the site and the nature of the obstruction have been disclosed in one of these ways, the further procedure is directed along the following lines:

The operative procedure can follow two fundamentally different paths. First is the radical etiologic procedure by which the stenosing lesion is removed and normal conditions or conditions closely approaching the normal are reestablished. Second is the symptomatic procedure by which the intestine is drained or short-circuited without attacking the pathologic lesion.

The radical etiologic procedure consists either in the removal of the obstruction itself, for example in the extraction of a foreign body blocking the gut, the division of a constricting adhesion, the extraction of the bowel from a constricting ring, the relief of an intussusception; or in the resection of the stenosed segment, for example, the resection of a twisted loop, a cicatricial stenosis or a tuberculous or carcinomatous segment. Symptomatic procedure consists either in an entero-enterostomy between the proximal and distal loops short-circuiting the obstruction or in the establishment of an intestinal fistula or an artificial anus in the region of the proximal loop.

In strangulation the radical procedure of removing the obstruction must be followed. In this condition the simple removal of the obstruction without intestinal resection is to be considered and preferred only in case the intestinal wall is still sound or capable of recovery. If the intestinal wall is already necrotic, resection is the only possible treatment. Whether in that instance, one elects primary resection or a preliminary eventration of the diseased loop depends upon the technical possibilities, the condition of the patient and the severity of the ileus. Eventration and drainage of the proximal loop are easier for the patient.

In obstructive ileus, on the other hand, both the radical as well as the palliative procedures are possible. The radical procedure of removal of the obstructive lesion is to be preferred if it seems surer and less severe than a palliative procedure. So, for example, the removal of a foreign body obstructing the lumen of the gut, or the freeing of a kinking adhesion is usually the simplest and the most dependable measure.

When the radical removal of the lesion in obstructive ileus is possible only by an intestinal resection, then the palliative procedure of short-circuiting the obstruction is to be preferred if it relieves the obstruction with equal certainty and if the nature of the lesion does not demand a resection. So, for example, an intestinal stricture (Fig. 258) or a clump of adherent intestinal

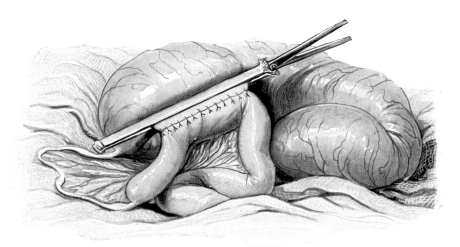

FIG. 258.   Treatment of a congenital stenosis of the small intestine by means of a side-to-side anastomosis between the proximal and distal loops. The proximal loop has been clamped off in order to prevent the escape of the accumulated intestinal contents during the performance of the anastomosis.

loops is usually short-circuited more simply and, in the long run, more surely by an entero-enterostomy than by attacking the causes of these lesions by freeing adhesions or by resecting the diseased loops. On the other hand, in obstructive ileus caused by a malignant disease (carcinoma, at times also tuberculosis), resection is to be preferred, not because of the danger of peritonitis, but because of the threat to life which the nature of the lesion involves in its further development.

Four procedures are at our command in the treatment of mechanical ileus: (1) removal of the obstruction with preservation of intestinal continuity, (2) resection of the intestinal segment bearing the lesion, (3) entero-enterostomy between the proximal and the distal loop, and (4) intestinal fistula or artificial anus proximal to the obstruction. If the gravity of the patient's general condition does not restrict the operation to the simplest procedure at the outset, one should proceed in the following manner in the various lesions concerned.

2. Treatment of Congenital Stenosis and Atresia of the Intestine

A congenital atresia of the small or large bowel is short-circuited by an entero-enterostomy (Fig. 258). The outlook after this operation is doubtful, because the newborn have little resistance to begin with, because an internal atresia is not diagnosed until late and because multiple congenital anomalies are frequently present which correspondingly enlarge the operation or because other malformations lessen the viability of the patient. In intestinal suture in the newborn the instruments for blood vessel surgery are used.

3. Treatment of Acquired Benign Cicatricial Stenosis of the Intestine

An acquired benign cicatricial stenosis of the intestine, such as may follow the healing of tuberculous, syphilitic, typhoid or dysenteric ulcers, is best short-circuited by an entero-enterostomy. (Gastrojejunal ulcers will be discussed later.) The removal of a cicatricial ring by longitudinal splitting and transverse suture as is occasionally recommended is more difficult and decidedly uncertain in its functional result, so that it is not recommended.

4. Treatment of Adhesions and Kinking of the Intestine

Adhesions between intestinal loops arise either after inflammatory diseases or after laparotomy where trauma and infection give rise to postoperative adhesions. They may lead to intestinal obstruction in a few days, or only after some time, under certain circumstances, only after years. The symptoms of acute postoperative ileus due to adhesions are the same as those of a postoperative incarceration which arises when a loop of intestine slips into an opening produced at operation; for example, after a gastro-enterostomy when a loop of small intestine slips in the ring formed by the stomach, the proximal jejunal loop and the spine.

The prophylactic measures employed to prevent postoperative adhesions have been by no means wholly successful. Our efforts in this direction are limited to handling the peritoneum with the greatest care, to avoiding mechanical, thermal, chemical and bacterial irritation as far as possible and to closing all surfaces denuded of peritoneum by carefully reuniting the peritoneal wound edges. The prophylactic introduction of medicaments, oils or special fluids, does not prevent the formation of adhesions. The constitutional tendency of some individuals often resists all our efforts in this regard. After the simplest laparotomy one patient will develop indissoluble adhesions, while another, after an extensive operation and severe inflammation, will have an abdominal cavity completely free of adhesions in a short time.

If the adhesions are limited in extent, they may at times be relieved permanently by simply freeing them (Fig. 259). However, the more extensive the adhesions and the more they involve broad surfaces, the more difficult it is to free them and the greater is the likelihood of their recurrence. If the bases of kinked intestinal loops can be brought together, the simplest procedure is to establish a by-pass by joining the proximal and distal limbs through a side-to-side anastomosis (Fig. 260). If a bundle of matted intestinal loops (accordion adhesions) can be isolated from the remaining sound intestine, the most effective procedure from the standpoint of permanence is the resection of the whole adherent mass.

The same is true for the treatment of the kinking due to adhesions which occurs occasionally at the splenic flexure, extremely rarely at the hepatic flexure, and which may lead to intestinal disturbances in the form of chronic constipation. Freeing the adhesions as a rule leads to new adhesions. An anastomosis between the proximal and the distal limb is the indicated procedure. In case of more extensive disturbances of the channel, which merge into Hirschsprung's disease, resection is the procedure of choice and is discussed under that subject.

Chronic adhesions in the abdominal cavity may assume such enormous proportions that all the intestinal loops are matted together into a single indissoluble mass (adhesion bellies), or are covered by a firm layer several millimeters thick ("icing intestines"). Such a condition usually presents an

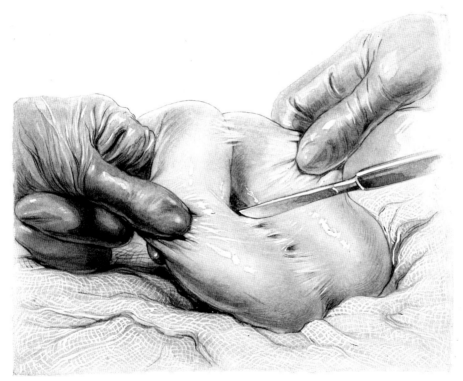

FIG. 259. Dividing adhesions between two loops of small intestine.

insurmountable obstacle to all attempts at operative relief. On opening the abdomen, it often is scarcely possible to find a free peritoneal cavity at any point. The gut can be isolated only for short distances and with the greatest difficulty and danger. Not much is gained by this, because the remaining mass of intestines cannot be untangled. The few loops which are freed with difficulty will readhere to one another in a short time. Short-circuiting by entero-enterostomy is rarely to be considered because of the extent of the adhesions and because of the difficulty or impossibility of finding a free

proximal and a free distal intestinal segment. Such patients, who have often
experienced many operations and for whom their continuing difficulties have
made life a burden, should be subjected to operation only in case of extreme

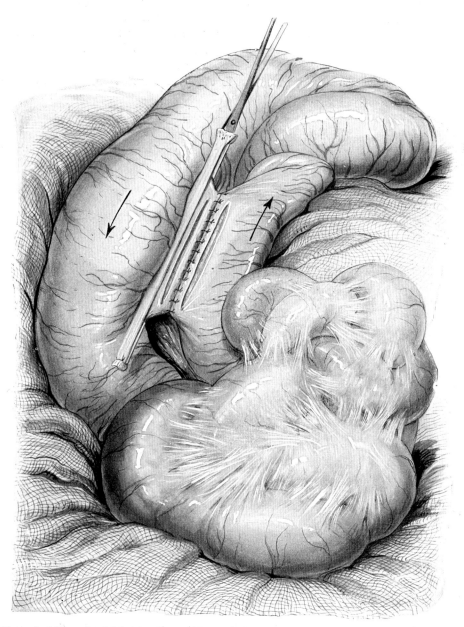

Fig. 260. Shortcircuiting of adherent loops of small intestine ("accordion" adhesions) by a
side-to-side anastomosis between the proximal and distal free loops.

necessity, for instance in a condition of acute ileus which threatens life. The
prevention of such a process is at present largely beyond our power; the cor-
rection of its acute results frequently so.

When signs of ileus arise immediately after a laparotomy, reoperation must not be long delayed. The abdomen should be reopened as soon as the diagnosis is made and simple postoperative gastric dilatation has been ruled out (Vol. I, page 48). The Roentgen ray with or without an opaque meal or enema renders excellent service in establishing the diagnosis. In such early cases the adherent loop can be freed largely by blunt dissection. Given a

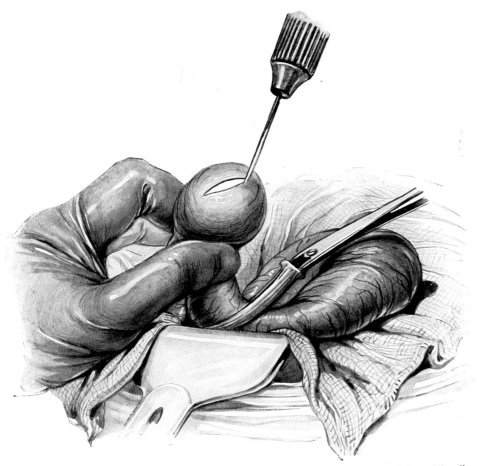

FIG. 261.   Removal of a gall stone from the small intestine through a small incision. The distended proximal loop has been blocked with an intestinal clamp.

recent incarceration, the pinched loop can usually be withdrawn without difficulty. The incarcerating opening is then closed by suture (Fig. 263).

5. MANAGEMENT OF FOREIGN BODIES WITHIN THE INTESTINE

Large foreign bodies obstructing the intestine, e.g., a large gall stone (Fig. 261), are as a rule removed by enterotomy. Only in case of ileus due to ascarides is this procedure not necessarily indicated. If the ascarides are scattered over long stretches of the intestine it is better to close the abdomen and to depend on the action of vermifuges to remove the obstruction. However, if a single large clump of ascarides distending the gut is present, its operative removal is advisable. For this purpose a small opening in the wall of the gut will suffice, through which the worms can be grasped and extracted singly (Fig. 262).

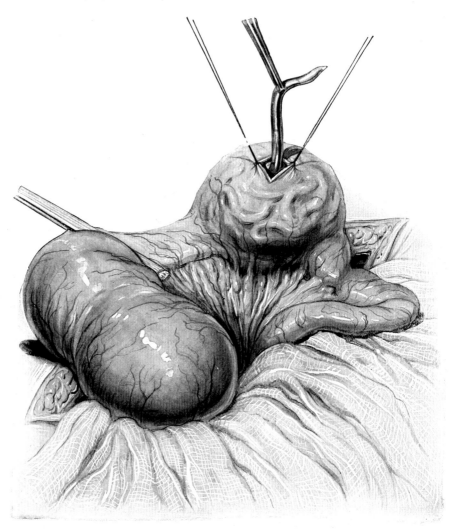

Fig. 262. Removal of a clump of ascaris worms, one at a time, from the small intestine through a very small incision. The proximal loop, distended with feces, has been blocked with an intestinal clamp.

6. Management of Tumors Compressing the Intestine from Without

A tumor not arising in the intestine but compressing the intestine from without is removed if possible. However in case of acute intestinal obstruction one usually has to abandon such a removal, which is frequently difficult and time-consuming, and be content with the establishment of fecal fistula. The removal of the tumor, if it is technically possible, is undertaken at a later date.

The circumstances are quite different in the case of a cyst. Here the pressure on the intestine can be removed instantly by a simple aspiration. External drainage will insure against a recurrent filling of the cyst and obstructive phenomena. If permanent external drainage of the cyst contents is not established, the cyst must be removed before its refilling can lead to further obstruction.

7. TREATMENT OF TUMORS OF THE INTESTINE (CARCINOMA, TUBERCULOUS TUMOR OF THE INTESTINE)

Carcinomatous and tuberculous tumors of the intestine assume a particular role in intestinal obstruction in that the state of obstruction existing at

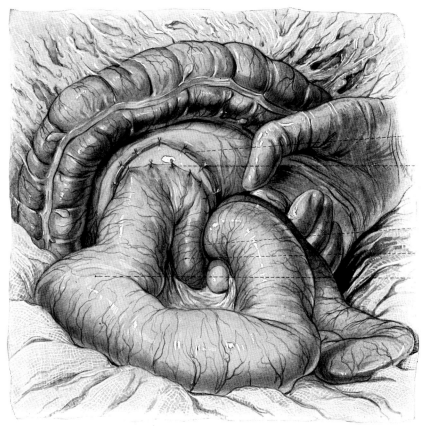

Slit in the transverse mesocolon

Anterior Lembert suture of the gastro-jejunostomy

Constricting ring

Duodeno-jejunal junction

Distended loop of gut between the gastro-jejunostomy and the site of constriction

FIG. 263. Freeing an obstructed loop of small intestine which after a gastrojejunostomy has slipped into the slit between the stomach and the jejunal loop leading to the gastro-jejunostomy. The finger is passed beneath the loop and pulls it gently out of the slit.

the moment is only a stage in an illness which in time will lead to death unless it is radically removed. In the choice of an operative procedure therefore the radical removal of the tumor must be considered in addition to the relief of the intestinal obstruction. In most cases primary resection is not advisable during a state of acute intestinal obstruction. One must therefore be satisfied with the relief of the acute ileus, either by eventration of the diseased loop or by an entero-enterostomy or by an artificial anus, leaving the removal of the growth for a second operation, provided that a resection is technically possible.

8. Treatment of Incarceration of the Intestine

Incarceration of an intestinal loop in a preexisting internal or external hernial orifice or in a constricting ring that has arisen within the abdomen must be relieved by dilation or incision of the ring, or by withdrawing the loop of intestine. If the incarcerated gut shows definite nutritional changes, primary resection or eventration of the affected loop is necessary. The hernial

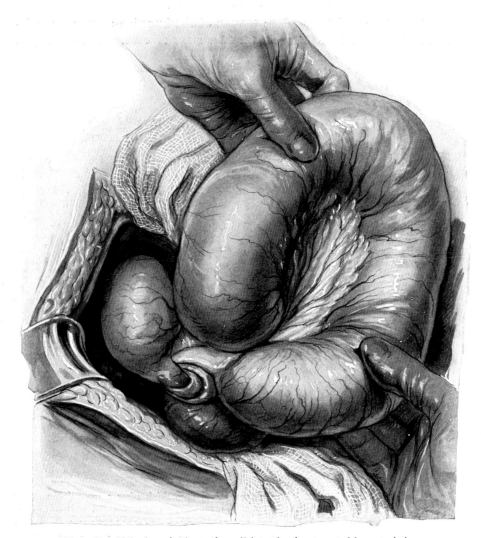

Fig. 264. Volvulus of a loop of small intestine is corrected by untwisting.

orifice should be closed by suture, provided that the removal of a constricting band does not also remove the orifice.

Postoperative incarcerations, which are not very rare occurrences, can usually be relieved if seen early by simply withdrawing the incarcerated loop (Fig. 263). Here, too, a repetition of the incarceration must be prevented by closing the hernial orifice.

The special procedures to be employed in the individual types of hernia, particularly the closure of the hernial orifice, will not be described in this volume.

9. Treatment of Volvulus of the Intestine

Twisting or torsion of a loop of intestine (most frequently a volvulus of the sigmoid flexure is concerned) is first treated by untwisting the bowel (Fig. 264) or by untying the knot. This simple procedure which reestablishes the original anatomical conditions existing prior to the production of the lesion, does not eliminate the danger of recurrence. Attaching the abnormally

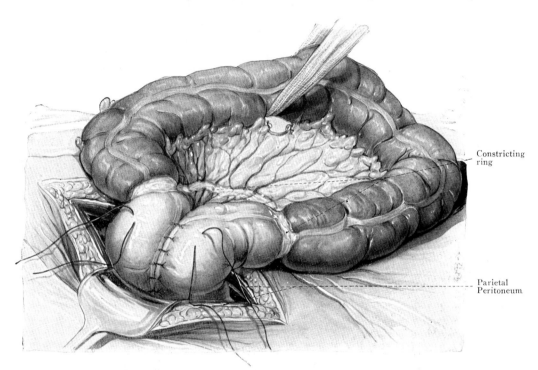

Constricting
ring

Parietal
Peritoneum

FIG. 265. Volvulus of the sigmoid flexure. After untwisting the loop it becomes evident that the intestinal loop, sharply demarcated from the normal bowel by a constricting groove, and its mesentery are gangrenous. The necrotic portions have been eventrated and a double-barrelled artificial anus is established.

mobile gut segments to the abdominal wall, to neighboring abdominal viscera or to each other is often not sufficient to prevent the recurrence of the lesion. Resection of the affected loop is the only sure method of preventing a recurrence. Resection, with or without eventration, is absolutely necessary if irreparable damage to the intestinal wall has already occurred (Fig. 265).

10. Treatment of Intussusception of the Intestine

The surgeon is often confronted with difficult decisions in the treatment of intussusception. An intussusception of the terminal ileum into the colon is the most common form of this lesion. As a rule the patients, frequently small children, have little resistance to withstand a major operation. The

attempt at reduction of the intussusception must not be made solely by traction on the intussusceptum but rather by pressure on the intussuscipiens and
the distal end of the contained intussusceptum (Fig. 266, the maneuver of
Hudson). The edema, which often greatly impedes the reduction, may at

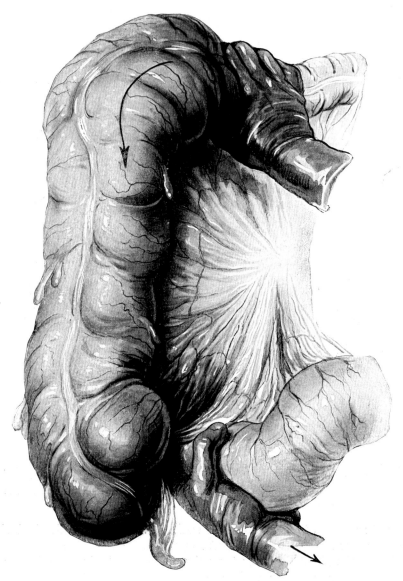

Fig. 266. Reduction of an intussusception by firm pressure in the region of the reflected end of
the intussusceptum and by gentle traction at the point of its entrance into the intussuscipiens.

times be removed to a large extent by prolonged even pressure. If reduction
is impossible, if the intestine tears, or if after successful reduction it shows
nutritional changes, a resection of the reduplicated segment is necessary, a
procedure which differs little from other forms of resection.

Only in extremely debilitated patients who can not be subjected to resection and in whom attempts at reduction of the intussusception have failed is an entero-enterostomy done between the intestinal loop just proximal to, and the loop just distal to the intussusception.   In the most unfavorable cases an artificial anus is established just proximal to the invagination.   An extension of the invagination and the escape of infected fluid is

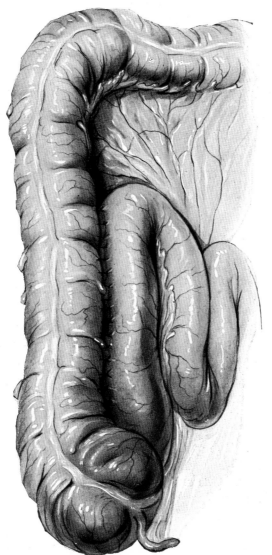

FIG. 267.   Double-barrelled type of fixation of the former intussusceptum and intussuscipiens to prevent a new invagination.

prevented as far as possible by a circular suture between the intussusceptum and the collar of the enveloping intussuscipiens.   The resection of the intestine, the reestablishment of the normal fecal channel and the closure of an artificial anus which may have been established are deferred until the general condition of the patient has improved sufficiently.

If the reduction is successful, recurrence may be prevented by suturing the affected intestinal segments together, side by side, for some distance (Fig. 267). If the invagination involved only the small intestine, fixation of any kind is not advisable.

11. Treatment of Chronic Constitutional Constipation. Cecum Mobile

In essence, chronic constipation is nothing more or less than a relative chronic ileus, localized to the region of the large bowel and due to atony or spasm of the large bowel. Experience has shown that this malady, if it has resisted all conservative measures, may be relieved surgically only by an extensive resection of the large bowel segment chiefly at fault. Entero-enterostomies or minor resections are unsuccessful.

Roentgen-ray studies should determine before operation in which part of the large bowel the chief delay in the passage of the feces occurs. This portion must always be included in the resection. Chronic constipation may be differentiated into an ascending-colon type and a descending-colon type, to which a sigmoid type may be added.

In the ascending-colon type, the cecum, the ascending colon and the right half of the transverse colon are resected and the terminal loop of ileum is anastomosed to the left half of the transverse colon (Fig. 268).

In the descending-colon type, the left half of the transverse colon and the descending colon as far as the first portion of the sigmoid are removed and the stump of the transverse colon is anastomosed to the upper portion of the sigmoid (Fig. 269).

In severe cases of the sigmoid type of colonic stasis the same procedure is used, the sigmoid being resected as extensively as possible, in addition to the descending colon and the left half of the transverse colon. Only in very mild cases is it good surgical technique to resect only the redundant portion of the sigmoid loop and anastomose the remaining portions.

Some authors consider the ascending-colon type of stasis to be the result of a functional disturbance of the descending colon and treat it in the same way as the descending-colon type of stasis.

Cecum mobile. The symptoms arising from cecum mobile, are largely those of chronic constipation although torsion of the cecum may give rise to more acute symptoms. The surgical treatment is similar to that of chronic constipation of the ascending-colon type. But occasionally at an operation undertaken for "chronic appendicitis" one finds an unusually large, moveable cecum which hangs down into the true pelvis like a large limp sack, and which is obviously the major cause of the patient's symptoms. In my experience this condition can be treated effectively, if it is treated surgically, only by resection of the dilated and abnormally mobile cecum, whereas all attempts at plication and suspension lead to failure. The resection must include the ileocecal valve, division of the terminal ileum on the one hand, and the ascending colon on the other. Depending on the conditions existing in the individual case, the proximal half of the ascending colon or the entire ascending colon and the hepatic flexure are resected. The proximal loop of ileum is then

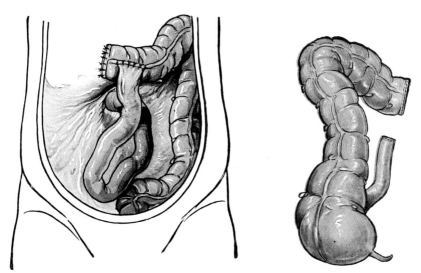

FIG. 268. Treatment of the ascending-colon type of chronic constipation by resection of the cecum, the ascending colon and half of the transverse colon and by anastomosis of the lower ileum with the remainder of the transverse colon.

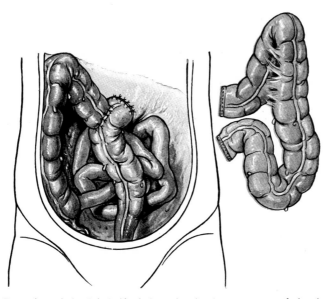

FIG. 269. Resection of the left half of the colon in the treatment of the descending-colon type of chronic constipation. Anastomosis of the end of the transverse colon with the remainder of the sigmoid.

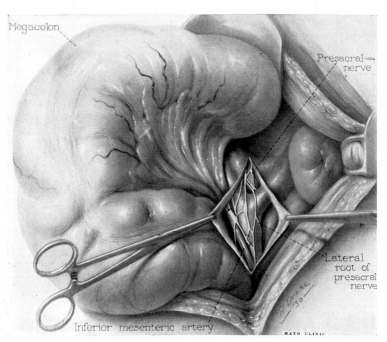

FIG. 269a.—(Case I). The field of operation. After division of the presacral nerve, the inferior mesenteric nerves were removed by dividing them at the points indicated. (Rankin and Learmonth Division of Surgery, Mayo Clinic.)

anastomosed with the remaining portion of the ascending colon or with the transverse colon.

Mention has been made above of the fact that chronic constipation is occasionally based on a pathologic kinking of one of the flexures of the colon. In such cases the lesion is corrected by freeing the adhesions, by a short-circuiting anastomosis, or by resection.

12. TREATMENT OF CONGENITAL MEGACOLON

The symptom complex of chronic atonic constipation is intensified in Hirschsprung's disease, which is characterized by an excessive dilatation and hyperplasia of the whole large bowel (congenital megacolon) or of the sigmoid alone (megasigmoid).

The first question is, whether the case at hand is one of idiopathic hyperplasia of the large bowel, a congenital megacolon in the narrower sense, or whether the dilatation of the large bowel is secondary to a partial obstruction at some particular point. Benign stenoses are located most frequently in the region of the sphincter ani or in the region of one of the transverse folds which project into the lumen of the rectum. If a stenosis exists, the only surgical treatment necessary is its removal. However, the closer the stenosis is to the anus, the more difficult is its permanent radical removal.

If the stenosis cannot be permanently overcome, then an artificial sigmoid anus is the only suitable measure. It is applied as a double-barrelled artificial anus, or as a terminal artificial anus, either after transsecting the gut and dropping the distal loop or with extirpation of the terminal gut. In so doing, the measures described previously under radical treatment of carcinoma of the rectum are applied.

If no stenosis is present, then a procedure is necessary in which the evacuation of the bowel through the natural anus is preserved. In my experience, a cure can be effected only by extensive resection of the dilated and lengthened gut. If possible, the resection should be carried so far that the remaining large bowel extends in approximately a straight line from the hepatic flexure to the anus. For this purpose three procedures must be considered: (1) primary resection and immediate reestablishment of intestinal continuity; (2) an eventration procedure with primary establishment of a double-barrelled artificial anus and with subsequent closure of the artificial anus, and (3) an invagination procedure. Personally, I consider primary resection the best, and an eventration procedure second best. Short-circuiting operations are useless.

(The author has failed to include the more recent contributions to this subject. Any adequate discussion of it must include the operations now being done on the abdominal sympathetic system. At this time I would evaluate these in comparison to the more radical procedures requiring resection as more physiological operations, carrying a lower mortality and likely to give a much more satisfactory end-result. (Fig. 269a.)

The operations which have just been described for the treatment of chronic constipation are now rarely done in this country. It is frequently possible by careful diet and medical regime to do just as much for these patients as one can do by resection and at the same time not subject the patient to the risk which extensive resections of the large bowel entail.

For some years surgeons in America, fired with the enthusiasm of Lane of Great Britain, carried out the procedures recommended by Professor Kirschner. Follow-up results were far from satisfactory and surgeons in the English speaking countries have nearly discarded resection of the colon for chronic constipation.

In those instances of chronic constipation in which the colon is dilated or in which chronic constipation is the result of true Hirschsprung's disease operations on the abdominal sympathetics offer a greater opportunity for relief of the symptoms. Rankin and Learmonth (Annals of Surgery, 1930, 92, 710) have published results which are indeed striking. I have tried the operation which they suggest with the most gratifying results.

There is little doubt but that overactivity of the sympathetic nerve supply to the colon results in dilatation of either the entire colon or of that portion whose nerve supply is affected. The sympathetic fibers when stimulated cause relaxation of the colonic musculature.

As first practiced either the right or left or both lumbar sympathetic chains were excised. This operation not only interrupted the sympathetic nerve supply to the distal colon, but also to one or both lower extremities. Rankin and Learmonth as a result of a closer anatomical study of this subject have suggested an operation which limits the nerve section to those fibers which supply the distal colon and rectum, and at the same time results in relaxation of the internal sphincter of the rectum.

The operation which they suggested provides for: (1) diminishing the dilatation of the colon, (2) leaving the motor nerves in control, (3) releasing the spasm of the internal sphincter of the rectum.

Occasionally frequency of urination is encountered after the operation, but this is not constant nor is it, as a rule, permanent. The operation does not affect the afferent nerves which have to do with reflex defecation.

The technic of the operation as suggested by these authors is as follows:

"*Technic of operation.*—Since the inferior mesenteric artery arises opposite the third lumbar vertebra, and the presacral nerve is to be found in front of the fifth lumbar vertebra, full exposure of these structures may be obtained through a left paramedian incision 15 centimetres long, and centered on the umbilicus. A self-retaining retractor is adjusted, and the table is tilted to the Trendelenburg position. The small bowel is packed off upward and to the right, so as to expose and pull upward the root of its mesentery; the attachment of the mesentery to the posterior abdominal wall is above the field of the operation, save when the bifurcation of the abdominal aorta is unusually high. An assistant draws the sigmoid colon to the left and slightly downward, to expose the bifurcation of the aorta. In rare cases, the root of the mesosigmoid may be displaced medially, in front of the fifth lumbar vertebra, when it must be mobilized by division of the right leaf of its peritoneum. The promontory of the sacrum is now identified, and in most cases it is possible to see the strands of the presacral nerve as they descend in the middle line, immediately under the peritoneum. The peritoneum is picked up in the middle line, and is incised vertically from the level of the promontory to the origin of the inferior mesenteric artery (Fig. 269a). The two edges of this incision are displaced by forceps to each side. The strands of the presacral nerve are not adherent to the membrane, and posteriorly they are separated from the great vessels by a layer of fine connective tissue. The nerve is first divided below, at the right border of the left common iliac vein; it is well to place a ligature on its distal end, as this is usually accompanied by a small artery. It is then raised upward by gentle dissection with cotton pledgets, and the branches which reach it from the fourth lumbar ganglia are divided on each side. Immediately below the bifurcation of the aorta, the connecting branches from the third lumbar ganglia are divided as they pass to join the nerve from beneath the common iliac arteries. When the nerve has been raised a little higher, its lateral roots, formed by the union of branches from the first and second lumbar ganglia, may be severed; the middle root is preserved if possible, to be used as a guide to the intermesenteric plexus. The trunk of the inferior mesenteric artery is now identified; by tracing upward the middle root of the presacral nerve the operator reaches the two large principal roots of the inferior mesenteric plexus, one on each side of the vessel, and joining it 1.5 centimetres below its origin. If the middle root of the presacral nerve cannot be used as a guide, the main trunks of the inferior mesenteric plexus will be found at the positions of five o'clock and seven o'clock with reference to the origin of the artery. They are large and easily isolated. About 2.5 centimetres of each are then resected; if any ganglionic mass is present on either, it must be included in the resected portion. Any subsidiary periarterial strands are then sought for and, if any are found, they are divided. Bleeding is not to be expected during this part of the operation. The inferior mesenteric vein is too far to the left to appear in the field. The incision in the posterior peritoneum is now brought together with a continuous suture of catgut, and the abdominal wound is closed in the usual manner."

When the right half of the colon is to be attacked the fibers going to this section of the bowel must be divided. Each case should be carefully studied before operation and a plan of operation drawn up for the individual case. I. S. R.)

In preparing the patient for operation, the emptying of the markedly distended bowel frequently presents difficulties. One must often resort to manual evacuation of the inspissated fecal masses. It is at times advisable to establish a cecal fistula as a preliminary measure. With the patient in the Trendelenburg position, the abdomen is opened by a midline incision beginning at the symphysis and the incision is prolonged as far as necessary in the direction of the ensiform process.

The intra-abdominal operation always begins with the mobilization of the large bowel. The freeing of the gut is usually easy in view of the great size of the structure. One small segment after another of the huge mesentery, of the gastrocolic omentum, and of the connective-tissue strands attaching the descending colon to the posterior abdominal wall is doubly ligated and divided. In mobilizing the descending colon, the dissection must proceed from the lateral toward the medial side. The mobilization must be continued until a well-nourished segment in the region of the hepatic flexure can be joined to a well-nourished segment of the intestine as it enters the true pelvis.

In **Primary Resection**, the intestine is divided at two points with the aid of the Petz suture instrument in the manner previously described, and the two remaining ends of the colon are anastomosed with each other, preferably end-to-end, otherwise end-to-side, and only in case of extreme necessity side-to-side.

If the **Eventration Method** is adopted, the proximal and distal limbs are sutured together for a considerable distance to form a double-barrelled anus, a procedure which, because of the large amount of material available, is never difficult. The mobilized loop of intestine is brought to the surface either through the midline main laparotomy incision or through a new left lateral rectus incision and is carefully sutured to the parietal peritoneum. In view of the enormous size of the eventrated loop, it is advisable to amputate it at once in order to relieve the patient promptly of a structure which is awkward and rapidly becomes necrotic. The amputation is best performed with the aid of the Petz instrument a few centimeters above the level of the skin. The after-treatment and the closure of the artificial anus are carried out in the manner previously described.

The treatment of Hirschsprung's disease by the invagination procedure of Grekow has been described and illustrated in detail on page 293. (Recently Sheldon and Kern have discussed the use of Parathormone (Collip's Parathyroid Hormone) in conditions simulating Hirschsprung's disease. I have had Dr. Kern treat one such patient for me with the most gratifying results. I. S. R.)

H. TREATMENT OF PARALYTIC ILEUS AND OF GENERAL SUPPURATIVE PERITONITIS

The operative treatment of paralytic ileus is only a part of the treatment of the acute general suppurative peritonitis underlying the ileus.

The treatment of general suppurative peritonitis consists of:

1. closure of the source of infection,
2. removal of the exudate and sterilization of the abdominal cavity,
3. drainage of the exudate, and
4. after-treatment.

1. Closure of the Source of Infection

The advances in the treatment of general suppurative peritonitis rest solely on early and well-directed surgical management. Among the measures which must be considered in this problem, the closure of the source of infection assumes the foremost place. It is the most important and indispensable part, in fact the basis of the entire treatment.

But the indication is not merely "the closure of the source of infection." It should be stated as "the immediate closure of the source of infection." The earlier the operation, the more favorable is the prognosis.

All patients, therefore, in whom a diagnosis of general suppurative peritonitis is made, should be operated on immediately, except of course the hopeless cases of which von Bergmann says, "I do not operate upon the moribund." These indications for operation also apply in children.

Exceptions to the above are gonococcal peritonitis originating in the female genitalia, which experience has shown will usually subside under conservative measures, and hematogenous or cryptogenetic pneumococcal peritonitis of children, in which in the absence of a localized focus of infection the closure of a source of infection is impossible. If, therefore, a diagnosis of gonococcal peritonitis or of pneumococcal peritonitis can be made with sufficient certainty and particularly if appendicitis can be ruled out, operation is postponed. If the diagnosis is in doubt, it must be established by an exploratory laparotomy. If the diagnosis of a pneumococcal or gonococcal peritonitis is established at the operation, the abdomen is closed without delay.

The entire operation, and especially the closure of the source of infection, must be carried out in the quickest and safest manner. The patient, who is frequently desperately ill, must be carefully protected against further strain to a circulation which is already near the breaking point. He is in immediate danger of "bleeding to death into his own vessels." The power of resistance of the peritoneum is impaired by every extensive abdominal operation, by trauma to the intestines, by traction on the mesentery, by chilling and by prolonged anaesthesia, and the impairment is proportional to the duration of the operation and the trauma inflicted. Greatest care and gentleness is the first rule in all these measures. "The less I did, the better my results became" (Heidenhain).

We should avoid all heroic procedures and content ourselves with the least that is possible to fulfill the indications originally postulated. We consequently use spinal anaesthesia if possible, since it is usually well borne. The abdomen is opened by an incision made immediately over the diseased organ if possible, in order to avoid touching larger portions of the abdominal cavity, but in all obscure cases the abdomen is opened by a midline incision below the umbilicus. The incision should be limited in extent, but large enough to permit unimpeded access and visibility for the operation, for not the length of the abdominal incision, but the nature of the procedures within the abdomen determine the magnitude of an operation. While in mechanical ileus eventration is proper for a prompt discovery of the site of obstruction, such a procedure is to be avoided at all costs in wide-spread peritonitis.

Closure of the source of infection is carried out technically either by closure of the perforation, or by the removal of the diseased organ, or its eventration, or by sealing it against the general abdominal cavity with packing, or by connecting it with the surface by means of drainage. In the latter case one can try to fortify the isolation of the infectious focus from the general abdominal cavity by bringing it up to the surface of the abdominal wall.

While in an operation for mechanical ileus the artificial evacuation of the overfilled intestine is often indicated, this measure is not indicated in paralytic ileus, because the intestine in most instances is already too severely damaged, and the general condition of the patient is too poor. On the other hand, in case of marked distension of a limited portion of the intestine, a prophylactic ileostomy may be considered. In most instances even this measure must be dispensed with and an intestinal fistula is deferred, pending further postoperative developments.

The following rules may be stated for the exclusion of individual foci:

An inflamed appendix and a Meckel's diverticulum should be removed.

A gangrenous or perforated gall bladder also should usually be removed if possible. If difficulties are encountered in the removal or if the patient's condition is poor, then drainage of the gall bladder (cholecystostomy) with walling-off of the general abdominal cavity by drainage is to be preferred.

Gangrenous or phlegmonous intestinal segments are resected or eventrated. Perforations of the stomach or intestine are closed. Inflammatory necrotic foci in the pancreas and other diffuse infectious foci are opened, sealed from their surroundings by packing and drained to the exterior.

Ruptured abscesses are drained and the general abdominal cavity is protected as far as possible by packing.

Recent Abdominal Injuries. The management of recent abdominal injuries is as a rule exceedingly difficult. This is particularly true of gunshot wounds, because there are usually numerous and often concealed injuries of

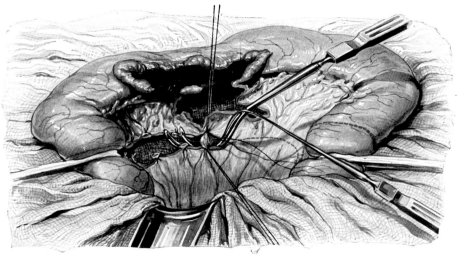

FIG. 270. Treatment of a fresh gunshot wound with laceration of a loop of small intestine and its mesentery by resection of the injured parts. The proximal and distal limbs of the gut have been closed with clamps. At each of the points of intended division a narrow tape has been passed around the intestine. The mesentery is being picked up in segments on an aneurysm needle, doubly ligated and divided. The dotted line indicates the intended line of division of the remainder of the mesentery and the intestine.

other abdominal viscera. It is a well recognized rule that the operative treatment of such injuries must not be delayed until the signs of peritonitis from perforation appear, but that all patients after blunt or sharp abdominal trauma must be opened at once if severe injury of the intraperitoneal viscera cannot be excluded. However laparotomy immediately after abdominal injury is not permissible during a state of shock, unless the shock is due to internal hemorrhage.

The abdominal incision is made over the organ suspected of having been injured. Since the location and extent of the injury are usually uncertain prior to the opening of the abdomen, a medium-sized midline incision is made as a rule. After opening the abdominal cavity and after the first cursory cleansing of blood and intestinal contents to permit inspection, bleeding vessels or gaping intestinal lacerations are provisionally closed with clamps. As soon as a view of the location and of the extent of the intestinal injury has been obtained, it must be decided whether the damage to the intestine can be closed by suture, or whether resection of the injured intestinal loops must be undertaken (Fig. 270). After intestinal suture the sutured segment must be short-circuited by an entero-enterostomy if too great narrowing of the lumen was caused by the suture.

After attention to all recognized injuries and after hemostasis there should follow a systematic revision of all the viscera. Injuries, especially of the posterior surface of the stomach, of the large bowel, and of the ureters, must be carefully looked for.

Unless packing is indicated for other reasons, for instance in order to control bleeding from an injured parenchymatous organ, and if one can depend on the intestinal sutures, the abdominal cavity is closed without drainage after an operation for a recent trauma.

2. Removal of the Exudate and Cleansing of the Abdominal Cavity

Since the fluid encountered on opening the abdomen in the presence of infection contains on the one hand the exciting causes of the suppuration and their toxins, and on the other hand the chemical protective substances and the cellular phagocytic elements produced by the body, it is by no means proven whether the removal of the fluid is an advantage or a disadvantage to the body. Practical experience, however, has shown that the thorough removal of the peritonitic exudate is advisable. If the fluid is to be removed the question arises, to what extent and by what method is this to be accomplished?

Technically, the evacuation of the purulent material, the "toilet of the abdominal cavity," is attempted by irrigation or by sponging and aspiration. Opinions differ as to the relative value of the two procedures. Each has its advantages and disadvantages, an analysis of which promptly shows that irrigation is obviously more advantageous in some cases, and sponging and aspiration in others.

Irrigation is used when the infection or the soiling probably involves practically all parts of the abdominal cavity and to the same degree, or in localized soiling if macroscopically recognizable particles cannot be removed quickly and completely by sponging and aspiration. In all other cases sponging and aspiration are used, especially if the infection of the abdominal cavity is obviously limited or unevenly distributed.

No special apparatus is required for irrigation. The idea of the irrigation is to play the stream on surfaces as large as possible and into every possible nook of the peritoneum in order to cleanse it mechanically. This is best accomplished by means of a large soft rubber tube the end of which is inserted repeatedly into numerous parts of the abdominal cavity as far as possible from the point of entry. The operator takes the tip of the rubber tube in one hand and guides it systematically between the loops of small intestine, into the true pelvis (Fig. 271), into both flanks, beneath the right and the left dome of the diaphragm, into the lesser peritoneal cavity or wherever else pus and intestinal contents are found. By this method the water or saline solution is forced through large segments of the abdominal cavity and cleanses them. Rougher attempts at cleansing, such as the barbarous procedure of brushing away de-

posits of fibrin, are to be condemned because they run counter to the fundamental rule of handling tissues gently. If one irrigates at all, it should be
done with large quantities of fluid, 10 to 30 liters. The temperature of the

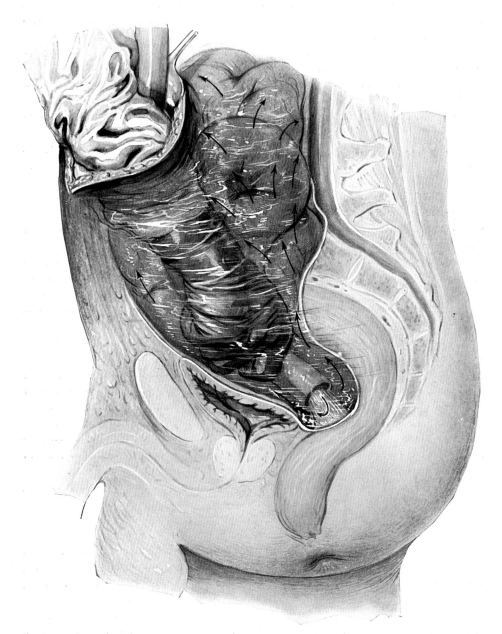

FIG. 271. Irrigation of the entire abdominal cavity in case of generalized suppurative peritonitis
by means of a tube introduced by the hand into the depths of the abdomen.

irrigating fluid must be carefully kept at about 40° C. At the end of the
irrigation the greater part of the fluid is permitted to drain off. (It is the
editor's opinion that more harm than good will as a rule result from irrigation.

In many instances the infection will actually become more widespread. I. S. R.)

Sponging and Aspiration. On the other hand, if the inflammation involves only a limited part of the abdomen or individual parts in an unequal degree, and it seems possible to remove the fluid without irrigation, coarse particles are removed with a dissecting forceps or a moistened sponge mounted on a holder. Visible collections of pus are carefully aspirated by suction or by well wrungout moist sponges introduced by a long sponge forceps. Prolapsing intestines and other viscera are carefully held aside with long spatulae during this procedure. The main quantity of the pus tends to accumulate by preference in certain pockets of the abdominal cavity, especially in the pouch of Douglas. Particular attention should therefore be given to these places.

Disinfection. It is a common practice to attempt to treat peritonitis by the introduction of disinfectants into the abdominal cavity. In addition to the disinfectant action, it is often sought to prevent absorption of the toxic peritoneal fluid by blocking the absorbing channels, or to prevent the formation of adhesions. The medicaments are either substituted for water in the irrigation or they are added to the irrigating fluid or are poured into the abdominal cavity at the end of the operation. Of the many substances which have been recommended I shall mention only ether, olive oil, camphor oil, hypertonic saline and glucose solutions, horse serum, Pregl's iodine solution, Dakin's solution, quinine derivatives, dyes, and pepsin hydrochloride. It is my belief that success in the treatment of peritonitis is not to be attained in attempts at disinfection of the peritoneal cavity, and I do not use such measures.

The attempts to prevent the development of postoperative adhesions by the introduction of medicaments have likewise been fruitless. Oil, human fat (Humanol), Pregl's iodine solution, amniotic fluid, and many others have been recommended. In the development of peritoneal adhesions, constitutional tendencies and infection, as previously mentioned, are obviously the factors of first importance. One patient after the slightest peritoneal irritation develops extensive adhesions that last a life time; while another may experience severe inflammation, or be subjected repeatedly to the trauma of operation, yet after a few weeks the abdomen looks as if it had never been touched. We know of no way as yet in which we can help these cases. It is obviously important to minimize trauma, both manual and chemical.

3. DRAINAGE OF THE EXUDATE

Just as in the routine treatment of an abscess a single evacuation of the pus is not sufficient but continued drainage must be provided for so, too, is it necessary to provide drainage in abdominal suppuration in the days after the operation.

It was firmly believed in the early days of the operative treatment of peritonitis that this was best accomplished by a most extensive tamponade, especially with Mikulicz drains, later by the insertion of numerous drains in as many places and as many directions as possible. Gradually, surgeons have become more and more conservative in this matter. Finally, Rehn closed the abdominal cavity except for a drain in the pouch of Douglas, through which he expected intra-abdominal pressure to force the pus as it collected in a pool at the bottom of the abdomen. (The normal intra-abdominal pressure is subatmospheric. I. S. R.) Then Rotter pointed out that it is impossible to drain the general abdominal cavity. The abdominal cavity seals itself completely against every foreign body and therefore against every drain within a few hours. After 12 to 24 hours the adhesions cannot be easily broken down, and a methylene blue solution no longer permeates them (Tietze). The little fluid which escapes from a drain inserted into the general abdominal cavity is in a short time nothing more than the secretion of the granulations of the drainage tract. The general abdominal cavity cannot be drained successfully for any prolonged period.

On the other hand, it is readily possible to place a focus of disease situated within the general abdominal cavity in communication with the exterior by means of a drain and in this way to make it possible for pus formed at that point to escape to the exterior through the drain.

Furthermore, it is possible to produce an artificial blockade between a localized infectious focus and the general abdominal cavity by the insertion of gauze strips (vioform) and eventually a natural blockade by the adhesions which form in a short time.

These facts and considerations have determined our procedure in actual practice.

(a) If it is possible at operation to exclude the primary focus of infection completely, and if we can be certain both of the absence of any existing focus of infection and that no secondary focus will develop, then the abdominal wound is closed completely even in severe infection of the abdominal cavity.

(b) If a focus of infection remains in the abdomen, or if the secondary development of a focus is to be expected which can initiate reinfection or maintain an existing suppuration, then that focus must be placed in communication with the exterior by a drain. This has nothing whatever to do with an attempted drainage of the general abdominal cavity. On the contrary, it is often advantageous to seal the general undrained abdominal cavity against the limited segment harboring the focus by means of packing surrounded by a rubber-dam wall.

The following are to be considered as such infectious or potentially infectious foci requiring drainage: walls of abscesses, necrotic tissue, granulating infected surfaces, foreign bodies, insecure closures of hollow organs, and to these must be added uncontrollable oozing.

It may be added that not every infectious focus must be drained. The body is often capable of handling insignificant infectious foci without drainage. This is however hard to predict. The final matter of drainage is a matter of the individual operator's personal experience which cannot be reduced to rules.

A few examples are offered to clarify further this viewpoint in the question, closure or drainage of the abdomen? In case of peritonitis due to a perforated peptic ulcer or to an intestinal perforation, if it is possible to close the hole in the stomach or intestine securely, the abdominal wound, after a successful cleansing of the abdominal cavity, is closed completely and without drainage, even in the presence of the severest infection with contamination of the general abdominal cavity. If in a case of diffuse suppurative peritonitis a gangrenous gall bladder had to be left in the abdomen, the infectious focus is isolated from the general abdominal cavity by means of packing and is drained externally. Similarly, in a case of general peritonitis if there remains a cavity lined with purulent, necrotic, phlegmonous, bleeding tissue after the removal of a suppurating appendix which caused the trouble, this infectious focus must be placed in communication with the exterior by a drain and under certain circumstances must be sealed against the general abdominal cavity by packing. I do not drain the general abdominal cavity however in either of the last two instances in spite of the most severe suppuration, either by a drain introduced into the pouch of Douglas or into any other parts of the abdomen. Drainage is also indicated when the source of infection has been excluded for the moment by the closure of an opening into the intestine, but the uncertainty of the closure makes a reopening of the source of infection possible or likely.

In view of the impossibility of draining the general abdominal cavity, the difference of opinion as to the form and the material of the drain is actually insignificant. Whether the drains be of rubber, glass or woven material, whether they are bare or covered or packed with iodoform gauze, none of them can drain the general abdominal cavity and no complicated devices are needed to evacuate pus which is constantly being formed by a local infected focus. The simplest, a rubber tube drain, is the best. Its diameter, length, lateral fenestrations, their size and position, are adjusted to the individual case. Because of its pliability it is least likely to occasion any danger of pressure necrosis.

Loose gauze packing can also for a time assist in evacuating fluids by its capillarity. But if an exit is to be kept open for fluid being produced constantly and in considerable quantity, and if all increase of pressure due to blocking is to be avoided, a drainage tube with its large channel undoubtedly gives better service than a strip of gauze, which after it becomes soaked acts only too frequently as a plug.

4. AFTER-TREATMENT

Any subsequent attempt at irrigation of the general cavity through a drain is not permissible, at best it is without effect. The general abdominal cavity, which promptly seals itself against the drain, is not reached by the irrigating fluid unless irrigation under high pressure separates the protective adhesions and thereby produces considerable damage. If a continuous production of pus takes place in a localized drained focus, the pus usually escapes through the drainage opening of its own accord. Only in deep cavities which cannot be opened at their deepest points by a counterincision, or in the later stages when necrotic bits of the wall of the abscess cavity are sloughed off, may careful irrigation occasionally be in order. Good services are also rendered in such cases by the instillation of glycerine, which by reason of its higher specific gravity and hygroscopic property forces out the pus.

Early or frequent manipulation of a drain is to be warned against. Such measures should only to be considered after a few days when firm adhesions have formed. The drains had best not be changed at all, but should be withdrawn bit by bit and shortened. Occasionally a thick drain may be replaced by a more slender one.

In other respects the after-treatment should be conducted with particular care according to the rules laid down in Vol. I, pages 47-49, and in this volume, pages 36-39.

The value of the Rehn-Fowler position, which was formerly much in favor, is no longer unqualifiedly admitted, since the spread of suppuration in the closed abdominal cavity does not take place simply according to gravity and because the elevation of the upper part of the body favors cerebral anemia if the circulation is failing. I therefore prefer the usual horizontal position, which is generally more acceptable to the patient.

In addition to stimulation of circulation, the improvement of the patient's general condition requires a free supply of fluid. Because of vomiting, the patient is unable to take water by mouth. The mucosa of the small intestine in peritonitis loses the power to absorb water; on the contrary, it secretes fluid into the gut in increased amounts. Fluid must therefore be administered by artificial means and with regard to the total 24-hour loss by all routes. Fluid is therefore given in the first place by rectal drip and by continuous intravenous infusion. In severe cases blood transfusion may also be of great value. (It is important in these cases to supply sufficient fluid to maintain an adequate fluid balance. In order to do this the loss of fluid by all measurable routes must be recorded and to this must be added an amount sufficient to make up for the loss through the lungs and skin. The loss through these latter two routes may at times equal the amount lost by the measurable routes. The continued loss of fluid by vomiting results in alkalosis. It is best to correct the dehydration with normal sodium chloride which will at the same time tend to correct the change in blood reaction. When there is an associated depression of circulation as the result of blood concentration from the loss of fluids into the tissues blood transfusion is invaluable. I. S. R.)

Stimulation of peristalsis is of great importance. In most cases there rapidly develops a paralytic ileus, with gaseous distention. The patients only too frequently perish, not from peritoneal sepsis but from a paralytic intestinal obstruction. Because of the vomiting which is frequently present, orally administered cathartics rarely produce the desired effect. As in the supplying of fluids, it is therefore necessary to resort to other modes of administration, enemata and smooth muscle stimulants, chief among which is pitressin. (We have been using as much as 1 cc. hypodermically every 2 to 4 hours for 48 hours in such a condition. I. S. R.)

The annoying and prostrating vomiting may be combated by gastric lavage and by "drying up the stomach" by means of a slender stomach tube with suction attached, introduced through the mouth, through the nose, or through a gastrostomy opening. A separate gastrostomy (Heller), which may be established primarily at the operation for the treatment of the peritonitis or may be performed secondarily, has the advantages that it completely relieves the stomach, that every inconvenience occasioned by a stomach tube can be avoided, and that the patient can drink as freely as he likes, effectively relieving the torturing thirst that otherwise accompanies the uncontrollable vomiting. (The same conditions can be attained by the use of a Jutte tube. I. S. R.)

A further operative measure which may be considered is the establishment of one or more Witzel fistulae in the small bowel as advised by Heidenhain.

This is done under local anaesthesia and according to the technique described on page 219. In desperate cases one may resort to multiple percutaneous aspiration of the gut as described on page 209.

I. TREATMENT OF PERITONEAL ABSCESSES

1. General Considerations

Localized intraperitoneal suppuration may arise in one of two ways. It can originate in a localized infected focus situated within the abdominal cavity cr in its wall, which has been prevented from involving the general abdominal cavity by the protective limiting adhesions of intestine or omentum or both or it may be the result of diffuse peritonitis which has been localized. The walls of these abscesses are formed by adherent abdominal viscera, the omentum, the stomach, the small and large intestine and their mesenteries, the liver, the gall bladder, the pancreas, the bladder, and the female genitalia. If the abdominal wall forms a part cf the wall of the abscess, the abscess is described as a mural one.

These abscesses may occur at any point within the abdominal cavity. Certain areas however are sites of predilection. For practical consideration abscesses are first divided into those which are situated above the transverse mesocolon and those which are below.

Of those encountered in the lower abdomen the most frequent etiologic factor is suppurative appendicitis. These abscesses frequently are found in the immediate neighborhood of the appendix, that is, in the right iliac fossa in front of the body of the ileum. They may also extend to the opposite side cf the abdominal cavity as a "horseshoe" abscess, whose midportion lies above the symphysis in front of the bladder and whose limbs lie more or less symmetrically in the right and left hypogastric regions. Of particular importance because of their hidden position are the collections at the deepest point of the peritoneal sac in the pelvis, the abscesses of the pouch of Douglas, which lie in the recto-uterine space in women and in the rectovesical space in men and press against the anterior wall of the rectum. In women they are frequently due to gynecologic infections. Abscesses in the above locations may also be the result of a Meckel's diverticulitis, and in the left iliac region and pelvis from a sigmoid diverticulitis.

Abscesses above the transverse mesocolon are often included under the collective term, subphrenic abscess. They may be subphrenic abscesses in the restricted sense, between the diaphragm and the liver, or they may lie between the liver and the transverse mesocolon. The upper space between the diaphragm and the liver is divided in the sagittal plane into a right and a left half by the falciform ligament, and into an anterior and a posterior half in the frontal plane by the coronary ligament of the liver. The upper space is therefore divided into four compartments: a right anterior, a right posterior, a left anterior and a left posterior subphrenic space. The lower space between the liver and the transverse mesocolon is divided into a right and left half by the falciform ligament. A loculated collection may occur in any of these six spaces. These abscesses may increase in size beyond their original confines and by contact infection or invasion of the neighboring structures frequently destroy the above mentioned anatomic boundaries with the formation of atypical abscesses extending over large areas.

Upper abdominal abscesses arising from appendiceal suppuration tend to collect in the right posterior space between the liver and the diaphragm, by extending toward the diaphragm behind and to the outer side of the ascending colon. Infections of the right kidney and the gall bladder may also give rise to collections in this region. Abscesses below the liver and on the right are usually connected with disease of the liver, the biliary tract, the duodenum, or the pylorus. Abscesses arising from the body of the stomach, the pancreas, the spleen and the left kidney occur chiefly in the left subphrenic space.

The diagnosis of subphrenic abscess may at times be difficult, because the abscess may lie largely beneath the ribs and in the depth of the abdomen where it cannot be palpated. The roentgenogram showing a high position of the diaphragm, a gas bubble in the subphrenic space, displacement of the bismuth-containing bowel, often gives corroborative information.

In many cases exploratory aspiration must be resorted to before a positive diagnosis can be made. The stomach must be emptied by the stomach tube before doing so. Aspiration may only be attempted at points where injury to the gastro-intestinal canal can be excluded. Such exploratory punctures are therefore usually made in the direction of the liver from behind or the side. Since the needle occasionally enters the pleural space, there is always danger of a resulting empyema thoracis. If pus is aspirated the abscess must be opened surgically at once in order to prevent, if possible, an infection of the pleural space. Frequently the pleural leaflets are tightly adherent or separated by a loculated exudate. After pus has been aspirated it is best to leave the needle in place to act as a sure guide during the operative procedure. (I believe that exploratory aspiration is only rarely indicated. It has been our practice that when subdiaphragmatic abscess was strongly suggested to resect one or two ribs posterolaterally under local anaesthesia and to pack against the unopened parietal pleura. Three to five days later the exploration can be done through an obliterated costophrenic space with a minimum danger of secondary pleural infection. Where the abscess is below the liver I believe it is safer to do an exploratory laparotomy than to explore through the abdominal wall with a needle. I. S. R.)

As soon as the definite diagnosis of an intraperitoneal abscess is made, evacuation is indicated. Although spontaneous cures do occur by absorption or by rupture to the exterior or into the stomach, the intestine, the bladder or the vagina, the danger of rupture into the general abdominal cavity is so great and is fraught with such dire consequences that we can not depend on the rare occurrence when recovery takes place without operation.

The chief point in the drainage of an intraperitoneal abscess is the avoidance of contamination of the general abdominal cavity. This is easily accomplished if the abscess is a mural one, and can be reached through the sealed portion without opening the general abdominal cavity. But difficulties are encountered when the abscess is not in contact with the abdominal wall or if a mural abscess cannot be approached from that side, so that the operator must go through the free cavity to reach the abscess. The procedure is then carried out in one or in two stages.

The single stage procedure is performed as follows. After the abdomen is opened, the general abdominal cavity is carefully walled off with gauze pads in the neighborhood of the abscess, so that even the smallest amount of escaping pus is immediately absorbed by the compresses and by an aspirating tube which should be constantly in the hand of an assistant. The abscess is first opened at a very small point and is at once aspirated with an electrically driven pump. Only after complete evacuation of the abscess is the opening enlarged. The cavity is sponged dry and is filled with a gauze roll. Irrigation of the abscess is contraindicated because the irrigating fluid can contaminate the general abdominal cavity. The gauze pads are then removed. In rare instances it is possible to suture the edges of the abscess cavity to the edges of the abdominal wound, thereby closing the general abdominal cavity and marsupializing the focus. One or more drains should be placed in the abscess cavity and led out through the abdominal wound.

In the two-stage procedure, the abdominal cavity is opened and the free space between the surface of the abscess and the abdominal wound is packed with vioform gauze so that a funnel-shaped space is made from the external wound to the abscess wall. It is often possible to suture the abscess wall to the parietal peritoneum in the region of the abdominal wound, thereby making the isolation of the abdominal cavity easier and more dependable. After a few days, when firm adhesions have formed walling off the free cavity, the abscess is opened and drained.

2. EVACUATION OF LOCALIZED APPENDICEAL ABSCESSES

Mural Abscess. If the abscess is a mural one, the attack is made on the mural side if this is possible. Such an approach in reality consists in what amounts to the drainage of an extraperitoneal collection. One must be prepared for an erroneous diagnosis. The operation can usually be performed under local anaesthesia. Otherwise one should select spinal anaesthesia, if no contraindication to this exists.

Depending on the point of attack, one of the typical abdominal incisions is selected, usually the gridiron incision or the lateral rectus incision. In order to obtain good exposure and free access, impeding muscles are more frequently cut across than in simple appendectomy. The incision continues layer by layer and the proximity of the abscess is signalled by the edematous state of the tissues. The edematous layer is incised very cautiously until pus is encountered. The pus is aspirated. The opening is carefully enlarged so that a finger can be introduced. The cavity is carefully palpated, its size is determined, and any shreds of tissue or fecoliths are removed. Any freeing of the limiting adhesions must absolutely be avoided.

The fear of opening the general abdominal cavity forbids any search for the appendix. Only if the appendix happens to come into view on opening the abscess or during the palpation is it removed. Otherwise, the appendectomy is postponed for a subsequent interval operation.

Drainage is provided by one or two rubber tubes which are brought out through the incision. If the abscess cavity proves to be very large and if it extends for some distance along the abdominal wall, a counterincision is made at the lowest point along the abdominal wall and a second large drainage tube is led out through it.

Such an extension of the abscess frequently takes place toward the right loin space where the counterincision is then made (Fig. 254). Also when the abscess extends along the anterior abdominal wall for some distance to the left, a second opening is made through the abdominal wall, for example in the "horseshoe" abscess described above. The greatest care must be taken not

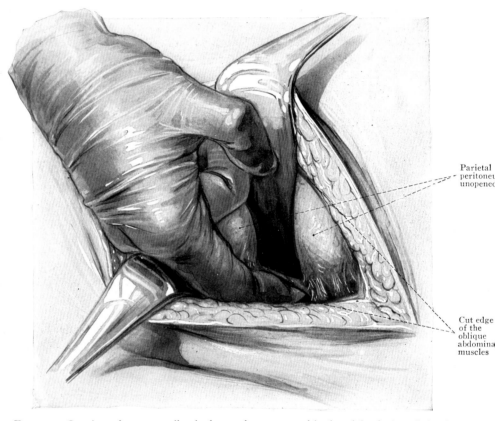

Parietal peritoneum unopened

Cut edge of the oblique abdominal muscles

FIG. 272. Opening of an appendiceal abscess in contact with the abdominal wall in the region of the right iliac fossa: the opening is made from behind, while the unopened peritoneum is retracted medially.

to break through the delicate adhesions which protect the free cavity. Occasionally an unexpected extension of the abscess well down into the pouch of Douglas is discovered by an operation from above. If it is deemed expedient the patient is then put in the lithotomy position and the abscess is opened through the vagina in the female or through the rectum in the male, counter-drainage being brought out through the abdominal wound.

The healing of the drained abscess can after several days be aided by careful irrigation of the cavity.

Iliopsoas Abscess. Abscesses resting on the iliopsoas muscle usually extend upward in the abdomen beyond the crest of the ilium so that they can be reached without opening the general abdominal cavity by an incision passing close to the anterior superior iliac spine. At times, however, the abscess lies so deep that the ilium extends higher than the abscess, and it can not be approached directly through the soft tissues of the abdominal wall. Nevertheless these abscesses can usually be reached without opening the general abdominal cavity. A fairly long incision is made close to the anterior superior iliac spine and parallel to the fibers of the external oblique muscle. Keeping to the outer side, one works down to the peritoneum, partly by blunt and partly by sharp dissection. The peritoneum is pushed away from the pelvic wall toward the midline with a sponge mounted on a forceps so that a deep cleft is formed between the iliopsoas muscle and the peritoneum, and a Langenbeck retractor is inserted into the cleft (Fig. 272). It is usually possible to feel the fluctuation of the abscess through the infiltrated wall by means of a finger introduced into the cleft. In the bottom of this cleft an incision is made from without inward or even from behind forward perpendicularly into the abscess wall, or an opening is bored into the abscess with a forceps or with the finger. After evacuation and drainage of the abscess, the cleft between the peritoneum and the pelvis must be packed widely, to prevent a phlegmonous retroperitoneal cellulitis.

If the free cavity is inadvertently opened before reaching a mural abscess, an inspection is made by sight and palpation to determine the extent of the abscess and the position of a possible point of contact with the abdominal wall. If the abscess is a mural one, it is opened in the manner previously described. If the abscess is in contact with the abdominal wall, the region of this point of contact is marked on the skin. I then close the laparotomy wound carefully and seal it with Mastisol and Billroth batiste. A fresh attack is then made on the abscess at the point where it was shown to be in contact with the abdominal wall.

If an appendiceal abscess is not in contact with the abdominal wall but lies within the interior of the abdominal cavity between the coils of intestine, the abdomen is opened over the apex of the collection. The abscess is then approached in one or two stages and drained in the manner above described for non-mural abscesses.

3. Evacuation of Abscesses in the Pouch of Douglas

Abscesses in the pouch of Douglas are opened preferably in the lithotomy position through the rectum or through the vagina. Theoretically, the abscess could also be opened through the connective tissue of the perineum. Experience has shown, however, that the approach through the two natural channels mentioned is simpler and is never followed by extension and it is therefore to be preferred. Before attacking an abscess in the pouch of Douglas, the bladder must always be emptied by catheterization. Aside from the fact that an operative injury of the bladder is thereby most easily avoided, many a supposed Douglas pouch abscess has been shown by this measure to be an overdistended bladder.

Evacuation through the Rectum. The rectal approach to the abscess can often be carried out with local anaesthesia of the sphincter by injecting one percent novocaine around it. The sphincter must be well dilated at the beginning of the operation. The bulge of the anterior wall of the rectum is brought into view by inserting suitable long blunt hooked retractors or a short proctoscope. If the bulging area is situated very high, it may often be drawn downward with one or two tenaculum forceps. The point of greatest protrusion is punctured with a long large-bore aspirating needle (Fig. 273). If clear fluid is obtained it is usually urine, an occurrence which can be prevented by thor-

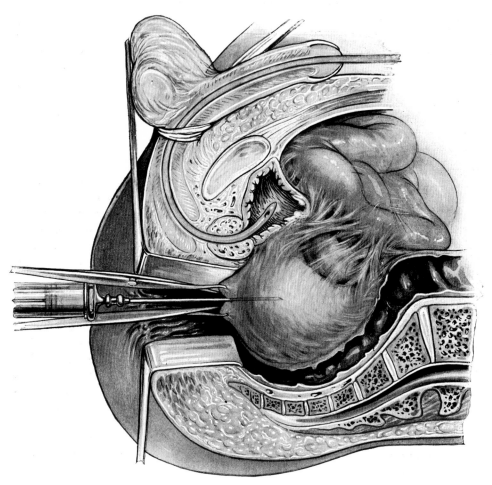

Fig. 273. Opening of an abscess in the pouch of Douglas through the rectum. After the bladder is emptied and the rectal sphincter dilated, the wall of the abscess is exposed by retractors inserted into the rectum. It is drawn forward with two tenaculum forceps and a diagnostic puncture is made with a large-bore needle and syringe.

oughly emptying the bladder routinely just before the operation. If urine is obtained at aspiration it is obvious that the needle has been carried too far forward, or that the mass is not a collection of pus. As soon as pus is aspirated, the needle is left in situ and an incision is made along the needle until pus flows freely out of the incision. The opening is enlarged with the aid of forceps and a drain without lateral fenestrations is inserted. The drain is fixed by a stout suture catching the edge of the abscess opening. The drainage tube is led out through the anus and is provided with safety pins.

In cutting through the anterior rectal wall, the injury of an artery can give rise to extremely troublesome bleeding, which, because of the deep position of the bleeding point, can at times be controlled only with great difficulty. Such bleeding can be particularly serious if it does not begin until after the operation is completed and the blood is held unnoticed in the large bowel, so that the bleeding is not discovered until a considerable amount of blood has been lost. In such cases the bleeding point must be sought for at once and must be controlled by ligation.

Evacuation through the Vagina. The evacuation of an abscess in the pouch of Douglas through the vagina is performed in a similar manner. Often no anaesthesia is necessary. The vagina is held open with a speculum and the bulge on its posterior surface is brought into view. The bulging area is caught on each side with a tenaculum forceps and drawn forward. An aspiratory puncture is made at the point of the most marked bulging and in the direction of the long axis of the vagina or diagonally backward. As soon as pus is aspirated, the evacuation and drainage of the abscess are carried out in the manner previously described.

An abscess in the pouch of Douglas may be extremely large, so that it can be palpated from above through the abdominal wall. Here it usually takes a horseshoe form, with its midportion above the symphysis and its limbs enclosing the bladder. In most of these cases evacuation from below is sufficient. If not, counter openings are made to right and left of the bladder. The opening of a "horseshoe" abscess through the abdomen has been described previously.

4. Evacuation of Subphrenic Abscesses

Anterior Approach. Low subphrenic abscesses, that is, those between the liver on the one side and the colon and transverse mesocolon on the other, usually present at the anterior abdominal wall below the rib margin. They can therefore be opened without difficulty in the manner described for an appendiceal abscess, whether they are mural, or whether a free portion of the abdominal cavity intervenes between the abscess and the abdominal wall. The abscess should if possible always be attacked at that point where it is presumably in contact with or close to the abdominal wall. Whether and where a second drainage opening is to be made, depends on the local conditions found at operation.

In approaching an anterior subphrenic abscess from in front when its location is uncertain and may be possibly above the liver, an incision along the costal margin is advised. The incision severs all layers of the abdominal wall down to the surface of the peritoneum which is spared for the moment. If pus is not encountered in the region of the outer surface of the exposed parietal peritoneum, the peritoneum is separated carefully from the under side of the costal margin by forcing the hand gently upward between the costal margin and the parietal peritoneum. In this manner it is at times possible to approach an abscess situated above the liver without opening the free abdominal cavity.

High subphrenic abscesses, that is those between the diaphragm and the liver, require a different approach for several reasons. In the first place, they are enclosed on all sides by the bony thorax. In the second place, they are roofed over in a dome-shaped manner by the diaphragm, and above this, by the pleural cavity. The direct approach must therefore include a rib resection and exposure of the lower portion of the pleural cavity. This raises the danger of pneumothorax and of pleural infection. In the back, where a high subphrenic abscess is usually attacked, the lower border of the pleural space is at the level of the 12th rib. Only the outer half of the 12th rib lies below the lower limit of the pleura.

These two peculiarities of the position of a high subphrenic abscess and the dangers which they involve must receive particular attention in the planning of the operation. The operation is best performed under local anaesthesia. It is advisable to empty the stomach with a stomach tube before the operation. The evacuation of the abscess may be carried out in two ways.

Transpleural Approach. This approach leads in a direct line from the exterior to the abscess (Figs. 274 and 275). After pus has been found by aspiration, the needle is left in place. Several inches of the rib just below the needle are resected. In most cases it is advisable to resect also a part of the rib above, or of the rib below, if the aspiration was obviously made in the upper part of the abscess. The intercostal muscles are picked up, ligated and divided at the points where the ribs were resected so that the parietal pleura is freely exposed in the full extent of the floor of the wound (Fig. 276).

Before proceeding farther, the presence of pus behind the exposed layer of tissue must be established with certainty. If the needle of a previous positive aspiration is not present as a guide, the location of the abscess must again be ascertained by aspiration (Fig. 276). With the patient lying on his sound side, the aspiration is occasionally not successful in spite of the presence of pus, since the pus will gravitate to the lower side if the abscess also contains gas. The fact that the tip of the needle is within the abscess cavity is then recognized either by the odor of gas escaping from the needle or by the aspiration of pus after shifting the position of the patient.

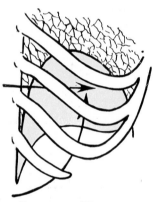

Fig. 274. The two approaches for opening a subphrenic abscess: transpleural and extrapleural. Diagrammatic.

After the location of the abscess in relation to the rib resection has been established, the further procedure depends upon whether the costal pleura is adherent to the diaphragmatic pleura or whether both pleural surfaces are free.

If adhesions are present, the indurated adherent double layer is incised along the needle and perpendicular to the long axis of the body, preferably with the electrosurgical knife, until the abscess is opened. The abscess is emptied by aspiration, sponged out, and under certain circumstances I have even cautiously irrigated it. The abscess cavity can be palpated with the finger and its interior may be inspected with the aid of an electrically lighted retractor. If necessary, the opening is enlarged downward to the most dependent portion, which procedure may require the resection of additional ribs.

If the costal pleura is not adherent to the diaphragmatic pleura, a fact which can easily be recognized by the gliding of one pleural surface over the other during respiration, there are two possibilities for further procedure.

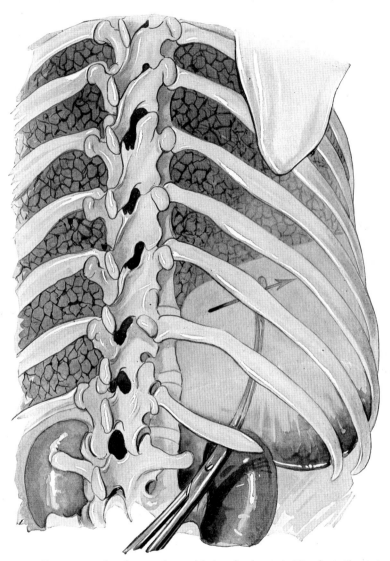

FIG. 275. Two approaches for opening a subphrenic abscess. The first, direct, *transpleural* route leads in the direction of the arrow through the obliterated costophrenic sinus; the second, indirect, *extrapleural* route leads to the abscess from below and posterior in the direction of the forceps.

If the evacuation of the abscess is urgent, the costal and the diaphragmatic pleura may be sutured together over an oval-shaped area. The individual sutures must overlap (Fig. 276). Since the delicate parietal pleura tears easily, it is advisable to use interrupted sutures with a round intestinal needle, since they hold better than a running suture. If the sutures cut through, one must prevent the entrance of air into the pleural cavity by firm pressure with sponges. The suture sealing the pleural space is then completed as carefully as possible. After the suture of the pleural surfaces which obliterates the costophrenic space at this site the two layers are incised within the sutured oval, preferably with the electrosurgical knife, until the abscess is reached. The further procedure takes place in the manner previously described. The closure of the pleural space by suture is however not really trustworthy in any case.

If on exposing the pleura an exudate is found in the pleural space, the clear character of which does not necessitate drainage of the cavity, the exudate is evacuated by an aspiratory puncture at a point above the operative field.

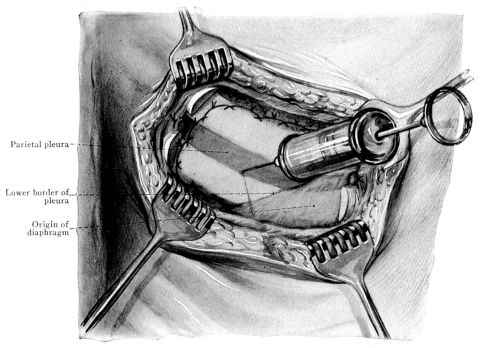

Parietal pleura

Lower border of pleura

Origin of diaphragm

FIG. 276. One-stage opening of a subphrenic abscess by the transpleural route. The two layers of the pleura have been united by overlapping sutures in order to avoid opening the general pleural cavity. The abscess is aspirated through the region within the circle of sutures.

Frequently, however, the fluid in the pleural space becomes secondarily infected and subsequently requires aspiration or even tube drainage.

If the evacuation of the abscess is not urgent, and this is by far the more favorable situation, and in the presence of non-adherent pleural surfaces, an attempt should be made to cause adhesions between them and thus obliterate the space at this site. The evacuation of the abscess is postponed until these have formed. Mechanical pressure and chemical irritation by packing tightly with vioform (or iodoform, I.S.R.) gauze or by the insertion of Baer's paraffin paste have proved to be the most satisfactory measures for the induction of the adhesions. The injection of irritant fluids into the pleural space (tincture of iodine) has not proved satisfactory.

Composition of Baer's Paraffin Paste. Solid paraffin (melting point 52° C) 75 g.; solid paraffin (melting point 43° C) 25 g.; neutral bismuth carbonate 1 g.; vioform 0.05 g. To this I add a tablespoonful of barium sulphate to make the paste more clearly visible in the roentgenogram.

To introduce the paste, the costal pleura is separated by gentle pressure from the chest wall for some distance around the operative site (Fig. 277). This mobilizes the pleura and the lung retracts, leaving a hollowed-out extrapleural space into which the paraffin paste or the vioform gauze pack is introduced with gentle pressure. The soft parts are sutured over this in layers.

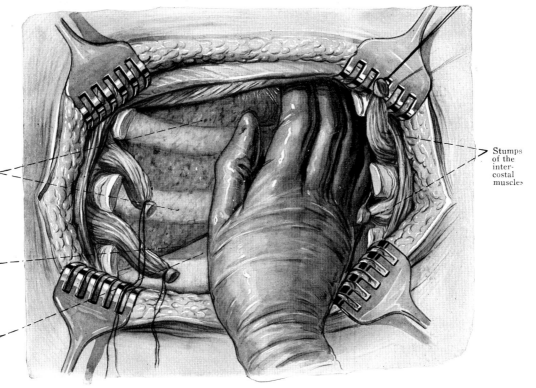

Parietal pleura through which the lung is faintly visible

Location of the lower lung margin during deep inspiration

Diaphragm

Stumps of the intercostal muscles

FIG. 277. Two-stage opening of a subphrenic abscess by the transpleural route. After removal of the interposing ribs and division of the intercostal muscles, the pleura is separated from the ribs by blunt dissection to permit the insertion of packing.

In this manner the costal pleura is pressed against the diaphragmatic pleura and both structures become adherent to each other in a short time with obliteration of the complementary space. Adequate adhesions may surely be counted on after five days. The paste or the packing is removed after complete opening of the wound. If no free pleural space is present in the line of incision, the adherent surfaces are incised and the abscess is evacuated and drained.

Infrapleural Approach. The second mode of approach to a high subphrenic abscess is from below, avoiding the bony thorax and the pleural space. (Fig. 274 and 275). An incision of considerable length is made through the soft parts at the lower border of the bony thorax along the 12th rib. As soon as the lower border of the 12th rib is exposed, the muscles attached to it are divided as is the fascia beneath the muscles. The operator then gently works upward with his finger or with a forceps on the inner aspect of the ribs in the direction of the diaphragm until the appearance of pus indicates the opening of the abscess (Fig. 275). The opening is enlarged by blunt or sharp dissection. The abscess is evacuated, explored with the finger, inspected and drained. Counteropenings are made if necessary. If no pus is found at first, the tip of the finger or of the forceps is carefully directed forward toward the liver so that the abscess is opened from behind.

A compromise is possible between the two procedures of direct and indirect approach. The outer half of the 12th rib lying below the lower border of the pleura is removed and the abscess may be approached from this point by dissection along the inner surface of the rib above.

In view of the uncertainty of predicting an obliteration of the lower pleural space, the uncertainty of the sealing of the pleural space by suture, and the danger of infection in going through the pleural space, even after the formation of adhesions, the extrapleural approach from below should be preferred, provided that the abscess is certainly present and large enough to be reached by blunt dissection. The transpleural route in the presence of a free pleural space always entails considerable danger of infection.

CHAPTER V

OPERATIONS ON THE RECTUM

A. ANATOMIC CONSIDERATIONS

The sigmoid merges imperceptibly into the rectum which in turn terminates at the anus (Fig. 278 and 279). The proximal portion of the rectum is called the pars ampullaris, and its termination, the pars analis.

While the sigmoid has a mesentery, the rectum is not so provided. The mesentery on entering the pelvis rapidly decreases in length and the colon, which after it loses the mesentery is called the rectum, is attached on its posterior aspect to the sacrum over a broad surface extending downward from the top of the third sacral segment. In contradistinction to this strict terminology of the anatomist, the surgeon often erroneously designates the colon as the rectum from the promontory of the sacrum down, and the free mesentery situated between the promontory and the third sacral segment he calls the mesorectum. Waldeyer uses the term pelvic colon (colon pelvinum) for the segment between the promontory and the third sacral vertebra, and the term mesopelvinum for the attached mesentery. There are, therefore, (1) the sigmoid with the free mesosigmoid above the sacral promontory, (2) the pelvic colon with the free mesopelvinum from the promontory to the third sacral vertebra, and (3) the rectum which has no mesentery and lies below the third sacral vertebra, including (a) the pars ampullaris above and (b) the pars analis in the region of the sphincter.

The Fasciae. The anterior and lateral surfaces of the rectum are covered with peritoneum farther down than is the posterior surface while below the pelvic floor the rectum is not covered with peritoneum. The peritoneum finally leaves the anterior and lateral surfaces of the rectum just above the level of the floor of the bladder, 6 to 8 cm. above the anal opening in the adult. At this point the peritoneum is reflected forward, in men onto the posterior surface of the bladder and in women to the uterus (Fig. 278 and 279). The pouch made by this acute angle of reflection is called the fold of Douglas. Beyond this point the rectum is enclosed on all sides only by the connective tissue of the true pelvis.

In direct contact with the rectum is the visceral layer of the pelvic fascia (endopelvic or rectovesical fascia) (Fig. 280). In addition, it encloses the prostate in the male and the cervix and the vagina in the female. In order to separate the rectum from these structures, this fascia must be divided. Otherwise, in the posterior approach, one is led around the prostate or around the vagina and the cervix uteri on the outer surface of the fascia. (This layer of the pelvic fascia passes down into the pelvis on the abdominal surface of the levator ani. It forms the fibrous part of the various pelvic ligaments which assist in holding the viscera in position. I.S.R.)

The perirectal connective tissue (rectal fascia) which lies outside of the visceral pelvic fascia is bounded by the levator ani. The levator ani, from its origins on the posterior surface of the body of the pubis, the spine of the ischium and the intervening white line, passes downward and toward the midline, converging toward the anus. This gives the fascia-bounded space

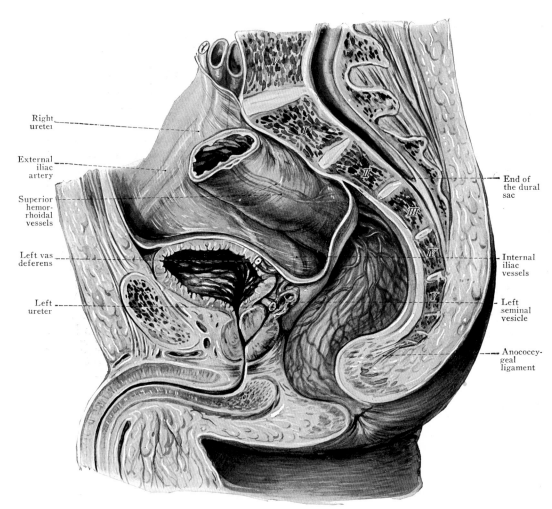

FIG. 278. Location of the pelvic viscera in the male. Semidiagrammatic sagittal section. The pelvic colon loses its mesentery, containing the superior hemorrhoidal artery, at the level of the third sacral vertebra and then becomes the rectum. The rectum is differentiated into an ampullar and an anal portion. The pouch of Douglas, which lies between the pelvic colon and the bladder, extends far down on the ventral (anterior) surface of the bowel. The ureter crosses the iliac vessels retroperitoneally. The vas deferens, passing upward and lateralward, crosses the ureter in an arch concave downward.

above it on each side, the subperitoneal pelvic fossa, a triangular shape with the apex pointing downward on frontal section. Corresponding to it and beneath the levator ani is a similar triangular space with its apex directed upward and bounded to the outer side by the ischium, the subcutaneous pelvic fossa or *ischiorectal space*.

External to the levator ani is the parietal layer of the pelvic fascia which covers the under surface of the levator and the muscles along the pelvic wall. The portion of the fascia which lies in direct contact with the external (inferior) surface of the muscle is therefore also called the external or inferior

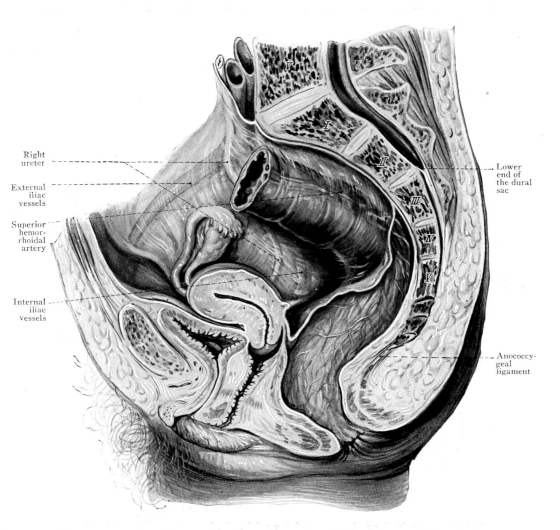

Right ureter

External iliac vessels

Superior hemor- rhoidal artery

Internal iliac vessels

Lower end of the dural sac

Anococcy- geal ligament

FIG. 279. Location of the pelvic viscera in the female. Semidiagrammatic sagittal section. The pelvic colon loses its mesentery, containing the superior hemorrhoidal artery, at the level of the third sacral vertebra and then becomes the rectum. The rectum is differentiated into an ampullar and an anal portion. The pouch of Douglas, which lies between the pelvic colon and the uterus, extends far down on the ventral (anterior) surface of the rectum. The ureter passes retroperitoneally over the iliac vessels and to the lateral side of the cervix uteri to reach the bladder.

diaphragmatic fascia (anal fascia). It must be divided to approach the levator and the rectum from below. On the upper (superior) surface of the levator ani a separate layer of the visceral fascia, the interal or superior diaphragmatic fascia (rectal fascia), may be distinguished.

The following layers, from without inward, are therefore found inside the bony pelvis: parietal layer of the pelvic fascia (anal fascia), levator ani, the perirectal connective tissue (rectal fascia) and the visceral layer of the pelvic fascia (Fig. 280 and 325).

The space in front of the rectum is bounded differently in the two sexes. In the male we find the bladder, the two seminal vesicles, the prostate and

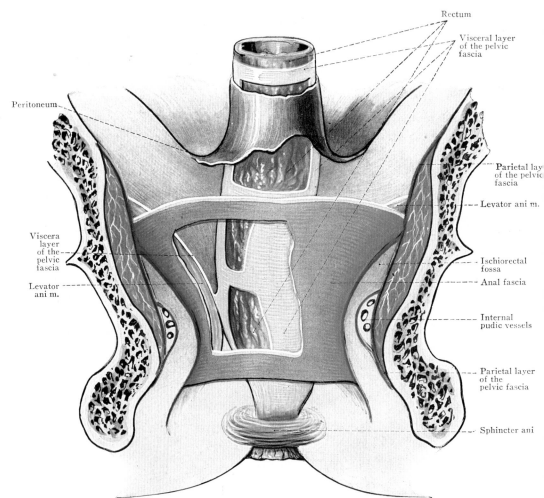

FIG. 280. The fasciae and muscles of the pelvis. In immediate contact with the rectum is the visceral layer of the pelvic fascia; it is reflected onto the medial surface of the levator ani. On the lateral surface of the levator ani lies the anal fascia. The wall of the pelvic inlet is clothed by the parietal layer of the pelvic fascia. The subperitoneal fossa is the space beneath the peritoneum covering the pelvic floor and above the levator ani, covered by the visceral layer of the pelvic fascia. Between the levator ani and the pelvic wall lies the ischiorectal fossa.

the membranous portion of the urethra (Fig. 278); in the female, the cervix and the full extent of the vagina (Fig. 279). All of these structures, including the rectum, are enclosed by the visceral layer of the pelvic fascia.

Just beneath the peritoneum and to each side of the rectum lies an important structure, the ureter (Fig. 343 and 344). It crosses the common iliac artery near its termination. Where the pelvic colon still possesses a mesentery, the ureter lies to its lateral side. It then dips diagonally downward, forward and toward the midline in the true pelvis and gains the ventral aspect of the rectum. Beneath the fold of Douglas it leaves the rectum, which here is surrounded on all sides by connective tissue, and converges toward the midline to reach the urinary bladder. Just before it empties into the bladder in the male, it crosses the vas deferens (Fig. 278).

Just below the place where the rectum is surrounded and reinforced by the muscle bundles of the levator ani coming from both sides, it is enclosed by the circular internal and external sphincters. The external sphincter borders on the bulbocavernosus and the superficial and deep transversus perinei muscles in front and is attached posteriorly to the coccyx by the anococcygeal ligament.

Blood Vessels. The sigmoid and the upper part of the rectum receive their blood supply from the inferior mesenteric artery, an unpaired branch of the aorta (Fig. 159). It gives rise to the left colic artery, the sigmoid artery and the superior hemorrhoidal artery. The superior hemorrhoidal artery reaches the rectum in the connective tissue behind it at the point where the posterior surface of the rectum becomes attached to the pelvic wall. It gives off paired branches which enclose the rectum symmetrically as they course forward and toward the anus (Fig. 278 and 279). The branches of this vessel supply the rectal mucosa as far as the anus and the rectal musculature as far as the region of the sphincter. Its branches do not anastomose with the nearby branches of the middle and inferior hemorrhoidal arteries which approach the lower end of the rectum from both sides in pairs and weave around the terminal rectum and the musculature of the sphincter (Fig. 159). The middle hemorrhoidal arteries are branches of the internal iliac arteries and the inferior hemorrhoidal arteries are branches of the internal pudic arteries. (The superior, middle and inferior hemorrhoidal veins however do anastomose with each other and provide a means whereby the portal and systemic venous systems meet. I.S.R.)

The greater part of the rectum is therefore dependent for its nutrition on the unpaired superior hemorrhoidal artery. Through the arcading branches of the sigmoid artery the superior hemorrhoidal artery possesses anastomoses with the vascular system of the inferior mesenteric artery higher up. The last anastomosis is formed by the sigmoidea ima artery (Fig. 159). If the main trunk of the superior hemorrhoidal artery is ligated above the origin of the sigmoidea ima, the superior hemorrhoidal artery continues to receive sufficient blood by way of this arcade. If, however, the trunk of the superior hemorrhoidal artery is ligated below this point, the distal gut is deprived of its blood supply and becomes necrotic. The point where the sigmoidea ima artery meets the superior hemorrhoidal artery is therefore called "the critical point" (Sudeck).

The unpaired middle sacral artery, the direct continuation of the aorta, lies in the hollow of the sacrum. It has nothing to do with the blood supply of the rectum.

The rectum is surrounded by a network of the interanastomosing superior, middle and inferior hemorrhoidal veins, which empty in part into the portal system and in part into the systemic venous system. At the anal opening these veins are arranged in a circle directly beneath the mucosa, and from them hemorrhoids may arise. This venous plexus may bleed profusely in case of rupture or when incised.

The lymph channels of the external anus empty into the inguinal lymph nodes, while the anal mucosa and that of the lowest portion of the ampulla are drained into the internal iliac nodes along the veins of the same name. The upper ampulla is drained into the sacral lymph nodes which lie in the mesosigmoid along the superior hemorrhoidal vessels and are in communication with the lymph nodes along the common iliac vein and the inferior vena cava. Aside from metastases in the more distant lymph nodes, carcinoma of the rectum tends to spread decidedly in an oral direction, so that a segment of gut immediately on the anal side of the lesion may be considered sound, while portions for a considerable distance on the oral side must be considered diseased. The most frequently involved lymph nodes of the immediate neighborhood lie along the superior hemorrhoidal artery (Westhues).

B. GENERAL TECHNIQUE OF OPERATIONS ON THE RECTUM

The healing of the wound of a rectal operation may be influenced unfavorably by various circumstances. Since the major portion of the rectum has no peritoneal covering and its blood supply is easily interfered with, rectal suture lacks the certainty and dependability of healing afforded by the marked adhesive power of the peritoneum in suture of other segments of the gastrointestinal tract. A more or less complete reopening of the suture line is therefore a common occurrence. Since the rectum is tightly surrounded on all sides by the adjacent connective tissue, it can be mobilized only by being dissected free of its surroundings and then only for a short distance, so that after the removal of even small segments, there may result an appreciable lack of material. Such a lack of material can only be obviated by the radical procedure of extending the mobilization of the gut as far as the sigmoid.

The blood supply of the rectum depends as has been stated largely on a single vessel, the superior hemorrhoidal artery. If this vessel is divided, kinked, squeezed or thrombosed, necrosis of the gut supplied by it invariably results. Since the paired vessels of the lower rectum do not anastomose with the vessels of the upper portion, nutritional disturbances of the lower portion can also easily follow circular mobilization. The bacterial flora of the terminal bowel are particularly virulent, so that there is increased danger of infection when this segment of the bowel is opened. Furthermore, inspissated fecal masses place a severe mechanical strain on sutures of the rectum.

The sphincter mechanism of the anus, on the one hand, is very easily stimulated reflexly, so that after operation painful tenesmus may frequently arise which may prevent even the passage of flatus and may also extend to the vesical sphincter. Through such a reflex anal closure the ampulla may become greatly distended and the rectal sutures may thus be subjected to great tension. On the other hand, the function of the sphincter is very sensitive so that it may suffer considerably directly, through pulling, crushing, dissection and division, and indirectly, through injury of the inferior mesenteric plexus and the sacral nerves. (The stimulus to defecation from the rectal ampulla passes over the sacral nerves. I.S.R.)

These unfavorable conditions necessitate particular measures of foresight in operations on the rectum and on the anus.

The bowel must be evacuated and cleansed as well as possible before operation. The rectum must be kept free of feces not only during the operation but for some days thereafter. One must therefore provide not only for the evacuation of the large bowel but also of the small intestine before the operation, and the rectum must be placed at rest functionally after the operation. The cleansing measures should however not be carried to extremes, out of consideration for the condition of the patient. The patient's bowel should be emptied every day for 2 or 3 days before operation but no cathartic should be given within 24 hours of operation. On the morning of the day before the operation a high cleansing enema or colonic irrigation, is given and on this same day two doses of 15 to 20 drops of tincture of opium, and the same dose of opium on the day of operation before the operation. The administration of opium is usually continued for from 3 to 5 days after the operation. Only after complete extirpation of the rectum is the splinting of the bowel by opium not required, since the structure requiring protection, the rectum, has been removed. If after stopping the opium there appear the signs of the first bowel movement, the passage of the inspissated fecal masses is made easier by giving an oil enema through a Nelaton catheter. After the first bowel movement has taken place, a soft mushy consistency of the stool is provided for during the next few days by means of mild cathartics and liquid petrolatum.

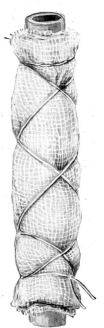

Fig. 281. Rectal tube wrapped with gauze.

If a rectal disease has caused such a marked stenosis of the bowel that a thorough evacuation is impossible before the operation, an intestinal fistula or an artificial anus should be established 1 to 3 weeks before the major operation. This is done in the sigmoid, or, if the sigmoid is to be used in the main operation, in the cecum. Through this opening the terminal gut is irrigated and cleansed daily. A few surgeons recommend the establishment of an intestinal fistula before every major rectal operation, especially those involving a partial resection of the rectum, in order to relieve the suture line.

Operations in the region of the anus are usually performed in the lithotomy position. In men the scrotum must be elevated by means of a sling passed under it and around the patient's neck. In operations on the rectum, the abdominal-suspension position is preferred, or a lateral position may be used. The details of these positions are described in Volume I. Peculiarities of position are mentioned under the individual operations.

Postoperative reflex spasm of the sphincter is prevented by its preliminary stretching. This may be done instrumentally or with the fingers. For instrumental dilatation, which is preferable because it can be accurately gauged, the dilators illustrated in Volume I, are employed. They must be thoroughly lubricated before introduction, as otherwise the delicate rectal mucosa may adhere to them and be torn. For digital dilatation both index fingers are used. After being covered with vaseline they are introduced into the anus and are crooked in such a way that they grasp the sphincter which is easily felt in the shape of a ring. The fingers are gently and cautiously pulled apart in a dorso-ventral direction to the extent that in adults one thumb can be inserted between the two fingers. Any excessive or brusque stretching of the sphincter is to be avoided, because it can lead to permanent incontinence. The sphincter should be gently stretched, not torn.

After some rectal operations it is advisable to insert a rectal tube, not too thick, 6 to 8 cm. long and wrapped on the outside with vaseline gauze (Fig. 281). It remains in place until the first bowel movement. Its insertion must always be preceded by dilatation of the sphincter. The tube facilitates the escape of flatus. In operations in the region of the rectum it also controls bleeding by pressure. As an alternative to suture to the anal skin, the tube can be held in place in the following manner: Two large safety pins are stuck through the projecting part of the tube. A gauze ring or a gauze compress incised on one side is placed between the safety pins and the skin. A piece of gauze with a small hole in the center for the egress of the tube is glued with mastisol to the skin in a wide circle around the anus and holds the tube back by means of the safety pins.

The bladder should be thoroughly emptied just before every major rectal operation and if necessary this should be done by means of catheterization.

After major rectal operations, I use an indwelling catheter for several days. This measure serves the purpose of placing the operative field at rest, which otherwise would be subjected to constant displacements by the successive distension and collapse of the bladder and the straining incident to forced urination. In addition, the indwelling catheter insures against an overdistended bladder. Urination is often difficult for several days after operation due to reflex spasm or to damage to the bladder nerves.

The girdle type of spinal anaesthesia is particularly suitable for extensive operations on the rectum because of the accurate way in which its extent and dosage can be limited. The steep Trendelenburg position which is so desirable in rectal operations, especially in the combined procedure, is advantageous in, and an integral part of this type of anaesthesia.

Minor operations in the more restricted region of the anus and dilatation of the anal sphincter may be performed under local anaesthesia, for which $\frac{1}{2}$ to 1 per cent novocaine is adequate. At a distance of 1 to 2 finger-breadths from the right and left sides of the anus, two symmetrically placed wheals are raised. They are joined by a subcutaneous zone of injection which encircles the anus. The lubricated left index finger is introduced into the anus beyond the sphincter. Through each wheal the needle is passed into the deeper tissues, injecting the anaesthetic solution as it goes, until the index finger in the rectum feels the tip of the needle and the escaping fluid as it raises a wheal under the mucosa (Fig. 282). Two similar injections are made, one in the anterior and one in the posterior commissure, the points of injection having in the meantime

become anaesthetic from the subcutaneous injection. The anus and the
sphincter are thereby enclosed by the anaesthetic solution after the four
injections in the shape of a truncated pyramid, the hypothetical apex of which
lies in the middle of the rectum about 6 cm. above its lower end. If the
high-pressure local-anaesthesia apparatus is used, the anaesthetization can be
completed within a minute or two.

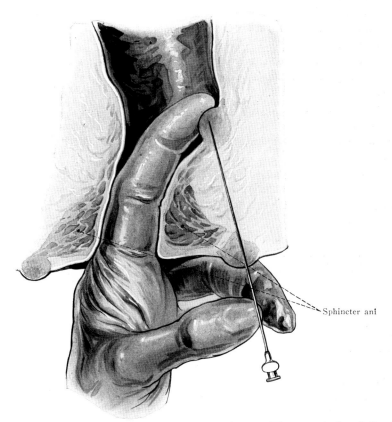

Sphincter ani

FIG. 282. Local anaesthesia of the anus and the anal sphincter. The anaesthetic solution is
injected in the form of a truncated cone around the anus and external to the sphincter. With
the tip of the left index finger inserted into the anus the surgeon recognizes the escape of the
fluid immediately beneath the mucosa.

C. TREATMENT OF INJURIES OF THE RECTUM

Injuries of the rectum may result either from foreign bodies which pierce
the rectum from without or from foreign bodies which gain access to the
interior of the rectum, usually through the anus, more rarely by way of the
proximal intestine, and which injure the bowel from within. Of particular
importance are injuries due to impaling on a pointed object. These are much
like stab and bullet wounds in that the wound is usually of small caliber, and
its course and length cannot be determined from the outside. The object
often reaches important and more distant structures to which the clinical
phenomena do not at first call attention. The strucures which are most liable

to such injury are the bladder, the urethra, the peritoneal cavity and its contents, especially the small intestine, and in women the vagina and the uterus.

Among the sequelae of such injuries the foremost are the dangers of infection, of hemorrhage and of damage to the function of the affected organs, notably the anal sphincter.

The extent of the injury must first be determined. It is important to determine whether the abdominal cavity has been opened or not. The further steps in this regard are based on the general rules for the management of abdominal injuries as set forth on page 330. The first principle is that if the possibility exists that the peritoneal cavity has been opened the diagnosis must be clinched by immediate laparotomy, instead of waiting for the first signs of peritonitis. The abdomen is opened through a midline incision above the symphysis. The wall of the rectum, the bladder, in women the uterus and the vagina, the small intestine and the other intra-abdominal organs are examined for injuries. Particular attention should be given to the region of the pouch of Douglas, which must be completely exposed and inspected. Every injury must be closed by double suture in the usual manner. If hollow viscera have been securely closed (and the contamination has not been too great. I.S.R.), the abdomen is closed without drainage in accordance with the general rules for drainage which have already been discussed.

In injuries of the rectum a rectal tube is inserted at the completion of the operation. In bladder injuries a permanent catheter is inserted either through the urethra or through a suprapubic cystostomy.

If the trauma does not involve the abdominal cavity, the region of the wound is exposed in the perineum. A wound involving the anus is first explored through the anus, a wound situated beside the anus is first followed outside the gut to its full extent. If in addition to the rectum there has been an injury to the bladder, the urethra or the vagina, but without involvement of the peritoneal cavity, the injury is taken care of from the perineum.

Depending on the degree of soiling and crushing of the tissues, the wound is "debrided" or sutured directly, with or without drainage. Particular care must be given to the repair of an injured sphincter.

In case of extensive injury to the rectum it is advisable to establish a double-barrelled artificial anus in the sigmoid, in order to protect the injured area temporarily from the feces and to put it at rest. If there is an associated injury to the bladder or urethra, the urine must be drained through a permanent catheter in the urethra or through a suprapubic cystostomy. If the latter method is used I attach the suprapubic drainage tube to a low pressure suction pump.

D. TREATMENT OF IMPERFORATE ANUS AND RECTAL ATRESIA

In congenital atresia the rectum is either completely closed or it empties in the form of a more or less narrow fistula through the perineum, the scrotum, or into the urethra, or bladder, into the vagina or into the fossa navicularis.

In the presence of a fistula, if the orifice is large enough to permit of adequate evacuation of the feces, the operation is postponed if possible for

2 to 3 years, until the child seems strong enough to stand so serious an operation. In the meantime attempts are made to dilate the fistulous tract with bougies. Only in case of a rectovesical fistula is prompt operation always necessary, since otherwise the child may quickly die of an ascending infection of the urinary tract.

Occasionally an imperforate anus is due merely to the presence of a delicate occluding membrane. Treatment is then simple, the membrane being pierced by a sound and the narrow opening stretched with small Hegar dilators.

The deciding factor in the end-result after operation is whether one has to deal simply with a short atretic stretch of bowel in the region of the anus (atresia ani) or whether a large segment of bowel is missing (atresia recti), two conditions which merge into each other without any sharp distinction.

Atresia ani is preferably treated by the dorsal route, whereas the abdominal approach is more satisfactory in atresia recti. (I have however operated on a case of atresia of the rectum in a 16-hour old baby by the perineal route with an excellent end-result. I.S.R.) It is therefore of the greatest importance to determine which of these conditions is present before beginning the operation. If the position of the end of the bowel is indicated by a bulging in the anal region, the diagnosis is easily made, and the perineal route only should be considered. If this is not the case, a roentgenogram with the child in an inverted position (Cackovic) will give the greatest aid in making an exact diagnosis. The gas bubble which collects in the end of the gut and which is demonstrable in the roentgen picture makes it possible to decide in most cases whether a procedure from below is possible or whether the abdominal route must be used.

The operation has three objectives: the establishment of an adequate means of evacuation of feces (indicatio vitalis), the establishment of sphincter function and the closure of a fecal fistula, if this is present.

I. DORSAL APPROACH

If the end of the gut is recognized by a bulge in the anal region, an incision is cautiously made in the median plane over the bulge. The infiltration of the operative field with novocaine and the use in part of the electrosurgical knife to lessen bleeding (which otherwise often occurs) will be found advantageous. The incision is carried toward the coccyx, rather than toward the perineum, so that the sphincter is divided only posteriorly if at all, and not also anteriorly. When the "rectal balloon," recognizable by the dark color of the black meconium within it, comes into view, it is not opened at once but is carefully freed on all sides until it can be brought to the normal anal region without tension. This is frequently impossible and the gut must then be sutured into the wound at a higher point.

The external wound is closed from its posterior angle up to the gut which has been sutured to the wound edge farther forward. The gut is incised, and the meconium, which is sterile, is evacuated. The bowel may be irrigated with saline solution. However, it empties itself spontaneously in most cases. The edges of the opening in the gut are attached to the skin margins by means of through-and-through sutures in such a way that mucous membrane everywhere borders on the skin.

If the end of the bowel cannot be located from below, then searching for the bowel and bringing it down to the wound by the perineal route usually constitute a procedure which is very uncertain in its results and which in many cases must be abandoned in favor of the combined approach. If signs of ileus have already appeared, and if the end of the bowel according to the roentgenogram is not in the immediate neighborhood of the perineum, a double-barrelled sigmoid anus should be established and the search for the bowel from below should be postponed until a later time. In the presence of a fistula or after the establishment of an artificial anus roentgenographic study with a barium enema will give valuable information concerning the position of the rectum and the type of subsequent operation to be employed, especially as to whether it is possible to bring the lower end of the gut down to the position of a normal anal opening.

The chief danger in the procedure from below in the male child is injury to the bladder or the urethra. One should therefore keep close to the sacrum throughout the operation. The location of the urethra is kept constantly in view by the introduction of a very small sound.

With the patient in the abdominal-suspension position, the operative field is infiltrated with an adrenalin-novocaine solution. A longitudinal incision is made in the median raphe, beginning at the upper end of the coccyx and extending forward far enough to divide the posterior half of the sphincter but not to divide it completely. It is best to remove the coccyx at once. Occasionally a cord of fibrous tissue will lead to the end of the gut. The incision is extended cautiously upward along the sacrum, a constant watch being kept for the dark-colored "rectal balloon." If an artificial anus is present, a semi-rigid sound is introduced into the distal limb of the sigmoid and gently pushed downward. It often furnishes a valuable guide for the further advance.

When the end of the rectum has been found from below, it is mobilized on all sides before it is opened (Fig. 283) and to such an extent that it is possible to bring it to the skin in the normal anal region without too great tension. To accomplish this, it is usually necessary to open the pouch of Douglas. This is done in the manner described in the dorsal operation for rectal carcinoma. After adequate mobilization of the mesosigmoid and the ligation of any bleeding points the bowel is delivered sufficiently and the pouch of Douglas is closed.

When the bowel has been sufficiently freed, the operative wound is made smaller, so that the point of exit of the bowel will come to lie as close as possible in the normal anal region. The gut is opened and sutured to the skin. The evacuation of the meconium can be aided by irrigation and suction.

If there is present an intestinal fistula communicating with the bladder, the urethra, the vagina or the body surface, the operation is carried out in the manner described, and in addition, the fistulous tract is tied off, divided and sutured as carefully as possible at the same time.

In case of a perineal or a vulvovestibular fistula, a circular incision is made around the fistulous opening. The skin incision is prolonged dorsally as far as

the normal anal region. The fistulous tract together with the lower end of the
bowel is freed on all sides and is transplanted into the normal anal region. If
the fistula is too narrow, it is split open as far as the normal bowel, the bowel
is pulled down and after the removal of the fistulous canal its lower end is
sutured to the normal anal region. As broad a perineum as possible is built up
in front of the newly made anus by transverse suture of the tissues.

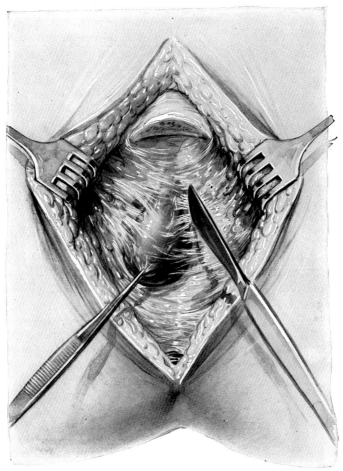

FIG. 283. Search for the end of the bowel through a dorsal approach in case of atresia
of the anus. The coccyx has been resected. The dark meconium-filled balloon of bowel is
visible through the connective tissue and is being dissected free.

2. COMBINED APPROACH

In a child with complete atresia there may be no bulging in the anal region
when the child cries or when pressure is made on the abdomen to give any
clue that the closed end of the bowel lies at not too great a distance from the
skin. Roentgenographic studies with the child in an inverted position may
also be negative in this regard. At the same time, there may be no external
intestinal fistula. Under these conditions, in view of the uncertainty of the
position of the lower bowel, the primary search for the end of the bowel from

below is usually abandoned. In view of the magnitude of the combined procedure, it is advisable first to establish a temporary double-barrelled artificial
anus in the left iliac fossa. This procedure is obligatory if the child already
shows signs of ileus, and is therefore greatly weakened, or if there is considerable abdominal distension. After the establishment of an artificial anus, the
second operation can be postponed for a number of weeks, months or even
years.

At the second operation, the abdomen is opened in the midline above the
symphysis after emptying the bladder and the end of the bowel is searched for
from above. This corresponds to the combined abdominosacral procedure for
the removal of a rectal carcinoma. When the gut has been found and if it
can be sufficiently mobilized so that its end can be displaced as far as the anal
region, the peritoneum of the pelvic floor is opened in a transverse direction
close to the sacrum and a forceps is pushed along the sacrum as far as the
anal region. An incision from the outside is made down on the tip of the
forceps and a second forceps is drawn from the perineal region into the upper
operative field by means of the first forceps. The second forceps then grasps
the end of the bowel and brings it down into the perineum. The peritoneum
of the pouch of Douglas is sutured around the gut where it passes through it.
The laparotomy wound is closed. The end of the rectum is opened and sutured
to the edge of the wound in the anal region.

The combined operation is carried out in a similar way if the attempt to
find the gut from the perineum has failed. After opening the peritoneum in
front of the sacrum the lower operative field is easily reached, so that the
formation of the tunnel to the anal region becomes simpler.

If it was possible to suture the intestinal opening into the normal position
and if an artificial anus had been established previously, the artificial anus
is closed in the manner described on page 251, as soon as the evacuation of
feces by the natural route has begun.

E. TREATMENT OF RECTAL PROLAPSE

In infants, prolapse of the mucosa of a minor degree usually corrects itself
spontaneously if the protrusion can be prevented for some time. After regulation of the bowels, the prolapsed gut is pushed back and the buttocks are
pulled together with strips of adhesive plaster so tightly that the child can no
longer force the bowel out. Three times a day the dressing is removed for
defecation. A nurse holds the buttocks together so that the feces escape between her gloved fingers while the prolapse is held back.

In adults, if there is only a very moderate protrusion of the mucosa (anal
prolapse), the condition is treated as are hemorrhoids, from which it can
often only with difficulty be differentiated. Single tabs are removed in the
manner there described. In an annular prolapse of the mucosa the Whitehead
operation is used.

If, however, larger portions of the rectal mucosa or the whole rectum
protrude from the anus, these procedures will not suffice and one of the following operations must be employed:

1. The Ring of Thiersch

The principle of the wire ring of Thiersch is to prevent the escape of the prolapse for a considerable time by narrowing the anal opening and thereby to give the sphincter and the pelvic floor a chance to recover. If the ring causes discomfort it may be removed after several months without difficulty and usually without a recurrence of the prolapse, because in the meantime the sphincter and the pelvic floor have become sufficiently strengthened and because a ring of scar tissue has formed in the neighborhood of the Thiersch

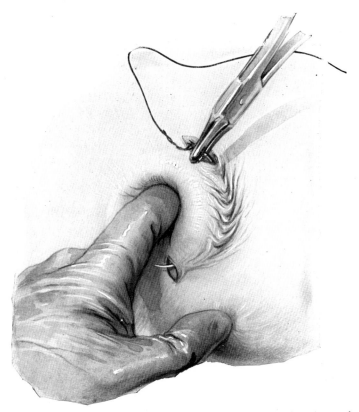

Fig. 284. Insertion of a Thiersch wire ring for the treatment of prolapse of the rectum. The wire is passed, under the protection of the finger inserted into the anus, between skin and mucosa by means of a needle introduced into a small incision in the anterior commissure and withdrawn from an incision in the posterior commissure.

ring and takes its place. The Thiersch ring is however likely to be successful only in small prolapses in adults, and in children.

The ring is inserted in the following manner (Fig. 284): With the patient in the lithotomy position, two short radiating incisions are made, one in the anterior raphe, the other in the posterior raphe, about 2 cm. from the anal opening. A large curved needle provided with a fairly strong rustless steel wire is introduced through the anterior incision, and is carried around the anus and brought out through the posterior incision. The surgeon's left index finger introduced into the anus guards against injury to the mucosa. In a similar manner the needle is carried on the other side from the posterior to the anterior incision. The two ends of the wire protruding from the anterior incision are now twisted together until in adults the first phalanx of the surgeon's index finger, and in children only the tip, can just pass through the ring. The remaining ends of the wire are cut off, the twisted ends are bent inward and the

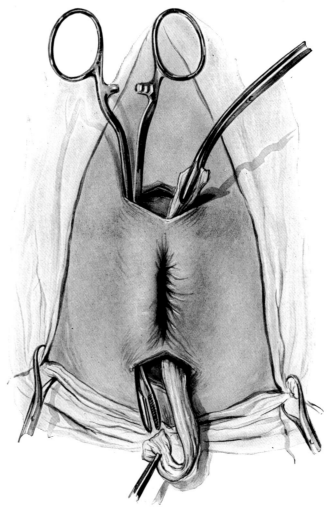

FIG. 285. Insertion of a fascial ring for the treatment of prolapse of the rectum. A strip of fascia has been passed from a small incision in the anterior commissure to a small incision in the posterior commissure through a tunnel just to the left of the anus between skin and mucosa. A forceps has been passed in a similar manner just to the right of the anus and is about to grasp the end of the strip of fascia to carry it back to the point of introduction.

two skin incisions are sutured over the buried wire ring and sealed with collodion.

The insertion of such a wire may lead to a number of difficulties. The ring may cut through the rectum. It may break and the sharp ends pierce the tissues and the gut. The tissues around the metallic foreign body may become inflamed and suppuration may ensue which may lead to fistula and the final extrusion of the ring. Even in the absence of these complications, the wire ring is best removed after a time, as it will eventually lead to them.

These complications can usually be avoided by the use of a pliable auto-plastic tissue ring, such as a strip of the fascia lata, instead of the foreign-body metal ring. The insertion of a fascial ring is carried out in a similar manner to that just described. After the small skin incisions have been made in the

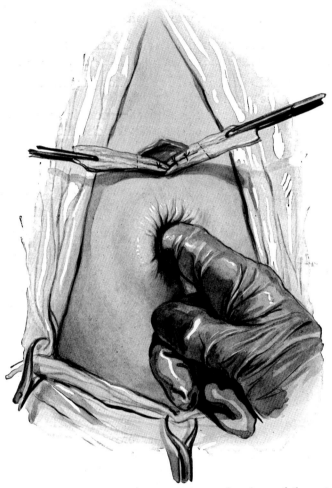

FIG. 286. Insertion of a fascial ring for the treatment of prolapse of the rectum. The two ends of the strip of fascia which encircles the anus are joined so that the resultant ring tightly hugs the index finger which has been introduced into the anus. The junction of the two ends of the fascial strip is effected by passing one end through a slit in the other, pulling the loop snug and suturing.

anterior and posterior commissures, the surgeon undermines the tissues beside the anus from the upper to the lower incision first on the left side, then on the right, by means of a forceps (Fig. 285). A strip of fascia lata of suitable length and about 2 cm. wide is removed. Its ends are grasped by the forceps tips protruding from the lower skin incision and are pulled out through the upper incision. A small slit is made near one end of the strip and the other end is pulled through it. Each end of the strip is grasped with a Kocher hemostat and pulled tight until the strip grips the finger in the anus in the manner above described. The ends of the strip are sutured together in this position (Fig. 286).

(In children, I have found the operation of separating the posterior portion of the anus and rectum from the sacrum and their soft tissue attachments as far as the sacral promontory and the subsequent packing of the cavity a very efficient one. In the adult the Moschcowitz operation of obliterating the pouch of Douglas has often given very satisfactory results. I. S. R.)

2. PERINEAL PLASTIC OPERATION

Larger rectal prolapses can often be treated successfully by a perineal plastic procedure which reinforces the pelvic floor, together with a narrowing and a suspension of the rectal canal.

To perform a posterior perineal plastic operation a curved incision is made around the posterior third of the anus at a distance of 2 cm. from it. A second incision is made perpendicular to the curved incision posteriorly in the midline and is carried beyond the coccyx. By freeing and retracting the two triangular flaps so outlined, the parietal layer of the pelvic fascia in the region of the posterior wall of the rectum is exposed above the internal sphincter as far as the coccyx. This is described in detail under resection of the rectum on page 411. It is usually advantageous to resect the coccyx and to extend the exposure of the rectal wall as far up as possible.

The muscle bundles of the levator ani converging toward the anus are freed from the rectum and pulled aside with blunt hooked retractors. After replacement of the prolapse, the posterior wall of the rectum is plicated in its long axis from the internal sphincter to high in the hollow of the sacrum by a row of interrupted silk sutures (Fig. 287). Each suture picks up a fold of gut wall on the right side and the left side, not including the mucosa. Tying the sutures narrows the lumen by forming a longitudinal inverted fold. The highest sutures are also passed through the sacral ligaments in such a way that when they are tied they elevate the posterior rectal wall.

The margins of the right and the left levator ani are sutured together in the midline over these plicating sutures (Fig. 287) distal to their original attachment. This forms a firm support, reenforcement of the pelvic floor, distal and dorsal to the rectum. The wound is closed by suture and without drainage.

In a similar but less extensive way a narrowing of the rectal canal and a transplanting of the levator fibers can be performed on the anterior side of the rectum through an anterior perineal incision. In the male, this exposure is carried out as in the exposure of the prostate by the perineal route; in the female, by splitting the rectovaginal septum.

3. AMPUTATION OF THE PROLAPSED PORTION

(A) AMPUTATION OF ALL LAYERS OF THE PROLAPSED RECTUM (VON MIKULICZ)

In an old or incarcerated prolapse which cannot be reduced because of adhesions or induration of its walls or whose reduction is not possible because of nutritional changes, resection of the prolapsed gut is the only treatment to be considered. The results of this operation are so good that the procedure is also to be recommended in other types of cases.

While the prolapsed rectum is pulled well down by two traction sutures, a transverse incision is made through its anterior (ventral) wall for half its

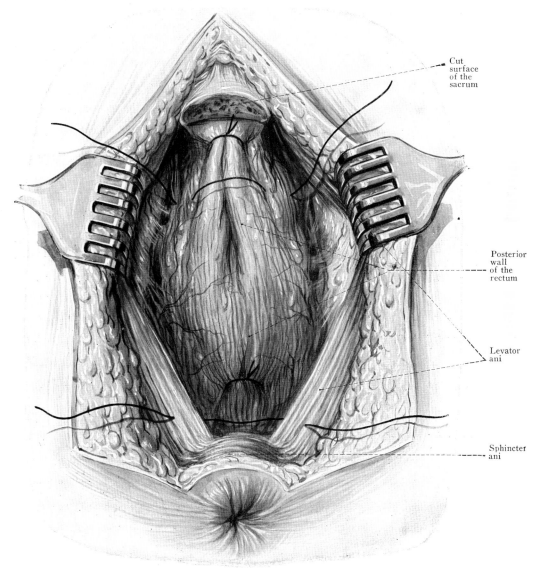

Fig. 287. Treatment of prolapse of the rectum by a posterior perineal plastic procedure. After resection of the coccyx and exposure of the rectum from behind, the posterior rectal wall is folded longitudinally by means of plicating sutures and the posterior margins of the right and left levator ani muscles are sutured together.

circumference and at a distance of 2 cm from the anus with the electrosurgical knife. The incision extends through all layers, mucosa, muscularis (Fig. 288), and if the pouch of Douglas is involved in the prolapse, through the serosa as well, opening the peritoneal cavity in the region of the pouch of

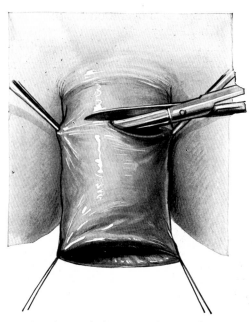

Fig. 288. Treatment of prolapse of the rectum by complete amputation (1). While the prolapsed portion is held taut by means of two traction sutures, its outer anterior wall is being divided transversely at a distance of 1 cm. from the anus.

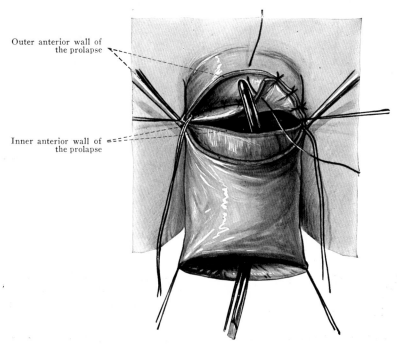

Outer anterior wall of
the prolapse

Inner anterior wall of
the prolapse

Fig. 289. Treatment of prolapse of the rectum by complete amputation (2). After joining the serous surfaces of the outer anterior wall and the inner anterior wall of the prolapse by means of a row of Lembert sutures, the inner anterior wall was also divided transversely. The cut edges of the two anterior walls of the prolapse are being joined by a row of interrupted sutures which include all three layers.

Douglas and exposing the serosa-covered anterior wall of the inner intestinal segment. Any intestinal loops or other viscera encountered in the peritoneal pocket are replaced in the abdominal cavity. Every bleeding vessel is carefully ligated.

The serosa of the divided segment protruding from the anus is sutured at a distance of 0.5 cm from the cut edge to the serosa of the anterior wall of the inner segment by means of interrupted Lembert sutures. Then the anterior wall of the inner segment is divided at the same level as the outer gut. The cut edges of the outer and the inner segments are joined by interrupted three-layer sutures (anterior Albert suture) (Fig. 289). The posterior wall of the inner gut is then divided (Fig. 290). In case of a large prolapse,

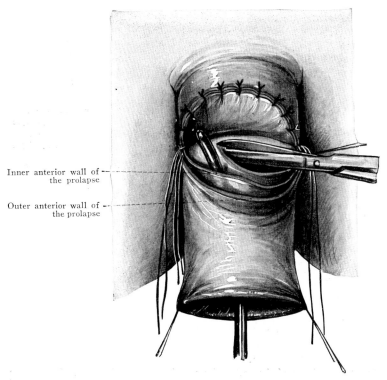

Inner anterior wall of the prolapse

Outer anterior wall of the prolapse

Fig. 290. Treatment of prolapse of the rectum by complete amputation (3). The inner posterior wall of the prolapse is being cut across at a distance of 1 cm. from the anus.

the mesosigmoid lies in the cleft so exposed. It is ligated and divided. At a distance of 0.5 cm from its cut edge the posterior wall of the inner gut is sutured to the serosa of the posterior wall of the outer gut (posterior Lembert suture). This completes the circular serosal suture. The posterior wall of the outer gut is then divided, removing the prolapsed intestine (Fig. 291). The cut edges of the posterior walls of the inner and the outer gut segments are joined by interrupted sutures including all three layers (posterior Albert suture). This completes the circuit of the three-layer suture.

The circular site of suture of the gut which has been united in this manner by two rows of sutures is now carefully replaced through the anus and above the sphincter. A small-bore rectal tube may be inserted to retain the bowel in position and permit the escape of flatus. The after-treatment is the same as that after a hemorrhoid operation.

(B) AMPUTATION OF THE MUCOSA OF THE PROLAPSED GUT (REHN-DELORME)

Since the resection of all layers of the prolapsed gut is a rather extensive and bloody operation which in many instances involves the opening of the peritoneal cavity, the efforts in the direction of a simpler and less radical procedure are justified. If the prolapse is reducible, the end may be attained

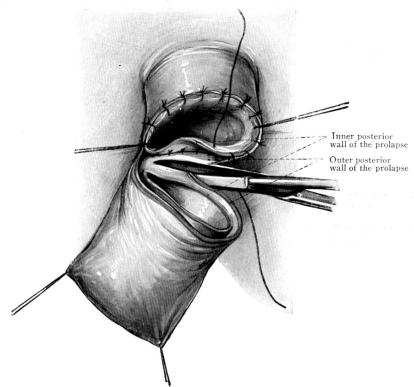

Inner posterior
wall of the prolapse

Outer posterior
wall of the prolapse

FIG. 291. Treatment of prolapse of the rectum by complete amputation (4). The serous surfaces of the inner and outer posterior walls of the prolapse have been joined by a row of Lembert sutures. The outer posterior wall is being divided and the cut edges of the outer and inner posterior walls are being joined by a row of interrupted sutures which include all three layers.

by merely amputating the prolapsed mucosa while the muscle layer and a possible serous coat remain intact.

The prolapse is pulled out as far as possible. The operation is made easier by injecting a novocaine-adrenalin solution under the mucosa which lessens the bleeding and helps to begin the separation of the mucosa from the muscular layer. A circular incision is made in the mucosa at the border between mucosa and skin. The edge of the mucosa is grasped with four Kocher hemostats in order to make even traction. The mucosa is dissected free from the muscle layer in a continuous everted tube (Fig. 292). The separation is

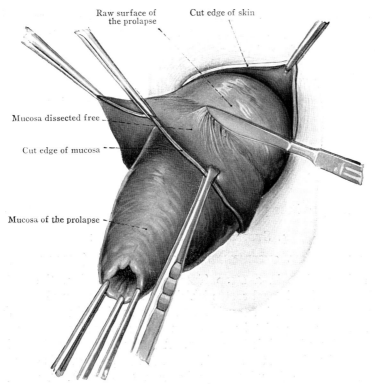

Raw surface of
the prolapse

Cut edge of skin

Mucosa dissected free

Cut edge of mucosa

Mucosa of the prolapse

FIG. 292.   Treatment of prolapse of the rectum by removal of the mucosa and by plication (1).
The mucosa is being dissected free from the surface of the prolapse.

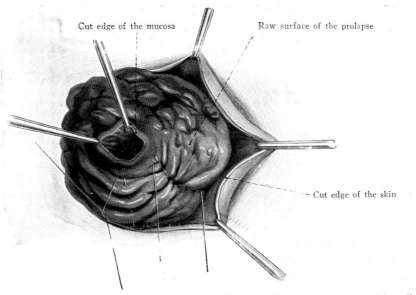

Cut edge of the mucosa

Raw surface of the prolapse

Cut edge of the skin

FIG. 293.   Treatment of prolapse of the rectum by removal of the mucosa and by plication (2).   After the removal of the mucosa, the prolapse is being shortened by means of plicating sutures in the long axis of the bowel.   The sutures should include the cut edges of the skin
and of the mucosa.

easy in the proper plane of cleavage, especially since the mucosa is much thickened as a rule. When the separation of the mucosa has reached the tip of the prolapse, the mucosal cylinder is cut across and removed.

The prolapsed muscle tube denuded of its mucosa is now provided in its long axis with a number of catgut sutures each of which passes through the skin at the base of the prolapse, picks up a number of superficial folds of the muscle and grasps the edge of the mucosa at the tip of the prolapse (Fig. 293). Depending on the circumference of the prolapse, 4 to 8 such plicating sutures are applied parallel to each other in the long axis of the gut. When these sutures are collectively pulled tight and tied, the muscle cylinder is folded up like an accordion and forced back into the anus. The plicated tube of tissue surrounding the anus forms a firm ring of scar tissue after healing and prevents the further escape of the prolapse.

4. Suspension of the Rectum

(a) intra-abdominal suspension of the sigmoid (colopexy, jennel)

With the patient in a steep Trendelenburg position, the abdomen is opened through a left lateral rectus incision. The descending limb of the sigmoid is put on stretch with considerable force so that the anus is markedly retracted. A flap of parietal peritoneum with a lateral pedicle is dissected free in the region of the left iliac fossa. A portion of the surface of the sigmoid is scarified and, with the sigmoid under tension, this area is sutured to the margins of the space denuded of peritoneum (Fig. 294). The loose peritoneal flap is attached to the surface of the gut by sutures (Rotter).

Kümmel recommends suturing the gut to the anterior longitudinal ligament just above the promontory. Care must be used to avoid the large vessels if this is done.

The sigmoid may also be attached to the abdominal wound (von Eiselsberg). The sutures closing the peritoneum of the laparotomy wound at the same time grasp the superficial layers of the intestinal wall which was previously scarified.

The end results of colopexy are in general not very satisfactory.

(b) suspension of the rectum from the sacrum (rectopexy, ekehorn)

A much simpler procedure is to fasten the rectum to the sacrum by way of a dorsal approach as proposed by Ekehorn. The measure is however applicable only for the treatment of prolapse in children.

The child lies on its right side and the surgeon stands at the back of the child, his left index finger in the rectum (Fig. 295), thus holding back the prolapse. He then introduces a large Reverdin needle to the right of the last sacral vertebra perpendicularly through the skin and the intervening soft tissues into the rectum, catches the tip of the needle with his left index finger and under guidance of the finger brings the needle out of the anus. A strong silk suture is threaded on the needle and needle and thread are withdrawn through the skin in the back. The needle is introduced a second time, but to the left of the last sacral vertebra, and is brought out through the anus in the same way. The other end of the silk thread is attached and is drawn out through the back. The two ends of thread are then tied over the sacrum. A small gauze sponge may be placed as a pad between the suture and the skin.

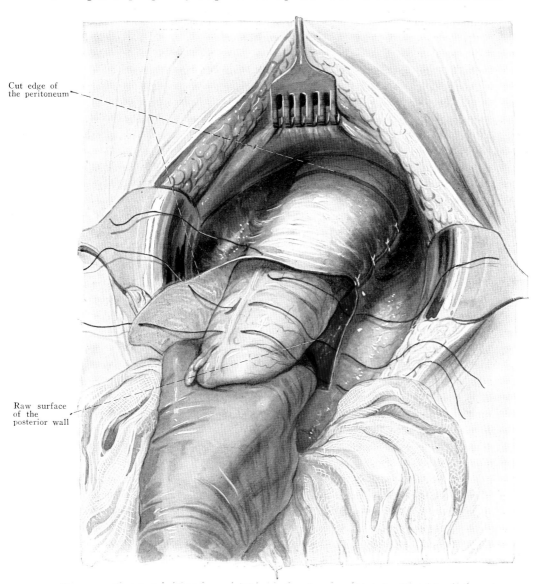

Cut edge of
the peritoneum

Raw surface
of the
posterior wall

FIG. 294. Treatment of prolapse of the rectum by suspension by the abdominal route. Through a left lateral rectus incision the peritoneum in the region of the left iliac fossa is dissected free in the shape of a flap which is being sutured in place again, over the sigmoid flexure, drawn forcibly upward. The sutures include the intestinal wall.

The suture is left in place for from 2 to 3 weeks, unless inflammation forces its earlier removal.

F. TREATMENT OF HEMORRHOIDS

The open operations for hemorrhoids require the careful preoperative and postoperative treatment previously outlined for operations on the rectum.

However, in a condition as common and as inconspicuous as hemorrhoids, and which by many is looked on more as a social handicap than as an actual disease, "treatment without incapacitation" has found many adherents. It is applicable, however, only in case of isolated small varices.

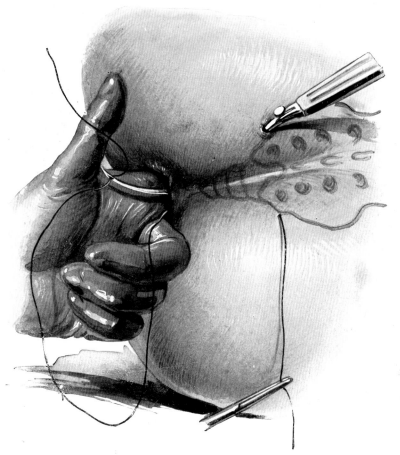

Fig. 295 Treatment of prolapse of the rectum by suspension to the sacrum. The one end of a long suture has been passed from within outward on the right side, just beside the last sacral vertebra. The other end of the suture, which is hanging out of the anus, is to be carried from within the rectum to the skin of the sacral region on the left with the aid of a Reverdin needle which has been thrust into the bowel and led out through the anus under the protection of the left index finger introduced into the rectum.

All operations on the hemorrhoidal veins should be performed in the lithotomy position.

1. Obliteration by Injection

The injection treatment is in my opinion suitable only for small isolated dilated veins. Moreover, the procedure is by no means as completely painless and harmless as it is often represented to be. It may lead to painful and progressive thrombosis and to abscess formation. In more extensive hemorrhoids the open operation is invariably to be preferred. The method of injection is similar to that used in the treatment of varicose veins.

The injection is carried out as follows: After the dilated vein has been well exposed (it is usually possible to draw it out by means of a Knapp suction glass), it is painted with a 5-per cent cocaine solution and is thoroughly lubricated with vaseline. It is punctured with an extremely fine hypodermic needle and 1 or 2 drops of a solution of phenol (0.5 cc., glycerine 10 cc.), or a similar amount of a solution of quinine and urethane, or 50 per cent glucose, are injected. The withdrawal of the needle is delayed for a few moments. Not more than 2 or 3 veins are treated at a single sitting, and no veins are injected which are immediately adjacent. (The method is not without danger. Extensive thrombosis and embolism may occur, as well as extensive necrosis. I. S. R.)

2. LIGATION

Ligation of the hemorrhoidal masses is comparable to injection as far as the insignificance of the disturbances caused by the operation is concerned. It is suitable for the rather polypoid hemorrhoids. It should be used only in case of isolated well-pedunculated nodules, but in a few clinics it is employed also in more extensive hemorrhoids. The individual dilated vein is pulled forward with a grasping forceps and is cocainized, unless the whole anal region has been injected with an anaesthetic solution. The mucosa is incised on both sides at the intended level of ligation. The nodule is transfixed with a needle carrying a silk suture, is tied off tightly on both sides with the silk (Fig. 296) and is excised just peripheral to the ligature with a scissors. This avoids all bleeding. The small raw surface resulting after the ligature sloughs off heals quickly under applications of zinc oxide ointment. It is much better to excise the nodules in the manner described than to wait for them to drop off after the pedicle becomes necrotic.

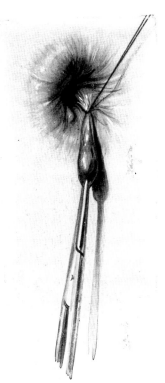

FIG. 296. Ligation of a hemorrhoid. The hemorrhoidal mass has been transfixed at its base with a silk ligature and is being tied off on both sides. It will be cut off peripheral to the ligature.

3. WIDE AMPUTATION

The operations which follow require local anaesthesia of the whole anal region by means of the injection method described above or general anaesthesia. Furthermore, the bloodless dilatation of the sphincter previously described must constitute the first step of the operation, since it brings deep-seated nodules into view and prevents a later spasm of the sphincter.

In the Langenbeck operation, still frequently used today, each individual nodule is grasped with a Luer forceps and pulled down, is grasped at its base and flush with the anus by a flat-bladed Langenbeck clamp, is crushed and is then removed flush with the clamp by means of a cautery after a moist compress has been placed beneath the clamp. The Langenbeck clamp is faced with ivory on its under surface to guard against burning of the adjacent tissue. After removal of the clamp there remains a seared ridge which is grasped with Kocher hemostats and is oversewed with a running catgut suture. In

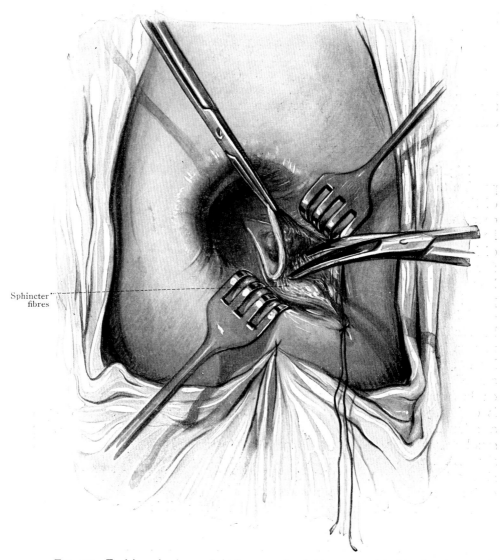

Sphincter fibres

FIG. 297. Excision of a hemorrhoidal mass. A whetstone-shaped incision has been made around the base of the hemorrhoid in the region of the skin and mucosa and radial to the anus. The mass is being excised, exposing the fibers of the external sphincter. The wound is closed by interrupted sutures.

removing a number of nodules, care must be taken that there remain sufficiently wide strips of normal mucosa between the seared areas, as otherwise a cicatricial stenosis of the anus might develop.

The results of the Langenbeck operation are not always satisfactory. Primary healing is rare because the wound edges, injured by the heat, tend to separate and slough off, with resultant broad wounds that heal slowly by granulation.

I personally, therefore, do not use the Langenbeck procedure, but prefer excision in the case of isolated, broad-based, sessile venous nodes. The individual venous node is grasped with two Kocher hemostats. An oval incision is made around its base in a radial direction so that one pole of the oval lies in the region of the skin and the other in the region of the mucosa. The dilated vein is dissected free, together with the attached skin (Fig. 297). The incision should at no point be carried deeper than to the external sphincter.

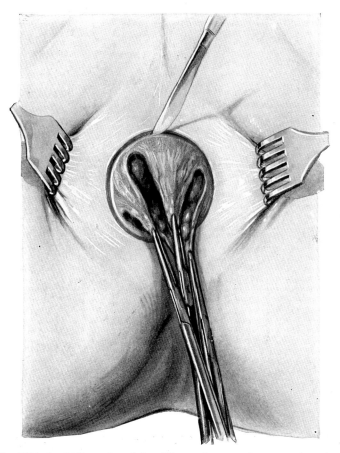

FIG. 298. The Whitehead Operation (1). The varicose anal mucosa is put on stretch by means of four Kocher forceps and a circular incision is then made at the mucocutaneous border.

The dissection is carried from without toward the anus. The outer tip of the oval skin segment is first grasped with a Kocher hemostat and put on stretch while sharp hooked retractors are inserted into the margins of the wound. As the dissection gradually progresses, the opposite edges of the wound are joined by deep-reaching catgut sutures which at the same time control the bleeding.

It is necessary in this operation also to take care that sufficiently wide undamaged stretches of tissue remain between the individual lines of suture, in order to avoid nutritional disturbances.

4. The Whitehead Operation

A circle of dilated veins that completely surrounds the anus can be removed most completely by the Whitehead operation. It also offers the best assurance against a recurrence of the hemorrhoids, which must always be

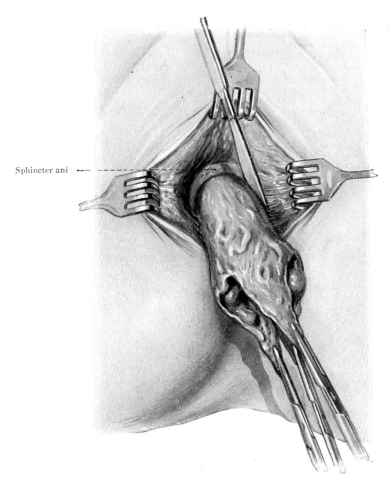

Sphincter ani

Fig. 299. The Whitehead Operation (2). The mucosal cylinder of the terminal rectum, including the veins, is being dissected free in a circular manner for a considerable distance, while the surrounding tissues are being forcibly retracted. During this procedure, the sphincter muscle comes into view; it must be guarded carefully.

reckoned with in the other procedures, since they remove only the isolated developed nodule and not the adjacent hemorrhoidal veins which have a tendency to become varicosed. The Whitehead operation gives excellent results if primary healing takes place. To accomplish this, there must be a sufficiently extensive dissection of the mucosal tube to permit the suture of the cut edge of the mucosa to the skin without tension. In the absence of primary healing, extremely unpleasant anal stenoses may arise. (This operation if skillfully done gives good results but it has so frequently resulted in stricture that at present it is not widely used in this country. I. S. R.)

After a careful dilatation of the sphincter, a circular incision is made around the anus just at the junction of skin and mucosa (Fig. 298). The hemorrhoids are within the circle. The outer skin edges are grasped with Elting forceps and the inner mucosal edges with four Kocher hemostats and are drawn in opposite directions. With a knife or scissors the mucosa and its attached venous plexus are freed from the sphincter (Fig. 299), the fibers of which are easily recognized by their concentric course around the anus. There is scarcely any bleeding if the dissection is in the proper plane and the delicate mucosal tube can easily be freed with proper technique, partly by sharp and

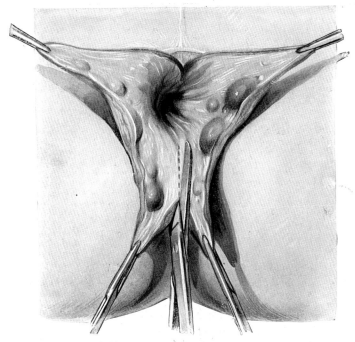

Fɪɢ. 300. The Whitehead Operation (3). The cylinder of mucosa which has been dissected free has been split longitudinally in the midline of the anterior wall and is being split posteriorly in the same manner.

partly by blunt dissection. The attachment is usually quite firm at the anterior commissure. The dissection must be carried up until the outer surface of the mucosal tube no longer shows any nodules of any size and until the free upper edge of the mucosal tube to be amputated at this level can be brought down to the skin edge without any tension. The segment to be freed measures 3 to 6 cm. in length. It is better to free too much than too little.

When the mucosal tube has been sufficiently freed, the four Kocher hemostats attached to its edge are shifted so that two are side by side at the wound edge of the mucosal tube on the anterior surface and two on the posterior surface. Between each pair of adjacent hemostats the anterior and the posterior walls of the mucosal tube are cut with a straight scissors (Fig. 300) so that the mucosal tube is split into a right and a left flap, each grasped at the corners by two Kocher hemostats. The base of the right flap is attached in front and behind to the edge of the skin wound with a catgut suture. The redundant flap of mucosa is cut off. All bleeding points are caught and ligated. The fresh mucosal wound edge is fastened to the skin wound edge with interrupted catgut sutures. *Careful coaptation* is necessary. The left half of the mucosal tube is now cut off and sutured to the skin edge of the other side in the same manner (Fig. 301). A light gauze dressing is applied to the anus. The insertion of a rectal tube is not necessary.

5. Treatment of Pruritus Ani

If the treatment of pruritus ani by conservative measures (Roentgen-ray irradiation) is unsuccessful, its operative treatment is often involved in that

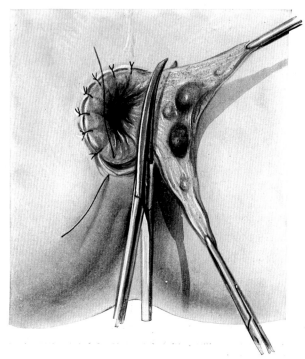

Fig. 301. The Whitehead Operation (4). The right half of the cylinder of mucosa has been excised and the edge has been sutured to the edge of the skin. The left side of the cylinder of mucosa is being excised in the same manner.

of hemorrhoids, of fistula, abscess or fissures in the region of the anus. In only a few cases is a separate operative treatment of the condition required. (This condition is a symptom-complex probably due to a variety of causes. In many instances the disease is undoubtedly a neurosis, but cutaneous changes are observed in long standing cases. I. S. R.)

The simplest procedure, and one which is adequate in most cases, is to undermine the area of skin which is pathologically hyperesthetic. On each side of the anus a curved incision encircling the anus is carried from the anterior to the posterior commissure (Fig. 302). The ends of the incisions however do not meet, a bridge of skin of sufficient size for the blood supply being left between them. The skin incisions are carried down as far as the external sphincter and the skin segments so outlined are freed from the subjacent tissues. The dissection must include the full extent of the pruritic skin. It can be carried inward as far as the anus as well as to the outer side of the incisions. After an adequate dissection the skin incisions are closed by suture.

If this simple procedure is not successful, the resection of the coccyx with its nervous connections, as proposed by Payr, is advised. The patient is placed

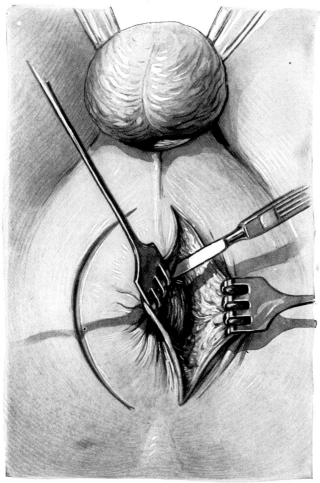

FIG. 302. Undercutting of the skin of the anal region for the treatment of pruritus ani. The skin for a considerable distance around the anus is dissected free temporarily from the underlying tissue, beginning from two lateral curved incisions.

in the abdominal-suspension position. An incision is made in the midline over the coccyx and carried toward the anus, ending in a ⋏-shaped incision, the limbs of which extend to either side of the posterior half of the anus. The posterior surface of the coccyx is exposed and the coccyx is separated from the sacrum by a transverse incision. A tenaculum forceps is inserted (Fig. 303) and the coccyx is pulled forcibly toward the anus and is freed from its bed with scissors. A sharp hooked retractor is inserted on each side into the lower angle of the wound. The connective tissue attached to the coccyx on the anal side is removed in connection with the coccyx so that a fair-sized mass of soft tissue remains at the tip of the resected bone. It contains the nerves which pass from the coccyx to the anal region. The wound is closed without drainage.

G. TREATMENT OF FISTULA IN ANO AND OF PERIRECTAL ABSCESS

The fistulous channel is often extensively branched and circuitous. Dilatations and lateral sacculations occur, and there may be several openings. In

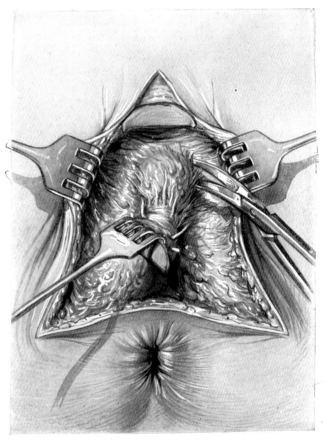

FIG. 303. Treatment of pruritus ani by extirpation of the coccyx. The coccyx, exposed from behind through a Y-shaped incision, has been separated from the sacrum and is being dissected out with the tissue containing the emerging nerves.

every anal fistula it must first be determined whether it is the drainage tract of a deep-seated focus of disease. If such a focus is present, it is useless to treat the fistula alone. On the contrary, the focus itself must be considered, since with its removal the fistula heals of itself. In view of the tuberculous nature of a large proportion of anal fistulae, the prospects of cure after an operation for a fistula are not always favorable. A cure is frequently not effected, or the lesion may recur.

The following types must be differentiated in the treatment:

Complete fistula in ano, in which the fistula opens at one end in the skin near the anus, and at the other into the rectum.

Incomplete external fistula, in which there is only an opening in the skin and no communication with the rectum.

Incomplete internal fistula, in which there is only an opening into the rectum while the skin shows no opening.

It is difficult at times to determine whether an external fistulous opening also communicates with the bowel. Simple probing, in view of the frequent twists and turns of the canal, often fails to answer this question. In case of doubt, an examination with the proctoscope should be made, at which it may be possible to see pus exuding into the rectum when pressure is made on the region of the fistula or to note the appearance of methylene blue injected into the external opening.

A further point of importance in operative procedure is whether the fistula lies inside or outside of the sphincter ani. Since the sphincter must always be protected in the operation, the operative field lies within the sphincter in intrasphincteric fistulae and outside of it in extrasphincteric fistulae. The differentiation between the two types of fistulae is not always simple. A valuable aid in this regard is the following procedure: The examiner introduces a finger into the anus and a probe into the fistula and notes whether the probe is made palpable or whether it disappears during a voluntary contraction of the sphincter by the patient.

The procedure of widely splitting the tract, formerly employed indiscriminately in all anal fistulae, should no longer be sanctioned, since in case of extrasphincteric fistulae it involves cutting the sphincter with possible serious damage to its function.

The operation is performed with the patient in the lithotomy position. Local anaesthesia is usually satisfactory. The sphincter is carefully dilated before the operation.

1. Treatment of Intrasphincteric Anal Fistula

In a complete intrasphincteric fistula a flexible grooved director or probe is introduced into the external opening and passed through the fistula into the rectum. The tip of the operator's left index finger catches the grooved director in the rectum, bends it back and leads it out through the anal opening (Fig. 304). In an intrasphincteric incomplete external fistula the tip of the grooved director is forced through the mucosa; in an incomplete internal fistula, through the skin. This converts an incomplete into a complete fistula. In an incomplete internal fistula it may be difficult to find the fistulous opening in the rectum. For this purpose the anus must be well held open by a speculum. Pressure on the region of the fistula usually makes the opening recognizable by the escape of pus.

The bridge of tissue picked up on the grooved director is divided, preferably with an electrosurgical knife. The cautery is to be preferred to an ordinary knife because the wound surfaces are so damaged by the heat that they heal quite slowly and from within outward. This tends to prevent recurrence. The floor of the fistula, exposed by the splitting, is scarified with the cautery or is excised with the electric loop. The sphincter must not be injured during this process. The cleft is held wide open with vioform or iodoform gauze. In the after treatment the packing is continued for as long a time as possible so that the wound will heal from the bottom. Healing may take many weeks.

The duration of the treatment may at times be shortened by excision with the knife and primary suture of the fistula. A grooved director is passed in the manner described. The bridge of tissue on the director is cut with a knife

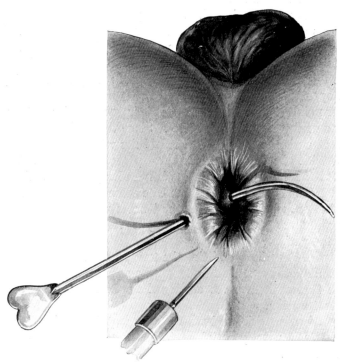

Fig. 304. Treatment of an intrasphincteric anal fistula by splitting. A grooved director has been passed through the fistula into the rectum and, after bending its tip, has been brought out through the anus. The bridge of tissue carried on the grooved director is about to be split by the electrosurgical knife.

and the resultant wound and the fistula are excised in a wedge-shaped piece. The wound is sutured in layers with catgut, beginning in the bottom of the wound so that no dead space remains. Unfortunately, because of the infected operative field, a smooth healing of the wound does not occur after this operation in a considerable number of cases. Often the wound reopens spontaneously or must be reopened.

2. TREATMENT OF EXTRASPHINCTERIC ANAL FISTULA

There is a particularly slight tendency to heal on the part of extrasphincteric fistulae because of the constant play of the sphincter and because of the marked tension in the ischiorectal fossa, bounded by the ischium and the bowel,

In extrasphincteric fistulae the procedures just described under intra-sphincteric fistulae are warned against, because their use would mean cutting the sphincter. A radical excision of the fistulous tract, together with its branches, external to the sphincter is indicated. In order to make the fistula with its usually numerous ramifications more easily recognizable, it is injected under considerable pressure just before the operation with indigocarmine solution.

After dilatation of the sphincter, an oval incision is made around the external opening of the fistula, with the long axis of the oval tangential to the anus (Fig. 305). The incision is continued a short distance beyond the ends of the oval. The incision should not be made too small. In case of necessity it can be enlarged at any time by a radiating incision to the outer side since there are no important structures in this region. The circumcised opening of the fistula is grasped with a Kocher hemostat or a Museux forceps and is put on tension. Sharp hooked retractors are inserted into the wound edges. The fistulous tract with its ramifications is dissected out of the sound

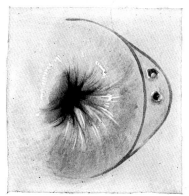

FIG. 305. Whetstone-shaped incision around the external openings of an extrasphincteric fistula in ano (1).

tissue as a closed structure if possible, using scissors or an electrosurgical knife (Fig. 306). The fistulous tract is recognized from without by the blue color of the injected dye solution visible through its walls and by its hardness in contrast to the soft perirectal tissue. An injury of the wall of the tract is easily recognized by the escape of the dye. In that case the wall is again grasped with Kocher hemostats and the dissection proceeds. Lateral branches and sac-culations are followed in the same way.

In this manner it is eventually possible to excise the entire fistula, like a malignant growth, out of the sound tissue. If the rectal mucosa is opened at the end of a complete fistula, the opening is promptly closed, the mucosa being inverted into the gut.

If the fistula has pierced the levator ani, the complete excision of the fistula may be very difficult or impossible.

The funnel-shaped wound resulting from the excision of the fistulous tract may be left wide open and packed, or it may be made smaller by sutures and a drain inserted, or it may be completely closed. At times the wound heals primarily after complete closure. If necessary the subsequent reopening of the wound, necessitated by infection, does not tend to cause any great damage.

The excision of the fistula as carried out by Moszkowicz and Kleinschmidt is done in the following manner: A curved incision concentric with the anus is made through the center of the opening of the fistula (Fig. 307). At the ends of this incision radial incisions are made to the outer side, and if necessary, to the inner side as well. The outer rectangular skin flap is dissected outward, and if an inner flap was also outlined, it is dissected inward. The core of tissue so exposed and which contains the fistula is thoroughly excised.

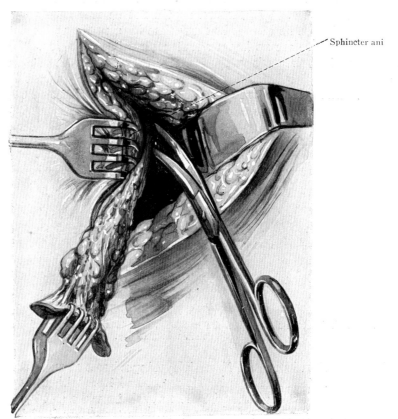

Sphincter ani

FIG. 306. Excision of an extrasphincteric fistula in ano (2). The fistulous tracts are followed and are excised together with the surrounding connective tissue.

Into the large resultant cavity the outer skin flap, and also the inner flap if one was formed, are infolded (Fig. 308). The flaps are fastened in the bottom of the wound by a few catgut sutures and by packing. If several fistulae are present, they are included in a single concentric incision if possible.

The treatment of a fistula between the rectum and the bladder is carried out by exposing the operative field from the abdominal cavity. Preparation and position of the patient correspond to the first step of a rectal operation by the combined approach. The bladder is drawn forward and the rectum pushed backward and the site of the fistula, which is usually enclosed in dense adhesions, is looked for. The tract is divided, resulting in an opening in the bladder and an opening in the rectum. Each opening is closed separately and as securely as possible by at least two rows of sutures. If possible, another abdominal structure, preferably the omentum, is fastened between the two points of suture so that they do not lie in immediate contact with each other.

If the suture of the rectum and bladder has been satisfactory, the abdo-

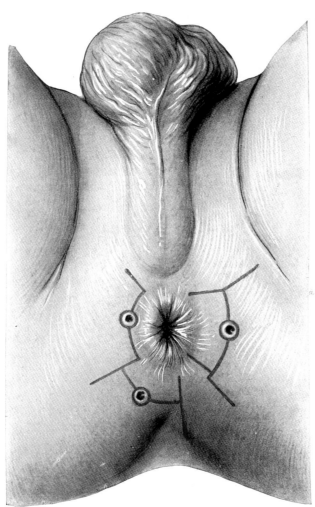

FIG. 307.   Excision of extrasphincteric fistulae in ano by the Moszkowicz-Kleinschmidt method (1). External incisions.

men is closed, otherwise, drainage is necessary. An indwelling catheter is inserted into the bladder and a rectal tube into the rectum.

In case of a fistula between the rectum and the male urethra, the site of the fistula is exposed and divided in the manner described for perineal prostatectomy. The opening in the rectum is carefully closed with a double row of sutures. The opening in the urethra is likewise closed as well as possible, but a dependable closure is often difficult because of the lack of material. By drawing together the tissue from the sides, as thick a dividing layer as possible is formed between the urethra and the rectum. An indwelling catheter is inserted into the bladder.

The treatment of rectovaginal fistulae will be discussed in the section on gynecology.

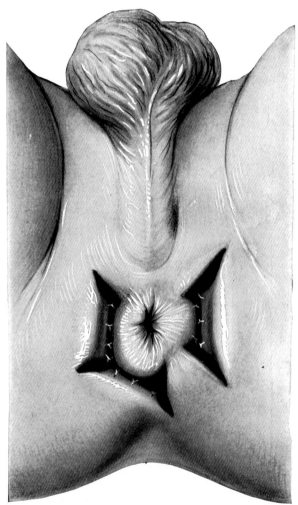

Fig. 308. Excision of extrasphincteric fistulae in ano by the Moszkowicz-Kleinschmidt method (2). The skin flaps have been folded inward into the depressions resulting from the excision of the fistulae.

3. Treatment of Pilonidal Cyst and Sinus

Although entirely different in origin, the pilonidal cyst is closely related to the fistula in ano in the manner of its operative treatment. The condition is the result of a congenital epithelial inclusion. It can be treated successfully only by complete excision of the lesion.

The patient lies on his side and turned a little on his abdomen, with thighs fully flexed, or he may be in the abdominal-suspension position, as described under amputation of the rectum. It is best always to inject the cyst or sinus with methylene blue before beginning the dissection. A longitudinal oval incision is made around the fistula and the dissection is carefully continued down to the sacrum, removing every part of the lesion which frequently has a number of lateral pockets. The use of the electrosurgical knife will be found of great advantage. As a rule the cyst runs to the tip of the coccyx or extends a short distance in front of the coccyx into the pelvis. In that case the coccyx must invariably be resected. Not until all diseased and scar tissue has been removed may the operation be considered completed.

In most instances it is better to pack the wound and permit its healing by granulation rather than to suture it, since its rigid walls can not be brought

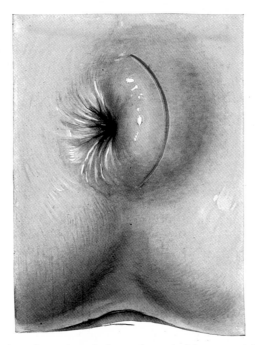

FIG. 309. Opening of a perirectal abscess by an incision concentric with the anus.

together dependably. (The method of Lahey which consists of transferring a lateral flap to the midline after the excision of the lesion is a very good one. I. S. R.)

4. TREATMENT OF ANAL FISSURE

Most anal fissures heal after dilatation of the sphincter, insertion of a rectal tube, ointment dressings and regulation of the bowels. If these measures fail, or if they seem unsuitable because of the size of the fissure, the ulcer, after dilatation of the sphincter, is either cauterized and packed or it is excised into sound tissue and the wound is closed with catgut sutures. If the wound reopens, it heals gradually by granulation. (It may be necessary to divide the rectal sphincters at one point to put the muscles at rest. I. S. R.)

5. TREATMENT OF PERIRECTAL ABSCESS

The operative treatment of perirectal abscesses follows the general rule of abscess treatment, wide incision of the abscess. The incision is made concentric with the anus (Fig. 309) to avoid the sphincter muscle which must not be injured. Any injury of the rectum must carefully be avoided. Depending on the position and size of the abscess, a curved incision through one-fourth to one-half of a circumference is made around the anus, at its side, or somewhat in front of, or behind it. The pus usually gushes out after a superficial incision. If this does not occur, sharp hooked retractors are inserted in the wound and the surgeon works deeper by sharp dissection parallel to the surface of the rectum. In doubtful cases an injury of the rectal wall can be avoided by introducing the left index finger into the bowel, and the male urethra is safeguarded by the introduction of a metal catheter.

After the abscess has been opened and the pus evacuated, and after the abscess cavity has been irrigated if that seems necessary, a search must be made in every case for a possible connection with the rectum. If such a connection is found, the bridge of soft tissue is split, provided that it does not contain any sphincter fibers. If sphincter fibers are present, nothing more can be done for the time being, since cutting the muscle fibers is out of the question and since any sutures which might be applied invariably give way in the suppurative operative field. The wound is drained and kept open by packing.

H. OPERATIONS ON THE INTERIOR OF THE RECTUM

All operations which are performed from within the rectum can effect at most the removal of a narrowly restricted lesion of the bowel. They can never be extended to procedures of greater magnitude or to operations which interrupt the continuity of the bowel. From this it is obvious that the objective of a procedure which is so limited to begin with cannot be the radical treatment of a malignant tumor as a rule. The procedure is therefore applicable only in benign lesions or in those malignant lesions in which from the start there is no thought of a radical removal and in which only a palliative treatment is intended.

Intrarectal operations may be carried out either through the anus or through an opening in the posterior rectal wall, with or without division of the sphincter.

1. Procedure through the Anus

The approach to the operative field through the anus is effected either with the help of the proctoscope or by wide separation of the anus with retractors. The use of the proctoscope does not require a dilatation of the sphincter. It deserves preference if the lesion in the interior of the bowel lies at a considerable distance from the anus, if the lesion is restricted to a small area, if no procedures requiring any considerable freedom of action, such as suturing or ligation, are necessary.

A wide separation of the anus is necessary, however, in case of lesions situated in the lowest segment of the rectum, in more extensive lesions and in measures which require a certain freedom of action for applying sutures or ligatures. If the approach through the anus is inadequate for these measures, posterior proctotomy is indicated.

The procedure with a wide separation of the anus begins with the gentle dilatation of the sphincter. The anus is then held open with sharp hooked retractors, or with long narrow retractors if higher portions of the bowel are to be approached, and the lesion is thereby exposed. Suitable illumination is essential for satisfactory work. This may be from an external source and directed over the left shoulder of the operator or by means of a light introduced into the bowel. By means of traction with suitable forceps catching

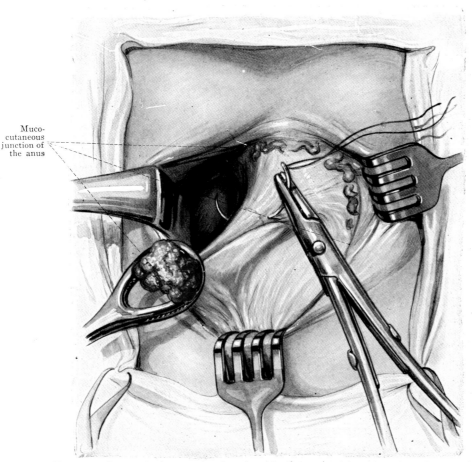

Muco-
cutaneous
junction of
the anus

Fig. 310. Removal of a rectal polyp through the anus. After dilatation of the sphincter, the polyp is pulled forward with a forceps, its base is transfixed with a mounted ligature, tied off on both sides and amputated distal to the ligation.

the lesion or its surroundings, the region of the lesion can often be brought down a considerable distance or can even be brought out through the anus.

Small benign polyps of the rectum can be removed in many cases through a proctoscope with a snare or with an electric loop. In dealing with larger growths proper treatment of the pedicle is essential, which requires a wide approach through the anus. The polyp is often hard to grasp, since if it has a long pedicle it may tip upward and get out of sight as well as out of the reach of the palpating finger. When the polyp has been found it is grasped with a suitable forceps and pulled down. The stretched pedicle is either simply ligated, or, what is safer and therefore advisable, is transfixed with a ligature and tied off on both sides (Fig. 310). The pedicle is cut distal to the ligature.

There is little point in attacking more than a single polyp by proctotomy, since multiple polyps usually involve the greater part of the large bowel in the form of an intestinal polyposis.

The treatment by electrocoagulation of rectal carcinomata which are no longer suitable for radical removal has attained considerable adoption in some quarters in recent years. It can be carried out either through the anus which is held open by specula or after a wide opening of the posterior wall of the rectum. In every case an artificial anus (sigmoid anus) must be established before electrocoagulation. When a non-metallic speculum or proctoscope is used, which provides, naturally, a less thorough exposure of the tumor than posterior proctotomy, the surface of the tumor after it has been exposed to view is shaved away bit by bit with the electrocoagulation loop. The operation can be greatly handicapped by bleeding. The mass of the tumor which cannot be removed in this manner is cooked and seared with a mass-coagulation electrode. Particular caution is necessary to avoid the bladder.

A rectal tube must be inserted after the operation for the drainage of secretions from the wound.

2. The Opening of the Posterior Wall of the Rectum in Its Upper Segment (Posterior Superior Proctotomy)

Posterior proctotomy may be carried out through a superior or an inferior exposure. In inferior proctotomy, the sphincter is divided in the posterior commissure, a procedure which is followed by a permanent weakness of the sphincter mechanism. Therefore, in spite of the fact that the operation as a purely soft-tissue procedure is simpler than superior proctotomy, the latter is to be preferred if possible, even though it involves resection of the coccyx and also of the 5th or even the 4th sacral vertebra. No permanent damage results from the removal of the bony segments mentioned.

In posterior superior proctotomy, after dilatation of the sphincter, a skin incision is made in the midline beginning above the coccyx or, if necessary, above the 4th sacral vertebra and ending 2 cm above the anus. The incision is deepened and the bone appearing in the upper angle of the wound is dissected free. The tip of the coccyx is elevated with tenaculum forceps, so that the soft tissues on the inner surface of the bone may carefully be separated from it without damaging the middle sacral artery. After the bone has been sufficiently freed it is removed with a Luer rongeur forceps. The exposed middle sacral artery running from above downward in the midline is picked up as high as possible and divided between ligatures. The anal fascia and the pelvic fascia on the under surface of the levator and forming the floor of the wound is incised exactly in the midline from above downward. The incision is gradually carried deeper and finally through the posterior wall of the rectum (Fig. 311).

The sphincter fibers appearing in the lower angle of the wound are spared. Both wound edges of the rectum are provided with traction sutures. These are drawn lateralward and further visualization is obtained with blunt retractors so that the operation in the interior of the rectum can be carried out directly under vision.

If the approach effected in this manner is inadequate, the wound may be enlarged upward with removal of more bone, or downward (inferior proctotomy) by division of the soft tissues, including the sphincter as far as the anus.

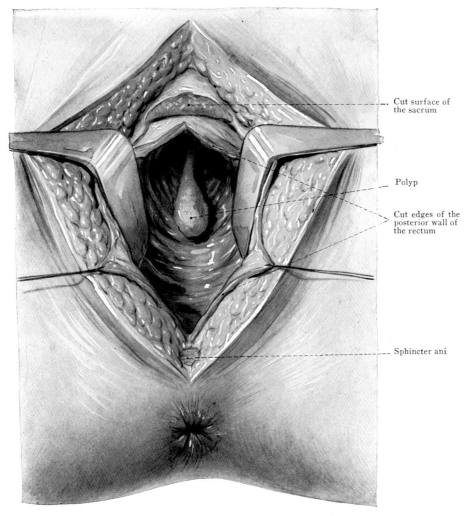

Cut surface of the sacrum

Polyp

Cut edges of the posterior wall of the rectum

Sphincter ani

FIG. 311. Posterior superior proctotomy. After the skin and soft parts have been divided in the midline, the coccyx and the lowest sacral segments are removed. The rectal wall has been split in the full extent of the wound and is retracted by traction sutures and retractors so that the polyp within comes into view. The uninjured anal sphincter is visible in the lower angle of the wound.

After completion of the procedure within the bowel the gut is carefully closed by three-layer interrupted silk sutures and by infolding catgut Lembert sutures.

The overlying fascia is also closed with interrupted catgut sutures, and the skin with silk sutures. A drain is placed in the upper angle of the wound. A small rectal tube is inserted into the anus for the escape of flatus.

3. THE OPENING OF THE POSTERIOR WALL OF THE RECTUM IN ITS LOWER SEGMENT (POSTERIOR INFERIOR PROCTOTOMY)

After the sphincter has been dilated, the skin, the sphincter, the levator ani and the rectum are divided exactly in the posterior commissure by an

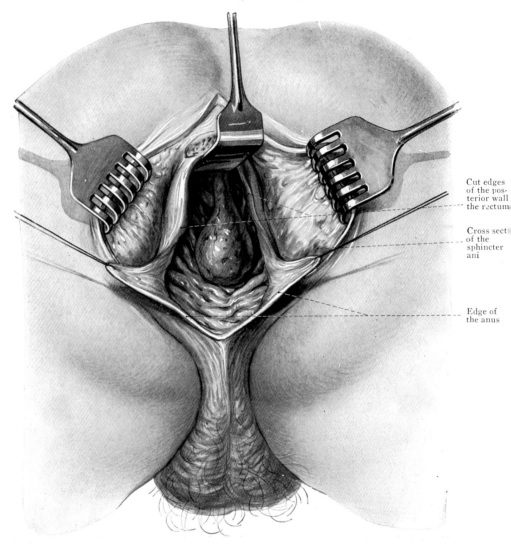

Cut edges
of the pos-
terior wall
the rectum

Cross sect
of the
sphincter
ani

Edge of
the anus

FIG. 312. Posterior inferior proctotomy. After the skin and soft parts have been divided in the midline, the coccyx and the lowest sacral segments are removed. Beginning at the anus, all the soft parts including the sphincter have been split upward into the rectum in the full extent of the outer incision. The wound is held open by means of traction sutures applied to the edges of the anal incision and by means of sharp hooked retractors. A large polyp is visible in the interior of the rectum.

incision which is carried as high as the tip of the coccyx (Fig. 312). The wound edges are drawn apart by hooked retractors, giving wide exposure to the ampulla.

If the exposure so effected is insufficient, the skin incision is prolonged over the coccyx or even over the last two sacral vertebrae. These bones are freed and removed with the Luer rongeur, and the fascia and the posterior rectal wall so exposed are split upward. This merges an inferior posterior proctotomy into the superior form.

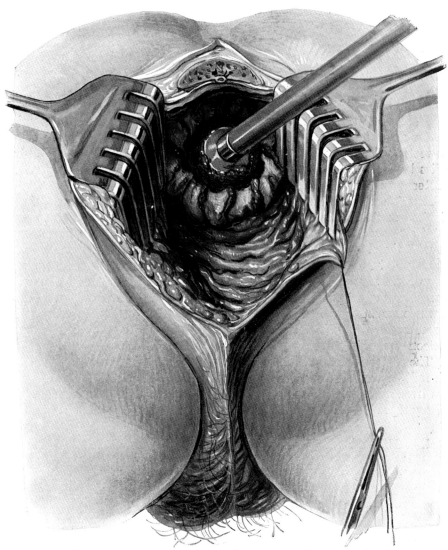

FIG. 313. Electrocoagulation of carcinoma of the rectum. The rectum has been opened by a combined inferior and superior posterior proctotomy. The cancerous growth has been removed partly by the electric loop and is now being coagulated and scarified with the coagulation electrode.

After the conclusion of the intrarectal procedure, a traction suture is inserted in each edge of the anus and the gut wall is closed with interrupted silk three-layer sutures and with interrupted Lembert catgut sutures. The subcutaneous fatty tissue and the divided muscles are also united by catgut sutures. The greatest care must be employed in the reconstruction of the sphincter. A drain is placed in the region of the coccyx. The remainder of the skin incision is closed. A small rectal tube is inserted into the rectum.

Even after primary healing of the wound the function of the rectal sphincter tends to show permanent damage.

Pedunculated tumors may be removed if their exposure is necessary through a posterior proctotomy after ligation of the pedicle in the manner described above under the peranal procedure. Broad-based sessile tumors are best removed by means of the electrosurgical knife. Bleeding vessels are ligated and the wound in the mucosa is carefully sutured with catgut. When in exceptional instances the removal of a malignant polyp by proctotomy seems possible, the base of its pedicle is excised by a longitudinal oval incision going through all layers of the rectal wall. The opening is closed by tier suture.

The broad approach to the interior of the rectum afforded by a combined superior and inferior proctotomy is admirably suited for the direct treatment of a rectal carcinoma which is no longer amenable to radical removal. This applies both to treatment by electrocoagulation and to treatment by radium and Roentgen ray.

After a sufficient exposure is obtained of the posterior rectal wall, the gut is incised and the tumor is exposed by means of retractors. The tumor is shaved away with the electrocoagulation loop or is excised from its surroundings with the electrosurgical knife. The portions of the tumor which cannot be removed in this way are cooked and seared with the mass-coagulation electrode (Fig. 313). In so doing, it is necessary to be mindful of possible damage to important neighboring structures, notably the bladder. Finally the whole wound area is packed so that the incision in the posterior wall of the rectum remains wide open. This makes it possible to repeat and complete the electrocoagulation treatment at a later time.

The tumor is exposed in the same manner for the purpose of treating it with radium and the Roentgen ray under the guidance of the eye. In most cases irradiation is combined with the electrocoagulation. Of course a preliminary sigmoidostomy should be performed.

I. EXTIRPATION OF THE RECTUM (RADICAL TREATMENT OF RECTAL CARCINOMA)

1. CHOICE OF METHOD

General Considerations. In the extirpation of the entire rectum or of one of its parts, the following procedures are recognized.

(In the following discussion Professor Kirschner uses the term "combined operation" in a very broad sense, in that it includes any operation which involves laparotomy and a dorsal or perineal approach. He includes in the term "combined operation" the making of an artificial anus plus what we are accustomed to look upon as the Kraske or the Lockhart-Mummery operations which in the stricter sense of the term are not combined operations.

The original Langenbeck operation which removed the growth from below has proven unsatisfactory in that it is too frequently followed by recurrence. This procedure was modified first by Kraske and then by Bardenheuer who increased the exposure by removing the coccyx and a portion of the sacrum.

In the latter procedures the peritoneum in the pouch of Douglas could be opened and a more extensive resection could be done. Although the end-results are better with this type of exposure, due to the possibility of a more adequate exposure, it was frequently impossible to remove the required amount of bowel and to dissect the lymph glands of the pelvis. When these procedures are used no attempt should be made to save the anus and its sphincters.

The complete abdomino-perineal operation as advocated by Jones, Lahey and Coffey in this country and Miles in England is without doubt the operation of choice. The patient must have a permanent abdominal artificial anus but the percentage of five-year cures is undoubtedly higher when a complete dissection can be made. I.S.R.)

(a) **Resection of the rectum,** in which an annular segment is removed and the proximal and distal ends of the rectum are reunited. Under rectal resection may also be included the "telescope" operation in which only the sphincter is preserved and the remainder of the rectum is removed.

(b) **Amputation of the rectum,** in which the terminal portion of the rectum including the sphincter is removed and the proximal gut segment is led to the surface with the establishment of an artificial anus. Under rectal amputation is also included that type of extirpation in which the whole rectum is removed, including the sphincter, as far as the promontory of the sacrum or even into the sigmoid.

Both procedures may be carried out "**from below,**" that is, through a dorsal (sacral) approach, with the additional modifications of a perineal and a vaginal approach, or they may be performed by a **combined procedure** from above and below, that is, by an abdomino-sacral or a sacro-abdominal approach. Under the combined procedure is understood primarily a single-stage operation in which the dissection of the diseased bowel is begun in the abdomen and is completed by the dorsal route at the same sitting. It can however be carried out in the reverse direction in one or in two stages. (In fact the majority of surgeons now favor the two-stage abdomino-perineal operation. I.S.R.)

In the choice of a method, we must consider the following viewpoints, which, it must be admitted, are not given the same values by different surgeons.

(c) **The immediate danger to life.** Extirpation of the rectum is always a formidable procedure that is often associated with circumstances that threaten life. The most important aspect to be considered is therefore the lack of danger and the safety of the operation. (I believe it is equally important to consider the end-results of each operation. I.S.R.)

Insecurity of the suture line in the rectum after resection in continuity, the danger of gangrene of the proximal gut segment which was brought down a considerable distance to reestablish continuity, the contamination of the wound and surrounding tissues in the event that the intestinal suture gives way and the associated danger of infection are arguments for amputation and against resection as far as the immediate danger is concerned.

The procedures which are carried out from below, especially the dorsal procedure, save the patient from an extensive laparotomy and a separate abdominal incision, in contrast to the combined procedure. The magnitude and the duration of the operation are materially lessened and the shock following extensive abdominal operations is largely avoided in this procedure. (Carefully done in two stages I do not believe shock is any greater after the combined operation than after the simple dorsal operation and the end-results after the combined operation are undoubtedly better. I.S.R.)

A particular advantage of the dorsal procedure from the standpoint of sparing the patient's strength has become evident in recent years. Only in this procedure is it possible to utilize the advantages of the electrosurgical knife in the crucial part of the operation, the dissection of the diseased bowel out of the true pelvis. These advantages are particularly valuable in the radical treatment of rectal carcinoma. They consist primarily in the avoidance of bleeding when the tissues are divided, in the resultant excellent exposure and in an increased accuracy of dissection. They further include the closure of the lymph channels by electrocoagulation, whereby the absorption of bacteria, and of the products of tissue necrosis from the large wound cavity is reduced. It is possible they may also include the destruction of carcinoma cells in and beneath the cut surfaces, a point which will be referred to later in detail.

The immediate reduction of the dangers of operation therefore for several reasons, in my opinion, is in favor of amputation with utilization of the dorsal procedure. There are certain disadvantages in the purely dorsal operation however.

(d) **The Radical Nature of the Procedure.** The operative treatment of rectal carcinoma is intended to rid the patient of a disease which if untreated or inadequately treated would lead to his relatively early death and usually under the most distressing circumstances. The operative procedures must therefore be evaluated from the aspect of permanent cure, which in our present state of knowledge runs parallel to the thoroughness with which invaded tissues are removed. That procedure would therefore seem the best in which the largest possible portions of the diseased rectum, the adjacent tissues and the associated lymph nodes are removed, without regard to any other considerations. These demands are best met by those operations which are not limited in their extirpation of the diseased tissue by other considerations, in that they unconditionally sacrifice the sphincter on the one hand, and on the other remove the lower bowel high up into the sigmoid, together with the lymph nodes and the lymph channels in the mesorectum and in the mesosigmoid. This means, therefore, amputation of the rectum by the combined procedure in its most complete form.

Just as it is considered an indispensable measure in removing a carcinoma of the breast to remove the lymph nodes in the axilla, so too it seems indicated to remove those lymphatic structures which experience has shown are most apt to be involved in rectal carcinoma. These are the lymph channels along the superior hemorrhoidal artery and the sigmoid artery. Their inspection and complete removal are possible only in the combined procedure.

Recent researches have shown that extension of the carcinoma takes place predominantly in an upward direction not only in the pararectal lymph spaces but also in the wall of the rectum itself. In the radical operation therefore not only should the lymph channels in the perirectal connective tissue and along the superior hemorrhoidal vessels in the mesentery be removed as high as possible but also the intestinal wall far proximal to the lesion. Although the division of the bowel at a distance of 2 to 3 cm. distal to the carcinoma may seem to be adequate, it is necessary to remove what appears macroscopically to be normal bowel for from 8 to 10 cm., better still from 12 to 15 cm. proximal to the lesion. The higher the resection, the greater are the chances for permanent cure. This consideration also argues in favor of the combined procedure which makes the proximal portion of the bowel accessible in a far greater degree.

The more extensively the bowel is removed proximal to the tumor to effect a radical cure, the more impossible does it become to reunite the proximal segment with the remaining anal segment. Radical excision results in an unbridgeable gap and thereby necessitates the removal of the anal segment. Amputation is therefore the more radical procedure from this viewpoint as well.

On the other hand, the possibility in the dorsal procedure of dissecting out the diseased rectum by means of the electrosurgical knife and the attendant probability of destroying carcinoma cells located in and beneath the cut surfaces are in favor of combining the abdominal and dorsal operation and against the complete dissection of the rectum from within the abdominal cavity.

Granted the removal of equally extensive zones of tissue, the question arises as to whether, in attempting to prevent the spread of carcinoma cells, it is more favorable to begin the extirpation of the tumor on its proximal side and to conclude with the perineal operation or to proceed in the opposite direction. I myself see no good reason why in the one-stage combined operation the distal portion of the dissection should not be done first, although I nearly always begin with the abdominal portion of the operation. The concept that the primary manipulation of the main tumor will mobilize cancer cells and cause them to be carried to points which will eventually be inaccessible seems to me to be based upon a too grossly mechanical viewpoint and not supported by practical experience. (While there may be no definite grounds upon which it may be unqualifiedly stated that the proximal portion of the operation should be done first, it does appear that such a plan is based upon sounder surgical principles and is I believe the choice of the majority of surgeons doing this type of surgery. I.S.R.)

In summary, for the radical removal of a rectal carcinoma I favor amputation as opposed to local resection, and the combined abdomino-perineal procedure as opposed to operation by the dorsal route alone.

(e) **The influence upon the subsequent social adjustment of the patient.** The social adjustment of the patient depends largely on the function of the rectal sphincter and the continence of feces and flatus. Those procedures may be considered less valuable by which control of fecal evacuation is lost or by which the evacuation of the feces is transferred to a point at a distance from the normal anal opening. In this respect resection in continuity would seem to have a decided advantage over amputation, for it is the only procedure in which the anal sphincter can be preserved. However, resection by no means always leaves the patient full control of his sphincter action. Because of the unfavorable conditions for healing under which it is placed, the suture line after resection frequently gives way and heals only after a long period of granulation. This frequently necessitates several secondary operations which entail a long stay in bed. In other cases healing never takes place and there remains a permanent dorsal fecal fistula or an intestinal stenosis. Therefore many patients after local resection are worse off in the end than after the primary establishment of an artificial anus. The poor results described are particularly frequent when the dorsal or perineal approach alone is used. Since partial resection procedures by the dorsal route require extensive mobilization of the proximal gut, nutritional disturbances are particularly

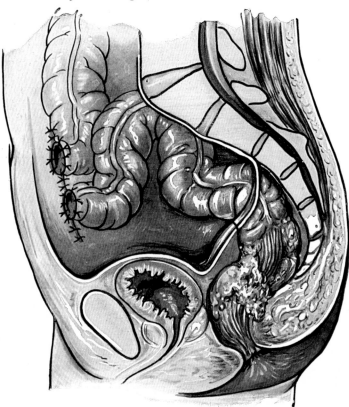

Fig. 314. Two-stage amputation of the rectum by the combined procedure with retention of an intestinal segment shortcircuited at one end. Conditions at the end of the first operation (diagrammatic). An abdominal anus has been established.

common after ligation of vessels where the operator is working without being able to visualize the entire field.

In spite of this, one repeatedly yields to the temptation to preserve a sound sphincter for the patient; the more so, the farther the carcinoma is situated from the anus, the easier and the more extensively the normal bowel above the tumor can be displaced downward, and the stronger the patient seems to be.

Patients with an abdominal artificial anus are undoubtedly better off than those with a sacral anus. They can cleanse the surroundings conveniently and carefully under guidance of the eye, which is difficult with a sacral anus. Soiling and leakage of fecal matter are more unpleasant between and on the buttocks than on the abdomen and bandages for receptacles for feces, or for closing devices, are more easily attached over the abdomen than over the sacrum. Finally, the attempts to effect by operative measures a voluntary control of an artificial anus have had appreciable results only in the abdominal anus. Therefore an abdominal artificial anus is preferable to a sacral anus.

Therefore for the patient's subsequent well-being, the preferable procedures are partial resection with preservation of the rectal sphincter or, if this is not possible, amputation with an abdominal artificial anus.

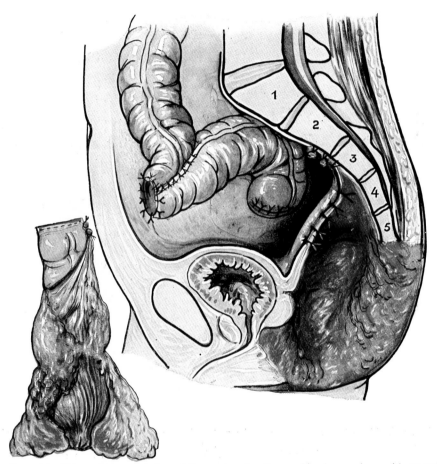

Fig. 315. Two-stage amputation of the rectum by the combined procedure with retention of a gut segment shortcircuited at one end. Diagrammatic. Conditions at the end of the second operation. The rectum has been amputated by the dorsal route. The terminal portion of the sigmoid has been closed blind and dropped into the pouch of Douglas. The abdominal cavity has been closed in the region of the pouch of Douglas without drainage.

If we again survey the manifold pros and cons of the various procedures, it is obvious that in most instances there are present a number of opposing irreconcilable indications, between which it is necessary to compromise. This will lead to various conclusions, on the one hand because individual cases will present different premises in regard to these indications, and on the other hand because individual surgeons will assign different values to these indications. Surgery in general, and all surgeons have experienced changes of opinion.

Practical Procedure. It is my belief that by dividing the combined procedure into two operations separated by a time interval it is possible to minimize the above-mentioned disadvantages of the combined procedure and to increase its advantages. I usually proceed in the following manner. In the first operation, the laparotomy, the abdominal cavity is inspected to determine the extent of the carcinoma and the presence of metastases, and an artificial abdominal sigmoid anus is established, with (Fig. 316) or without (Figs. 314

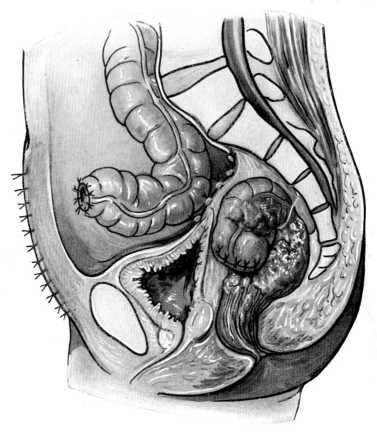

FIG. 316. Two-stage amputation of the rectum by the combined procedure with complete removal of the gut distal to the abdominal anus. Conditions at the end of the first operation. Diagrammatic. The sigmoid has been divided. Its proximal end has been sutured into the abdominal wall as a terminal abdominal anus. The descending limb has been closed blind and buried beneath the pelvic peritoneum which has been closed over it.

and 318) transsection of the sigmoid. At the second operation, which is performed at a later date, an amputation (Figs. 315 and 317) or a resection (Fig. 319) is performed by the dorsal route. After a resection, there follows as a possible third stage the closure of the artificial anus (Fig. 320).

In such a division of the combined procedure, the most important part of the whole operation, the removal of the diseased rectum from the true pelvis, is carried out by the dorsal route instead of through the abdomen as in the single-stage combined procedure. It is a matter of opinion whether such a procedure in its entirety may still be designated a combined procedure or whether it should rather be called a sacral procedure with a preliminary inspection of the abdominal cavity and establishment of an abdominal artificial anus.

This subdividing of the combined procedure into several stages has the advantage of conserving the patient's strength. I consider it the safest of all the procedures.

Furthermore, the drainage of feces through the artificial anus insures thorough evacuation of the bowel before and immediately after the main

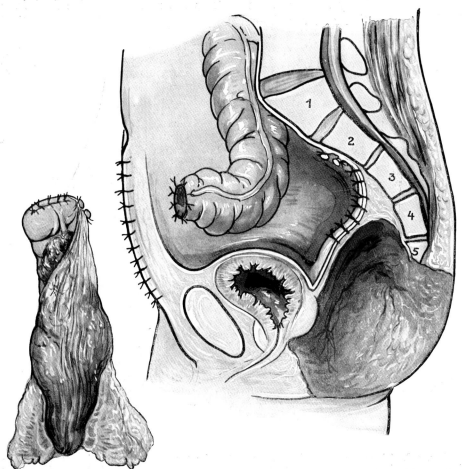

Fig. 317. Two-stage amputation of the rectum by the combined procedure with complete removal of the gut distal to the abdominal anus. Diagrammatic. Conditions at the end of the second operation. The rectum and the attached portion of the sigmoid which had been extra-peritonealized have been amputated by the dorsal route.

operation. As a result of the fact that the carcinoma is placed at rest and spared from mechanical irritation by means of the artificial anus, the extent of the lesion and the inflammatory infiltration into the surrounding tissues are often materially lessened, so that cases, which originally were considered to be no longer suitable for a radical operation in view of the patient's general condition and of the local findings, appear to be operable after a time and can be subjected to a radical operation successfully.

The danger of infection of the abdominal cavity is greatly reduced by dividing the operation into two stages. In the abdominal part of a two-stage combined procedure the intestine can be carefully handled. In the dorsal operation, the peritoneal cavity is opened to only a limited extent. In case of resection it is securely closed before opening the bowel, and in amputation it is closed immediately after the transsection and suture of the rectum. It is highly improbable that the blind closed stump of the transsected sigmoid which was replaced in the abdominal cavity could reopen.

The preliminary artificial anus protects the sacral operative field from fecal contamination and affords a mechanical protection to the intestinal

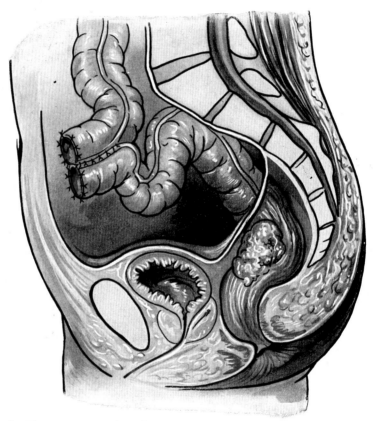

Fig. 318. Three-stage resection of the rectum by the combined procedure (1). Conditions at the end of the first operation. Diagrammatic. A double-barrelled abdominal anus has been established.

suture line after resection. Also, while in the single-stage combined procedure the important part of the operation, the freeing of the diseased rectum from the surrounding tissues is done by way of the abdomen, largely by blunt dissection and without the electrosurgical knife, this part of the operation in the two-stage combined procedure is performed from below and can be carried out almost exclusively with the electrosurgical knife.

It may seem that the removal of the tumor cannot be as extensive when the combined procedure is divided into two stages. The dissection of the bowel and the ligation of the mesentery no longer take place from above under the guidance of the eye, but are carried out from below in a restricted operative field. It is possible, however, to limit this disadvantage to a large extent by a number of special maneuvers.

In the first stage, the laparotomy, it is determined whether suspicious glands are present in the region of the mesentery, in front of the promontory or in front of the spine. If so, the combined procedure is carried out as a single-stage operation with its particular advantages in such cases, or else

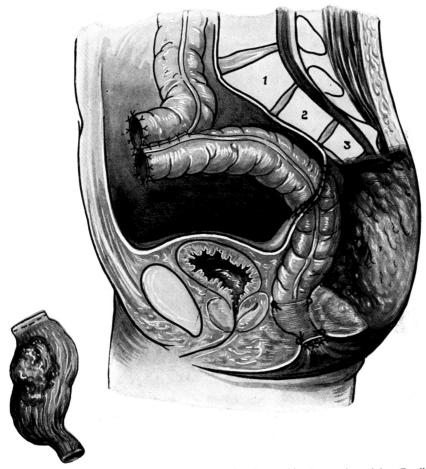

FIG. 319. Three-stage resection of the rectum by the combined procedure (2). Conditions at the end of the second operation. Diagrammatic. The diseased segment of the rectum has been resected and the proximal portion of the sigmoid has been led out through the anus, according to the "telescope" procedure.

the two-stage combined procedure is modified in the following manner: During the laparotomy, the sigmoid is divided under guidance of the eye, and the distal end after ligation and division of its mesentery is buried beneath the peritoneum of the pelvic floor. The extent of the operation can be as great as is desirable and is thus carried out under guidance of the eye in doubtful cases.

Furthermore, it is important when the dorsal operation alone is done to free the bowel from the bone by blunt dissection as high as possible. The bowel, the retrorectal connective tissue and the mesentery are separated by blunt dissection close to the bone and the free mesentery is divided high up and close to the bowel. The high pressure local anaesthesia apparatus which I have described is of inestimable service in this procedure. That much can be accomplished in this direction has recently been emphasized by Goetze. If in addition the pouch of Douglas is opened widely, it becomes possible to obtain a fairly good view into the abdominal cavity.

The advantage of the single-stage combined procedure, in being able to ligate the mesenteric vessels under guidance of the eye and consequently to

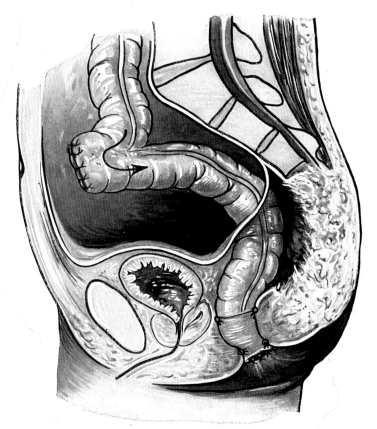

Fig. 320. Three-stage resection of the rectum by the combined procedure (3). Diagrammatic. Conditions at the end of the third operation. The double-barrelled abdominal anus has been closed.

assume responsibility for the viability of the bowel which is to be buried in the pelvis, is lost in the two-stage combined operation where a sigmoid stump is left distal to the artificial anus. (In the two-stage combined operation of Jones or Coffey this disadvantage is not present. I. S. R.)

A particular advantage of the two-stage combined procedure in my opinion is the ability to typify, in all forms of rectal carcinoma, the operative procedure and the fixed succession of its various single steps follow one another as steps along the same way. The decision at which point to end the total procedure is deferred to the last minute when the deciding local conditions and the state of the patient can best be surveyed. Whether only a palliative operation, in the form of an abdominal artificial anus, or a radical operation should be done and whether resection or amputation are best suited are decisions which can follow sequentially, and any further operative step can be performed later, even if originally it had been planned to end the operation at an earlier stage.

In the light of these considerations I always proceed as follows: In every case of rectal carcinoma, I begin with the first step of the combined procedure which ends with the establishment of a double-barrelled abdominal artificial anus (Fig. 314 and 318), whether the case seems radically operable, or whether as a result of the local extent of the tumor or because of intra-abdominal metastases it seems no longer radically operable.

If in a radically operable carcinoma there are found suspicious glands in front of the spine, in the mesorectum or in the mesosigmoid, the artificial anus is formed preferably by dividing the bowel. After closing the stump, dividing its mesentery, and removing the suspicious glands (Fig. 316) the distal end is dropped into the pelvis and the peritoneum closed over the stump as completely as possible. The proximal end of the sigmoid is then carried to the exterior in the form of a terminal artificial anus of the abdominal wall. The dorsal part of the operation (Fig. 317) in such a case can be performed immediately or at a second sitting as an amputation.

If, after the establishment of the double-barrelled artificial anus, or after the establishment of a terminal artificial anus, the case seems inoperable, the operative procedure has reached its conclusion, temporarily or permanently. But if the case proves to be radically operable at the time, the method just described may be used or the second step may consist of amputation a week or more later by the dorsal route. In a doubtful case, provided that the bowel did not have to be transsected at the first operation, the decision as to whether an amputation (Fig. 315) or a resection (Fig. 319) is to be performed can be deferred to the last moment. If an amputation is performed, the abdominal artificial anus must remain; and if a double-barrelled type of anus is established, the distal short blind segment of gut remains in the body permanently (Fig. 315) since it is not possible to remove the sigmoid up to the colostomy by the dorsal route. However if a resection is performed (Fig. 319), the abdominal artificial anus is allowed to remain, so that functionally the conditions of an amputation exist. Not until the lower gut segment has healed without a fistula and is freely patulous, is the abdominal artificial anus closed (Fig. 320).

The freeing of the rectum, by careful anatomic dissection and conscientious adherence to the measures later to be described, can be performed without material difficulty if the carcinoma has not invaded the surrounding structures. In the latter instance the mobilization of the gut may encounter great or insuperable obstacles. Injuries to the rectum and to neighboring organs, above all to the bladder, may result. Provided that radical operation should not be abandoned in such a case, it is advisable to conclude the operation in the simplest way, in particular, to abandon a difficult and uncertain resection in favor of an amputation of the rectum with preliminary, simultaneous or subsequent establishment of an abdominal artificial anus. The electrosurgical knife has greatly widened the limits of operability.

The use of electrocoagulation has greatly widened the scope of our attack upon carcinomata which by anatomic dissection are no longer operable, and this is particularly true in case of the rectum. The procedure to be used has been described on page 396; it must be preceded by the establishment of an artificial anus. If metastasis has taken place to the inguinal nodes, it is in my opinion no longer radically operable, just as in the case of any other distant metastasis.

Spinal anaesthesia is particularly suitable for the radical operation for rectal carcinoma. The sacral procedure may however be performed satisfactorily under local anaesthesia. The rectum is injected on all sides with ½ percent novocaine, ¼₀ percent percaine solution by means of a high-pressure local anaesthesia apparatus. The injection should also be carried high behind the sacrum and, after resection of the coccyx and sacrum, into the epidural space of the sacrum. The injection exerts a dissecting effect by means of its hydraulic force. In case of necessity, the injection can be carried higher within the pelvis as the operation proceeds.

In the dorsal operation, the abdominal-suspension position with the lower extremities abducted, described and illustrated in Vol. I, page 64, offers the best approach. If in this position respiration is not free and quiet, the patient is placed on his left side and a bit forward on the abdomen, which is raised by placing a large pillow beneath it, with the hip- and knee-joints each bent at approximately a right angle. The perineal and the vaginal procedures are performed in the lithotomy position (Vol. I, page 62). The abdominal part of the combined procedure must be performed in an exaggerated Trendelenburg position (Vol. I, page 61), since the success of this operation depends entirely on keeping the small bowel completely out of the operative field during the operation.

The bladder must be emptied immediately before the operation and kept empty after operation by introducing a permanent catheter.

2. The Operation from Below (dorsal, sacral, perineal or vaginal approach).

The technique of radical operations attacking the rectum from below has been materially aided in recent years by the use of the electrosurgical knife. It has almost eliminated the excessive bleeding, for instance, during the opening of the venous plexus which surrounds the anus, which otherwise interfered with visibility and added greatly to the postoperative shock. Small vessels do not bleed at all when divided by the electrosurgical knife, the large vessels can usually be grasped before being cut, because of the excellent visibility in the dry wound. Large sections of the buttocks may be incised in a few moments in this manner without difficulty. This primary hemostasis which is accomplished with any properly made apparatus is not, of course, permanent. At the conclusion of the dissection the wound must be carefully inspected for bleeding points and packing must be used. The slow primary healing of skin wounds which have been made with the electric knife is ordinarily considered a disadvantage, but this is not the case in operations for rectal carcinoma where primary healing of the large packed wound cavity is not expected. A further advantage of the electrosurgical knife lies in the fact that after its use the immediate and later convalescence is smoother. This is due obviously to the closure of the lymph spaces effected by the electrosurgical knife, so that the entrance into the body of the products of tissue necrosis, which are always present in large wound cavities, and of bacteria and their toxins is retarded.

It is debatable whether electrocoagulation also has a deeper effect in destroying carcinoma cells. The fact remains that the advantages of electrical operating as described have placed us in a position to attack successfully and with the hope of prolonged freedom from recurrence, rectal carcinomata which were considered inoperable according to criteria that obtained until recently. The hope for a permanent cure of rectal carcinomata removed in this manner is enhanced by the fact that the large granulating wound cavity offers for a long time a free approach for inspection, for the subsequent electrical extirpation of local recurrences and for the superficial and deep application of radium. In view of these advantages I use the electrosurgical knife routinely in the dorsal or perineal part of the operation.

In order still further to check the bleeding and to obtain the full advantages of a bloodless procedure, I inject the operative field freely, especially in the region of the anus, the natal fold and the dorsal and ventral aspects of the coccyx and sacrum, with a $\frac{1}{2}$ percent novocain, $\frac{1}{40}$ percent percaine solution, even if I am not operating exclusively under high pressure local anaesthesia.

I consider the dorsal approach to be the standard procedure of the operative methods attacking the rectum from below. If another approach is selected, it must be justified by a particular peculiarity of the case, and even then it is largely dependent on the individual surgeon, for any aspect of a case which seems to justify the perineal or the vaginal procedure can be overcome by the proper adaptation of the operation by the dorsal approach.

The perineal procedure (Lisfranc, Dieffenbach) may be chosen if the growth has developed especially anteriorly and has involved the region of the urethra, the prostate or the bladder. Obviously a rectal carcinoma which already involves the urethra or the bladder is fundamentally to be considered inoperable, because the resection of these organs exposes the patient to great hazards and after a long and painful illness is usually followed by an early recurrence. The same holds true for an invasion of the sacrum by the tumor. Conditions are somewhat more favorable in an involvement of the prostate. If the removal of the posterior portion of the prostate without opening the urethra is sufficient to remove the tumor, this operation does not particularly increase the difficulty of the procedure. Even the complete removal of the prostate with the urethra traversing it is not excessively dangerous and often heals without leaving a permanent urinary fistula.

Relatively least harmful is the involvement of the female genitalia, in which the vaginal procedure of Rehn can be used. The female genitalia can be removed wholly or in part in connection with the rectum without thereby enlarging the operation to threatening proportions and without decidedly lessening the expectancy of a permanent cure. It is always better to remove the genital organs extensively in a suspicious case than to place the radical nature of the operation in doubt by allowing them to remain.

If the dorsal approach is selected, it is advisable to remove the coccyx in all cases (Kocher) and, if there is the slightest interference, the two lower sacral vertebrae as well (Kraske). These measures do not greatly extend the operation and no noticeable deformity is produced. The freedom of movement, the visibility during the operation, and the possibility of a high removal of the lymph glands and the bowel are greatly increased. I therefore remove these bone segments almost routinely. On the other hand, it is not advisable to go higher than the 4th sacral vertebra in the removal of the sacrum, since otherwise permanent disturbances in the emptying of the bladder may result, and since, from the 3rd sacral vertebra up, the possible opening of the dural sac carries with it the danger of a meningitis.

The safeguarding of the urethra in the male is facilitated by the introduction of a metal catheter. However I do not use this routinely. If doubts arise in an individual case as to the position of the urethra, a catheter can be inserted during the course of the operation.

(A). AMPUTATION OF THE RECTUM FROM BELOW, WITH ESTABLISHMENT OF A SACRAL ANUS

To repeat once more, this procedure is the simplest and the safest form of radical removal of a deep-seated rectal carcinoma, but it is fraught with a number of disadvantages so that it is by no means the procedure most to be recommended.

(1). *Amputation of the Rectum by the Dorsal Approach.*

Depending on whether only the last or also the next to the last sacral vertebra is to be removed, the skin incision begins over the vertebra in question, extends exactly in the midline to the anus and passes around the anus at a distance of about 2 cm. in the shape of a longitudinal oval (Fig. 321). The loose skin in the region of the anus is put on stretch during this procedure by means of sharp hooked retractors inserted into the unbroken surface adjacent to it. If there is any suspicious infiltration in the region of the anus, the incision is carried correspondingly farther at these points. Large portions of the natal cleft may be removed. As soon as the skin around the anus has been completely divided, the rosette of skin around the anus is closed tightly by means of strong silk sutures over a small sponge inserted into the anus. The instruments used for this purpose are then put aside. The sutures are left long so that traction can be made on the gut by means of them and they are caught together with a hemostat (Fig. 322).

The incision is deepened to the bone in the midline while sharp hooked retractors are inserted on both sides. The dorsal and lateral aspects of the bone are dissected free. In doing this, the origins of the coccygeus muscle and the anococcygeal ligament are divided. The bone is lifted forcibly with a four-pronged sharp hooked retractor (Fig. 322) and the soft parts are pushed away from the ventral surface of the coccyx and the lower sacrum by blunt dissection with a periosteal elevator and a sponge mounted on a forceps. This is done to avoid premature injury to the middle sacral artery which runs from above downward in the midline in this region.

If a considerable part of the sacrum is to be removed (Kraske), the posterior and anterior sacrosciatic ligaments with the attached bundles of the

gluteus maximus are nicked or divided. The coccyx and the lower segment
of the sacrum freed on all sides in this manner are removed with a powerful
Luer rongeur and the fibrous tissue strands attached to the resected piece of
bone are divided. Bleeding from the bone is checked by packing.

The floor of the dorsal incision gaping in its full length is formed by a

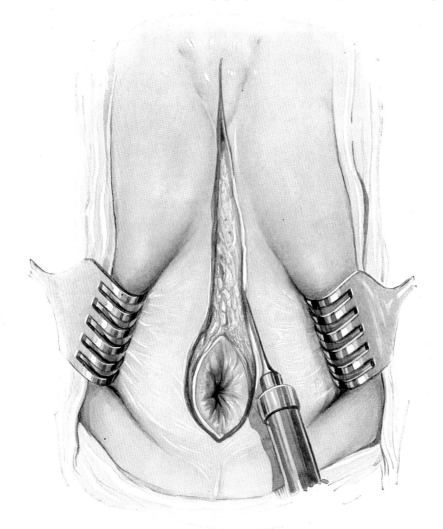

FIG. 321. Amputation of the rectum by the dorsal route. The skin incision is made in the
midline from the region of the third sacral segment to the anus, encircling the latter. The anal
region is being held apart with sharp hooked retractors to put the skin on stretch.

tough fascial layer, the parietal pelvic fascia. On its surface and close to the
bone the middle sacral artery passes downward. If the vessel was not previously injured, a ligature is passed around it below the divided edge of the bone
and tied and the vessel is divided below the ligature. The transverse incision
is now carried quite through the parietal pelvic fascia (Fig. 323). This fascia
is attached in the midline to the levator ani beneath, and this in turn is
attached to the visceral layer of the pelvic fascia and to the posterior wall of

the rectum. Since these structures can scarcely be separated from one another in the midline, a longitudinal incision that is slightly diagonal outward is made on each side, beginning above at the ends of the transverse incision and carried toward the anus, through the fascia and the levator to the posterior wall of

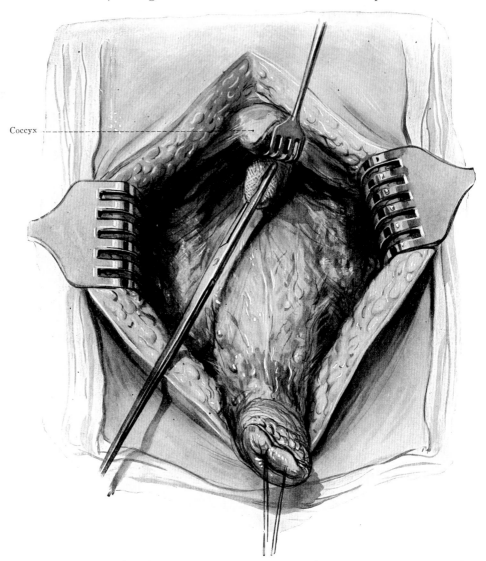

Coccyx

FIG. 322. Amputation of the rectum by the dorsal route (2). The incision has been carried down to the anal fascia. The coccyx is freed from its surroundings. The anal opening has been closed by sutures and their ends have been left long.

the rectum. This outlines an approximately rectangular flap consisting of fascia and levator ani, pedunculated and attached to the rectum at its anal end (Fig. 323).

The dissection is now carried forward, first to one side, then to the other of the flap, at the side and along the surface of the rectum in the cleft between the parietal and the visceral layer of the pelvic fascia; in the direction of the bladder, prostate and urethra in the male, and toward the vagina in the female.

This procedure is carried out parallel to the median longitudinal incision and in its full length, always beginning at the level of amputation of the sacrum

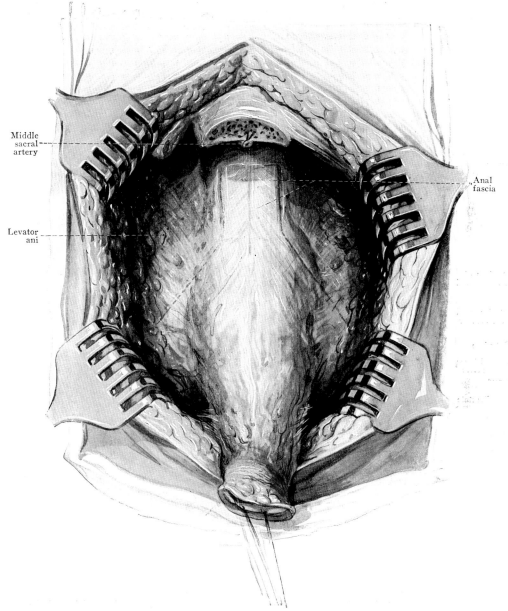

FIG. 323.   Amputation of the rectum by the dorsal route (3).   After resection of the coccyx and the last two sacral segments and after ligation of the middle sacral artery, the anal fascia and the levator ani are incised.   The dotted line indicates the intended continuation of the incision.

and ending only at the incision carried around the anus.   For this purpose the rectum is put on stretch in its long axis by means of the sutures closing the anus and sharp hooked retractors are inserted into the sides of the rectum and into the lateral walls of the wound.   The rectum is not only pulled to one side but is twisted on its long axis at the same time, so that the cleavage space previously mentioned is gradually unfolded and rolled up, first on one side, then on the other. In this dissection the fibers of the levator ani which are always easily recognized are divided at right angles to their course, uncovering the visceral layer of the pelvic fascia which encloses the rectum and the

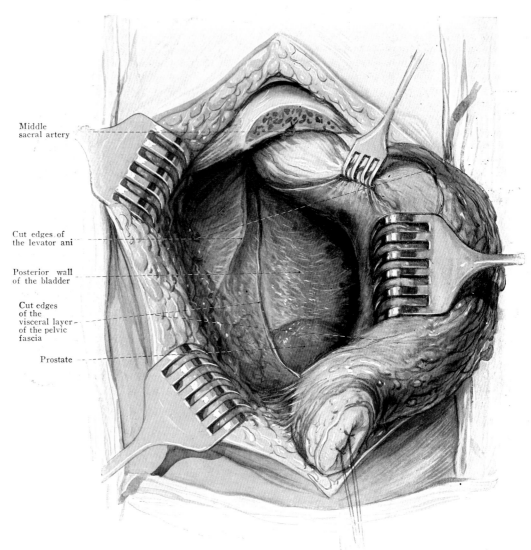

Middle
sacral artery

Cut edges of
the levator ani

Posterior wall
of the bladder

Cut edges
of the
visceral layer
of the pelvic
fascia

Prostate

Fig. 324. Amputation of the rectum by the dorsal route (4). After the division of the anal fascia and the levator ani on the left side, the rectum has been rolled over toward the right. After the division of the visceral layer of the pelvic fascia the rectum will be freed from the prostate, the seminal vesicles and the bladder.

prostate and the seminal vesicles or the vagina. On the levator ani a number of vessels are encountered running transversely. These are branches of the middle hemorrhoidal artery. They are caught and ligated. With the division of the levator ani, connection is established between the subperitoneal fossa and the ischiorectal fossa. The visceral fascia is also divided in a longitudinal direction parallel to the gut, since otherwise on its outer surface the surgeon would be led around the prostate or the vagina (Figs. 324 and 325). The outermost line in which this fascia may be divided in order to gain access to the space between the rectum on the one hand and seminal vesicles or prostate, or vagina, on the other, is marked in the male by the vessels of the vesicoprostatic plexus running parallel to the rectum. In the female the operator can always assure himself of the borderline between rectum and vagina by inserting a finger into the vagina.

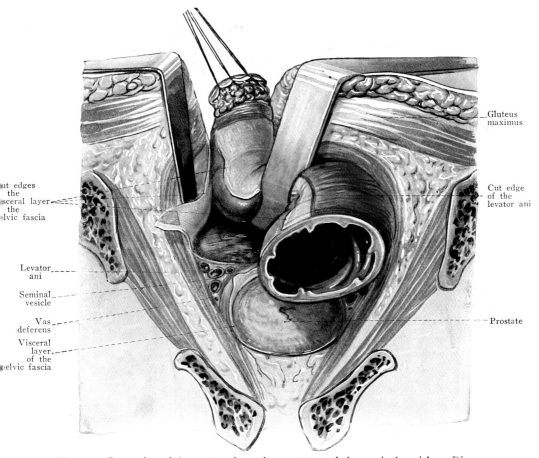

Fig. 325. Separation of the rectum from the prostate and the seminal vesicles. Diagrammatic. The skin, the anal fascia and the levator ani have been divided on the left. The visceral layer of the pelvic fascia has also been incised so that the rectum can be freed from the left seminal vesicle and from the prostate.

After the proper plane of cleavage has been opened, in doing which the high-pressure local anaesthesia apparatus is useful, the rectum can be separated from the seminal vesicles and prostate or the vagina. This brings the left and the right pararectal operative fields into communication with each other. The characteristic longitudinal course of its superficial musculature helps guard the rectal wall against accidental injury. In case of doubt this longitudinal musculature should be exposed.

The fibers of the anal sphincter which are exposed by the dissection in the lower region of the wound are avoided, the incision passing around them, so that they remain attached to the rectum. This is made easier by vigorous retraction with sharp hooked retractors.

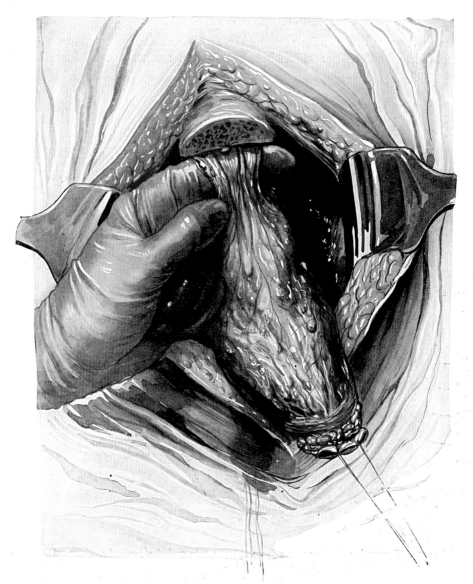

Fig. 326. Amputation of the rectum by the dorsal route. The rectum has been freed from the sacrum. The mesentery of the lower sigmoid (mesopelvinum) which contains the branches of the superior hemorrhoidal artery, is picked up on the finger and will be divided in segments between double ligatures.

The annular dissection of the anus, begun in the region of the skin at the start of the operation, is quite simple, especially freeing it from the urethra. The anus is pulled backward first on one side, then on the other, by means of the sutures closing the anus. Sharp hooked retractors are inserted in the outer wound edge and the rectum is grasped with forceps in the region of the ischiorectal fossa. The lateral attachments and the connection between the external sphincter and the bulbocavernosus muscle are divided, at times with considerable bleeding from the large venous plexus. While the rectum is pulled sharply backward and upward, it is separated in the male from the membranous urethra, whose position in case of doubt is made clear by the

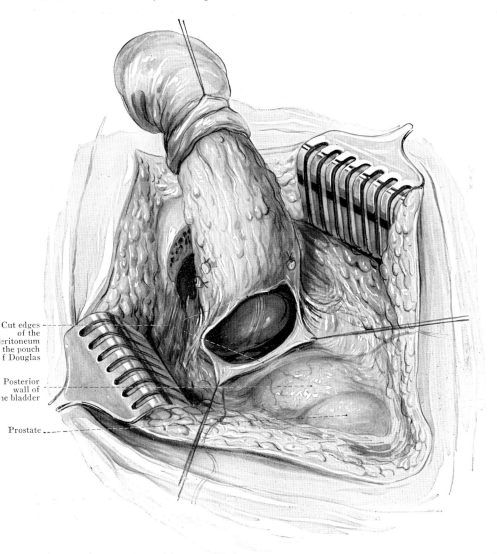

Cut edges
of the
peritoneum
the pouch
f Douglas

Posterior
wall of
he bladder

Prostate

Fig. 327. Amputation of the rectum by the dorsal route (6). The rectum has been completely freed in the anal region and from the prostate and bladder and has been reflected upward and backward. The pouch of Douglas has been opened in the region of the highest portion of the anterior rectal wall. The anus has been enclosed in a small rubber bag. (The posterior wall of the bladder has been drawn too large in the picture; it is often barely to be seen.)

insertion of a catheter. The separation is continued between the rectum and the prostate, the seminal vesicles and the posterior wall of the bladder. In this way the operative field is reached from in front. In the proper layer of cleavage this separation proceeds with ease.

In the female, the external sphincter is separated from the bulbo-cavernosus muscle by a transverse incision and the posterior wall of the vagina is freed from the rectum. In order to be more certain of the boundary, the surgeon can palpate the posterior vaginal wall by a finger inserted into the vagina, and can prepare the tissue for the dissection by means of the hydraulic force of a high-pressure local anaesthesia apparatus. The described mobiliza-

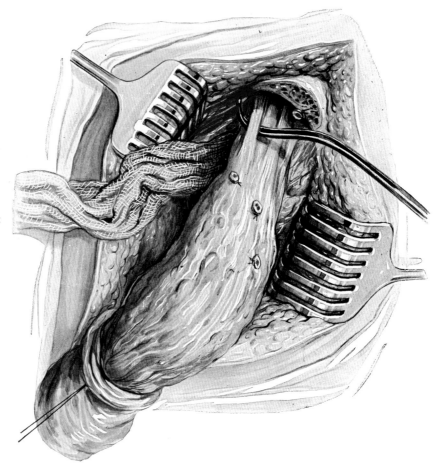

FIG. 328. Amputation of the rectum by the dorsal route (7). In continuation of the ligations of the mesopelvinum the mesosigmoid is also brought down. It is picked up on an aneurysm needle and divided in segments between double ligatures.

tion of the rectum may of course be performed by working alternately on the two sides, freeing a little at a time.

The dorsal operation for freeing the lower segment of the rectum which has here been described as proceeding from above downward may also be performed in the reverse direction. The anus is first freed on all sides, and the dissection is then carried upward as described under the perineal method.

Only in the exceptional case and only with a carcinoma located immediately above the anus will the degree of mobilization of the rectum as described above, be adequate for an amputation in sound tissue and for the

establishment of a sacral anus. However, in view of the extensive spread of
the carcinoma in an upward direction, it is not sound surgery to be too sparing
of tissue in the amputation. If, however, the mobilization is considered adequate, the rectum is pulled out as far as possible and is sutured into the upper
angle of the skin incision. The protruding segment is amputated (Fig. 329).
The wound distal to the artificial anus is closed by wire sutures or by silk
sutures and a drain is inserted in the region of the former anus (Fig. 330).

In most cases, however, the mobilization of the gut must be continued
higher.

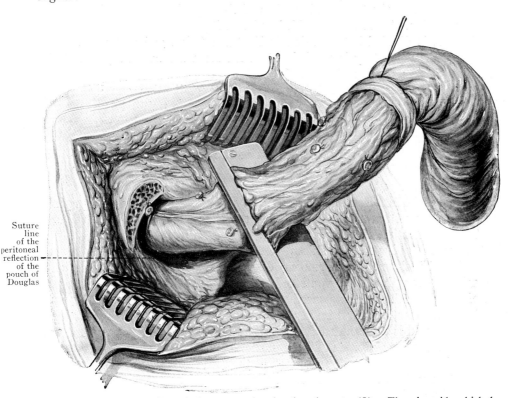

Suture
line
of the
peritoneal
reflection
of the
pouch of
Douglas

Fig. 329. Amputation of the rectum by the dorsal route (8). The sigmoid, which has
been freed from its mesenteric attachments, has been pulled far down and sutured to the free
edge of the peritoneum, thereby closing the abdominal cavity. The remainder of the bowel is
amputated with the aid of the Petz suture instrument.

When the freed terminal portion of the rectum is pulled forcibly backward and upward out of the wound, the thin peritoneum of the fold of Douglas,
moving with each phase of respiration, appears in the region of the highest
freed point of the ventral surface of the bowel and between it and the bladder
or the vagina. The peritoneal fold is grasped with two long surgical forceps
and is incised in the coronal plane close to the rectum (Fig. 327). The resultant opening is enlarged beside the rectum by dividing the peritoneum to the
right and left, remembering that its line of attachment to the gut runs backward and upward. Since the pelvis of the patient is elevated and with its
dorsal surface uppermost, no intestinal loops protrude in spite of a wide opening of the pouch of Douglas. On the contrary, on the entrance of air into the

abdominal cavity the intestines gravitate toward the liver. A gauze pad, made secure in the usual manner, is pushed into the peritoneal opening to protect the abdominal cavity from contamination and to prevent the protrusion of intestinal loops in case of straining.

While the anterior wall of the rectum is made accessible for a considerable distance by the opening of the pouch of Douglas, the posterior wall, which is broadly attached to the sacrum, is still inaccessible. It can however be pushed away from the sacrum fairly high up by blunt dissection. If traction is now made on the rectum, the lower part of the mesorectum and the mesosigmoid containing the terminal branches of the superior hemorrhoidal artery is put on tension. The mesosigmoid, insofar as it prevents the mobilization of the sigmoid, is divided between double ligatures (Figs. 326 and 328). The division of the mesentery is carried out as far from the bowel as possible in order not to endanger its nutrition.

Goetze has recently pointed out that the mobilization can be carried higher if after the removal of the sacral segments the parietal layer of the pelvic fascia is first separated by blunt dissection from the bone to a point above the promontory and the abdomen is not opened until this point is reached. This opening is first made just to the right of the bowel. At the same level an opening is made to the left of the bowel and a loop of gauze is passed around the gut. By means of the gauze loop the gut is pulled downward and is mobilized by a high division of its mesentery and by a subsequent division of the peritoneal fold in the bottom of the pouch of Douglas.

The mobilization of the gut is complete as soon as it is possible to bring the tumor well out beyond the skin, preferably over 15 cm., in the upper angle of the dorsal incision. As a rule no difficulty is encountered in materially increasing the length of the eventrated sound segment by extensive mobilization of the sigmoid. In this procedure the proximal gut must show no nutritional disturbances, but must have a fresh rosy appearance.

The sigmoid is then pulled downward and backward, the gauze compress is removed from the abdomen and the peritoneal opening is closed by suturing the free edge of the parietal peritoneum of the fold of Douglas tightly around the gut at its point of emergence from the peritoneal cavity with interrupted sutures (Fig. 329).

The extensive wound, after a careful inspection for any bleeding points, is packed with vioform gauze and the ends of the packing are brought out in the region of the former anus. The gut is carried through the upper posterior angle of the wound. The wound edges distal to the point of exit of the bowel are brought together for a distance of 3 to 4 cm. by means of two through-and-through wire sutures and by silk coaptation sutures so that the open upper angle just permits the unobstructed exit of the gut and the lower open angle the egress of the strips of vioform gauze and a drainage tube. The circumference of the gut is sutured to the skin at its level of exit (Fig. 330). Finally, or else just before the gut is sutured to the skin, the rectum is transsected somewhat above the level of the skin because it tends to retract (Fig. 320). The cut edges of the rectum are further attached to the neighboring skin by means of through-and-through interrupted sutures.

If the proximal gut after mobilization shows any disturbance of its circu-

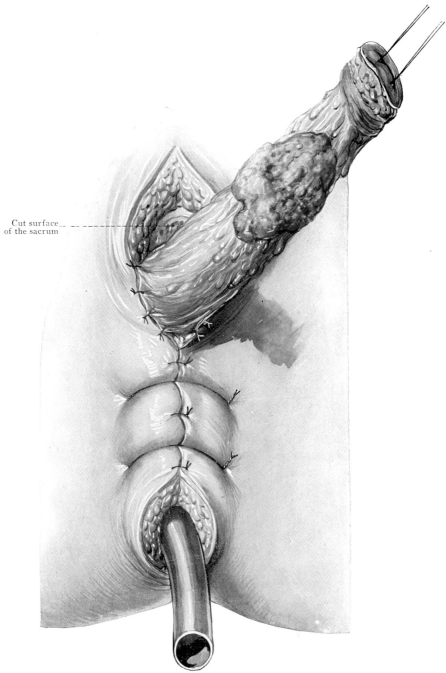

Cut surface
of the sacrum

Fig. 330. Amputation of the rectum by the dorsal route. Establishment of a sacral anus. The caudal portion of the dorsal wound has been closed by suture. A drainage tube has been placed at the former site of the anus. The bowel, which has been brought out through the cranial portion of the wound, is sutured to the skin edge and will be amputated at the skin level.

lation, recognizable by a bluish discoloration, its possible necrosis must be reckoned with. The attempt can then be made, by continuing the ligation and division of the mesosigmoid, to bring down a higher and more adequately nour-

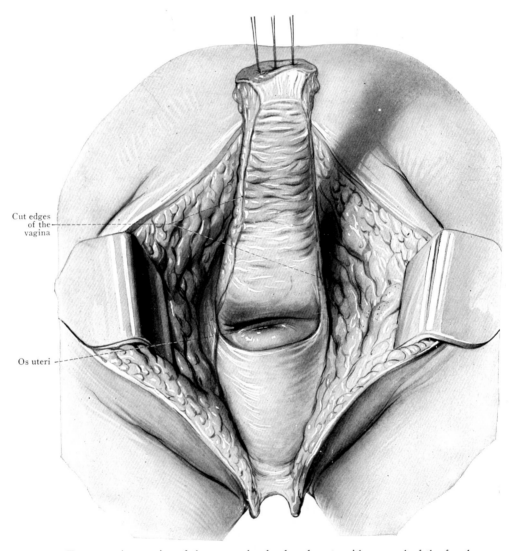

Cut edges of the vagina

Os uteri

FIG. 331. Amputation of the rectum by the dorsal route with removal of the female reproductive organs (1). The dorsal incision, which begins in the region of the sacrum, has been extended onto the posterior vaginal wall which has been divided on the right and left as far as the cervix. The posterior vaginal wall in the form of a broad strip remains attached to the rectum which has been extensively mobilized.

ished segment of the gut. If this is unsuccessful, the operation is extended into a sacro-abdominal procedure and the proximal gut is brought out of the abdominal cavity in the form of an inguinal artificial anus. The gut is divided in the dorsal operative wound above the carcinoma by means of the Petz suture instrument. The distal portion is removed. The proximal end is covered with a condom and is replaced in the abdominal cavity. The pouch of

Douglas is then carefully closed from below by suture.   The sacral wound is packed with vioform gauze.   The patient is turned on his back and placed in

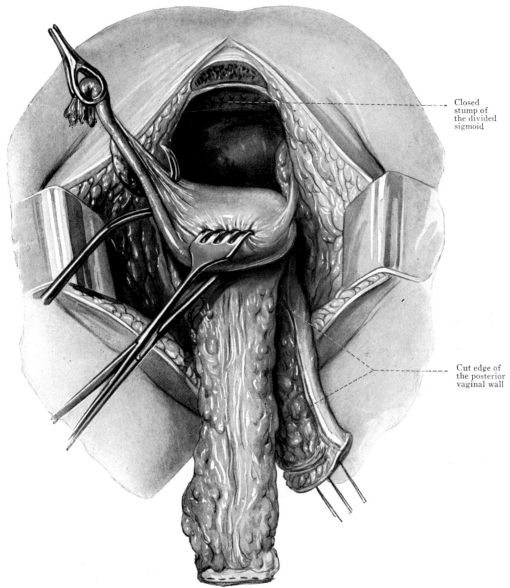

Closed
stump of
the divided
sigmoid

Cut edge of
the posterior
vaginal wall

FIG. 332.   Amputation of the rectum by the dorsal route with removal of the female reproductive organs (2). The rectum has been extensively freed.   To the distal portion of its anterior surface is attached the posterior wall of the vagina.   The sigmoid has been divided. The lesion has extended into the uterus.   The uterus and the left adnexa are pulled down by forceps and their attachments to the surroundings are picked up on an aneurysm needle and divided.

an exaggerated Trendelenburg position.   The abdomen is opened by a low left lateral rectus incision.   The gut is mobilized to the necessary degree from above, and a well-nourished segment is carried to the surface through the lower angle of the wound to form an inguinal artificial anus. The security of the suture of the pouch of Douglas as applied from below is determined from above. The laparotomy wound is closed up to the point of emergence of the artificial anus.

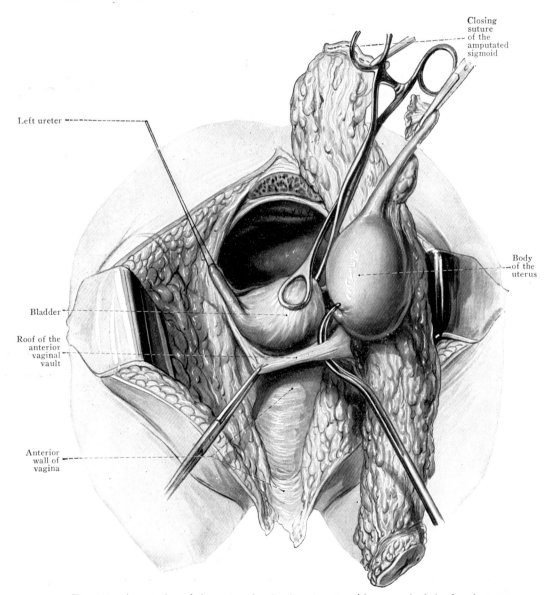

Fig. 333. Amputation of the rectum by the dorsal route with removal of the female reproductive organs (3). The uterus and the left adnexa have been freed. The bladder is put on stretch with a round grasping forceps. The left ureter is drawn aside by means of a ligature. The anterior vaginal vault is picked up in segments on an aneurysm needle and divided between double ligatures.

If at the end of the dorsal operation the proximal segment of intestine shows nutritional disturbances and the patient's general condition no longer permits the performance of the sacro-abdominal procedure described above, there is nothing to do but to bring the gut down as far as possible, to close the pouch of Douglas, to amputate the carcinomatous portion and also the part showing nutritional disturbances. A large rubber tube is tied into the proximal end of the gut and is led to the exterior while the gut remains in the dorsal wound, well surrounded by vioform gauze. As soon as the patient has sufficiently recovered, the proximal gut is brought out as an abdominal artificial anus at a secondary laparotomy.

The Simultaneous Removal of the Female Genital Organs. If the female genital organs must also be removed because of carcinomatous involvement, the surgeon will find the approach to the operative field in the direction, dorsum-rectum-female genitalia, preferable as a rule, to the procedure in the reverse direction by the vaginal route as described in a later section. The operation is begun in the manner just described, but the incision encircling the rectum is continued into the vaginal vestibule. If a part of the vagina is diseased and is to be removed, the incision forks and passes through the posterior vaginal wall, around the diseased area (Fig. 331). The best plan in such a case is to remove the whole posterior vaginal wall as far as the cervix. The part of the vagina included in the incision remains attached to the anterior wall of the rectum.

The mobilization of the gut is begun dorsally in the manner just described, in that the gut is freed from the hollow of the sacrum after the resection of the bone segments. The peritoneal cavity is opened at a point where the gut is not attached to the uterus by carcinomatous tissue. The mesentery is ligated and cut step by step and the sigmoid is drawn down and divided. Its proximal end is sutured into the wound as a sacral artificial anus, or, in case an abdominal artificial anus had been established beforehand, it is closed and dropped into the abdominal cavity.

Through the opening into the peritoneal cavity the uterus is grasped with a forceps and, together with the attached distal segment of the rectum, is lifted out of the wound (Fig. 332). As the tissues are put on stretch they are divided between ligatures. The adnexa may be removed at the same time, or they may not be removed depending on the findings at operation. The ureters, which pass close to the cervix of the uterus as they converge in their course downward and forward from above and behind, must be carefully guarded. In this manner, the anterior surface of the eventrated uterus is eventually reached (Fig. 333). At this point the anterior vaginal wall is divided and the bladder is dissected free. The anterior vaginal fornix is now divided in its full circumference and the whole dissected mass, consisting of the gut and the female genital organs, is removed, together with any part of the posterior vaginal wall that was included in the original incision.

The abdominal cavity is closed securely, the bladder as a rule being drawn into the large gap resulting from the removal of the genital organs.

(2) *Amputation of the Rectum by the Perineal Approach (Lisfranc, Dieffenbach, Lockhart-Mummery).*

The location of the carcinoma on the anterior wall in the region of the anal segment of the rectum may justify the use of the perineal approach in the male. The patient is placed in the lithotomy position. The midline incision begins at the base of the scrotum, which has been elevated by a suitable bandage, encircles the anus and is continued in the midline to a point over the coccyx (Fig. 334). The coccyx should be removed at the beginning of the

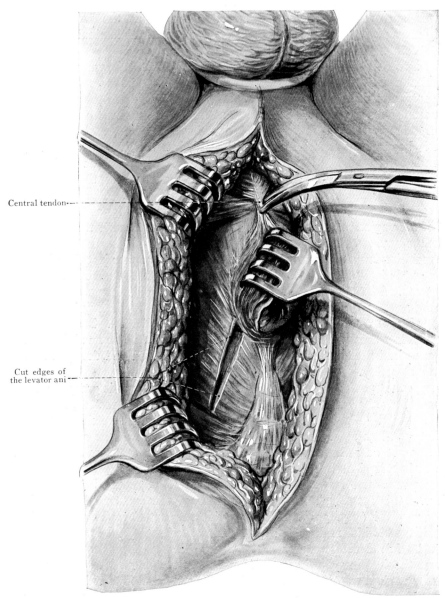

Central tendon

Cut edges of
the levator ani

FIG. 334. Amputation of the rectum by the perineal route (1). The midline incision which encircles the rectum extends from the central tendon to beyond the coccyx. After exposure of the muscles of the pelvic floor the levator ani has been incised on the left side. The central tendon is cut with the scissors.

operation in the manner previously described. The incision is deepened in its anterior portion as in the performance of a perineal prostatectomy. The external sphincter is separated from the bulbocavernosus muscle by a transverse incision through the central tendon (Fig. 334). The anus is closed by suture in the manner described and is pulled sharply backward. The surgeon works down between the bulbous urethra and the anterior surface of the rectum until he reaches the membranous urethra, the prostate and the seminal vesicles (Fig. 335). While these structures are pressed forward and the rectum backward, their separation is carried upward; if possible, to the extent that a portion of the posterior bladder wall is separated from the rectum.

Sharp hooked retractors are inserted into one side of the skin incision encircling the rectum to retract the anus and the sphincter to one side and the fat of the ischiorectal fossa to the other side, so that dissection of the rectum may be continued dorsally along the side of the anus from the anterior wound. The levator ani soon appears and is divided (Fig. 334). The same procedure is carried out on the other side of the rectum.

The rectum which has been freed anteriorly and on the sides is now pulled forward. Posteriorly, the anococcygeal ligament and the parietal pelvic fascia which are thereby put on stretch are divided. Farther up, the rectum can be freed from the hollow of the sacrum by blunt dissection.

When the anus and the lower portion of the rectum have been freed on all sides in this manner, there follows, if necessary, the opening of the pouch of Douglas anterior to the rectum so that the mesosigmoid may be pulled down, ligated and divided. The operation is then concluded in the manner described under the dorsal procedure.

The perineal procedure therefore differs from the dorsal procedure only in that it is carried out in a ventral-dorsal and an anal-oral direction whereas the dorsal or sacral procedure, in the main, is carried out in the reverse direction.

(3) *Amputation of the Rectum by the Vaginal Approach (Rehn, Gersuny)*

If the posterior vaginal wall or the uterus is involved by the carcinoma, these structures are removed wholly, or in part, together with the rectum. In such a case the operation may be started in the region of the vagina and continued dorsally. The female genitalia may, however, be removed by the usual dorsal approach as described previously on page 425.

In the vaginal procedure the patient is placed in the lithotomy position. The vagina is held open by lateral retractors and the incision begins in the region of the cervix. It extends either along the midline of the posterior wall of the vagina, or, if a part of the vagina is to be removed, it forks and runs more or less close to the right and left margins of the posterior wall of the vagina to the vestibule, in this way including the lesion. The best plan is to include the whole posterior wall of the vagina between two parallel longitudinal incisions (Fig. 331). From the vestibule the incision forks to both sides of the anus and ends over the tip of the coccyx which is resected at the beginning of the operation. Since plenty of room is afforded by the opening of the vagina, the length of the incision posteriorly is adequate as a rule. Otherwise it can be lengthened in that direction by resecting part of the sacrum.

The wound edges are separated with sharp hooked retractors. The dissection proceeds from the vagina backward and upward, first on one side, then

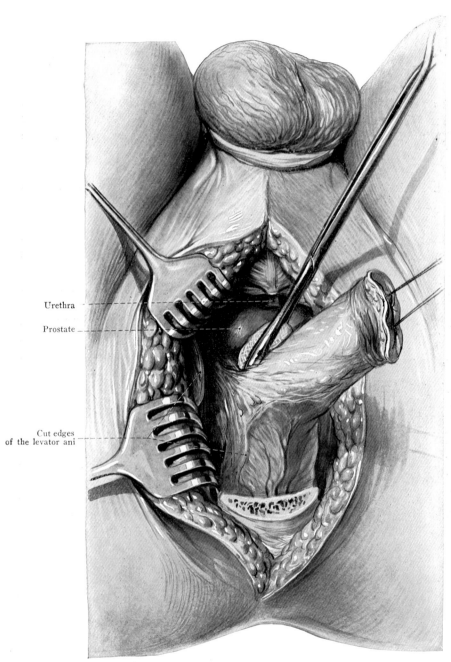

Urethra

Prostate

Cut edges
of the levator ani

FIG. 335. Amputation of the rectum by the perineal route. The coccyx has been resected and the central tendon and the levator ani divided. The rectum is being freed from the prostate by blunt dissection. The membranous portion of the urethra is in view.

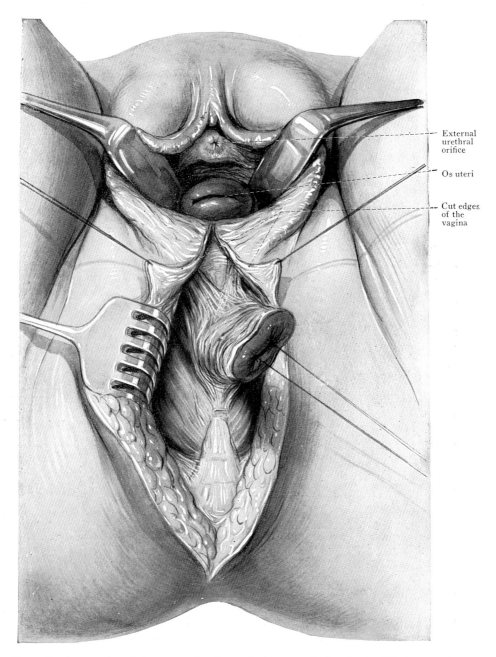

External
urethral
orifice

Os uteri

Cut edges
of the
vagina

FIG. 336. Amputation of the rectum by the vaginal route. Patient in the lithotomy position. The midline incision which encircles the rectum has exposed the coccyx in its posterior angle and anteriorly has been carried through the midline of the posterior vaginal wall as far as the cervix. The muscles of the pelvic floor have been exposed.

the other, at the side of the anus which was closed by suture at the beginning of the operation and at the side of the rectum into the ischiorectal fossa (Fig. 336). In this way the lower end of the rectum is gradually freed antero-posteriorly on both sides. After the division of the anococcygeal ligament the posterior surface of the rectum is freed from the sacrum by blunt dissection. Finally, the fold of Douglas appears high in the wound on the anterior surface of the rectum, at which point the peritoneum is opened. After the abdominal cavity has been opened, the amputation of the bowel, after ligation and division of the mesorectum and the mesosigmoid, is completed in the manner described in the preceding section.

The vagina, whether it was simply split or whether its posterior wall was removed, is either sutured at the end of the operation after the closure of the abdominal cavity or it is packed, together with the large wound cavity.

If on the other hand the uterus, or the uterus and adnexa, are also to be removed in the vaginal procedure, the incision through the posterior wall of the vagina is continued around the cervix within the vaginal vault and the anterior fornix is opened between the uterus and the bladder. Through this incision the anterior vaginal wall, whose removal is probably never necessary, is separated from the uterus. Through the opening in the anterior vaginal vault the uterus is caught with a suitable forceps and is pulled downward together with the adnexa, the exposure being similar to that used for a vaginal hysterectomy. All tissue strands that become taut are picked up on an aneurysm needle and are divided between ligatures, thus gradually freeing the internal female genitalia. Particular attention must be paid to the ureters and the posterior wall of the bladder in this procedure. The ureters in this region enclose the neck of the uterus as in the limbs of a fork as they converge downward and forward (Fig. 279). They therefore lie a little above and to the side of the dome of the vaginal vault. If there is any question as to the position of or danger to a ureter, it is better to expose it by dissection than to wait until it has been injured.

The whole mass of tissue which has been dissected free, consisting of the anus, the rectum, the posterior wall of the vagina, the uterus and the adnexa, is now attached only to the gut itself as it emerges from the abdominal cavity. The gut is further mobilized by blunt dissection from the sacrum and by ligating and dividing the mesorectum and the mesosigmoid step by step, and is pulled downward.

After the amputation of the rectum, removing that structure and the attached female genital organs, the operation ends either with the establishment of a sacral artificial anus, or, if an abdominal artificial anus had been previously established, with the closure and burial of the proximal gut in the abdominal cavity.

In every case the peritoneal cavity is carefully closed by suture, as a rule after fastening the bladder into the large gap resulting from the removal of the female genital organs, taking care that the ureters are not damaged.

(B) RESECTION OF THE RECTUM FROM BELOW

(1) *Resection of the Rectum by the Dorsal Approach*

The exposure of the rectum by the dorsal route for the purpose of a resection is very similar to the exposure for the purpose of amputation. It differs from it in the one chief point that in a resection the distal segment of the rectum surrounded by the sphincter remains undisturbed. The freeing of the gut above this point and the mobilization of the sigmoid are performed entirely in the manner above described. In amputation of the rectum when a portion of the sigmoid is left behind, the distance from the point of division of the gut to the angle of the wound at the lower end of the sacrum is usually shorter than the distance in rectal resection from the upper gut transsection

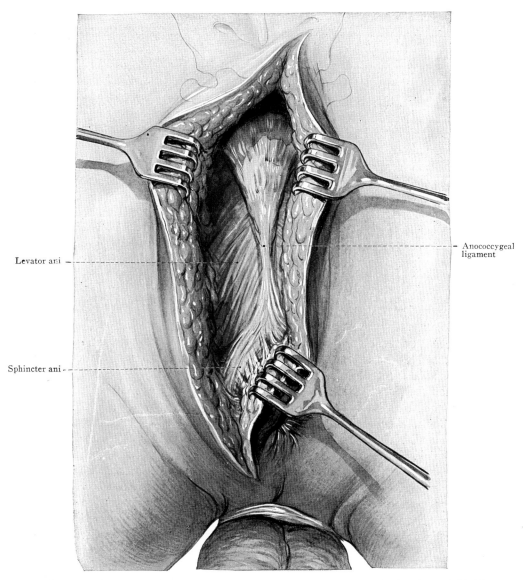

Levator ani

Sphincter ani

Anococcygeal ligament

FIG. 337. Resection of the rectum by the dorsal route (1). The skin has been divided by a curved incision concave to the right, beginning at the right side of the spinous process of the second sacral segment, continuing toward the left, passing the anus on the left and extending to the anterior raphe. The coccyx, the anococcygeal ligament, the levator ani and the sphincter ani have been exposed.

to the lower transsection line or to the anus. Furthermore, in a resection several additional centimeters of gut are necessary for the intestinal suture. Resection therefore actually necessitates a more extensive mobilization of the proximal sigmoid if any permanent results are to be hoped for.

Resection from below is performed almost exclusively by the dorsal route. The patient is placed in the abdominal-suspension position or on the right side. The skin incision is made either exactly in the midline from the third sacral vertebra to a point 2 cm. behind the anus (Kocher), or it passes in a curve, convex to the left, from the right side of the second sacral vertebra across the midline to the left, past the anus, and ends in the midline about 2 cm. in front of the anus (Voelker, Fig. 337). The second incision affords a better view and is therefore preferable.

The skin flap outlined by the incision is dissected free to the right beyond the midline. The dissection is halted in the lower segment by the sphincter ani and the anus. In the course of the dissection of the flap the coccyx and the lower part of the sacrum appear in the upper part of the wound (Fig. 337). These structures are freed in the manner described under rectal amputation, with preservation of the middle sacral artery. The coccyx and the 4th and 5th sacral vertebrae are removed with the Luer rongeur. A suture is passed around the middle sacral artery and the vessel is ligated and divided. If the incision does not reach high enough, it is prolonged along the side of the sacrum by nicking the gluteus maximus muscle and the greater and lesser sacrosciatic ligaments.

The anococcygeal ligament and the parietal pelvic fascia are divided transversely just below the cut edge of the bone. In the upper part of the wound the diagonally coursing fibers of the levator ani are divided, first on the left, then on the right, between hooked retractors inserted into the rectum and into the lateral wall of the wound (Figs. 326 and 328). The attachments of this muscle are divided as far from the bowel as possible, because the nerves to the sphincter run close to the bowel. In the lower angle of the wound the sphincter ani comes into view. It is preserved. After the division of the levator ani the visceral layer of the pelvic fascia appears. The cut edges of the levator are pulled apart with sharp hooked retractors and the rectum is thereby turned on its long axis. The visceral fascia is divided first on the left side, then, after shifting the retractors, on the right side, and is freed from the rectum which can be recognized by its longitudinal musculature (Figs. 324 and 325). In freeing the visceral pelvic fascia from the rectum in front, the operator keeps close to the longitudinal musculature of the bowel and gradually separates it first on the left side, then on the right, from the seminal vesicles, prostate and bladder in the male, and from the vagina in the female. This frees the rectum on all sides and a rubber tube is passed around it. By means of the rubber tube the rectum can be retracted in any direction, facilitating its further mobilization. Strands of tissue attached to the bowel are doubly ligated before being divided.

The circular dissection of the rectum is extended toward the anus until only the part of the rectum in the region of the sphincter ani remains in connection with the surrounding tissue (Fig. 338). The tissues are always divided as far from the bowel as possible in order to safeguard the nerves to the sphincter.

When the circular dissection of the gut has been carried down far enough, its further mobilization is undertaken in the direction of the abdominal cavity.

After the transverse division of the anal fascia and the levator ani on the

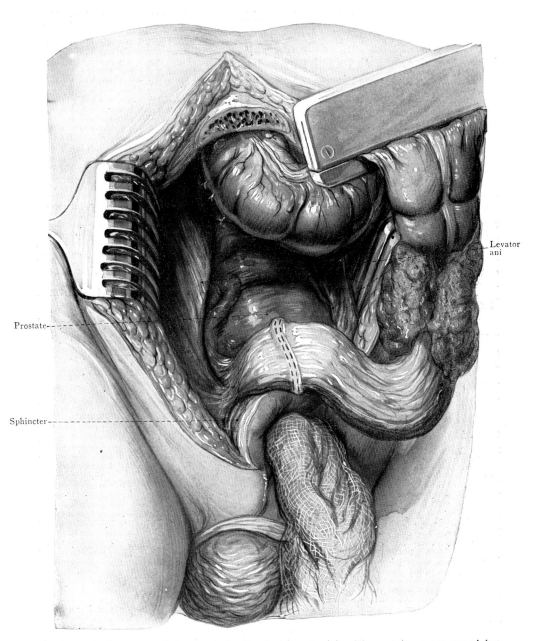

FIG. 338.   Resection of the rectum by the dorsal route (2).   The rectal segment containing the lesion has been freed on all sides from its attachments.   The pouch of Douglas has been opened, the mesosigmoid divided and the sigmoid brought down to a considerable extent.   The rectum has been closed just above the sphincter ani and is closed above the tumor by means of the Petz suture instrument.

posterior surface of the bowel, the gut is easily separated from the anterior surface of the sacrum by blunt dissection.   This blunt dissection is continued on both sides of the gut.   As soon as the anterior surface is reached, the peritoneal fold of the pouch of Douglas appears above the exposed posterior surface of the bladder or of the vagina.   The peritoneum is opened and is divided close to the bowel in front and at the sides where its attachment rises diagonally upward and backward.

The further mobilization of the gut by ligation and division of the superior hemorrhoidal artery and of the mesosigmoid is carried out in the manner described under amputation of the rectum. The vessels are ligated as far from the gut as possible, with preservation of their arcades and mindful of the critical point of Sudek. The mobilization is continued until a well-nourished and obviously entirely normal cross-section of sigmoid above the carcinoma can be joined without tension to a well-nourished normal cross-section of gut below the carcinoma. It must be remembered that the gut may be considered normal just below, but only a considerable distance above the macroscopic limit of the carcinoma.

If it is impossible to mobilize the sigmoid sufficiently from below, or if the mobilized segment shows nutritional disturbances, then either an amputation with establishment of a sacral anus is performed or it becomes necessary to resort to one type of the combined procedure. In this case a midline laparotomy is performed and the gut is either mobilized sufficiently from above to make possible resection and suture, or it is amputated and an abdominal anus is established.

If it is possible to mobilize the proximal bowel sufficiently from the sacral wound, the gut is drawn far out and the pouch of Douglas is closed carefully around the sigmoid at its point of exit by interrupted sutures (Fig. 338). The cavity of the wound is packed with compresses to limit its contamination as far as possible during the succeeding portion of the operation. The bowel may be grasped above and below each of the two points of intended transsection by clamps, four in all. It is divided between the pairs of clamps, freeing the diseased segment. Every trace of escaped intestinal contents is carefully sponged away and the remaining gut lumens are carefully cleansed with dry sponges.

It is preferable to close the bowel above and below the lesion with the aid of the Petz suture instrument (Fig. 338) and to carry out the transsection between the pairs of rows of clips with a scissors. The use of the apparatus which makes the application of clamps unnecessary is, however, made difficult at times by the depth of the wound.

Three procedures come into consideration for the purpose of reestablishing the union between the proximal and the distal gut end: (1) circular suture, (2) the "telescope" procedure of von Hochenegg, and (3) the "telescope" procedure by the Whitehead method.

Resection with Circular Suture. The sphincter is cautiously dilated. The suture is performed end-to-end in the manner described under intestinal suture: End-traction sutures are applied before beginning each suture line. A posterior Lembert suture, a posterior three-layer Albert suture, an anterior three-layer Albert suture and an anterior Lembert suture are introduced. A third outer Lembert suture line is added if possible. If the ends of the bowel were closed by means of the Petz suture instrument (Fig. 339), the edges bearing the clips are removed in the course of the anastomosis. If the gut was closed with clamps, the clamps are removed after the completion of the suture. Any tissue in the neighborhood which is available is brought close and attached by suture over the line of anastomosis to protect it and relieve it of tension.

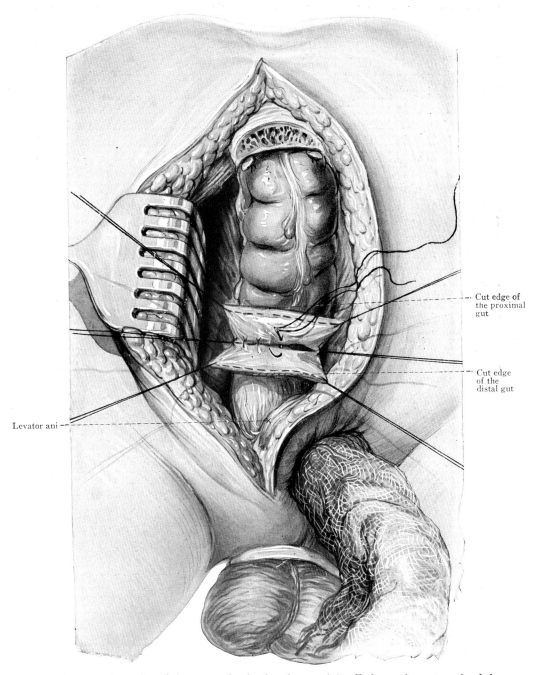

Cut edge of
the proximal
gut

Cut edge
of the
distal gut

Levator ani

Fig. 339. Resection of the rectum by the dorsal route (3). End-to-end anastomosis of the gut ends. After resection of the segment included between the two rows of Petz clip sutures, the proximal and distal ends of the rectum, each closed with a row of Petz clips, are joined by posterior interrupted Lembert sutures.

The anastomosis must be especially protected in this way from the packing with which the wound is now loosely filled.

The soft-tissue flap formed by the skin incision is folded back and fastened into its old bed by a number of interrupted sutures.

In the suture of the rectum, intestinal surfaces are joined which in part or in whole lack a peritoneal covering. The feces in the rectum are highly infectious and solid in consistency. The proximal end of the intestine frequently shows nutritional changes. For these reasons circular rectal suture is only too frequently insecure. Careful dilatation of the sphincter, the use of opium and restriction of food intake in the first few days after the operation help to safeguard the anastomosis. For these same reasons it is frequently advisable to establish a temporary intestinal fistula in the descending colon or the cecum before the operation, in order at least to divert gas and feces and prevent them from producing tension at the line of suture. In spite of these measures, fecal fistulae frequently develop which as a rule do not close spontaneously and may even resist stubbornly operative attempts at their closure.

In order to increase the security of the anastomosis of the two intestinal ends, to lessen the possible dangers of the development of gangrene of the segments, and to shorten the long duration of the operation with its dangers of shock, a number of modifications of the technique of resection of the rectum have been proposed, among which the eventration procedure of Küttner has received the widest adoption. Küttner divides resection into two separate operations with an intervening time interval. He concludes the first stage at the point where the carcinomatous segment has been sufficiently mobilized so that the normal bases of the loop can easily be brought together after the closure of the abdominal cavity and the diseased loop can be eventrated through the sacral wound. Depending upon whether gangrene develops, the eventrated loop is amputated 1 to 4 days later, under the pretext of changing the dressing, and the two cross-sections of gut remaining in the body are immediately anastomosed end-to-end in the wound by means of two or three circular layers of interrupted silk sutures in the usual way. Frequently general anaesthesia is unnecessary, morphine alone sufficing. By this technique, Küttner has in a few instances observed primary healing, whereas the fistulae, which as a rule develop even after this operation, eventually heal spontaneously.

I do not use this method at present. Since I operate upon my patients under the girdle type of spinal anaesthesia or under high-pressure local anaesthesia, I seldom encounter severe shock in the radical operation for rectal carcinoma. I have seen severe sepsis follow the eventration procedure, the sepsis arising from the gangrenous loop remaining in the cavity. If I were compelled by the development of shock to end the operation abruptly and to abandon the time-consuming anastomosis, I would at least amputate the mobilized and eventrated intestine with the aid of the Petz instrument, a procedure that is over in half a minute.

The "Telescope" Procedure (Hochenegg). The outlook for healing without the development of a fistula is greater with the "telescope" procedure of Hochenegg. The sphincter is cautiously dilated after the excision of the diseased intestinal segment. The cut edge of the anal stump, from which the

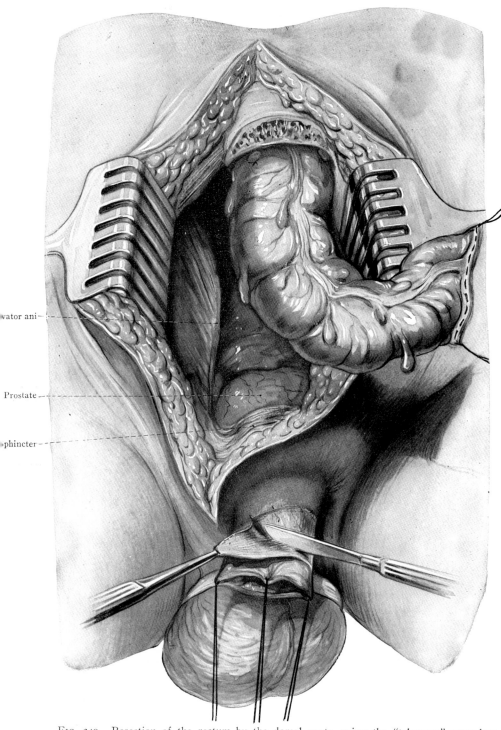

vator ani

Prostate

phincter

Fig. 340. Resection of the rectum by the dorsal route, using the "telescope" procedure. The rectal segment of gut included between the rows of Petz clips has been resected. The free end of the anal segment with its Petz clips has been trimmed off and the anal segment turned inside-out by bringing it out through the anus with the aid of three traction sutures. The mucosa of this segment is removed with the exception of a ring about 2 cm. wide, next to the anus.

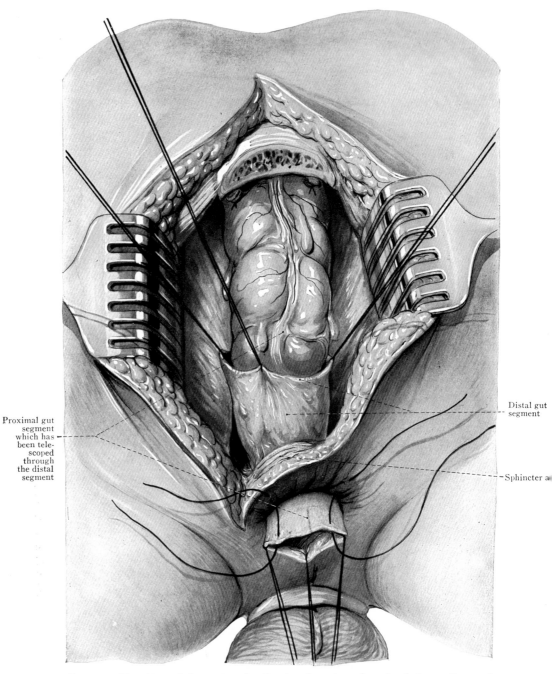

Proximal gut
segment
which has
been tele-
scoped
through
the distal
segment

Distal gut
segment

Sphincter a

FIG. 341. Resection of the rectum by the dorsal route, using the "telescope" procedure.
The anal gut segment after being denuded of its mucosa has been reinserted through the anus to
its original position.   The proximal sigmoid—the sigmoid, closed with Petz clips—is pulled
through the anal segment and the anus to the exterior.   The cut edge of the sigmoid is sutured
to the skin in the region of the anus.

clamp, or the Petz clips, has been removed, is provided with three equidistant traction sutures which are carried out through the anus. By pulling on these sutures the end of intestine is turned inside out and projects from the anus with the mucosa on the outside. A solution of adrenalin is injected under the mucosa which is then carefully dissected away, beginning at a distance of 2 cm. from the anus, so that the outside of the everted gut with the exception of the 2 cm. wide strip consists of a continuous raw surface (Fig. 340). The reason for leaving the narrow ring of mucosa in the immediate neighborhood of the anus is that the nerve endings concerned with the reflexes involving the closure and the opening of the anus are found in this region. The end is then pulled back through the anus into its original position in the operative wound by means of the three traction sutures.

The cut edge of the proximal end or, if the gut is closed with Petz clips, its immediate vicinity is likewise provided with three traction sutures. These traction sutures are led through the distal segment and out through the anus. Traction is now made downward on the three traction sutures of the proximal end and upward on the three traction sutures of the distal end. This causes the proximal gut to slip through the distal segment and its cut end appears outside of the anus, while the anal segment extends quite a distance upward over the surface of the proximal gut segment (Fig. 341). The transsected end of the proximal segment is fastened to the circle of mucosa at the anus by means of interrupted sutures. The free margin of the anal segment is attached all around to the outer surface of the proximal segment by suture. The operative wound is packed lightly with gauze, the soft-tissue flap is folded back into place and is fastened by a few sutures.

"Telescope" Procedure according to the Whitehead Method. The resection procedures described so far have the disadvantage of dividing the bowel within the dorsal wound so that infection of the wound can hardly be avoided. I have found the following clean and technically quite simple procedure very serviceable. The rectum is freed down to just above the anus in the manner described but is not at this time divided. Leaving the dorsal operative field, I next perform a typical Whitehead operation on the anus (page 378). The separation of the rectal mucosa from the musculature is carried upward until the region of the upper wound is reached on all sides. The musculature is then divided so that the cleft between the mucosa and the musculature communicates with the upper wound. As soon as the gut has been freed completely from the anus in this manner, it is pulled down through the anus until its diseased segment lies well outside of the anus. The segment is amputated a short distance distal to the anus and is sutured to the edge of the skin wound around the anus.

The "telescope" procedure is so dependable that failures of the suture are only rarely observed, and then as a rule only in case of nutritional disturbances of the proximal gut. It ought always to be used, therefore, when sufficient material is available and this type of operation is attempted. It is only to be regretted that even after perfect healing, complete continence is rarely achieved, due to the unavoidable damage to the sphincter and to the nerves of the sacral plexus supplying it.

(2) *Resection of the Rectum by the Vaginal Approach*

Resection of the rectum, less easily than amputation, may also be performed by the vaginal approach in the female. The posterior wall of the vagina which is well exposed by a speculum is split in the midline from the cervix to the vaginal entrance. At the point where the incision reaches the perineum it forks and passes a short distance beyond each side of the anal opening. The completed incision has the shape of an inverted Y. Both vaginal flaps are dissected free to right and left from the underlying tissues, and held with sharp hooked retractors. This brings the anterior wall of the rectum into view. The rectum is freed above the sphincter ani on all sides and a rubber tube or a strip of gauze is passed around it. The dissection is continued and the bowel gradually freed from its attachments in front and on the sides, with division of the levator ani, until the pouch of Douglas appears above. Posteriorly the rectum is freed from the hollow of the sacrum by blunt dissection. After the opening of the peritoneum the operation is carried to completion in the same manner as in the dorsal resection procedure.

The surgeon will find the dorsal approach more satisfactory in most cases, and equally as serviceable as the vaginal method in all cases of resection.

(3) *Appendix: Treatment of Fecal Fistula and of Stenosis of the Rectum following Resection of the Rectum*

If a fecal fistula develops after resection of the rectum, it is first necessary to wait for the main portions of the large operative wound to heal and for the fistula to become smaller. During this time the development of a rectal stricture must be prevented by bouginage and by the use from time to time of an indwelling rectal tube. If in spite of this a marked stenosis of the gut develops and if the fecal fistula becomes very annoying to the patient, he will often be most benefited by the subsequent establishment of a permanent abdominal artificial anus. The short-circuited lower bowel distal to the artificial anus may either be allowed to remain, or it may be removed subsequently by one of the methods used for amputation of the rectum.

If an attempt is to be made to close the fistula with preservation of the lower bowel and the natural anus, this task will be made easier and more likely to succeed by the establishment of a temporary abdominal artificial anus. In case the attempt to close the fistula is unsuccessful, the double-barrelled abdominal anus may be allowed to remain as a permanent anus.

The first step in the treatment of an intestinal fistula is the removal of the stenosis beyond it. If bouginage is unsuccessful, open operation must be resorted to. After spreading the anus open widely with blunt retractors, the stenosis is divided on the sides with a knife or is widened by dissecting out the scar tissue until a free straight passageway is made to the upper part of the bowel. The epithelialization of this wound channel can be attempted by keeping a rubber tube in it for a number of weeks. The rubber tube may be provided with Thiersch grafts in the manner described and illustrated in Vol. I, page 397, before placing it in the freshened stenosed segment. The tube is fastened in situ for 10 to 14 days. In every case bouginage must later be resumed.

Pedicled skin flaps rarely lead to a dilatation of the stenosis because of the lack of material and the unfavorable conditions in the narrow funnel-shaped wound.

It is futile to attempt to close the fistula until the stenosis has been removed. Simple freshening and suture of the fistula is never successful. Covering the fistula by means of a large pedicled skin flap from the neighborhood offers a good prospect of closure (Fig. 342). The skin around the fistula is

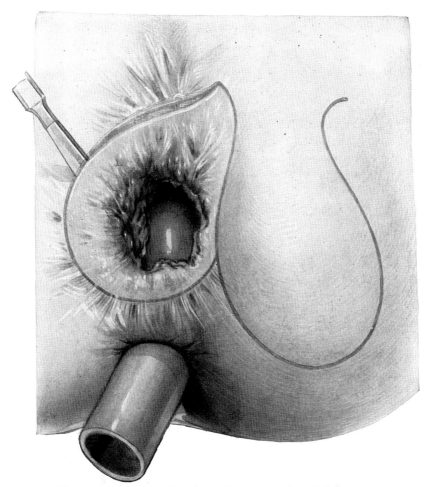

Fig. 342. Closure of a fecal fistula arising after a resection of the rectum. A stout tube has been inserted into the terminal bowel. An incision is made around the fistulous opening. The skin flap intended for the closure of this wound is outlined in red in the illustration.

dissected free and the flap is turned inward, and sutured into the denuded area. These attempts are not always successful. Often enough the establishment of a permanent abdominal anus terminates the time-consuming efforts to close the fistula.

In chronic inflammatory stricture of the rectum due to lues, gonorrhoea, tuberculosis or a lymphogranulomatosis, the establishment of an artificial sigmoid anus may also at times be the last resort for the relief of a condition which severely taxes the patient. To remove the torturesome tenesmus and to prevent the progress of the disease process it may even be necessary to perform an amputation of the rectum by the combined procedure, which is carried out in the manner described under carcinoma of the rectum.

3. The Abdomino-Sacral Procedure (Quénu)

(In the English speaking countries the Jones, Coffey, Miles, or Lahey technique is usually employed. These operations are alike in their general principles and are carried out as amputation operations. I. S. R.)

In the combined procedure, the gut segment to be removed is usually attacked from above through a laparotomy and then from below by the dorsal approach or by one of the other procedures from below as previously described. As a rule the operation is begun with the laparotomy and the abdominal wound is closed, with the exception of an abdominal artificial anus which may have been established, after the complete performance of the abdominal operation. The patient is then turned over and the lower operation is performed at once or this may be postponed until a later time, the abdomino-sacral or abdomino-dorsal procedure. The operation can however be begun below and concluded with the laparotomy, the sacro-abdominal or dorso-abdominal procedure. The last mentioned is frequently an emergency measure when an operation begun from below cannot be completed in this manner. The prognosis is naturally made less favorable by such an enforced change in the plan of operation. Changing back and forth between the upper and the lower operative field, is a measure which is highly questionable because of the unavoidable danger to asepsis. It should therefore be avoided if at all possible.

The combined operation can be carried out as a one-stage or a two-stage operation. The chief considerations mentioned on page 402, will again be emphasized at this point. In the one-stage operation, the emphasis lies on the abdominal part of the procedure, because the mobilization of the rectum is performed as far as possible from the abdomen, while the dorsal part of the operation consists, in case of amputation, only in the excision of the anus requiring but a few minutes, and in case of resection in the transsection and suture of the gut. (This is not always done. In the one or two-stage abdomino-perineal operation the sigmoid, below the colostomy, and the pelvic colon are extraperitonealized. The dissection below the pelvic floor need not be done from the abdominal approach. I.S.R.) In freeing the rectum from the pelvis from above it is not possible to use the electrosurgical knife. The tumor-bearing segment and the part of the operative field first under the suspicion of metastasis must be carefully freed. On the other hand, the combined one- or two-stage operation offers the greatest hope for a permanent cure, at least theoretically, because it is as radical as anatomic limitations permit. Its disadvantages are the magnitude of the procedure and, in the obese, the difficulty of the technique. Weak or excessively fat patients can therefore not be subjected to it as a routine measure. In case of a high-lying carcinoma the combined procedure alone is to be considered, since, in the operation from below, the approach and the visibility are too limited.

In the two-stage procedure, the mobilization of the gut in the initial abdominal part of the operation may be carried only to a point where no nutritional disturbances are to be feared. (The vascular supply to the bowel which is to be removed at the second stage must be preserved or necrosis with spreading infection will result. I.S.R.) The emphasis of the procedure therefore falls upon the second dorsal stage of the operation. The two-stage procedure however has these advantages: The electrosurgical knife can be used almost exclusively in the crucial part of the operation, the dissection of the diseased gut out of the pelvis. The division of the operation into two stages with an intervening space of time greatly lessens the demands upon the strength of the patient. This type of procedure, of all the methods of the radical treatment of rectal carcinoma, appears to be the one in which the sum of radicality plus sparing of the patient is greatest.

(A) SINGLE-STAGE COMBINED PROCEDURE

In the majority of cases the goal of the one-stage combined procedure is the extensive amputation of the terminal gut (amputation of the rectum, extirpation of the rectum). The combined procedure may however be carried out as a resection, by completing the operation by the "telescope" method.

A purely abdominal procedure, that is, the performance of the entire operation from the abdominal cavity alone, is possible only when the gut segment distal to the tumor remains in the body with its proximal end closed and buried extraperitoneally in the pelvis. This in turn is possible only in case of a very high-lying carcinoma, in which the gut at its lower line of transsection can still be reached and securely closed from above. Such lesions are more apt to be in the sigmoid than in the rectum. At any rate, one should always think of this procedure when the laparotomy discloses a high-lying rectal carcinoma or a low-lying sigmoid carcinoma.

The advantage which the laparotomy offers in the combined procedure for the search for intra-abdominal metastases should always be fully utilized. In this connection, one should not forget to palpate the liver. It will prevent many a purposeless intestinal resection or amputation.

(1) *Mobilization of the Gut through the Abdomen*

The bladder is carefully emptied and a rectal tube is inserted. After the induction of the girdle type of spinal anaesthesia, I have the patient placed in the Trendelenburg position, head toward the source of light, legs bent down at a right angle, so that any further exaggeration of the Trendelenburg position is possible at a moment's notice. For this purpose there must be an operating table especially constructed for an exaggerated Trendelenburg position. I use a table of my own design which holds the patient securely by the legs just above the ankles. The midline from the symphysis to the umbilicus and the region above Poupart's ligament on the left intended for a possible artificial anus are marked with a dye. The surgeon, standing at the left of the patient, opens the abdominal cavity by an incision reaching from the symphysis at least to the umbilicus. At the symphysis the incision is carried down to the bone, avoiding the bladder. The recti are nicked on both sides of the incision close to the symphysis. The abdominal wound is widely opened by means of a self-retaining retractor.

While traction is made on the rectum anchored in the pelvis, an attempt is made to palpate the tumor from above and to determine its extent and mobility. The abdominal cavity, including the liver, is then searched for metastases. If radical resection or amputation no longer seems feasible, an artificial anus is established at the indicated point in the left inguinal region.

If it appears that the tumor can be radically removed, all the abdominal viscera with the exception of the rectum and the sigmoid are displaced toward the liver and carefully walled off with large moist sponges, while the patient is gradually raised to an exaggerated Trendelenburg position. The isolation of the operative field is of considerable importance in the conduct of the operation. The walling off must be so dependable that it will not be disturbed in the event of straining or gagging by the patient. Under no condition should loops of small bowel or the cecum be visible or protrude. The true pelvis and the whole of the white line must lie freely exposed distal to the compresses.

In the female a long silk suture is passed around each tube. A heavy clamp is attached to the ends of each thread and hangs out at the sides of the wound. In this manner the adnexa can be held out of the operative field satisfactorily.

If the sigmoid is fixed by adhesions on the left, it is put on stretch and is freed by dissection. This can usually be done with ease and without bleeding, until the sigmoid hangs freely by its mesentery and can be drawn over to the right.

If amputation of the rectum has been decided upon as a single stage operation it is advisable as the first operative measure to ligate both internal iliac arteries, since this greatly lessens the bleeding during the freeing of the rectum from the pelvic wall. However, if a resection of the rectum is planned, the ligation of these two vessels should be omitted, since they give rise to the middle and inferior hemorrhoidal arteries supplying the rectum.

To ligate the internal iliac artery the sigmoid is first drawn to the left. As a rule it is not difficult on the right side of the pelvis to find the bifurcation of the common iliac artery just below the pelvic brim where the internal iliac artery dips down into the true pelvis (Fig. 343). The peritoneum is carefully pulled upward and lateralward, and at the point where it is reflected onto the sigmoid it is incised from the fold of Douglas toward the vertebral column. Posteriorly the incision extends into the peritoneum of the mesosigmoid, however without injuring the vessels visible beneath. The lateral cut edge of the peritoneum is retracted upward and outward and is undermined. This denudes the right internal iliac artery of peritoneum (Fig. 344). If the lateral cut edge of the peritoneum is on too much tension, it is further divided at this point by an incision perpendicular to the artery, and the right-angled flaps so formed are dissected free. The internal iliac artery is freed on all sides, partly by blunt, partly by sharp dissection, and with extreme care to avoid the accompanying vein. The ureter must also be kept in mind as it crosses the vessels at this point. It is just visible through the peritoneum and may at times be recognized by its worm-like contractions. It is exposed for a short distance and displaced lateralward (Fig. 344). An aneurysm needle with a catgut ligature is passed around the internal iliac artery from within outward, avoiding the accompanying vein on the inner side, and the vessel is tied. **A left-handed** aneurysm needle is necessary for the ligation of the right internal iliac artery. If the artery is sclerotic, the ligature must not be pulled too tight, lest it cut through.

With the sigmoid drawn to the right, the peritoneum is incised on the left in a similar manner and the left internal iliac artery is ligated. Here, too, the vein lies on the inner side of the artery.

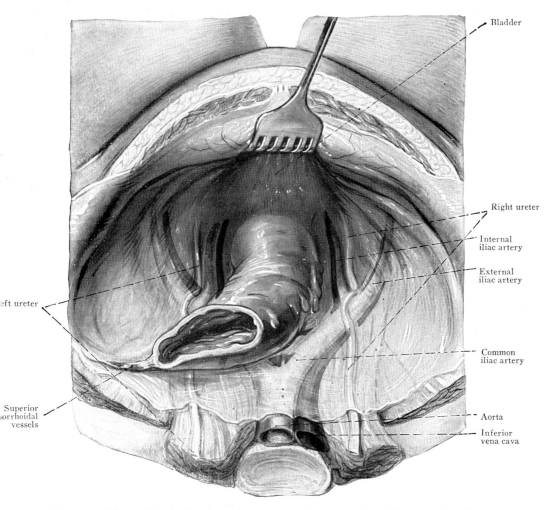

Fig. 343. View of the pelvic floor from the abdominal cavity. The mesosigmoid approaches the gut from the left side. The ureter courses retroperitoneally in front of the great vessels to the bladder. The bladder is drawn forward by means of a retractor, exposing the space of Douglas.

A hooked retractor is inserted into the posterior wall of the bladder or of the uterus just above the fold of Douglas and the bladder (Figs. 343 and 344) or the uterus is drawn well forward and upward. At the same time, the sigmoid is retracted backward. This puts the peritoneum on stretch as it extends from the posterior surface of the uterus or bladder to the gut and clothes the pelvic floor. The peritoneum is incised in the bottom of the pouch of Douglas. The incision ends on each side in the incisions made for the ligation of the internal iliac arteries. By these incisions, the peritoneum of

the pelvic floor surrounding the rectum at its entrance into the lower pelvis
has been divided on all sides in the form of a lyre. The middle section of
the lyre lies in the pouch of Douglas, the two limbs embrace the gut and run
upward toward the base of the mesosigmoid on both sides of the spine.

The two limbs of the lyre are now prolonged as far as the dome of the
sigmoid loop on each side of the mesosigmoid, avoiding for the time being the

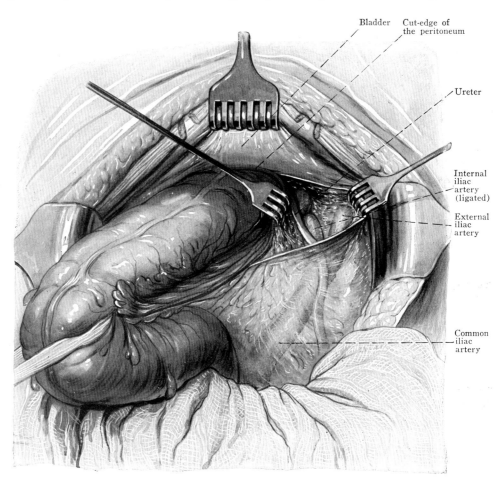

FIG. 344. Extirpation of the rectum by the combined procedure. The abdominal cavity
has been opened by a midline incision above the symphysis. The sigmoid has been caught up on
a strip of gauze and drawn to the left. The peritoneum of the pelvic floor has been split over
the iliac vessels on the right. The continuation of the incision onto the right side of the mesosigmoid and onto the reflected fold between the rectum and the bladder has been outlined in
red in the illustration. The right internal iliac artery has been ligated, care being taken to
avoid any injury to the ureter.

vessels in that structure (Fig. 344). For this purpose the mesosigmoid is put
on stretch by traction on the sigmoid, which was reflected toward the left,
and the incision is carried through the peritoneum on the right side of the
mesosigmoid without injuring the vessels. The vessels on the right side of
the mesosigmoid as they lie exposed in the incision are picked up individually
on an aneurysm needle, doubly ligated and divided. This is done as close to

the spine as possible and always medial to any glands demonstrable in the mesentery. Any single glands situated along the spine are removed separately. Later the line of division shifts to the free mesentery and is continued to the dome of the sigmoid loop.

In a similar way the sigmoid is pulled to the right and the same procedure is carried out on the left side of the mesosigmoid. This produces an opening in the mesosigmoid through which a rubber tube or a strip of gauze is passed (Fig. 344). In this manner the vessels of the mesosigmoid are divided between ligatures alternately on the right and the left and the gut is gradually freed to the extent which seems necessary. Above, this is as far as is necessary to bring the proximal end of the bowel easily to the site selected for the artificial abdominal anus. Below, it is to the point where the sigmoid loses its mesentery and becomes the rectum, which lies against the sacrum.

The dissection of the rectum from the depths of the pelvis follows. By continuing the mobilization it is possible to separate the rectum without difficulty from the sacrum and even the coccyx by blunt dissection. However this freeing of the posterior wall is usually not carried beyond the coccyx until later, when the dissection has made the necessary progress on the other aspects of the bowel in the region of the pelvis.

In order to free the lateral aspects of the rectum in the pelvis, the sigmoid and rectum are pulled first to the right, then to the left, and the dissection proceeds parallel to the bowel down into the pelvis through the peritoneal incision encircling the gut. The connective tissue here encountered is so loose that one can proceed downward quickly. For this purpose the lateral edge of the peritoneal incision attached to the pelvis is retracted lateralward and the rectum is pulled medialward by the hand. The exposed connective tissue is separated with a sponge mounted on a forceps. Denser fan-shaped strands of connective tissue which run in the frontal plane between the rectum and the pelvic wall on the right and left are ligated if necessary and divided with a long scissors, whereupon the rectum can be pushed away from the pelvic wall. Bleeding is rarely encountered, due to the preliminary ligation of the internal iliac artery. Should bleeding occur nevertheless in unligated strands, the vessels are caught with hemostats and ligated. In this manner the dissection proceeds downward, and the resultant deep pockets on the right and left sides of the rectum as well as the pocket between the rectum and the sacrum are constantly brought into communication. The transverse strands of connective tissue are divided with the scissors. The ureter, which was exposed during the ligation of the internal iliac artery, may be exposed and freed from this point to its entrance into the bladder at any time if it seems to be in danger.

Only on its anterior surface, that is, below the pouch of Douglas, is the rectum more firmly attached to the bladder and the prostate or to the uterus and vagina and here it must be freed by sharp dissection. For this purpose the bladder or the uterus is drawn forward and upward and the rectum is pushed backward with a specially shaped spatula covered with a thin layer of gauze and with a crescentic notch at the end (Fig. 345). In the cleft so formed one proceeds with a long scissors, alternately cutting the short bridges of connective tissue as they are put on stretch and separating the remainder by blunt dissection. As the depth of the operative field steadily increases, a scissors about 25 cm. long becomes necessary.

In the attempt to connect the pocket made along the anterior surface of the rectum with those on its sides, a number of coarse, fan-shaped strands of connective tissue extending from the rectum to the lateral wall of the pelvis are made taut. They can be picked up on the finger and are divided with the long scissors. This does not usually result in any bleeding. If so, the bleeding vessel is caught with a hemostat and ligated.

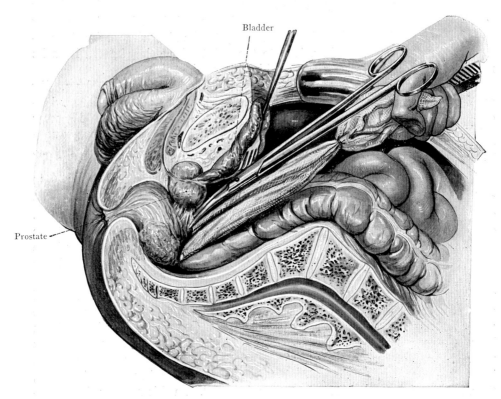

Fig. 345. Extirpation of the rectum by the combined procedure. Freeing of the anterior wall of the rectum from the prostate. Semidiagrammatic sagittal section. The posterior wall of the bladder is pulled upward with a sharp hooked retractor and the rectum is pushed backward with a spatula the end of which has a crescentic margin so that the fibrous tissue connections between the prostate and the rectum are put on stretch. They are divided with a very long scissors.

This circular dissection of the rectum is carried out by alternately dissecting on the right side, then on the left, in front, and behind the bowel. In this way the gut is gradually freed on all sides from its attachments. It is surprising how far down this dissection of the rectum can be carried from above. In patients who are not too fat it may be continued until the posterior surface of the bladder and of the prostate or the posterior wall of the vagina is freely exposed and until the anterior surface of the coccyx can be palpated. The rectum is now attached only by the sphincter mechanism and the skin of the anus and can be grasped in its full circumference from above all the way to the anus without any obstruction. Further progress from above is blocked by the funnel-shaped levator ani as it runs from the sides of the pelvis to the sphincter area and forms the floor of the pelvis.

It is a matter of opinion and custom whether the dissection of the rectum from above should be carried to this extreme. It is further determined in the individual case by the accessibility of the lower pelvis and the extent of the lesion. The freeing of the lowest section of the bowel is of course also relatively easy from below, after the proper plane of cleavage has been opened from above. Usually the dissection is continued from above as long as it proceeds without great difficulty. If an amputation is planned, it is necessary to carry the dissection to the point where the anal segment of the rectum after the transsection can be dropped into the pelvis and the roof of peritoneum can be completely closed over it.

If in the female the genital organs are involved by the carcinoma, the uterus and adnexa are also freed from above. This is done as follows: These structures are included in the lyre-shaped peritoneal incision, the middle portion of which is located between the uterus and the bladder, while its lateral extensions encircle the adnexa on their lateral sides. The bladder is drawn forward and the uterus is pulled backward. The cervical region is then separated from the bladder and the anterior vaginal vault is opened. The adnexa are pulled upward and toward the midline and the strands of tissue which are made taut on the sides and which contain the uterine arteries are doubly ligated and divided. (The ureters must be carefully exposed and guarded so as not to damage them. I.S.R.)

If the vagina can be completely preserved, the uterus is freed from the anterior, lateral and posterior vaginal walls until the anterior wall of the rectum is reached. Here the separation is continued between the posterior vaginal wall and the anterior wall of the rectum. If the posterior wall of the vagina is diseased, the anterior fornix is opened and the anterior vaginal wall is divided in sound tissue with scissors from above downward on the right and left as far as may be necessary. Care must be taken of the ureters while working at the sides of the vaginal fornix.

Should the occasion arise, no difficulties are involved in removing the adnexa on one side only, while the adnexa of the other side and the uterus are preserved. A detour of the lyre-shaped incision is carried around the diseased adnexa on their outer side and returns between the lateral wall of the uterus and the adnexa to the fold of Douglas. In deepening this incision, the broad ligament is doubly ligated and divided.

After the dissection of the gut has been completed, the decision between amputation and resection of the rectum must be made in those cases in which the possibility of resecting the gut and reestablishing its continuity still exists, and in which amputation is therefore not certainly indicated from the start. Resection with reestablishment of continuity is contingent on the presence, proximal to the lesion, of a sound and well-nourished segment of intestine which can be drawn to the anus without tension. The part of the sigmoid which most nearly meets this condition is measured by first measuring the distance from the anus to the fixed point of the loop, and then laying off this distance on the gut. If the loop is long enough, resection with reestablishment of continuity can be undertaken. Otherwise, amputation or resection without reestablishment of continuity but with establishment of an artificial anus is performed. Valuable information as to the suitability of the sigmoid loop for preservation of continuity can at times be obtained prior to operation by means of roentgen-ray studies with a barium enema.

(2) *Continuation of the Single-stage Combined Procedure as an Amputation of the Rectum*

(a) **The Termination of the Laparotomy.** The funnel-shaped wound surrounding the rectum in the true pelvis is packed tightly with compresses. The ligation of the mesosigmoid is carried upward on both of its sides to the site of the intended division of the gut. At this point the gut is completely freed for a distance of about 5 cm. After the operative field has been carefully walled off, the sigmoid is divided so that its proximal end can be drawn to the left inguinal region without tension. If possible, the division should be performed with the aid of the Petz suture instrument and between the two rows of clips, otherwise between two circular ligations. A condom is pulled over each intestinal stump and tied, unless in a given case it seems safer to invaginate the closed end of the gut by means of a Lembert suture.

If the carcinoma is situated rather high so that after the division of the sigmoid above the lesion a sound, completely free gut segment distal to the carcinoma can be reached from above, the gut is again divided at this point in the same manner and the gut segment bearing the carcinoma is removed. In such a case we are really dealing with a carcinoma of the lower sigmoid rather than with one of the upper rectum. The anal segment of the rectum can then be permitted to remain in the body permanently, provided that it can be dependably closed from above with Lembert sutures. This procedure is nothing other than a resection of the diseased gut segment without reestablishing continuity and with establishment of an abdominal artificial anus.

A very dependable closure of the end of the anal segment of the rectum and its thorough burial in the bottom of the pelvis is accomplished in the following manner: After the compresses have been removed from the pelvis, a sound made of thick fused copper wire and bent to form a loop at the end, is introduced through the anus into the rectum by an assistant who need not be scrubbed up. In an emergency a Babcock sound may be used (Vol. I, Fig. 513, page 459). After the division of the intestine, the end of the sound is advanced to the closed end of the gut. The surgeon, who can feel the wire loop through the wall of the gut, passes a heavy silk suture through the gut and the loop of the sound. The thread is tied. The assistant then carefully withdraws the sound. This pulls the divided end of the anal segment of the gut into the interior of the intestine like an inverted finger of a glove. The surgeon can then easily apply a row of sutures over the buried end, and if need be, a second or even a third row (Fig. 346). The assistant will have little trouble in pulling the tied end of the gut down far enough to cut the suture holding the sound so that the sound can be withdrawn. The end of the gut may also be buried from above alone, without the use of a sound, simply by means of Lembert sutures.

In every case, after the removal of the compresses from the pelvis, the cut end of the anal segment of the rectum, guarded by a condom or Lembert sutures against escape of intestinal contents, is buried deep in the pelvis. For this purpose it is important that the insertion of a rectal tube is not forgotten at the beginning of the operation, to permit the escape of the contents of the bowel. It is our rule to insert a rectal tube before every abdominal operation.

The peritoneum is sutured without a gap over the entrance to the lower pelvis, like the roof of a tent. This is usually accomplished quite easily, since the peritoneum is very elastic and the posterior lower surface of the bladder or the uterus and adnexa can be used to help in the closure. The closure must be absolutely tight. If any gaps remain, there is not only the danger of an ascending peritonitis, but it is also possible that a loop of small intestine may be caught, with resultant intestinal obstruction. Should complete peritoneal closure be impossible, which has never occurred in my experience, the bottom of the wound in the pelvis should be walled off by a vioform gauze pack which should later be carried out through the dorsal wound and removed through it after several days.

After the pelvic floor has been securely reconstructed in this manner, the self-retaining retractor is removed from the abdominal wound and the proximal end of the divided sigmoid is brought out as a terminal artificial anus in the left inguinal region in the manner previously described. The left side of the abdominal wall is elevated. The layers of the abdominal wall are divided at the point previously marked for the location of the abdominal anus, the proximal end of the sigmoid is drawn through the opening and is carefully sutured inside and outside to the peritoneum and the skin. The gut may be opened at once or preferably after 1 or 2 days.

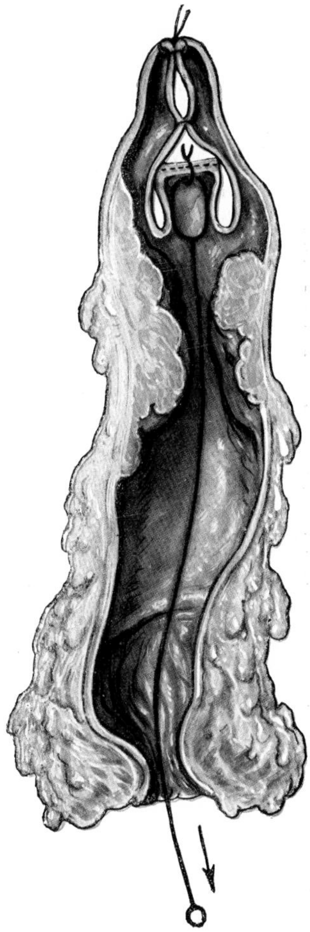

The midline abdominal incision is closed and securely dressed, so that the dressing will not slip when the patient is turned on his abdomen.

(b) **The Dorsal Operation.** If, as is the rule, the carcinoma was left attached to the lower segment of the bowel it must now be removed. The patient is placed in the abdominal-suspension or the lateral position customary for the dorsal approach and the operation is completed as an

Fig. 346. Invagination of the end of the transsected sigmoid in amputation of the rectum by the combined procedure. Diagrammatic. A sound with a ring-shaped end is i n s e r t e d through the anus and is fastened to the distal stump of the divided gut by a through and through suture. By means of the sound the end of the gut is invaginated like the finger of a glove. The invaginated end is closed, step by step, by suture.

amputation of the rectum by the dorsal route. The operation is performed essentially in the manner described for this procedure on page 410. The procedure is however much easier and can be more quickly performed, since in a short time the upper operative field is reached and since the dissection of the rectum has already been carried out in large part from above.

The dorsal operative field is infiltrated with a novocain-percain-adrenalin solution. Although the completion of the operation from the perineum, after a preliminary extensive dissection from the abdomen, can be performed by a simple incision around the anus, it is nevertheless advisable to resect the coccyx in every case. Its removal does no harm, it greatly enhances the visibility, sureness and speed of operating, and the drainage from the wound cavity is particularly good through the large dorsal wound.

The anus is closed by suture. The skin incision begins over the coccyx and encircles the anus. The skin is dissected away with the aid of sharp hooked retractors, and the coccyx is exposed and resected. By deepening the incision around the anus, the sphincter is freed. In so doing, considerable fat from the ischiorectal fossae on the sides is included and the vessels approaching the gut from both sides are ligated before being divided. If after ligation of the middle sacral artery the parietal layer of the pelvic fascia and the levator ani below the sacrum are incised in a transverse direction, the upper operative field is usually reached and the rectum, already freed from above, found. While the rectum is retracted to the right and the wound edge to the left, the freeing of the rectum is carried downward on the left side as far as the sphincter ani. The fibers of the levator ani are divided in the dissection. The same procedure is carried out on the right side.

The upper end of the rectum which lies free in the hollow of the sacrum is pulled down and brought out of the wound and is used as a handle in the rest of the dissection. A moist compress is placed in the large wound cavity against the peritoneal suture line, applied from above and clearly visible at the bottom of the pelvis. All strands of tissue made taut by traction on the rectum are divided between ligatures. In the region of the bladder caution must be used to avoid the ureter, which may hang far down if it was extensively mobilized during the laparotomy. The freeing of the anterior surface of the rectum, especially the separation from the prostate and urethra or from the vagina, can be performed easily and quickly under traction on the rectum and the appropriate use of retractors. This frees the rectum which was previously divided in the abdomen and it is removed.

After the removal of the compresses introduced toward the abdominal cavity, the large wound cavity is drained and packed lightly with vioform gauze. No suture is necessary. An indwelling catheter is inserted into the bladder.

After two days at the most a small opening is made in the abdominal artificial anus. A few days later the anus is more widely opened.

The vioform gauze is permitted to remain in the lower wound for 6 to 10 days in case of an aseptic course. It is then gradually removed. Under irrigation treatment the large wound tends to heal quickly. While the wound is healing, it may be treated by applications of radium, radium needles or by the Roentgen-ray.

(3) *The Continuation of a Single-stage Abdomino-sacral Operation as a Resection of the Rectum with Reestablishment of Intestinal Continuity*

(a) **The Termination of the Laparotomy.** If after the abdominal mobilization of the gut the above-mentioned conditions required for resection with the reestablishment of intestinal continuity are fulfilled, the operation may be concluded in that manner.

The intestine is freed as previously described. The compresses are removed from the pelvis and the mobilized bowel is entirely displaced into the bottom of the pelvis in such a way that the sigmoid runs in a straight line to the floor of the pelvis and the anterior surface of the sacrum. It is important that the bowel shall be able to empty itself during this procedure through a rectal tube which was inserted before beginning the operation. In spite of this it is at times difficult (but never impossible) to pack the bowel into the bottom of the pelvis in case of a small pelvic cavity and a very large sigmoid. At the point where the bowel passes through the peritoneum of the pelvic floor the peritoneum is carefully closed around the bowel by suture. The bladder or the female genitalia are usually drawn close for the suture. The closure must be absolutely tight on the one hand, and on the other it must not constrict the gut or its mesentery as they pass through into the lower pelvis. After the removal of all compresses the laparotomy wound is completely closed and a dressing is securely applied.

(b) The Dorsal Operation. This can be carried out by one of two methods.

The "Telescope" Procedure. If the rectum was mobilized so extensively from above that it has been freed on all sides from its surroundings to just above the sphincter, the upper operative field can be reached from below and the rectum completely freed by the procedure described under the modified Whitehead operation on page 378. For this procedure the patient is placed in the lithotomy position, the region of the anus is injected with an adrenalin-novocain solution and an incision is made around the anus at the junction of skin and mucosa. The surgeon works upward on all sides between the mucosa and the sphincter of the anus (Fig. 347), and finally cuts through the posterior wall in the lower operative field in the direction of the coccyx. In this way he enters the upper operative field. Once this has been opened at a single point, it is not difficult to separate the rectum on all sides and to complete the communication between the lower wound and that produced from above. As soon as the last connection has been divided, the carcinoma-bearing rectum prolapses out of the anus for a considerable distance. Since the gut is fairly heavy, it must be supported in order to avoid undue tension on the meso-sigmoid and should be brought out through the anus only to an extent which will not result in too great a strain on the vessels of the mesentery. Care must be taken that the gut and the mesentery are not twisted on their long axis.

In order to drain the large wound cavity in the lower pelvis of accumulated wound secretions, a forceps is inserted through the anus at the side of the rectum and a counter incision is made down on its point to one side of the midline just below the coccyx. The incision is enlarged to provide adequate room for drainage. In case of insufficient room, the coccyx may be resected. Through this opening a stout drainage tube is pulled from the outside into the wound cavity within the pelvis.

At the point where the gut emerges without tension from the anus, it is sutured to the edge of the skin wound surrounding the anus. Two or 3 cm. below this point the gut is closed by means of the Petz suture instrument and is divided between the two rows of clips, proximal to the carcinoma. This removes the carcinoma-bearing rectum. The proximal tip of the bowel projecting from the anus is once more fastened to the skin in the neighborhood

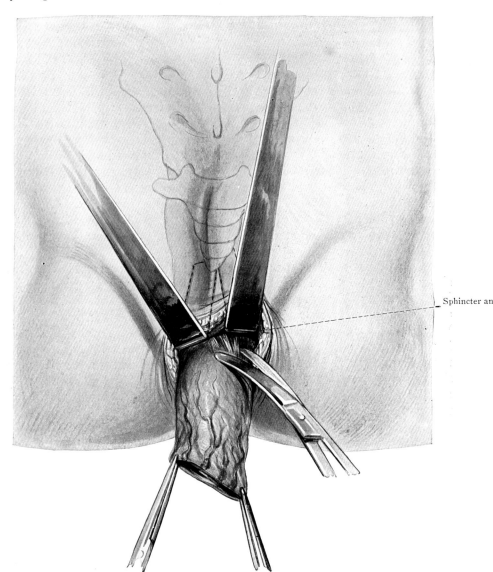

Sphincter an

FIG. 347. Resection of the rectum by the combined procedure. The rectum has been extensively mobilized through the abdomen as far as the anal region. Through an incision carried around the anus from below, the rectum is then freed from its surroundings, in particular from the sphincter ani. The tips of the Langenbeck retractors actually lie within the upper operative field. The last fibrous tissue strands separating the lower from the upper operative field are cut with the scissors.

of the anus by a few sutures. It may be opened at once or after several days.

   The Resection. If the bowel could not be freed on all sides as far as the sphincter in the course of the laparotomy, the laparotomy wound is closed and the patient is placed in the abdominal-suspension or the lateral position.

A skin incision is made in the midline, beginning just above the coccyx and ending 2 cm. above the anus.   In the manner previously described under resection of the rectum by the dorsal approach, the coccyx and if necessary also a portion of the sacrum are resected in the upper end of the wound, the middle sacral artery is ligated and the parietal layer of the pelvic fascia and the anal fascia are incised just below the edge of the bone.   This opens the upper operative field.   Proceeding from above downward, the surgeon mobilizes the rectum, passes a strip of gauze around it as soon as possible, and frees it from its attachments in the manner described under resection of the rectum. Since the proper planes of cleavage have already been opened from above, the mobilization is as a rule not difficult, even on the anterior side.   As soon as the gut has been freed on all sides to just above the sphincter in the manner described, it can be doubly divided, above and below the carcinoma.

The reconstruction of intestinal continuity takes place either by end-to-end anastomosis or by the "telescope" procedure after removal of the anal mucosa, as described on page 439 under resection by the dorsal route.   An end-to-end anastomosis is reenforced as well as possible by oversewing the adjacent tissues.   The wound cavity is packed lightly with vioform gauze.

If it becomes evident in the procedure from below, that the proximal end of the rectum, pulled down through the anus or exposed behind and intended for an end-to-end anastomosis, is insufficiently nourished, then the ideal procedure would be to reopen the laparotomy wound and to perform an amputation of the rectum with establishment of an abdominal artificial anus.   However, in view of the long duration of the operation and the demands upon the patient's strength entailed, this is rarely the course taken.   In most instances the alternative is chosen of bringing the proximal gut to the surface through the dorsal wound with the formation of a sacral anus, for it is usually possible to bring a well nourished part of the bowel to the surface in the upper angle of the dorsal wound.

If exceptionally even this is impossible, the gut is amputated in sound tissue and a large rubber tube is tied into its end and is brought out through the wound.   This insures the evacuation of the feces for the time being.   As soon as the patient has recovered sufficiently, an abdominal artificial anus should be established.

If the gut becomes necrotic after resection, for even an initially well-nourished gut may later become necrotic from thrombosis of the mesenteric vessels, the remaining sound proximal end is drawn out behind as a dorsal anus, if it is long enough.   Otherwise, the feces are permitted to drain unhindered into the dorsal wound cavity or an attempt is made to evacuate the feces temporarily through a large rubber tube inserted into the gut.   An abdominal artificial anus must be established secondarily as soon as possible, with or without the removal of the distal gut segment.

(B) MULTIPLE-STAGE ABDOMINO-SACRAL PROCEDURE

The two or three-stage combined procedure should, if possible, be the routine procedure.   At the first operation, the laparotomy, the abdominal cavity is inspected as to the possibility of a radical operation by determining the extent of the tumor and the possible presence of metastases, and an artificial anus is established, while the diseased bowel remains in situ. At the second operation, performed in a week or later, the rectum is amputated or resected (or the abdomen may be reopened and the distal portion of the sigmoid may be dissected free and placed beneath the pelvic peritoneum. I.S.R.).

(a) The abdominal part of the procedure is carried out according to the principles already given, by simply establishing a double-barrelled artificial anus (Figs. 314 and 318) after inspecting the abdominal cavity. The dorsal procedure consists either in the amputation of the rectum and the blind closure of the end of the proximal gut (Fig. 315), so that the short segment of gut which is situated between the abdominal artificial anus and the point of amputation and which is short-circuited on one side remains permanently in the body; or the dorsal part of the operation may consist in the resection and the reestablishment of intestinal continuity (Fig. 319). The closure of the artificial abdominal anus follows later (Fig. 320). (b) In the abdominal part of the operation the bowel is transsected in the region of the sigmoid (Fig. 316), the proximal limb is led to the surface as a single-barrelled abdominal anus, the distal limb is closed blind, and is buried under the peritoneum of the pelvic floor, after an extensive removal of the mesentery, tied off close to its base. The dorsal part of operation then consists in the complete excision of the terminal bowel distal to the point of division (Fig. 317). This procedure is used especially in the presence of suspicious glands in the mesentery.

(1) Two-stage Combined Amputation of the Rectum

(a) Leaving behind an intestinal segment short-circuited on one side.

(1) *Abdominal Part of the Operation (Fig. 314).* The abdominal cavity is opened preferably by a low left lateral rectus incision. However, if difficulties in the inspection of the abdominal cavity are to be anticipated, a midline incision below the umbilicus may be selected. The abdominal cavity after being opened is searched for metastases, not forgetting the liver, and the possible extension of the carcinoma to the pelvic floor, the bladder or the uterus is looked for. A particularly careful search is made for any suspicious glands in the mesosigmoid and in front of the spine. Only if no suspicious glands are encountered in these places is the operation continued in the intended manner as a two-stage procedure without division of the bowel; otherwise the combined procedure is carried out in one or two stages and with division of the sigmoid.

If the operation is to be completed in this manner, a double-barrelled artificial anus is established by the usual technique as described on page 234. The gut is brought to the surface through the lower angle of the lateral rectus incision, or, if the abdomen was opened in the midline, through a new opening in the left iliac fossa. The artificial anus is placed high in the sigmoid loop, so that in the dorsal operation the operator will have sufficient bowel at his disposal to bring down, and also to close the divided bowel. The abdominal incision is closed without drainage.

(2) *Dorsal Part of the Operation (Fig. 315).* After the wounds of the first operation have healed, the artificial anus has been shown to function perfectly in both directions, and the short-circuited rectum has been cleansed by

irrigations from above and below, the second stage of the operation, the dorsal amputation, is undertaken after 1 to 3 weeks, or even after months if the operability of the tumor does not become evident until later. The freeing of the rectum proceeds exactly in the manner described under primary sacral amputation on page 410. If the carcinoma is situated quite low, it occasionally becomes unnecessary to open the pouch of Douglas, since the cross-section of the remaining gut segment need not be brought to the surface but can be left in the bottom of the wound. One should however be radical in this direction and always in dividing the bowel should keep a good distance above the carcinomatous portion in view of the danger of cancerous involvement of the lymphatic structures in that region. Nearly always, therefore, the pouch of Douglas is opened in the manner described under amputation and a large segment of the sigmoid is brought down after its mesentery has been ligated and divided.

When the bowel has been freed sufficiently, it is brought out of the wound and divided. This frees the rectum and it is removed. The end of the proximal segment is closed securely with a Petz suture instrument or three-layer sutures reinforced with Lembert sutures and returned to the abdominal cavity. The slit in the peritoneum is closed tightly by suture. The wound cavity is packed with vioform gauze. It is unnecessary to attempt to make the wound smaller by means of sutures.

(b) Complete Extirpation of the Rectum.

(1) *Abdominal Part of the Operation (Fig. 316).* The first stage of this procedure, which is usually begun with the intention of carrying out the combined procedure without transsecting the bowel, is performed in exactly the same manner as was described in the previous section for the first stage of the two-stage combined procedure without transsecting the bowel. If suspicious glands are found in the mesosigmoid or in front of the spine, and the case nevertheless still seems suitable for a radical operation, then the combined procedure is carried out, either in a single stage or in two stages with division of the bowel.

In the latter instance the sigmoid is freed of its mesentery for a distance of several centimeters at as high a point as possible and is transsected with the aid of the Petz suture instrument. Each end of the divided bowel is enclosed in a condom. The proximal end is laid aside for the moment, while the surgeon turns his attention to the dissection and management of the distal gut segment.

The parietal peritoneum surrounding the bowel at its point of entrance into the lower pelvis is incised in the shape of a lyre, as described under the single-stage combined procedure on page 446. The internal iliac arteries, however, must not be ligated, in consideration of the blood supply of the bowel which is to be left in the body for the time being. The distal end of the sigmoid is now put on stretch so that its mesentery is taut and the gut is pulled forward, away from the spine. The connective tissue can be separated from the bone partly by blunt dissection, so that the anterior surface of the lumbar spine and of the upper sacrum is dissected clean. In continuation of this procedure and with a suitable deepening of the lyre-shaped incision the gut is freed in the direction of the anus as far as the level of the lesion permits.

In most cases it will be possible to divide the bowel, which has been freed for a considerable distance in this manner, a second time with the aid of the Petz suture instrument at a point distal to the first division. In this way a normal redundant piece of the sigmoid is removed. In each case, whether this second transsection is possible or not, the end of the remaining distal gut segment is buried with a Lembert suture. In doing this, it will be found particularly advantageous if this closure is carried out by invagination by means of a wire sound introduced through the anus, as described under single-stage combined amputation on page 450. It is necessary to make sure that the invaginated gut is well nourished. If this is not absolutely certain, the operation must be carried out in a single stage.

The distal bowel, which was closed blind, is dropped and the peritoneum is carefully closed over it in the manner described under single-stage combined amputation on page 451. If the stump of the bowel cannot be buried under the peritoneum, it is allowed to remain just above it but this is much less satisfactory.

The proximal limb of the divided sigmoid is brought to the surface as an abdominal artificial anus in the left inguinal region through the lower angle of the lateral rectus incision, or through a separate incision, in case the abdomen was opened in the midline. The rest of the abdominal wound is closed.

The sphincter is stretched. A stout drainage tube is inserted into the anus to afford free drainage for any wound secretion that may be formed in the rectum. This concludes the first stage of the operation.

(2) *Dorsal Part of the Operation (Fig. 317).* The second stage, which in case of assured and adequate nutrition of the buried intestine is usually undertaken within a week or at times even later, is performed in exactly the same manner as a primary dorsal amputation of the rectum. But since the bowel has already been divided and has usually been buried beneath the peritoneum, the operation is limited to the area below the pouch of Douglas. The dissection is carried on until the transsected bowel as a closed structure drops into the operator's hand. If, in so doing, the peritoneum is inadvertently or purposely opened, it must again be carefully closed at the end of the operation. After an amputation the wound is packed in the usual manner without applying any sutures.

(2) *Three-stage Combined Resection of the Rectum with Reestablishment of Intestinal Continuity*

(1) *The Abdominal Part of the Operation (Fig. 318)* is like the procedure described under two-stage combined amputation with an intestinal segment short-circuited on one side and left behind. But particular attention must be given to these points: the artificial anus must be in as high a loop as possible; the double-barreled segment must be as long as possible so that the sigmoid can later be brought down without difficulty and to the extent necessary to reestablish the continuity of the intestine, so that the closure of the artificial anus can be carried out with ease.

(2) *The Dorsal Part of the Operation (Fig. 319)* corresponds to resection

as described on page 430. The whole situation is, however, more favorable in the combined procedure for the following reasons: The short-circuited lower bowel, which remains in connection with the abdominal artificial anus, can be thoroughly emptied and cleansed by irrigation before the operation. The feces are entirely excluded from the operative field and from the intestinal sutures both during the operation and in the course of the after-treatment. Because of the presence of the artificial anus it is always possible to shift over to an amputation of the rectum with terminal closure and consequent unilateral short-circuiting of the lower bowel. The resection and the reestablishment of continuity can be carried out with end-to-end anastomosis, with the "telescope" procedure or by the modified Whitehead technique, as already described.

(3) *Closure of the Abdominal Artificial Anus (Fig. 320).* If the site of the resection has healed without a fistula and if the terminal bowel shows no stenosis, the double-barrelled artificial anus is closed in the manner described on page 253.

CHAPTER VI

OPERATIONS ON THE GALL BLADDER AND THE BILE PASSAGES

A. INTRODUCTORY REMARKS

1. ANATOMIC AND GENERAL CONSIDERATIONS

The gall bladder is differentiated into the fundus, the body and the neck. The tip of the fundus usually projects beyond the edge of the liver at the point where the lateral edge of the right rectus muscle is attached to the costal margin. From this point the gall bladder runs along the under surface of the liver in a ventro-dorsal direction. As a rule the gall bladder is closely attached to the liver by a layer of connective tissue and the peritoneal cover-

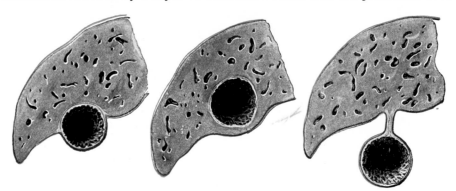

Fig. 348. Various positions of the gall bladder in relation to the liver. (a) Lateral apposition. (b) Intrahepatic position. (c) Free gall bladder connected with the liver by a peritoneal reduplication.

ing of the liver passes over the free surface of the gall bladder, the transition being sharply defined as a reflected fold (Fig. 348 a). After this peritoneal fold has been divided, the gall bladder can usually be freed from the liver without considerable bleeding. Preceding inflammation and abscess may prevent separation without annoying hemorrhage. Occasionally the binding layer of connective tissue is drawn out into a free mesentery clothed on both sides with peritoneum (Fig. 348 c). In very rare instances the gall bladder lies within the liver parenchyma (Fig. 348 b), so that it can be reached from the outside only after splitting a more or less thin layer of liver tissue (intrahepatic gall bladder).

The neck of the gall bladder merges without a clear-cut borderline into the cystic duct (average length 4 cm.) which turns off toward the median plane and after a varying distance joins the hepatic duct (Figs. 349-351). The cystic duct is usually quite twisted or angulated and in its interior has a number of spiral folds of mucosa, the valves of Heister, so that probing of

460

the duct is often impossible, even though it be patulous. The junction of the cystic duct with the common hepatic duct may be at right angles, or more usually, at an acute angle after the two structures have travelled parallel for some distance. The cystic duct may run behind the common hepatic duct and after a spiral course empty into its posterior or even into its left side. On raising the gall bladder by its fundus, the cystic duct is not as a rule put on

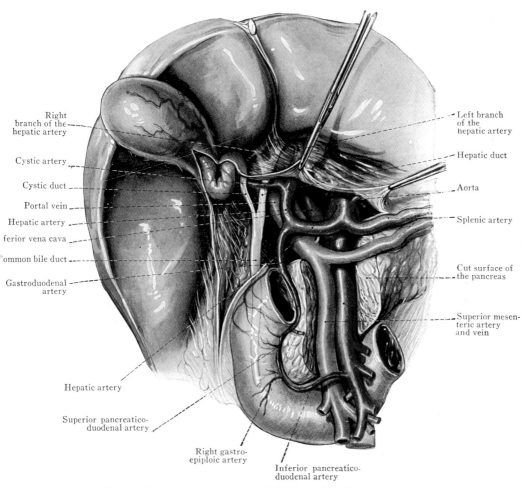

Right
branch of the
hepatic artery

Cystic artery

Cystic duct

Portal vein

Hepatic artery

ferior vena cava

ommon bile duct

Gastroduodenal
artery

Hepatic artery

Superior pancreatico-
duodenal artery

Right gastro-
epiploic artery

Inferior pancreatico-
duodenal artery

Left branch
of the
hepatic artery

Hepatic duct

Aorta

Splenic artery

Cut surface of
the pancreas

Superior mesen-
teric artery
and vein

FIG. 349. The blood vessels in the region of the liver, the bile ducts and the pancreas.

stretch. This occurs only when the neck of the gall bladder is grasped and retracted outward just above its transition into the cystic duct (Fig. 357).

The route of the bile from the liver to the duodenum begins in the intra-hepatic bile ducts, which converge in the portal fissure to form the right and left hepatic ducts coming from the corresponding lobes of the liver (Figs. 349-351). These join to form the common hepatic duct which runs as far as the junction with the cystic duct where the common bile duct begins. The common bile duct lies at first above and to the right side of the duodenum, and after it has passed diagonally behind the second portion of the duodenum in the retroperitoneal space, empties into the duodenum together with the pancreatic duct at the papilla of Vater. The opening in the papilla may be in the form of a common channel or two separate channels. The papilla of Vater lies on the dorsal side of the duodenum about at the junction of its vertical with its lower horizontal limb (Figs. 361 and 367).

The common bile duct as it runs free through the peritoneal cavity forms the right border of the hepatoduodenal ligament. Posterior to this free edge the examining finger passing from right to left can find the foramen of Winslow, if this is patulous, and thus enter the lesser peritoneal cavity. Several fingers can be introduced into this opening from the right, picking up the free edge of the hepatoduodenal ligament. In this manner this portion of the common bile duct can be palpated on all sides between the thumb and the index finger as far as the portal fissure (Fig. 363). The retroduodenal portion of the common bile duct can be palpated and inspected only after mobilizing the duodenum (Fig. 366). It usually runs a short distance through the substance of the head of the pancreas, but more rarely it passes behind the head of the pancreas.

In order to mobilize the duodenum, an incision is made through the peritoneum of the posterior abdominal wall just beside and parallel to the lateral wall of the descending limb of the duodenum. The duodenum is freed from the posterior abdominal wall by blunt dissection and is carefully reflected to the left. After mobilization of the duodenum the papilla of Vater can also be palpated between the fingers. It can be inspected only from the interior of the duodenum after making a longitudinal incision through the anterior wall (Figs. 367 and 371).

In the hepatoduodenal ligament there are situated, in addition to the common bile duct, the hepatic artery to the left of and on the same level as the common duct; and between the two but deeper, the portal vein (Figs. 349, 350 and 351). The hepatic artery divides in the portal fissure or even sooner into a right and a left branch for each lobe of the liver. In case the division is closer to the duodenum the right branch may turn sharply to the right and pass close to the neck of the gall bladder where it can easily be unintentionally injured. If one approaches the hepatoduodenal ligament from in front and the right, one first reaches the common bile duct and does not run the danger of injuring one of the other two structures. (Anomalies of the gastroduodenal, hepatic and cystic arteries and the cystic and right hepatic ducts are so frequent that these structures should be visualized before ligating and dividing any structures in this region. The ligation of the hepatic artery may result in the death of the patient, while trauma to the common hepatic ducts may result in bile peritonitis, a permanent fistula or stricture. I.S.R.) Nevertheless, mistakes can occur if the operative field lies very deep, if there are adhesions, or if the patient strains as a result of poor anaesthesia. In case of doubt it is advisable to aspirate the structure believed to be the common bile duct with a fine needle and syringe before opening it.

Unfortunately the common bile duct is covered on its ventral side, the one toward the operator, by a fairly close network of small thin-walled veins, the venous plexus of Zuckerkandl, from which troublesome bleeding can occur in exposing the common duct. However, the small veins can usually be pushed aside or can be picked up and divided between ligatures.   The common bile duct is also crossed by a few unimportant arteries which in exposing the duct must be carefully ligated before being divided in the interest of good visibility of the operative field.   Aside from these small vessels and the cystic artery, the common duct can be exposed from the duodenum to the portal fissure as a rule without injury to larger vessels or other important structures.

The cystic artery arises either from the hepatic artery or from the right branch of that vessel.   In most cases it passes behind the bile ducts from left to right to the gall bladder (Fig. 350), crossing behind either the common

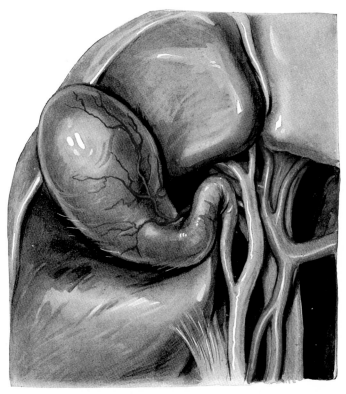

FIG. 350. Component parts of the hepatoduodenal ligament (free margin of the gastro-hepatic omentum). The cystic artery passes dorsal to (behind) the hepatic duct to reach the gall bladder.

hepatic duct itself or the right hepatic duct.   In 30 percent of cases, however, it runs in front of the bile passages (Fig. 351), so that it may easily be injured in exposing them, particularly the hepatic duct or the right hepatic duct.   The vessel, which may at times bifurcate early into two arteries of equal size, reaches the cystic duct, to which it is attached by connective tissue and fat, and runs in two branches to the dome of the gall bladder.   The artery can be separated from the cystic duct, whose convolutions it does not follow, after splitting their common peritoneal covering and it should be ligated separately from the duct before it is divided (Fig. 357).

The ligamentum teres runs in a reduplication of the peritoneum from the umbilicus to the umbilical notch of the liver, situated in the median plane.   It

forms the free margin of the falciform ligament which runs in a sagittal
direction and in the median plane to the diaphragm. In case of marked relaxation of the diaphragm, e.g., in deep anaesthesia, the liver drops after dividing
the ligamentum teres and incising the first part of the falciform ligament (Fig.
352). In spite of this, the liver can be raised and tipped over the costal
margin in only a fraction of cases (Fig. 353). This depends largely on the
contour of the costal margin and the shape of the liver.

The gall bladder lies in the immediate neighborhood of a number of
organs which also possess a serous covering. Below it lies the transverse

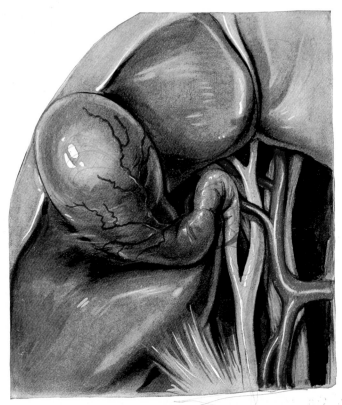

FIG. 351. Component parts of the hepatoduodenal ligament (free margin of the gastrohepatic omentum). The cystic artery passes ventral to (in front of) the hepatic duct to reach
the gall bladder.

colon with the mesocolon and the hepatic flexure. To the left are the stomach
and the first portion of the duodenum. The space above is limited by the
under surface of the right lobe of the liver. In inflammatory processes arising
in the gall bladder or in the neighboring bile passages, the inflammation can
extend to these adjacent organs and can give rise to adhesions (Fig. 353), to a
conglomerate tumor, to abscess, or the gall bladder may rupture into an adjacent viscus, resulting in a fistula between the bile passages on the one hand
and the stomach, duodenum, small or large intestine on the other. Aside
from the great danger of peritonitis during the formation of such a fistula,
there is the immediate danger of the passage of large gall stones, while later

there usually arises a chronic ascending infection of the bile passages by way of the internal fistula. The connection between the liver and gall bladder may become so fibrotic that a clean separation of the gall bladder from the liver becomes impossible. It must then be practically dug out of the liver. Abscess formation between the liver and gall bladder may also make dissection difficult.

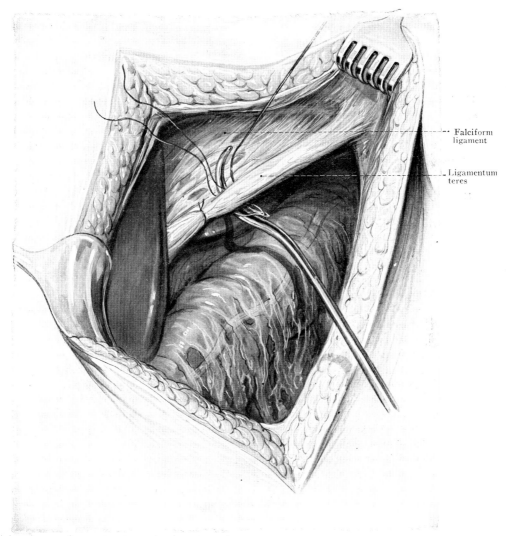

Fig. 352. Dividing the ligamentum teres. The ligament is made taut by elevating the umbilicus. It is picked up on an aneurysm needle and will be cut between two ligatures.

The exposure of the gall bladder, its neighborhood, and the bile passages is particularly difficult in the case of a shrunken gall bladder in which the gall bladder and the adjacent organs are fused into a solid mass of scar tissue in the midst of which lies the fibrotic gall bladder with its tightly enclosed stones.

An adequate approach to the biliary system is possible through several of the abdominal incisions described earlier in this volume. I prefer a right lateral rectus incision extended into a median costal margin incision with partial or complete division of the right rectus (page 18). The midportion of this incision is made first. Only after one has determined the position of the gall bladder, the mobility of the liver and the type of procedure to be

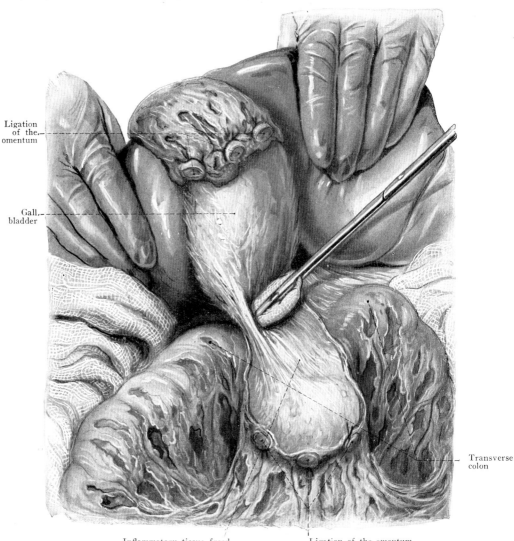

Ligation of the omentum

Gall bladder

Transverse colon

Inflammatory tissue freed from the gall bladder

Ligation of the omentum

FIG. 353. Exposure of the gall bladder. The liver is elevated and tipped over the right costal margin by an assistant's hands placed on each side of the gall bladder. Firm adhesions between the greater omentum and the fundus of the gall bladder have been divided between ligatures. Loose adhesions between the transverse colon and the body of the gall bladder are separated with a sponge mounted on a forceps.

undertaken, is the incision extended upward or downward. Many operators choose a midline incision above the umbilicus, which in case of necessity can be enlarged by a transverse incision beginning at the lower angle and dividing the right rectus. In my opinion the approach afforded by this incision is inconvenient. Kehr employed and popularized the "wave" or "Z-incision" (page 19), which begins at the xiphoid process, runs in the midline to a point half way between the xiphoid and the umbilicus, then divides the right rectus diagonally downward and ends at the outer margin of the right rectus as a lateral rectus incision of varying length. The right costal margin incision is also frequently employed (page 31). I used it for a long time. The access is good but there is considerable danger of postoperative hernia. (This has not been my experience. We have used it routinely in my clinic for several years and have found that postoperative hernia is rare if the incision is properly closed. I.S.R.)

When the abdomen has been opened in the midline above the umbilicus for a supposed gastric or duodenal lesion, the necessary room is then obtained if necessary by dividing the right rectus muscle. Appendicitis and gall-stone disease are also frequently confused. If the appendix was approached through a low lateral rectus incision, the incision can easily be continued upward as far as the costal margin and along the costal margin toward the xiphoid process. On the other hand, if a lateral gridiron incision was used, it is better to close this incision and to make a fresh incision over the gall bladder region than to damage the abdominal wall severely by cutting across the lateral abdominal muscles.

Access to the deep bile passages is made easier by accentuating the lumbar lordosis. To produce this position, the patient is placed on an air cushion before the operation. If difficulties are encountered, the cushion is inflated after the induction of anaesthesia and is deflated before suturing the abdominal wound. In order to assist in bringing down the liver and displacing trouble-some loops of intestine out of the operative field, the surface of the operating table can be so set that it slopes downward from the head end toward the foot and from the right toward the left. If spinal anaesthesia is being used the elevation of the head end is automatically ruled out. When general anaesthesia is used the operator had better stand on the left side of the patient than on the right as generally preferred, since with the patient in a left lateral position the operator has better access from the left and a better view of the deep bile passages.

Since complete relaxation of the abdominal walls is necessary for exposing the liver and the deeper bile passages, I prefer the girdle type of spinal anaesthesia in operations on the biliary system.

The operation for gall stones can be very simple, but it can also confront the operator with the most difficult problems of technique. Annoying, and occasionally almost insuperable difficulties may arise in operations on the biliary system from obesity; the presence of many pericholecystic adhesions; a firm consistency of the liver, which prevents dislocating the liver from beneath the costal margin and tipping it up, and poor relaxation of the abdominal wall associated with marked straining of the patient.

Most patients with gall-stone disease, as previously mentioned, carry with them the results of preceding attacks in the form of adhesions or distortions of the affected organs, in the form of scar tissue contractions or even internal fistulae. All these circumstances as well as the aforementioned frequent anatomic anomalies make it obvious that the exposure of the individual structures, especially the deep bile passages, can be unusually difficult and nearly or entirely impossible without damage to neighboring structures. Therefore even the more experienced operator in spite of every precaution will occasionally make errors or inflict unintended injuries.

2. INDICATIONS FOR OPERATION

Surgery of the bile passages and the gall bladder is in the majority of instances resorted to for gall-stone disease. Less frequent causes for operation are conditions which may or may not have been due to gall stones, such as suppuration, injury, congenital malformations or neoplasms.

The indications for operation are stated very differently by individual operators. There is unanimity at least on the point that acute conditions threatening life, in the form of inflammation spreading to the general abdominal cavity or to the portal vein, demand immediate operation. With the indications so stated that operation is practically the last resort to ward off an otherwise imminent death, it is obvious that the operation comes too late in many instances. The unfavorable result of such an operation is not to be blamed on the surgeon but to the delay of operation. In general, therefore, surgical practice has been accorded a much broader field.

In gall-stone disease the best and most radical view point demands operation following the first definite gall-stone attack. This opinion is based primarily on the following facts: Gall-stone disease does not clear up spontaneously. The dangers and the difficulties of operation become progressively greater with each attack, since every attack leaves anatomic changes behind it and the attacks, the associated changes in other viscera, and increasing age gradually undermine the patient's powers of resistance. The prospects of cure are steadily lessened by the progressive anatomic changes, changes which eventually may not be entirely remediable. Operation for gall stones performed early in a symptom-free interval is relatively not dangerous. The mortality should not exceed 5 per cent. Expectant treatment is in itself associated with danger to life. Finally, the operation usually cures the patient in a few weeks and at a slight cost, while otherwise he commonly faces an ailment that is costly and may last for decades. These considerations are so urgent and impressive that it seems justified to advise operation in a fairly young patient, otherwise well and with good resistance, as soon as there is no doubt of the presence of cholelithiasis.

Most operators take an intermediate position in regard to the surgical indications, in that they subject to operation only those patients who have had repeated attacks, in whom medical and Spa treatments have had no success, and in whom the severity of the attacks has frequently and materially impaired the patient's capacity for work and enjoyment.

Nor is there any unanimity on the question as to whether it is permissible to operate during an acute attack in the absence of a particularly urgent indication, or whether one should wait for a symptom-free interval. Experience has shown that the technique of the operation in an acute attack is not materially more difficult than in the interval. I am therefore of the opinion that as soon as one has definitely decided that an operation is indicated, one should not sacrifice the advantage of preventing further serious complications. This does not mean that the patient is immediately placed on the operating table. A few nights' sleep with the aid of narcotics, a satisfactory evacuation of the bowels, the appropriate preliminary treatment of the heart if this is indicated, a return to a normal body temperature and the subsidence of liver damage are advantages which counterbalance a delay of a few days, unless the severity of the condition makes immediate action desirable.

Chronic common duct obstruction by stones requires special discussion. It is impossible to be too emphatic in opposing the view point which, in the uncertain hope that a lodged stone will pass of itself, permits such a patient to lie for weeks or even months and which turns to surgical intervention only after the appearance of fever and chills or the obvious failing of the patient. The chances for the spontaneous passage of a lodged stone are very slight after 2 weeks. At the same time the resistive powers of the patient are rapidly diminished and the liver injury greatly increased. Therefore in complete obstruction of the common duct by stone, operation should not be delayed more than 2 weeks.

Jaundiced patients, as experience has shown, have an increased tendency to bleeding during and after operation. Hemostasis must therefore be carried out with particular care in these patients. The tendency to bleeding should also be lessened as far as possible by appropriate preliminary treatment as described in Vol. I, in which connection attention is called especially to calcium chloride, vitamine D, and the alpine sunlamp. (It would be a serious omission if I failed to point out that the most important measure in the preoperative preparation is the use of glucose. This may be given by mouth, but it probably is best given intravenously in a 5 or 10 percent solution. From 50 to 100 grams should be given every 24 hours for 3 or 4 days prior to operation. There is no good evidence that any calcium deficiency exists in obstructive jaundice and the editor considers its use superfluous. Glucose will do more to control bleeding than will calcium. If postoperative bleeding occurs blood transfusion should be resorted to. I.S.R.) The best prophylactic measure as well as the best treatment of hemorrhage is blood transfusion. The compatibility of donor and recipient must be determined, in my opinion, not only by the blood groups of donor and recipient, but by the absence of agglutination and hemolysis of the donor's blood in the recipient's serum and of the recipient's blood in the donor's serum as determined macroscopically on a glass slide.

Occasionally an acute insufficiency of the liver follows an operation on the biliary system, notably in long-standing common duct obstruction, especially if it has led to a hydrops of the bile passages, with the formation of white bile; or in severe infection of the liver. In this condition the patient may soon after operation develop symptoms very similar to those of shock, or else may soon become somnolent and present a picture not unlike that of uremia. Either condition is combatted most effectively by the liberal administration of glucose, partly intravenously and partly by mouth. At the same time 10 or 20 units of insulin may be given daily. (It has as yet not been proven that insulin is absolutely essential. I.S.R.)

In carcinoma of the biliary system the chances of permanent cure by operation are not good, so that a certain hesitancy in operating is understandable. However the very fact that the preoperative differentiation between cholelithiasis and carcinoma is very difficult and mistakes occur again and again, speaks in favor of operation, quite aside from the fact that early operation may disclose conditions which are peculiarly favorable to resection. If carcinoma produces common duct obstruction, prompt operation is always indicated, since in many instances it may at least rid the patient of the most distressing symptom of the disease, itching.

The question, as to whether after an uncomplicated operation on the biliary tract the abdomen may be closed without drainage ("ideal cholecystectomy"), is not answered unanimously at the present time. The circumstance that after a properly completed operation on the biliary system there remains no active infectious focus within the abdominal cavity and that bleeding has been completely controlled would argue for complete closure of the wound, in line with the fundamental principles governing the indications for drainage which I have previously discussed. As a matter of fact, we can unfortunately not be certain after an operation involving the opening of the bile passages and the mobilization of the gall bladder that a source of infection will not arise subsequently. Every suture of the biliary system, including the stump of the cystic duct as well as the common bile duct, is liable to some uncertainty because of the lack of peritoneum-covered material for closure, in contrast to the closure of intestinal segments. In the bed of the excised gall bladder, bile may escape from the tiny bile ducts which were opened and delayed bleeding may occur from the vessels of the liver parenchyma.

I, therefore, consider it better to insert a drainage tube in all cases and a small strip of vioform gauze packing in most cases. I have never seen any harm come from these measures. On the contrary, I have frequently benefited by them, as shown by the frequent escape of bile from the drainage tube during the first few days after the operation. (Although there is some difference of opinion on the question of drainage after cholecystectomy I believe the advice given in the preceding paragraph to be sound. I.S.R.)

The postoperative treatment after an uncomplicated operation on the biliary system differs in no respect from the measures employed after every other major laparotomy. If severe and continued vomiting follows the operation, a Jutte tube should be employed. If the postoperative course is uncomplicated, the packing, if this has been used, is removed in 4 or 5 days. The drainage tube is shortened daily and is completely removed on the sixth to eighth postoperative day.

The individual operations on the biliary tract have various objectives depending on the disease in question, and these objectives may frequently be reached by different routes. Nevertheless a number of constantly recurring principles can be set up, which will serve as the chief guide of procedure in most operations on the biliary tract and which are usually carried out in the same or in similar ways. Aside from the removal of all stones, three demands in particular are repeatedly being made on the operator: (1) treatment of infection within the biliary tract and in its surroundings, (2) establishment of free drainage into the intestinal tract of the bile formed in the liver, and (3) prevention of recurrence of the original disease. The individual operative measures attempt to achieve at times only one of these objectives, at times two or even all three.

B. OPERATIONS ON THE GALL BLADDER

1. Opening of the Gall Bladder (Cholecystotomy)

Cholecystotomy has as its object the single evacuation of the contents of the gall bladder. This operation only rarely comes into consideration at the present time as an independent procedure. The single evacuation of the gall bladder can rarely prevent the recurrence of infection or the reforming of gall stones, while this goal can be attained with considerable likelihood by cholecystectomy. However, if cholecystectomy is permanently or temporarily contraindicated by technical difficulties, by the poor condition of the patient or by a severe infection, cholecystotomy with temporary drainage of the gall bladder to the exterior is the next best procedure.

On the other hand, cholecystotomy plays an important role as an operative measure immediately preceding other operations on the biliary tract. In such cases it is always carried out as the first operative step if the size of the gall bladder impedes the approach to the deeper lying parts. This is above all the case in hydrops of the gall bladder, in empyema, in a gall bladder excessively filled with stones, or in marked distension of the gall bladder due to common duct obstruction. In every case the early evacuation of the gall bladder is indicated if there is danger of rupture and escape of pus when the damaged wall of the gall bladder is grasped or lifted.

After the neighborhood of the gall bladder has been carefully walled off with moist compresses, the wall in the region of the fundus is grasped with two Kocher forceps and is elevated. If the gall bladder is overdistended and friable it may be impossible or unwise to apply the forceps. A trocar and cannula attached to an electrically driven suction pump is introduced into the gall bladder and its contents are evacuated. The cannula must be quite large so that a very viscid fluid can flow through it. When the gall bladder is completely emptied, the cannula is withdrawn. The puncture wound is enlarged, so that the interior of the gall bladder is sufficiently accessible. Any remaining fluid is removed with sponges. Any gall stones present are removed with a gall-stone scoop or forceps. Stones lodged in the cystic duct can be milked upward by external pressure with the thumb and index finger (Fig. 354). Occasionally the whole mucosa can be removed as a necrotic sac, or a plug of fibrin can be extracted in a coherent mass.

After completely emptying the gall bladder, if a further operative procedure on the biliary system is to follow, the gall bladder is packed loosely with a piece of gauze and the opening is closed with a few stout sutures that grasp the entire wall. The suture ends are left long and furnish a valuable hold for lifting the gall bladder (Fig. 357).

If in the exceptional case cholecystotomy is an independent procedure, the opening in the gall bladder wall is closed as is an intestinal opening, first by a three-layer catgut interrupted suture and then by an invaginating sero-muscular suture.

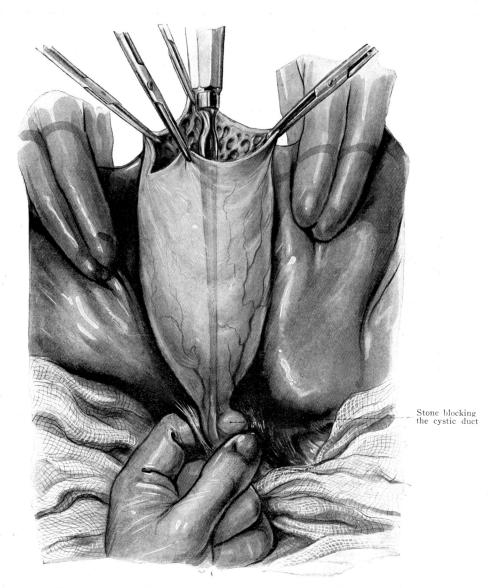

Stone blocking
the cystic duct

FIG. 354. The removal of gall bladder calculi by cholecystotomy. The fundus of the gall bladder has been opened. The wound edges are held apart with Kocher hemostats while the gall bladder is emptied with a gall-stone scoop. An obstructing stone at the beginning of the cystic duct is forced toward the scoop with the fingers of the left hand.

2. ESTABLISHMENT OF AN EXTERNAL BILIARY FISTULA (EXTERNAL CHOLECYSTOSTOMY)

Drainage of the gall bladder after a preliminary evacuation is looked on by most surgeons as an emergency measure, to be employed, in the presence of stones or inflammation, if the removal of the organ is inadvisable because of extraordinary technical difficulties, the poor condition of the patient or the severity of the infection. In this regard, drainage of the gall bladder is a very salutary procedure. It ought to be used more frequently than is commonly the case in old decrepit patients and in the severe acute infections.

By a few, the temporary drainage of the gall bladder is considered the procedure of choice in gall-stone disease. The proponents of this view claim for this procedure that it effects a cure of the inflammation of the gall bladder and of the catarrhal conditions causing the stones; that it is less dangerous; that in contradistinction to cholecystectomy, it preserves an organ, whose functional significance in a chemical sense and in the mechanical regulation of the entrance of the bile into the intestine can not be summarily denied. For reasons to be explained later, I can not subscribe to a view that fundamentally opposes cholecystectomy in gall-stone disease.

An emergency cholecystostomy may occasionally be performed for a second reason. If in a patient with common duct obstruction it is impossible to remove the obstruction or to establish a communication between the distended bile passages and the gastro-intestinal canal because of excessive technical difficulties or the poor condition of the patient, an external biliary fistula in the form of a cholecystostomy can give the patient a great deal of relief as well as relieve the liver of the greatly increased ductal pressure.

The technique of the operation is the same as that just described for cholecystotomy, including the evacuation of the gall bladder contents. Instead of closing the opening in the fundus of the gall bladder at the end of the operation, it is sutured all around to the parietal peritoneum of the abdominal wound. (I never suture the gall bladder to the peritoneum unless I desire permanent drainage. I.S.R.) A large drainage tube is inserted into the gall bladder and led to the outside (Fig. 355). The neighborhood of the gall bladder is walled off from the general abdominal cavity by gauze packing. The remainder of the abdominal incision is closed. If, as is usually the case, the cholecystostomy is being performed in the presence of a severe infection of the gall bladder, the walling-off of the general abdominal cavity must be correspondingly extensive and carefully performed. This is accomplished by a gauze barrier that completely separates the whole free side of the gall bladder and the cystic duct from the remainder of the abdominal cavity.

Since, after the gall bladder has been sutured to the parietal peritoneum in the manner described, the surface of the gall bladder is separated from the skin surface by the thickness of the abdominal wall, a lipped fistula rarely results and the opening usually closes spontaneously as soon as the drain and the packing are removed.

It may be desirable to make the fistula a permanent one, as in the treatment of an irremovable obstruction of the common bile duct. (In such instances I prefer to anastomose the gall bladder to the stomach or duodenum. I.S.R.) In that case the opening in the gall bladder is sutured to the skin edge of the abdominal incision, after the parietal peritoneum has been sutured at a deeper level to the peritoneal covering of the gall bladder. The epithelium of the skin and the mucosa then grow together and the opening persists as a lipped fistula.

3. ESTABLISHMENT OF AN INTERNAL GALL BLADDER FISTULA (CHOLECYSTENTEROSTOMY)

The communication of the gall bladder with the exterior as just described is an emergency measure, since the resultant lack of bile in the intestine greatly impairs digestion and the persistent external drainage of bile is a constant

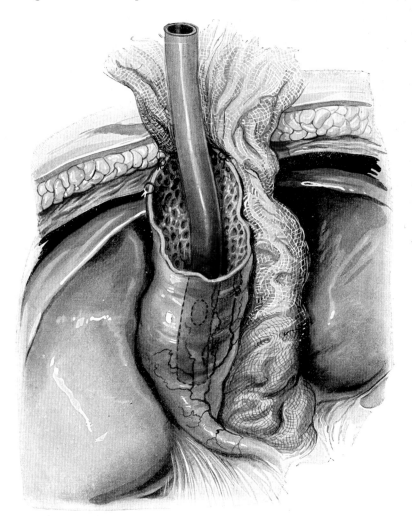

FIG. 355. External drainage of the gall bladder (cholecystostomy). The cut edges of the opened fundus of the gall bladder have been fastened by sutures to the edges of the abdominal wound. The surroundings have been guarded by gauze packing. A drainage tube leading to the exterior lies within the gall bladder.

source of annoyance to the patient. In case of an irremovable common duct obstruction it is therefore preferable to direct the bile into the digestive tract through an internal fistula. If the obstruction is in the immediate neighborhood of the papilla of Vater, as is most frequently the case in a carcinoma of the papilla or of the head of the pancreas, a choledochoduodenostomy is performed. However, if this procedure is very difficult, or if the obstruction is in the region of the common duct at some distance from the duodenum, it is preferable to anastomose the gall bladder to some other point of the intestinal canal, provided that the passage from the liver to the gall bladder is intact. A patulous condition of the channel from the liver to the gall bladder may be recognized, among other ways, by the distension of the gall bladder with bile and by the constant and continued flow of bile after the gall bladder is opened.

The gall bladder can be more or less safely anastomosed with the gastro-intestinal canal in three places, the stomach, the duodenum and the upper jejunum.

Anastomosis to the duodenum is the most natural, since in that case the bile reaches that part of the intestine which is normally accustomed to receive it. However, it is often quite difficult to bring the fundus of the gall bladder in contact with the anterior wall of the duodenum without tension. Furthermore, the delicate wall of the duodenum is less suited for suture than the strong wall of the stomach, so that a duodenal fistula occasionally develops, which must be looked upon as a serious complication.

The establishment of an anastomosis with the jejunum is a fairly involved procedure. A suitable loop must first be brought into the upper abdomen in an antecolic position, or it must be brought up by a retrocolic approach through openings in the transverse mesocolon and the gastrohepatic omentum. In addition, an entero-enterostomy between the bases of the loop in the lower abdominal space is recommended.

There are no such technical difficulties in anastomosing the gall bladder with the stomach. Experience has also shown that the introduction of the bile into the relatively bacteria-free stomach continues to be very well tolerated both by the stomach and by the biliary tract. Cholecystogastrostomy is therefore probably the procedure most to be recommended, provided that there is no obstacle to the emptying of the stomach into the intestine. This should not prevent the occasional use of the other two types of anastomosis, especially the duodenal, if the conditions are particularly favorable.

The first step in the establishment of an anastomosis between the gall bladder and the stomach corresponds to the procedure in cholecystotomy. After the gall bladder is emptied of its fluid and solid contents, the fundus is sufficiently freed from the liver so that it can easily be brought in contact with the anterior wall of the pyloric antrum. If possible, a fold of the anterior wall of the stomach is picked up within a clamp (Fig. 356). The opening previously made in the gall bladder can be used for the anastomosis. In many cases sufficient material will be available to make the anastomosis at another point, especially if the fundus of the gall bladder was previously freed to some extent from the liver. If it is possible to apply a clamp on the cystic-duct side of the anastomosis, the suture will be facilitated by blocking the otherwise troublesome flow of bile. Otherwise, one attempts to keep back the bile as long as possible by lightly packing the neck of the gall bladder.

The anastomosis itself is performed by the suture technique usually employed in the anastomosis of two intestinal segments. The delicate structure of the overdistended gall bladder wall constitutes a material difficulty, so that

it is scarcely possible at times to apply a sero-muscular suture without punc-
turing the mucosa. It is often advisable to use the instruments for blood
vessel suture in such cases. The posterior serosal suture is first applied with
interrupted silk sutures. The stomach and the gall bladder are then opened
with the electrosurgical knife. Next comes the posterior three-layer suture

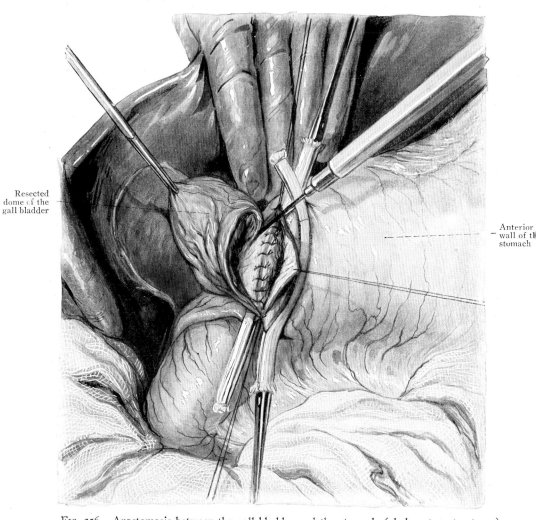

Resected
dome of the
gall bladder

Anterior
wall of the
stomach

Fig. 356. Anastomosis between the gall bladder and the stomach (cholecystogastrostomy).
A fold of the anterior wall of the stomach and the fundus of the gall bladder have been picked
up with intestinal clamps. Both structures have been joined by a posterior row of Lembert
sutures, and after being opened, by a posterior Albert suture. The redundant dome of the gall
bladder is cut away with the electrosurgical knife.

with interrupted catgut sutures (Fig. 356). The anterior wall of the gall
bladder is then also divided, removing the dome of the gall bladder. The
anastomosis is completed by the anterior three-layer suture and the anterior
sero-muscular suture. The stomach may be attached to the adjacent wall of
the gall bladder and to the surface of the liver by a few sutures.

    If the fundus of the gall bladder can not be sufficiently mobilized, the anastomosis between the gall bladder and the stomach may be performed side-to-side, as in the case of two segments of intestine, by simply making a linear opening in the dome of the gall bladder and without the removal of a part of the gall bladder.

If the anastomosis between the gall bladder and stomach has been accurately performed, the abdomen may be closed without drainage. Otherwise, a gauze pack and a drainage tube are inserted.

4. CHOLECYSTECTOMY

General Considerations. Cholecystectomy is the most frequent operation on the biliary tract. According to the prevailing view, gall stones are formed exclusively, or nearly so, in the gall bladder. Therefore the removal of the stone-forming organ would seem to be the surest measure of preventing the recurrence of gall stones. For most surgeons, consequently, the removal of the gall bladder is an essential part of the routine operation for gall-stone disease.

The controversy as to whether cholecystectomy or cholecystostomy is the operation of choice in cholelithiasis has been a very long one. Some surgeons believe that the routine removal of the gall bladder is an unnecessary mutilation of the body. They claim that the gall bladder has an important chemical function and a mechanical role in the distribution of the bile after the manner of a pressure chamber. They claim, too, that the reformation of calculi is prevented by prolonged external drainage of the gall bladder. These arguments can all be adequately answered. A thousand-fold experience has shown that no recognizable disturbances are caused by the loss of the gall bladder. The organ which the surgeon removes is no longer a sound gall bladder with a normal function, but a diseased viscus whose normal function is lost. If any damage to the body results from the removal of the gall bladder, it is trifling and is still the lesser of two evils. To be sure, it cannot be denied that gall stones may form in the deep bile passages after the removal of the gall bladder, but this is unusual. Personally, I hold to the principle of the removal of the gall bladder in cholelithiasis.

The removal of the gall bladder is also occasionally indicated in the absence of gall stones. This is true of those cases in which all the chemical manifestations of cholelithiasis are present and the gall bladder wall is evidently damaged, but in which in spite of the most careful exposure and search of the biliary tract no stones are to be found, and in which the inspection of other organs coming under suspicion (stomach, duodenum, pancreas, right kidney, hepatic flexure, appendix) produces no explanation of the symptom complex. The operator is then brought back to the gall bladder by a process of exclusion. Frequently the key to the existing complaints is furnished by a thickening of the gall bladder wall, adhesions with its surroundings, an enlargement of the organ, its unusual position or an obstructive kinking of its neck. It would be peculiar indeed if a mucosa-lined organ like the gall bladder, even aside from its uncertain attachments and its narrow tortuous outlet, would be exempt from inflammations and obstructions in the absence of stones. There is, therefore, scarcely room for doubt of the existence of gall bladder disease without gall stones. Nevertheless, the removal of a gall bladder without stones always has an unpleasant savor for the surgeon. In many such cases the histologic examination or the finding within a fold of Heister of a small cholesterin stone which could not be palpated from the outside, provides a delayed solace.

In rarer instances the removal of the gall bladder is demanded by a neoplasm or by disease due to specific organisms, as in typhoid carriers.

In case of injuries of the gall bladder, its removal is as a rule the simpler and safer procedure, as compared with the suture of the damaged organ.

I do not consider it proper to remove the gall bladder at the beginning of the operation as is usually done. I am of the opinion that the removal of the gall bladder should constitute the final step of the intraperitoneal portion of the operation, after the condition of the lower bile passages has been determined and corrected. Given a free passage between the liver and the gall bladder, the presence of the gall bladder in the body is a valuable asset to effect the passage of bile into the intestine by short-circuiting the common duct with a cholecystenterostomy, and undue haste in removal may thwart later efforts. It is impossible to predict whether the exposure of the lower bile passages will not disclose to one's surprise an irremovable neoplasm or a congenital or an acquired stenosis, and there is no unconditional guarantee against an irreparable, unintentional injury to, or an erroneous division of the common duct. The short-circuiting of the common duct by anastomosing the gall bladder to the intestinal tract may provide a welcome escape from such difficult situations. Furthermore, the gall bladder affords an excellent handle to raise the liver, to put the cystic duct on tension and to pull forward the deeper-lying bile passages, and we should not deprive ourselves of it too soon. Finally, in many cases hemorrhage from the liver bed after the freeing of the gall bladder hinders the work in the bottom of the wound. The objection that a large gall bladder may obstruct the approach to the deeper operative field may be met by the fact that the gall bladder can be emptied and made smaller without difficulty by a cholecystotomy. Because of these considerations I routinely defer the removal of the gall bladder to the end of the operation.

The gall bladder may be removed either in the direction from the fundus to the cystic duct or from the cystic duct to the fundus (retrograde). The difficulties of cholecystectomy lie in the exposure of the cystic duct and in its proper separation from the common duct and the right hepatic duct. Mistakes in this direction may lead to extremely annoying injuries, to the serious matter of a division of one of these passages, or they may lead to leaving behind a considerable portion of the cystic duct which in turn may give rise to the new formation of stones. If the anatomic relations at the junction of the cystic duct with the common duct cannot be exposed easily, completely and quickly, the freeing of the gall bladder in the direction from the fundus toward the cystic duct is to be preferred, because the cystic duct can be freed more simply in this direction and leads the surgeon directly to the common duct. One should make it a rule in cholecystectomy to examine the resected structure at once for the presence of a bile duct, in order to be able to repair immediately any injury which might have occurred.

Whichever direction is selected, it is always advisable to ligate the cystic artery first. This vessel usually runs dorsal (Fig. 350), more rarely ventral (Fig. 351) to the hepatic duct, lateralward to the left side of the cystic duct and runs along the gall bladder toward the fundus. In case of extensive adhesions in this region, which make it desirable to free the gall bladder in the direction from the fundus toward the cystic duct, the preliminary ligation of the cystic artery must of course be dispensed with.

Cholecystectomy in the Direction Fundus-Cystic Duct. The procedure in this direction, with or without a preliminary ligation of the cystic artery, is carried out in the following manner:

The right lobe of the liver, at times after division of the ligamentum teres and of the falciform ligament, is tipped upward over the costal margin as far as possible. Any existing adhesions of the gall bladder are divided. Adherent organs can usually be pushed aside by blunt dissection, otherwise the adhesions are dissected free with the knife or divided between ligatures. The neighborhood of the gall bladder is walled off with packing and a gauze roll is introduced into the foramen of Winslow.

If the gall bladder is excessively distended, if it contains pus or if its wall is severely damaged, the operation begins with a cholecystotomy and the packing of the emptied gall bladder (Fig. 371). The opening in the fundus is closed by heavy sutures, the ends of which are left long and serve as a useful handle in the further procedure (Fig. 357).

If the cystic artery is to be ligated first, an advisable step, it is not possible to make the neck of the gall bladder sufficiently taut simply by traction on these threads or on a clamp grasping the fundus. To accomplish this it is necessary to proceed gradually along the wall of the gall bladder to the neck with blunt grasping forceps and to lift it forcibly by each succeeding segment (Fig. 357). The peritoneal reduplication in the region of the cystic duct which is thereby put on stretch is cautiously incised parallel to the duct. The division of the serosa and of the subserous fat is usually possible without bleeding. The edges of the peritoneal wound are picked up with hemostats and are pushed back to right and left with a mounted sponge. With the additional cautious use of the knife it is possible to catch sight of the cystic duct and to its left can usually be found the cystic artery. As soon as the removal of the gall bladder is decided upon, the artery is picked up on an aneurysm needle, doubly ligated and divided (Fig. 357).

The cystic duct is pulled forward by means of a strong silk suture or a forceps and is followed further in the direction of the common duct, until the point where the cystic duct empties into the common duct has been reached. In this procedure one must remember the frequent protracted parallel course of the two structures and the frequent spiral twists of the cystic duct. Then follows in a routine procedure the inspection and the treatment of the lower bile passages as described in the following sections. Not until these measures have been completed does the surgeon again turn to the removal of the gall bladder. (The surgeon must be extremely careful in ligating the cystic artery that he does not damage the hepatic artery, since ligation of the latter artery will result in a progressive hypoglycemia and death. I.S.R.)

In order to lessen the parenchymatous and venous bleeding which usually arises during the separation of the gall bladder from the liver, it is advisable thoroughly to infiltrate both the peritoneal fold reflected onto the gall bladder and the portion of the liver covering the gall bladder with adrenalin solution (10 drops of a 1:1000 solution to 100 cc. of salt solution). This also tends to

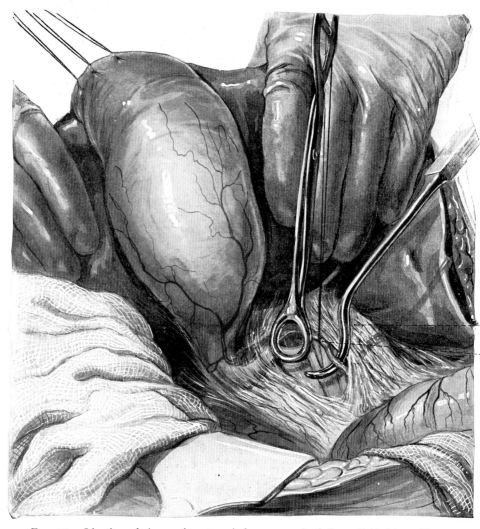

Left
branch
of the
hepatic
artery

Cystic
artery

FIG. 357. Ligation of the cystic artery before removal of the gall bladder. The serous covering of the hepatoduodenal ligament has been split in the region of the cystic artery. The cystic duct, the adjacent portions of the common and hepatic ducts and the cystic artery have been exposed. The cystic duct is elevated with a forceps. The cystic artery has been picked up on an aneurysm needle and ligated on one side.

open the plane of cleavage and facilitates the freeing of the gall bladder. The injection renders the peritoneal covering edematous and the surface of the liver grows pallid.

The separation of the gall bladder from the liver is carried out in different ways, depending upon the variations in its attachment as described above in the section on anatomy. If the gall bladder possesses a more or less free mesentery, this is put on stretch, is picked up in sections with an aneurysm needle, is ligated and cut with a scissors. If, as is the rule, the gall bladder presents a broad surface to the liver, and if it has a normal peritoneal covering

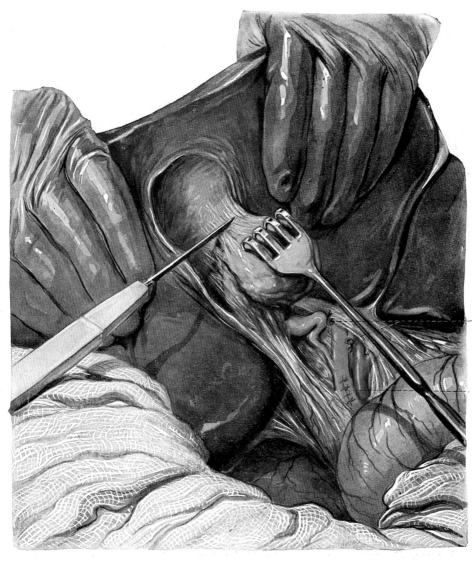

Stumps of
the cystic
artery

Suture line
of the
opening of
the com-
mon duct

FIG. 358. Removal of the gall bladder (cholecystectomy) in the direction from the fundus toward the cystic duct. After inspection and resuture of the common duct, the cystic artery was cut between ligatures. The line of reflection of the peritoneum from the gall bladder to the liver has been incised all around and the connective tissue strands joining the gall bladder to the liver are divided with an electrosurgical knife while the gall bladder is retracted forcibly with a sharp hooked retractor.

which can easily be stripped off, the peritoneum is incised in the middle in the long axis of the gall bladder and is dissected back on both sides in the form of two flaps. If, as is most usually the case, the peritoneal covering can not be removed easily, the peritoneum is incised on each side along the reflected folds and along the reflected fold at the junction of the liver edge and the fundus. From these incisions the gall bladder is freed partly by blunt, partly by sharp dissection. If the gall bladder is completely enclosed by liver tissue, the cover-

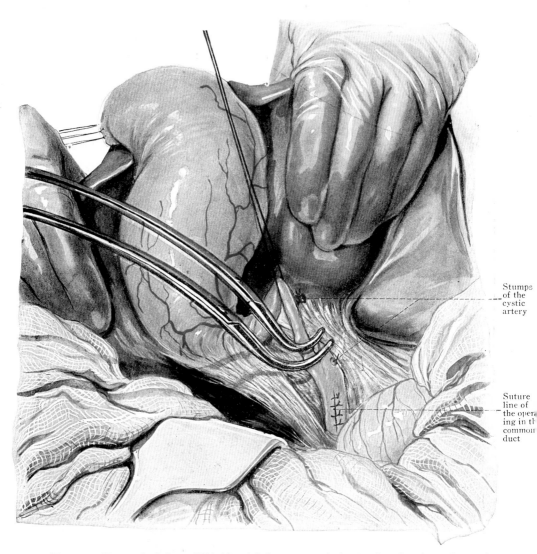

Stumps
of the
cystic
artery

Suture
line of
the opening in the
common
duct

Fig. 359. Removal of the gall bladder (cholecystectomy) in the direction from the cystic duct toward the fundus. The gall bladder and the common duct have each been opened, inspected and closed. The cystic artery was then cut between ligatures. The exposed cystic duct has been grasped with two clamps with concentric curvatures and will be divided between the clamps in the line marked in red.

ing parenchymatous layer is split at its thinnest point in the long axis with the electrosurgical knife and the gall bladder is separated on all sides.

If the proper plane of cleavage has been found and if the gall bladder and the liver are drawn apart (Fig. 358), the separation usually presents no difficulties and the blood vessels situated between the liver and the gall bladder can be doubly ligated before being cut. Frequently the separation proceeds so very easily in the proper plane, that the gall bladder can be freed with the finger and almost jumps out of its own accord. Yet after severe inflammations and in markedly shrunken gall bladders an anatomical separation between

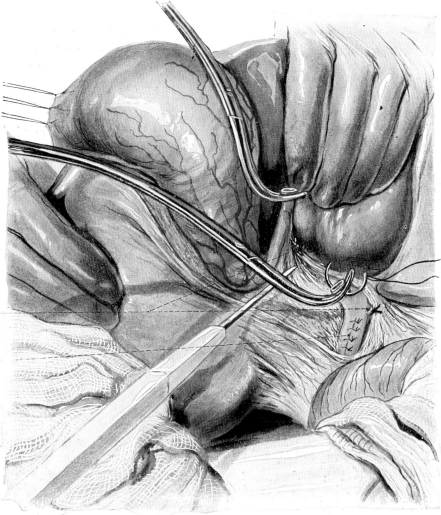

Stumps of
the cystic
artery

Suture line
of the
opening of
he common
duct

Fig. 360. Removal of the gall bladder (cholecystectomy) in the direction from the cystic duct toward the fundus. After the cystic duct is divided, the proximal end is pierced with a suture and ligated. Traction is made on the distal end and the connections between the gall bladder and the liver are divided with the electrosurgical knife. Any visible vessels are ligated before being cut.

the liver and the gall bladder may be difficult or impossible since the boundary of the gall bladder, after the destruction of its own wall, is formed by the liver or by inflammatory tissue. In that case the removal of the gall bladder is performed more in the manner of a liver resection, in that the diseased mass is cut out of the liver tissue with the electrosurgical knife.

The closer the dissection in the direction from the fundus to the common duct approaches the common bile duct, the broader the peritoneal reduplication enclosing the cystic duct becomes. It finally spreads out in the shape of a fan toward the common duct on the left and the portal fissure on the right. These peritoneal folds are picked up with an aneurysm needle and doubly ligated before being cut, since they usually contain blood vessels. In dividing the peritoneal fold on the left, care must be taken not to injure the right hepatic duct, which often lies quite close to it.

Finally the gall bladder is attached only by the cystic duct. The cystic duct is caught just above its entrance into the common duct with a small curved clamp constructed like a kidney-pedicle clamp. A second clamp similar to the first but with a shorter radius of curvature is applied to the duct just peripheral to the first (Fig. 359). The duct is then divided between the two clamps with a sharp knife, freeing the gall bladder.

A strand of catgut on a fine needle is passed through the stump of the cystic duct just under the first clamp (Fig. 360). The ligature is tied around both sides and the clamp is removed. The ligated stump of the cystic duct is buried if possible by interrupted Lembert sutures. The split edges of the peritoneal covering of the cystic duct and the peritoneal reduplications which were divided in freeing the cystic duct are sutured together to cover the stump.

Retrograde separation of the gall bladder is carried out in a similar manner. The cystic artery is exposed, ligated and divided. The cystic duct is exposed with particular care and is divided between the two small clamps as above described (Fig. 359). Before the body of the gall bladder is freed, the central stump of the cystic duct is taken care of. This is done in the manner above described by transfixing, ligating and burying it. Considerable traction is made on the peripheral clamp so that the band-like attachments of the cystic duct to its surroundings are put on stretch. They are doubly ligated and divided in the manner described. The gall bladder is then firmly retracted outward and is freed from the liver in the usual way and removed.

The manner of handling the gall bladder bed in the liver tissue is not of major significance. The chief concern is hemostasis, which must be made as dependable as possible. If the bleeding cannot be completely checked in this manner, a strip of vioform gauze is packed against the liver tissue and brought to the surface. If it was possible to separate the peritoneum from the gall bladder in two flaps, they are sutured together again so that the wound bed is peritonealized. If it can be drawn together conveniently, a wedge-shaped wound in the liver is closed with catgut sutures. If there is the slightest difficulty in covering the raw liver surface, it is better to forego suture and to pack the wound with vioform gauze than to waste time over attempts at suture, or to injure the adjacent liver tissue with suture and the cutting-through of sutures, which can only lead to further troublesome bleeding.

C. OPERATIONS ON THE BILE PASSAGES

1. The Opening of the Bile Passages (Choledochotomy, Hepaticotomy)

Choledochotomy serves the purpose of determining the site and nature of such foreign bodies as stones, ascarides, retained drainage tubes, which may be present in the interior of the large bile passages, and of their subsequent removal, or it may be used in finding and correcting stenoses of the bile passages, notably in the region of the papilla of Vater.

The common duct is the sole natural channel by which the bile is conducted from the liver to the intestine. As previously stated, one condition of all operations on the biliary tract is that a free drainage of bile into the intestine is insured. The fulfillment of this condition therefore demands an extremely careful examination and treatment of this channel. The fact that a patient has never experienced the symptoms of a common duct obstruction up to the time of operation does not warrant the assumption that there is no obstructive process in the region of the common duct, and in particular, that no stones are present. A careful examination of the common duct is therefore necessary in every case.

External inspection of the biliary system often gives valuable information in this direction. If the wall of the gall bladder is unchanged and elastic, if the gall bladder is not over-distended and can easily be squeezed empty, there can be no obstruction to drainage between the gall bladder and the papilla of Vater. If the common duct is thin and its wall not over-stretched, the bile passage distal to this point must be patulous. However, it must not be concluded from these observations that no foreign body or no stenosis is present in the bile duct, since such conditions frequently do not produce jaundice.

Palpation of the bile passages from without cannot give dependable knowledge of the state of their interior. To be sure, the free portion of the common duct can easily be palpated between the thumb and the fingers introduced into the foramen of Winslow. But in other segments this type of examination fails more or less. In the region of the portal fissure the bile passages can be palpated only with difficulty, and the ducts within the liver cannot be felt at all. Yet at these very points movable stones have a tendency to hide themselves. Palpation of the retroduodenal portion of the common duct often does not give unequivocal findings even after mobilization of the duodenum, since both the duodenal wall and the tissue of the pancreas lie between the palpating fingers. The results of palpation are particularly uncertain in the region of the head of the pancreas which is often surprisingly hard. Thus it is possible on the one hand that even fairly large stones in the region of the papilla of Vater may escape detection from without, and on the other hand, that induration from inflammation, a carcinoma or lymph nodes in the head of the pancreas may feel like calculi.

The best means for determining the conditions in the interior of the large bile passages with certainty is to open the common duct and to examine them from within. In every gall-stone patient there is a possibility of the presence of stones in the lower bile passages. Their absence can only be determined with any certainty after opening the common duct. Overlooking a stone may have the direst consequences. Therefore choledochotomy is becoming more and more (Lahey) an essential part of every routine gall-stone operation and may be omitted only because of particular technical difficulties or in case of absolutely certain conditions and clear-cut results of an external examination. Since I have been examining the interior of the common duct in almost every operation for gall stones for many years, I have been able time and again to determine the presence of stones in cases in which neither the disease picture nor the external examination of the bile passages gave any clue to their presence. I am convinced that, as a result of the usual failure on the part of most surgeons to examine the interior of the lower bile passages routinely, many stones are overlooked and that herein lies the reason for the development of numerous "recurrences."

The opening of the common duct of course becomes unavoidable when the presence of a stone, a foreign body, or the existence of a stenosis or other anomaly has been established by the external examination or by the presence of jaundice.

The common duct may be opened at one of four points; in the segment above the duodenum where it is freely exposed in the region of the hepatoduodenal ligament, in the segment behind the duodenum after mobilization of that structure, in the segment within the head of the pancreas, and in the papilla of Vater after opening the duodenum.

THE OPENING OF THE BILE PASSAGES ABOVE THE DUODENUM (SUPRADUODENAL CHOLEDOCHOTOMY. HEPATICOTOMY)

For the reasons given under the description of cholecystectomy, the opening of the common duct in properly conducted operations for gall-stone disease frequently follows immediately after the exposure of the cystic duct and precedes the removal of the gall bladder. Consequently, the operation of choledochotomy is performed exactly like the beginning of cholecystectomy as above described up to the point where the cystic duct is exposed and is surrounded with a thick silk ligature. The surgeon has an excellent handle in the gall bladder and in the silk ligature around the cystic duct by means of which he can put the common duct on tension in the depth of the wound and he is led directly to the common duct by the cystic duct.

The incision previously made in the peritoneal covering of the cystic duct is continued over the common duct which lies at the right border and in the most superficial layer of the hepatoduodenal ligament, as described under anatomic considerations on page 462. In splitting the peritoneal covering of the common duct care must be taken of the venous plexus of Zuckerkandl. Its vessels can usually be recognized and may either be pushed aside or cut between ligatures.

The common duct, exposed in this way for a short distance, is inspected and, after introducing the left index finger into the foramen of Winslow, is palpated between the thumb and finger from the portal fissure to the duodenum.

Before opening the common duct, its neighborhood is once more carefully walled off with packing. A gauze roll is again introduced into the foramen of Winslow after withdrawing the palpating finger. In difficult cases there may be some doubt as to whether a given structure really is the common bile duct. It is better before incising the supposed common duct to aspirate it with a fine needle than to take a chance of confusing it with the portal vein or some other structure. The result of the aspiration settles the matter. Occasionally the very dark color of some biles which may simulate blood is deceptive.

I open the common duct through a separate longitudinal incision in the anterior wall a few centimeters below the opening of the cystic duct. I use a separate incision not merely because I do not divide the cystic duct until after the choledochotomy is finished but because I feel that a new incision at a

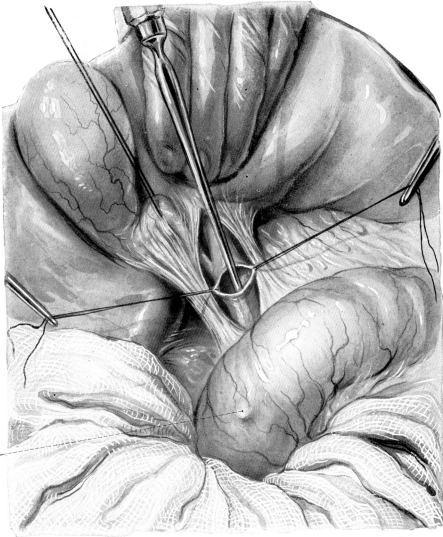

Bulging of the anterior wall of the duodenum produced by the tip of the gall-tone spoon which has been passed through the papilla of Vater

FIG. 361. Opening of the common bile duct above the duodenum (supraduodenal chole-dochotomy). Probing of the papilla of Vater. While the cystic duct, which had been picked up on a ligature, was put on stretch, the peritoneal covering of the common duct was split and the common duct opened. The edges of the common duct wound are held apart by two traction sutures. A gall-stone scoop which was inserted into the common duct has passed through the papilla of Vater and its tip is bulging the anterior wall of the duodenum outward.

distance from the opening of the cystic duct affords a simpler approach and can be better managed with less danger of stricture. The internal examination of the deep bile passages is also simpler through a lateral opening in the common duct than through the stump of the cystic duct, from which it is not always possible to probe the bile passages in the direction of the liver. The

incision is made between two fine traction sutures applied to the anterior wall
of the common duct with a very fine needle and held by forceps. An assistant
at once applies the mouth of a suction tube to the opening and aspirates the
escaping bile. Its amount, color and clearness should be carefully noted.

The internal examination of the bile passages from the opening in the
common duct is carried out in the following manner: Traction is made on the
two traction sutures so that the small opening in
the common duct gapes (Fig. 361). The interior
is explored first in the direction of the liver and
then toward the duodenum with a metal probe
or a small gall-stone scoop made of flexible copper
(Fig. 362). If its progress is impeded, the instrument is bent into a different shape and the attempt
is made with the greatest caution to advance it in
a new direction. If a stone is felt, an attempt to
grasp and deliver it is made with a gall-stone
scoop of proper size or with a slender forceps, or
else to milk it toward the opening between the
left thumb and the left index finger, the latter
being introduced into the foramen of Winslow
(Fig. 363). It is often possible to grasp a stone
which constantly eludes the instruments if it is
held tightly from without with the fingers of the
left hand and forced into the grasp of the instrument within the duct. The right and left hepatic
ducts must be probed and evacuated separately
after being individually identified.

If the bile passages contain a thick grumous
material, if numerous bits of stone come out, or
if a previously recognized stone disappears in the
depths of the liver, a Nelaton catheter provided
with a 10 cc. syringe is introduced into the common duct and the bile passages are washed out
with a stream of salt solution.

The lower bile passages can be cleansed in
this manner in most cases. If a stone cannot be
moved in spite of every effort, there remains the
last resort in the supraduodenal portion of the

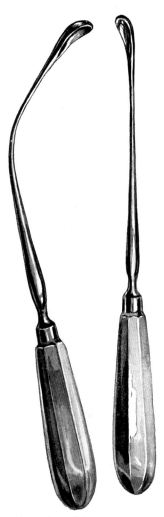

FIG. 362. Gallstone scoop
with flexible shank.

duct of cutting directly down on the stone. This
can also be done if the stone is in a hepatic duct.
Serious difficulties may really arise only in
the retroduodenal and papillary segments of the common duct. Here, too,
an attempt is first made to find and remove the stone in the manner described.
It is frequently possible to remove calculi in this region by these simple measures. The treatment of these parts of the common duct is however not to be
considered as completed until it is possible to pass the probe through the
papilla of Vater into the duodenum with ease. It is often possible to tell that
the probe has passed the papilla by a definite jerk and by the fact that the

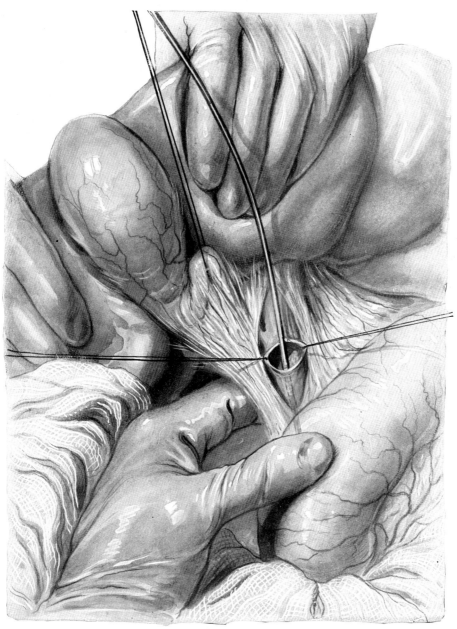

Fig. 363. Opening of the common bile duct above the duodenum (supraduodenal chole-dochotomy). Removal of a stone from the papilla of Vater. The common duct has been opened according to the directions given under Fig. 361. The retroduodenal portion of the common duct and the papilla of Vater have been grasped between the left thumb and index finger, the latter inserted into the foramen of Winslow. In this manner the position and the movements of a gall-stone spoon introduced into the interior of the common duct can be directed and guarded in the attempted evacuation of a stone lodged in the papilla of Vater.

probe can now be passed on for some distance without resistance and that its tip pushes the anterior duodenal wall forward (Fig. 361) and can be felt directly beneath it.

Occasionally these simple measures are not effective, since conditions here offer much more difficulty than in the region of the free portion of the common duct. Not only can the retroduodenal and papillary segments of the common duct not be palpated adequately, but their direction is anatomically inconstant and may be altered by preceding inflammation and contraction of the bile duct, and of the head of the pancreas. The lumen may be narrowed. The papilla of Vater may offer considerable resistance to the probe even under normal conditions, as a result of its small caliber and the contraction of its sphincter. It is often impossible to tell either by means of a probe in the interior or the palpating fingers on the outside whether one is dealing with a firm scar, a tumor or a stone. All use of force must be avoided, since the bile duct and the posterior wall of the duodenum may be punctured in this way, giving rise to a retroduodenal cellulitis and peritonitis.

The best procedure is to pick up the common duct on the left index finger, place the thumb lightly against it anteriorly and push the probe forward in the direction of the papilla under the guidance of these two digits (Fig. 363). With great patience one attempts to remove the calculus or to pass the stricture. It may be necessary to probe in several directions and with instruments of various kinds, forms and curvatures. If in this way a stone is located in the retroduodenal or the papillary segment, it is attacked after mobilization of the duodenum.

If the removal of the obstruction or the probing of the papilla does not succeed in this manner, it is possible to test whether the papilla is patulous by injection. A Nelaton catheter is introduced into the common duct toward the papilla, the edges of the opening in the common duct are held together tightly with surgical forceps and some hydrogen peroxide solution is injected with a Record syringe. If the papilla is patulous, the duodenum becomes distinctly distended in a few seconds as a result of the development of an oxygen foam and gives a tympanitic note on percussion. If the papilla is not patulous, these phenomena are not demonstrable and all the foam comes out through the opening in the common duct. The test can be made in a similar manner with saline solution. Even if the papilla is shown to be patulous by the injection test, it must be proved that it is patulous for instruments of fair-sized caliber.

If it is at all possible to pass a probe into the duodenum, the papilla may be dilated. An olive-tipped sound, whose stem is made of flexible copper (Fig. 364) so that it can be bent into any shape, is introduced with great care and followed by others of gradually increasing size. Each passage of the tip of the sound through the papilla is signalled by a slight resistance as it is inserted and withdrawn and the tip of the sound can be felt in the duodenum through its anterior wall.

If it is impossible to pass the papilla with instruments of sufficient size, or if the nature of an encountered obstruction remains unclear, the diagnosis of the underlying disease or the establishment of an anastomosis between the common duct and the intestine must be undertaken by one of the procedures to be described later.

After the lower bile passages have been evacuated and rendered adequately patulous, I close the supraduodenal opening in the common duct without drainage in most cases. For the reasons given under the description of choledochostomy on page 496, I very rarely use the opening for the establishment of drainage. The wound in the common duct is closed in the following way: The wound edges are brought together with fine interrupted catgut sutures. This suture line is buried as completely as possible by joining the edges of the reflected peritoneal covering with Lembert sutures (Fig. 359 and 360). In view of the uncertainty of this closure, the site of the suture is always drained to the exterior by means of a thin rubber tube, preferably in the form of a focal drainage, as described and illustrated under drainage of the stump of the appendix. This is performed by threading a drainage tube

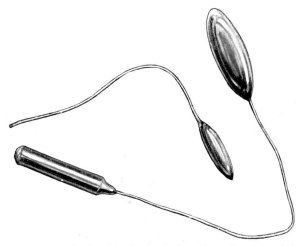

Fig. 364. Olive-tipped sounds with flexible shanks for the blunt dilatation of the papilla of Vater.

over a thread of the closing suture left long for the purpose and by pushing the tube into the bottom of the wound over the taut thread as a guide. The tube is held in place by catching the thread in a slit made in the wall of the tube at its outer end.

In a routine gall-stone operation the closure of the common duct is followed by the removal of the gall bladder.

THE OPENING OF THE COMMON BILE DUCT BEHIND THE DUODENUM (RETRO-DUODENAL CHOLEDOCHOTOMY)

If the attempt to remove a retroduodenal obstruction and to probe the papilla is unsuccessful, the problem can often be solved by exposing the retroduodenal segment of the common duct by mobilization of the descending limb of the duodenum. The peritoneum of the posterior abdominal wall is incised just beside and parallel to the lateral [right] duodenal border. The duodenum is separated from the posterior abdominal wall from the lateral side toward the midline by blunt dissection (Fig. 365) and is pulled to the left and forward with a retractor. This makes the retroduodenal portion of the common duct attached to the duodenum accessible as it runs diagonally medialward and downward.

This segment, the ampulla of Vater and the lateral part of the mobilized duodenum can now be picked up on the left index finger and palpated between

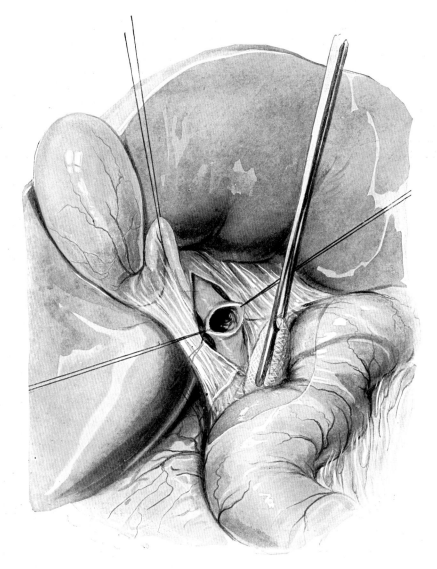

FIG. 365. Mobilization of the duodenum for the exposure of the retroduodenal portion of the common duct. The peritoneal covering of the posterior abdominal wall has been incised along the right border of the descending limb of the duodenum and the duodenum is pushed away from the posterior abdominal wall and toward the left by means of a sponge mounted on a forceps.

thumb and forefinger and can be treated just as was the free segment of common duct. It may then be possible to remove stones that could previously not be dislodged and to pass a probe into the duodenum.

If in spite of this a stone in the retroduodenal portion of the common duct cannot be removed, an incision is made directly down on the stone (Fig. 366) and it is squeezed out or delivered with a forceps or a gall-stone scoop through the opening so made. From this new opening a further attempt is made to probe and dilate the papilla.

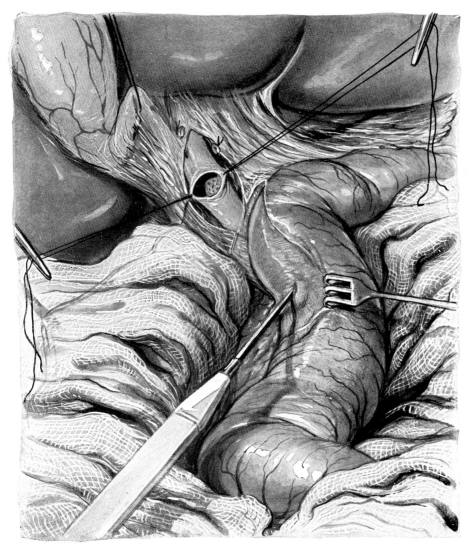

Fig. 366. Retroduodenal choledochotomy. Continuation of conditions of the preceding illustration. After the duodenum has been mobilized, an incision is made upon a stone lodged in the ampulla of Vater.

The opening in the retroduodenal segment of the common duct is closed with a double layer of interrupted catgut sutures according to the Czerny method of intestinal suture. The duodenum is replaced and is sutured into its old bed by suture of the peritoneal edges along its right side. The point of suture of the common duct, now once more retroduodenal in position, is drained to the exterior by focal drainage if there is any doubt as to the security of the suture.

THE OPENING OF THE COMMON BILE DUCT BY OPENING THE DUODENUM
ANTERIORLY (TRANSDUODENAL CHOLEDOCHOTOMY)

In case of an obstruction located at the papilla itself which cannot be
removed from an opening in the supraduodenal or the retroduodenal segment

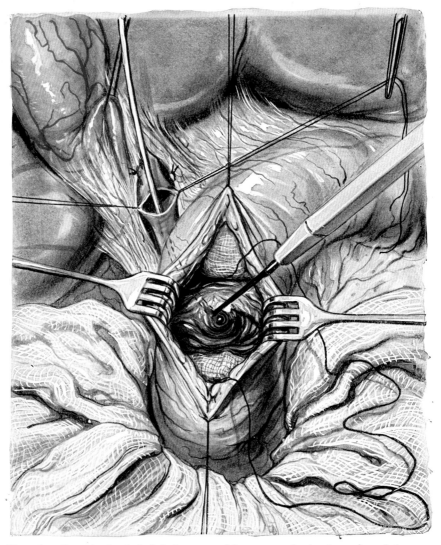

Fig. 367. Transduodenal choledochotomy. After a supraduodenal opening of the common
bile duct the anterior wall of the duodenum has been divided by a longitudinal incision at the
level of the papilla of Vater. The proximal and distal limbs of the duodenum have each been
closed with a tampon tied to a long thread. An incision is made down on the tip of a probe
introduced through the common duct and lodged beside a stone in the papilla of Vater.

of the common duct, or the nature of which is uncertain, there remains as a last
resort the exposure of the papilla by opening the duodenum.

Since the supraduodenal opening of the common duct always precedes
this operation, the approximate position of the papilla can be determined by
pushing a probe against it from this opening. The anterior wall of the duo-

denum is provided at the proper level with two traction sutures and is incised between them in the long axis with the electrosurgical knife. The bile-stained froth which escapes from the duodenum is carefully aspirated and sponged away. Gauze sponges are introduced into the proximal and distal limbs of the duodenum to prevent the further escape of intestinal contents. These sponges are joined by a long silk thread to guard against their being unintentionally left behind (Figs. 27 and 367).

The papilla of Vater is located by pushing the probe in the common duct against it. The nature of the existing obstruction can now be determined. If it is a stone, it is either removed by manipulation or the tissue surrounding it is split so that it can be withdrawn (Fig. 367). After the latter procedure and in case of stenosis of the papilla, the opening is dilated by a plastic operation, internal choledochoduodenostomy, which will be described on page 500.

At the conclusion of the intraduodenal procedure, the gauze sponges which were introduced into the gut are withdrawn by means of the attached silk thread and the intestinal incision is closed by a two-tier Czerny suture. The wound in the supraduodenal segment of the common duct and the wound in the retroduodenal segment, if present, are also closed in the manner previously described.

The abdominal cavity is drained in every case.

2. ESTABLISHMENT OF AN EXTERNAL FISTULA OF THE BILE PASSAGE (CHOLEDOCHOSTOMY AND HEPATICOSTOMY)

Permanent or long-continued drainage of the common duct may be established externally in the form of an external choledochostomy or it may take place into the intestine. For external drainage the hepatic duct may also be used (external hepaticostomy). The connection with the intestine may be established either by an anastomosis between the lower part of the common duct and the duodenum; or it may be effected, after opening the duodenum, by a plastic dilatation of the papilla of Vater in the form of an internal transduodenal choledochoduodenostomy.

In the case of infection of the lower bile passages and of the intrahepatic bile ducts, as recognized, in addition to the clinical manifestations, by the turbidity and purulent nature of the bile escaping from the opening in the common duct, it is necessary in accordance with general surgical principles to provide for free drainage of the infectious material over a long time. The measures intended for this purpose practically coincide with those for establishing the drainage of the bile. The bile, whether normal or infected, may be conducted into the gastro-intestinal tract or to the exterior. It is undisputed that in case of normal bile and patulous bile passages there is no indication for choosing or adding an unnatural channel to the exterior.

On the other hand, if the bile is infected, most surgeons consider it necessary to drain the common duct externally for a time (external choledochostomy). I believe this view to be erroneous. In most cases of severe infection of the lower bile passages there is usually an interruption or marked impairment of the natural drainage. In my opinion the reestablishment of natural drainage is the best means of combating the infection and possesses decided advantages over an unnatural drainage of the bile to the exterior.

Therefore I believe that an external choledochostomy is to be considered only if the establishment of free drainage of the bile into the intestine either as a temporary or a permanent measure is unsuccessful, impossible, or uncertain because of technical difficulties or because of the poor condition of the patient. It is an additional safety valve when a threatening lesion summarily requires immediate and adequate drainage of the bile at any cost; for example, in severe infectious jaundice, in prolonged jaundice with severe damage to the liver cells, in acute pancreatitis, or in certain injuries of the bile passages.

The following reasons are advanced to support this viewpoint in opposition to the more liberal indications for drainage of the common duct. The distance which the bile has to travel from a lateral opening in the common duct to the exterior is longer than the natural route to the duodenum. External drainage is against gravity. The bile must run uphill while the patient is on his back or must be assisted by suction drainage. In the other instance, the bile flow is with gravity. The peristalsis of the common duct assists in carrying the bile to the duodenum, while a rigid rubber drainage tube has no propulsive power. External choledochostomy creates an external biliary fistula which may not close spontaneously and may result in stricture. Internal drainage gives permanent conditions from the very first day. External drainage of the bile robs the patient of an important secretion which plays an important role in the intestine. With drainage of bile into the intestine the patient experiences its full benefit from the first day. The old claim that with external drainage stone fragments will later be discharged is based on very rare and accidental occurrences. Certainly no larger stones will pass through a medium sized drainage tube than can be evacuated into the intestine through the natural channel.

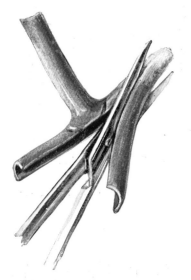

Fig. 368. T-tube. The short limb of the T-tube is converted into a trough by splitting it longitudinally.

I therefore consider drainage of the common duct as still generally practiced today to be an obsolete and unphysiologic procedure carried down through the years, a procedure from which modern biliary surgery should finally be freed. In my own fairly extensive experience in biliary surgery, years pass without a case in which external drainage of the common duct is necessary. I have seen no disadvantages in my conservative procedure.

The lateral opening made in the supraduodenal part of the common duct is used for the establishment of an external choledochostomy when this is necessary. The drainage is best carried out with a Kehr T-tube, since this also permits the passage of the bile into the duodenal portion of the common duct and best prevents an angulation of the common duct. The T-tube must be tested as to its quality before being used. In order to facilitate the removal of the T-tube and to prevent pressure ulcers, the short cross-piece of the T-tube is cut in half in the long axis so that it forms an open trough (Fig. 368). The two arms of the cross-piece are kept short, but they must be long enough to give the drain a sure hold in the common duct. Under no condition should the distal limb of the tube reach as far as the duodenum. The ends are pointed in order to make their introduction easier. After both limbs of the T-tube have been inserted (Fig. 369), the opening in the common duct is

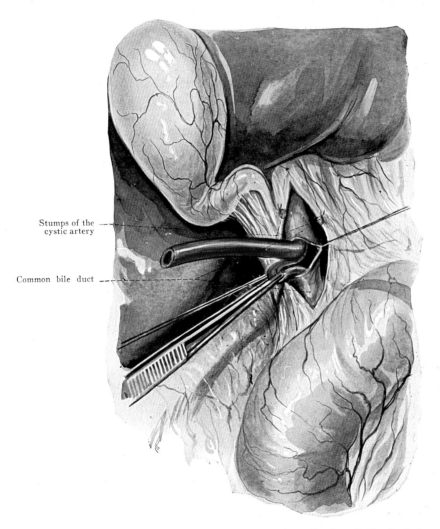

Stumps of the
cystic artery

Common bile duct

FIG. 369. Drainage of the common bile duct with a T-tube. A T-tube is inserted into the common duct through a supraduodenal opening, the edges of which are held apart by two traction sutures. One limb of the T-tube lies toward the liver, the other is inserted toward the duodenum.

closed by suture up to the point of exit of the drain, so that no bile can flow beside the drain into the abdominal cavity.

If a T-tube is not available, the drainage of the common duct may also be carried out with an ordinary narrow rubber tube. The tube is provided with an elongated lateral opening a few centimeters from one end. A small mark is made 1 cm. farther along in the direction of the other end. The tube is inserted into the proximal segment of the common duct. The mark on the tube serves as a guide in this procedure. Since such a simple tube easily changes its position, it is not sufficient to close the opening of the common duct around the tube, but the tube must be tied with a catgut ligature the ends of which are then fastened by suture to the wall of the common duct.

The common duct drain is sealed against the general abdominal cavity by means of a small pack of vioform gauze or a cigarette drain and the tube and drainage are carried out through the abdominal wound. The tube is also fastened to the abdominal wall and to the dressing by suture. A Hartert drop suction may be attached to the end of the tube projecting from the dressing (Vol. I, Fig. 241). If progress is satisfactory and the symptoms of disease subside, the tube may be clamped off from time to time after 8 to 10 days. If the clamping is well borne, if the jaundice and the signs of inflammation subside, and if the feces continue to be brown, the drainage tube is removed.

A straight tube slips out easily under gentle traction, while a T-tube occasionally is lodged a bit more tightly. If the removal of the T-tube causes any difficulty, light traction is used. The tube then usually slips out in a short time.

If there is a free communication between the liver and the intestinal tract, the biliary fistula resulting after the removal of the drain closes in a few days.

If the tube breaks during the attempt to remove it, which is a most annoying occurrence, and a piece remains deep in the abdomen, the fistula is immediately stretched and an attempt is made to grasp the piece left behind. If this is unsuccessful, there is nothing to do but to enlarge the drainage tract by incision, a procedure which is usually performed in the manner of a fresh laparotomy similar to an operation for recurrence.

3.   Establishment of an Internal Fistula of the Bile Passages into the Duodenum (Choledochoduodenostomy)

If it is impossible to remove an obstruction encountered in the lower bile passages, it is necessary to supply a new exit for the bile, and if possible into the intestine. We have considered one such way in the operation of cholecystenterostomy as previously described on page 474. This pathway, however, is unnatural, it at times does not last permanently, it results more easily in cholangitis, and it can be used only in case of free communication between the hepatic bile ducts and the gall bladder.

Since most obstructions are located in the region of the papilla of Vater, it seems more natural, simpler and surer, if these cannot be removed, to short-circuit this short impassable stretch by making an anastomosis between the lower common duct and the duodenum or if possible to remove the obstruction by a plastic enlargement of the opening of the papilla.

ESTABLISHMENT OF AN INTERNAL FISTULA OF THE BILE PASSAGES INTO THE DUODENUM FROM WITHOUT (EXTERNAL CHOLEDOCHODUODENOSTOMY)

The common duct can be anastomosed to the duodenum from the outside without making a large opening into the gut. Such an anastomosis gives excellent permanent results. It is therefore by far the best procedure.

Such a short-circuiting of the papilla of Vater has one disadvantage. The action of the sphincter muscle regulating the flow of bile is lost, so that the bile constantly flows in an unregulated stream into the duodenum and the infectious organisms of the intestine can ascend more easily into the bile passages and the liver. Even though this disadvantage may commonly not give rise to clinical manifestations, these considerations would argue that the papilla should not be short-circuited without an urgent reason. It is only to be used if the lower portion of the duct or the papilla is impassable or if there is reason to believe that they will become so.

The technique of external choledochoduodenostomy is as follows: If the opening made in the common duct for the examination of the lower bile pas-

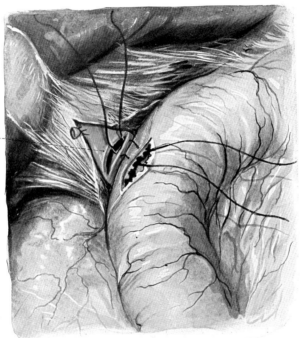

Common bile duct

Fig. 370. Establishment of an internal biliary fistula between the common bile duct and the duodenum *from without* (external choledochoduodenostomy). The peritoneum along the right margin of the duodenum has been incised and the duodenum freed a short distance from the subjacent structures. The duodenum and the retroduodenal portion of the common duct have been opened and the posterior Albert suture is applied.

sages is located close enough to the duodenum that it can be used for the anastomosis of the two structures, this advantage should be noted, instead of first closing the opening and then opening the common duct at another point. Occasionally the duodenum may be sufficiently mobilized so that it can be joined to a common duct opening which is located at some distance to begin with. In most instances it will be necessary to make a new opening at another point in the common duct, unless a choledochoduodenostomy was considered in the first place and therefore the opening was made particularly close to the duodenum.

If the duodenum was not previously mobilized for the inspection of the retroduodenal portion of the common duct, a small incision is made at the lateral edge of the duodenum through the peritoneal reflection close to the posterior abdominal wall and parallel to the line where the common duct disappears behind the intestine. The posterior wall of the duodenum is freed from its bed for a short distance by blunt dissection and is turned over toward the left. If it is easy to get at the line of reflection of the common duct from the duodenum, it will be unnecessary to apply a posterior Lembert sero-muscular suture which otherwise is carried out with fine interrupted silk sutures. If the common duct is narrow, it is opened in its long axis; if it is wide, it is opened transversely for a distance of about 1 cm. as close to the duodenum as possible. The duodenum is also opened transversely at a point opposite this opening (Fig. 370). The two openings are joined by extremely fine interrupted catgut sutures in the form of a posterior and an anterior three-layer Albert suture. Then follows an anterior Lembert sero-muscular suture with fine interrupted silk sutures. In view of the small size of the structures involved, it is advisable to use bloodvessel suture instruments. The mobilized duodenum is returned to its old bed and is fastened by interrupted sutures. A small piece of omentum may be fastened over the operative field to protect the suture line.

An idiopathic common duct cyst, a congenital lateral outpouching of the common bile duct, is treated in a similar manner, that is, by establishing a communication with the duodenum. The difficulties of the procedure lie in exposing the local conditions and in establishing the diagnosis. When the lesion has been properly recognized, it is usually easy to anastomose the cyst with the duodenum because the large mobile wall of the cyst can usually be placed beside the duodenum without difficulty.

ESTABLISHMENT OF AN INTERNAL FISTULA OF THE BILE PASSAGE INTO THE DUODENUM BY OPENING THE ANTERIOR WALL OF THE DUODENUM (INTERNAL TRANSDUODENAL CHOLEDOCHODUODENOSTOMY)

The procedure is the same as that described on page 495, under transduodenal choledochotomy and found to be the site of a benign stenosis or if the development of such a stenosis is to be feared.

The procedure is the same as that described on page 495, under transduodenal choledochotomy up to the point of exposing and splitting the papilla. Attention was called in the description of that operation to the necessity of preventing the recurrence of a stenosis or an obstruction of the papilla by means of special plastic measures. This is accomplished by internal choledochoduodenostomy.

A probe is passed through the papilla from a supraduodenal opening in the common duct, or from the duodenum, in case a supraduodenal choledochotomy was not performed. The papilla is split with an electrosurgical knife for a distance of about 2 cm. The incision is made in the direction of the liver through the part of the papilla bulging forward into the duodenum, that is, through that portion where the duodenum and the common duct run nearly parallel to each other for a considerable distance. The resultant wound edges of the common duct and the duodenum are joined to each other with fine interrupted catgut sutures (Fig. 371).

Resection of the papilla of Vater because of a papillar carcinoma is fundamentally nothing more than an extended internal transduodenal choledochotomy. A probe is pushed against the papilla from a supraduodenal choledochotomy opening and the papilla is made accessible by opening the duodenum in the manner above described. The carcinoma is picked up with

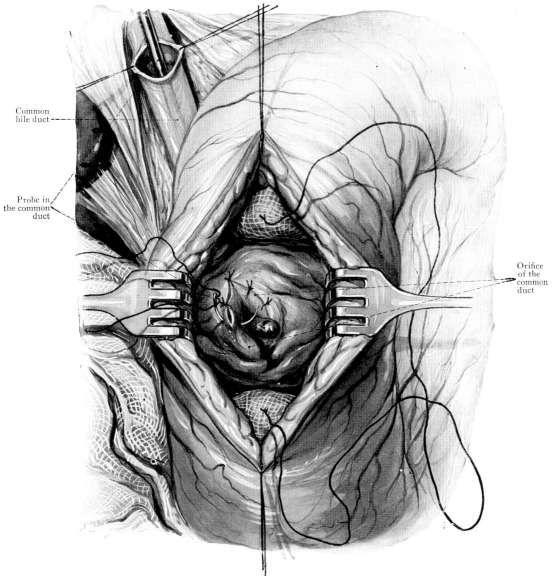

Common
bile duct

Probe in
the common
duct

Orifice
of the
common
duct

FIG. 371. Establishment of an internal biliary fistula between the common bile duct and the duodenum *from within* (internal transduodenal choledochoduodenostomy). The duodenum has been opened and the papilla of Vater has been split upward on a probe introduced through a supraduodenal opening in the common duct. The wound edges of the duodenum and the common duct are joined by interrupted sutures.

Kocher hemostats or with a Museux forceps and an incision is made around it with the electrosurgical knife. As soon as the wall of the duodenum and of the common duct is divided for a short distance, the two wound edges of the mucosa of the duodenum and of the common duct are joined with fine interrupted catgut sutures (Fig. 372). In this manner the incision is gradually carried around the whole circumference of the carcinomatous papilla, with attendant suture of the wound edges, step by step, until the lesion is freed

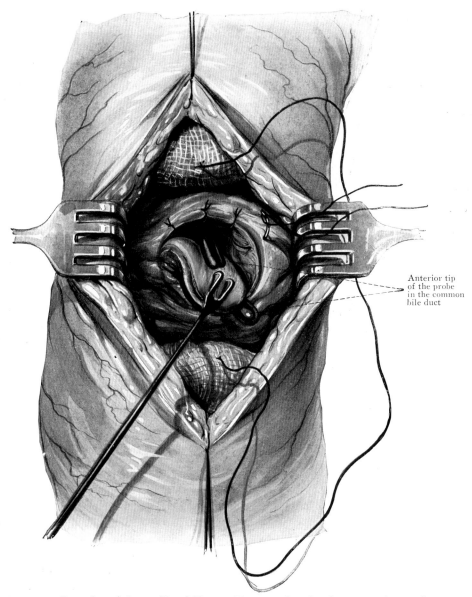

Anterior tip
of the probe
in the common
bile duct

FIG. 372. Resection of the papilla of Vater. The procedure has been started according to the description accompanying the preceding illustration. A circular incision is made around the papilla and the resultant wound edges of the duodenum and the common duct are joined by interrupted sutures. A probe introduced through the common duct into the duodenum facilitates orientation.

and removed. The probe in the common duct is of aid in making certain that the cut edge of the common duct is united all around to the duodenum and without stenosis.

The incision in the anterior wall of the duodenum is closed in the usual way.

4. SUTURE OF, AND PLASTIC OPERATIONS ON THE BILE PASSAGES
CLOSURE OF AN OPENING IN A BILE PASSAGE

Suture of the walls of bile ducts follows the fundamental principles of intestinal suture laid down by Czerny. A three-layer Albert suture with catgut is first applied and then an infolding Lembert suture with silk. Interrupted sutures are used as a rule. In case of a fairly long suture line the three-layer suture may be applied as a running suture. Because of the delicate nature of their walls and because of the danger of stenosis of the bile passages, which have a small caliber to begin with, the proper application of sutures often meets with difficulties and the surgeon must at times be content with an imperfect performance of the suture. The use of the instruments for blood-vessel suture often simplifies the procedure.

Bile Peritonitis. The escape of a small amount of bile into the abdominal cavity is in itself not a condition that is rapidly fatal but the extensive leakage of bile into the cavity leads to bile peritonitis. The mortality of bile peritonitis is materially greater under conservative treatment than with operation. Therefore every injury or spontaneous perforation of the bile passages or the gall bladder leading to the flow of bile into the abdominal cavity demands immediate operation.

If the injury was not inflicted at operation, it may be very difficult to find the point of injury, especially if fibrinous adhesions have already developed. Garrè advised the injection of air into the gall bladder, after which the point of injury may be recognized by the escape of the air from the point of perforation.

When the opening is found, the ideal treatment is closure by suture in the manner above described. If simple suture cannot be carried out because of the size of the defect, one of the various plastic procedures for bridging the gap, as described below, must be used. If difficulties are encountered, especially if an infection is already present, the insertion of a drain to conduct the bile to the exterior is often the simplest procedure. In that case the general abdominal cavity must be carefully walled off.

If the point of escape of the bile cannot be found, the common duct should be drained, and drainage of the part of the abdominal cavity in which the injury presumably lies established, the remainder of the cavity being walled off with packing.

Considerable portions of the walls of the bile passages, especially of the common duct, are occasionally lacking, for example after an unintentional operative or traumatic injury, in an extensive acquired cicatricial stenosis, in congenital aplasia or as a result of resection of part of the wall for carcinoma. In such cases four different procedures are available:

1. Direct anastomosis of the remaining parts of the common duct by suture,
2. Implantation of the remainder of the hepatic duct into the intestinal tract,

3. Insertion of a temporary prosthesis,
4. Insertion of a permanent prosthesis.

DIRECT ANASTOMOSIS OF SEGMENTS OF THE BILE PASSAGES

If at all possible the defect is closed by direct suture, whether it is a case of a lateral defect or a break in continuity. In the latter instance an attempt is made to free both ends of the bile duct from their surroundings for a short distance in order to make it easier to bring them together. Because of the small size of the structures it is often absolutely necessary to use the instruments for blood-vessel suture. If the suture threatens to cause a stenosis of the bile duct, it is applied over a rubber tube of appropriate diameter, and the tube is allowed to remain in position for a time as a temporary prosthesis. A T-tube is best suited for the purpose, in which case the long limb leading to the surface serves less to drain the bile than to act as a handle for the subsequent removal of the prosthesis.

ANASTOMOSIS BETWEEN THE STUMP OF THE HEPATIC END OF THE BILE DUCT AND THE GASTRO-INTESTINAL CANAL

If it is impossible to close a defect in the common duct by suture in this manner, and that is usually the case if a duodenal common duct stump suitable for suture can no longer be made available, then the next procedure to be tried is the direct implantation of the hepatic stump of the common duct into the intestinal tract. For this purpose the surgeon should first consider the duodenum. But since the mobility of the duodenum, even after it has been mobilized as previously described, is rather limited, it is often impossible to bring it close enough to the stump of the common duct. Occasionally the pyloric portion of the stomach can be brought close enough to the hilum of the liver and may then be used to receive the bile. However the upper jejunum possesses the greatest mobility. A suitable loop is brought to the region of the liver, preferably through an opening in the transverse mesocolon, the intestine being carefully sutured to the edges of the slit in the mesocolon. An antecolic position of the loop is less advantageous. The anastomosis of the bile duct is made either with the apex of a jejunal loop, in which case it is advisable to join the bases of the limbs of the loop by an entero-enterostomy, or an intestinal loop is short-circuited on one side, so that after the transsection of the intestine the proximal loop is implanted end-to-side into the distal loop, the distal loop is closed blind and is brought up to the region of the liver for the anastomosis with the common duct (Fig. 373).

The performance of the anastomosis between the hepatic stump of the common duct and the selected intestinal loop is simple and follows the usual rules of intestinal suture, provided that it is possible to expose a hepatic stump of the common duct suitable for suture. If difficulties arise in the anastomosis, the suture may be applied over a temporary rubber prosthesis which is carried into the intestine.

The surgeon is confronted with a most serious situation when it is impossible to find an extrahepatic bile duct in the region of the portal fissure. There is nothing left to do but to connect the intestine with a wound made in the liver, in the hope that the bile escaping from the liver wound will continue to empty into the intestine and in a sufficient quantity (cholangio-enterostomy) to be of some use and to relieve the jaundice.

In some cases the extremely distended bile passages are visible through the surface of the liver in the form of vesicles in the region of the portal fissure. In that case such an area is selected for the incision into the liver. Otherwise,

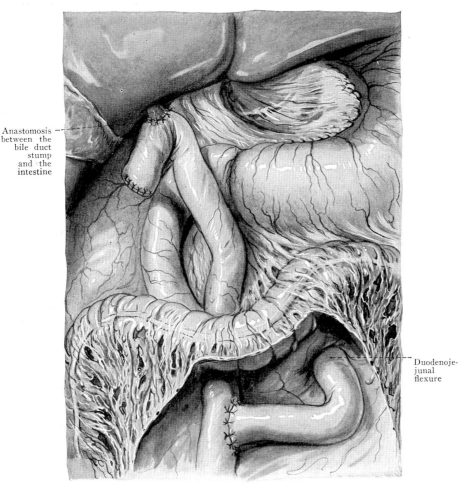

Anastomosis between the bile duct stump and the intestine

Duodenojejunal flexure

FIG. 373. Anastomosis of the end of a bile duct with a loop of small intestine short-circuited on one side. The jejunum has been divided 30 cm. beyond the duodenojejunal flexure and the proximal limb implanted end-to-side into the distal limb 50 cm. beyond the point of transsection. The distal limb has been closed blind and brought up through an opening in the transverse mesocolon to the hilum of the liver and there anastomosed with the end of a bile duct.

a region of the liver is chosen which does not lie in the neighborhood of the large liver vessels and where the intestinal segment selected for the anasto-mosis, usually the stomach, can be applied to the liver surface without tension. First the stomach or intestinal wall is fastened with interrupted sutures to the part of the liver to be opened (Fig. 374). An incision about 2 cm. long and 2 cm. deep is then made into the adjacent part of the liver with the electro-surgical knife. If the bleeding is not marked, a Korn forceps may be cau-tiously introduced into the bottom of the wound to enlarge it by blunt dissection. The segment of the stomach lying opposite the incision in the liver is also opened with the electrosurgical knife and the anterior edge of the gastric opening is fastened to the anterior edge of the liver wound with interrupted catgut sutures.

The procedure is highly uncertain both as to mortality and functional results. There is great danger of the development of an external intestinal fistula. It should be used only as a very last resort.

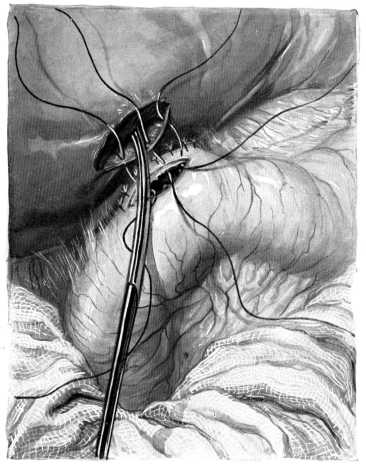

Fig. 374. Anastomosis of intrahepatic bile ducts with the duodenum (cholangioduodenostomy). An opening in the anterior wall of the duodenum is sutured to an opening in the under surface of the liver. The opening in the liver is brought into as extensive a connection as possible with the intrahepatic bile passages by probing with a Korn forceps.

Goetze recommends the following plastic procedure in such cases: The mass of scar tissue in the region of the opening in the bile passage or of the liver wound on the under surface of the liver is carefully dissected free, especially in its lower segment. The point of exit of the bile from the liver or the stump of the hepatic duct is enlarged by passing sounds, so that the beginning of its intrahepatic course can be well determined. The surgeon introduces a small button-tipped knife, with the blade forward (upward) and slightly outward, deep into this opening and splits it forward (upward) and slightly outward, where there is no danger of injuring vessels, for a distance of 2 cm. or even farther, depending upon the position of the branching of the main hepatic duct or of the right hepatic duct. This causes a wound about 2 cm. long to gape out of the scar-tissue opening on the under surface of the liver (Fig. 375). Its ventral wall is formed by the three-cornered wound in the liver parenchyma and its dorsal wall by the hepatic duct, enlarged in its

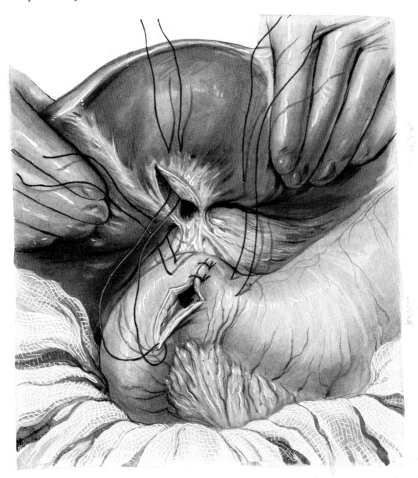

FIG. 375. Anastomosis of the end of a bile duct with the duodenum by means of a plastic procedure. A triangular flap has been formed from the anterior wall of the duodenum. A bile duct in the region of the hilum of the liver has been slit open and the flap of duodenum is drawn into it by means of a suture passed through the tip of the flap. The duodenum will be sutured to the under surface of the liver.

intrahepatic portion. Next, a small triangular flap 2½ cm. long and 1½ to 2 cm. wide at its base is formed out of the full thickness of the anterior wall of the duodenum, the tip of the flap pointing toward the liver. The resultant large opening in the duodenum is at once made smaller by a few transverse sutures so that it is of the proper size for anastomosis with the bile duct. A stout catgut suture is passed through the tip of the duodenal flap and each end of the suture is passed separately from within outward through the wall of the split hepatic duct with the aid of a large needle. The two ends of the suture which have been brought out on the under surface of the liver are tied together. This pulls the little duodenal flap into the split hepatic duct and the flap forms the mucosa-clothed anterior wall of the new canal for the bile. The slit in the liver is closed as well as possible over the buried flap with transverse sutures.

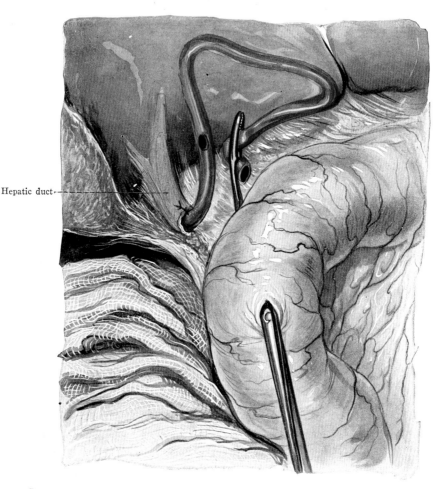

Hepatic duct

FIG. 376. Bridging a defect in the common bile duct by a temporary rubber prosthesis. One end of a rubber tube has been inserted into the end of the hepatic duct; the other has been grasped by a forceps which has been passed through the anterior and the posterior walls of the duodenum. By withdrawing the forceps the rubber tube is led through the duodenum. The rubber tube has a lateral opening intended for the interior of the duodenum.

The adjacent part of the duodenal wall is fastened on both sides to the under surface of the liver by additional sutures.

Such a plastic flap procedure may also be employed to effect bile drainage by using the stomach or a loop of the upper jejunum. (The danger of subsequent peritonitis is very great. I.S.R.)

INSERTION OF A TEMPORARY PROSTHESIS

A less advantageous but occasionally safer procedure is to abandon the establishment of an immediate direct organic connection between the hepatic

ducts and the intestine in favor of the insertion of a temporary rubber prosthesis. Its use is based upon the experience that the epithelium of the bile
passages seems to possess a definite, although somewhat limited capacity for
growing over granulating surfaces in time, provided their extent is within
reasonable limits, and forming a satisfactory substitute for the lost portion of
the wall in this manner. The edges of the defect in the common duct, provided

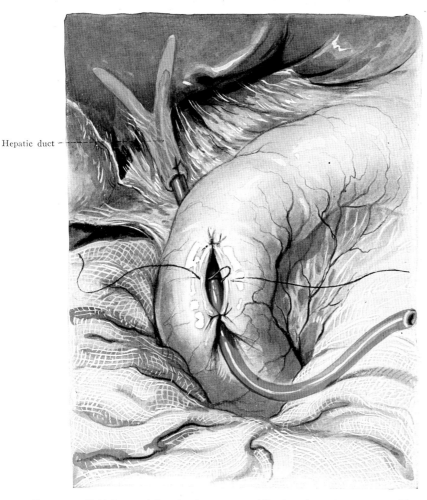

Hepatic duct

FIG. 377. Bridging a defect in the common bile duct by a temporary rubber prosthesis.
The rubber tube has been led through the duodenum by the withdrawal of the forceps, the lateral
opening in the tube lying within the bowel. The tube as it leaves the intestine is fastened securely
to its surface by means of a Witzel canal.

that a hepatic and a duodenal stump of the duct can be freed, are brought as
close together as possible and the remaining interval is bridged with a tube of
not too small a caliber which is inserted for some distance into each end of
the common duct. Here again the T-tube can be used to advantage. A piece
of omentum is sutured over the site of the plastic operation, insuring a tight
closure.

Such a temporary prosthesis can be left in place for months, during which time the rubber tube is irrigated from time to time to prevent the formation of concretions. In view of the usually long time during which the prosthesis is to be retained, the quality of the rubber must be tested carefully before it is used.

A T-tube may be used as a prosthesis even when no portion of the common duct remains attached to the duodenum so that one end of the prosthesis filling the gap must be inserted directly into the intestine. One end of the horizontal limb of the T-tube then lies in the common duct and the other in the duodenum.

It is preferable in such a case to use a simple rubber tube and to lead it to the exterior again after its insertion into the duodenum. This is done in the following manner: After one end of the rubber tube has been inserted into the hepatic end of the common duct and fastened in place, the duodenum is opened by a stab incision in its anterior wall. A slender Korn forceps is introduced into the opening and is forced out through the posterior wall of the duodenum in the direction of the common duct. The jaws of the forceps grasp the free end of the tube inserted into the common duct (Fig. 376) and pull it into the intestine, through it and out again anteriorly. The tube coming from the common duct now enters the duodenum through its posterior wall and leaves it through the opening in its anterior wall. Traction is made on the tube and the anterior wall of the duodenum is pushed back so that the part of the tube within the duodenum is drawn outside of the intestine. This segment is provided with a lateral opening and is then replaced within the intestine by relieving the traction. The tube as it emerges from the intestine is fastened to its anterior wall for a distance of about 3 cm. by forming a Witzel canal (Fig. 377) and is brought to the surface through the abdominal incision.

Since the duodenum is not very well suited for the plastic procedure of forming a Witzel canal because of the poor quality of its peritoneal covering and because of the danger of stenosis, the tube has been occasionally led from the interior of the duodenum through the pylorus into the stomach and thence to the exterior through a Witzel fistula.

The prosthetic tube is left in place for weeks or months, depending on the size of the defect. It can usually be removed easily by traction. If a patulous organic bile passage to the stomach or intestine has been formed, the external fistula resulting after the removal of the prosthesis will close in a short time.

5. Insertion of a Permanent Prosthesis

If the gap between the two ends of the common duct is very large or if the full length of the duct has been lost, a gradual bridging of the gap by epithelium after the insertion of a temporary prosthesis is very unlikely.

If it is impossible to anastomose a segment of the intestinal tract, the stomach, the duodenum or a loop of the upper jejunum directly with the stump of the bile duct in the fissure of the liver in the manner above described, the insertion of a permanent prosthesis that shall remain in the body for life must be resorted to. Experience has shown that such a prosthesis made out of good rubber can perform its function for years without disturbing the patient's health. Nevertheless its use remains a questionable emergency procedure that is to be advised only as a last resort.   One end of a tube of suitable size made of the best rubber is fastened securely into the proximal end of the common duct by catgut sutures.   The other end is introduced into the stomach or duodenum through a small opening in the nearest point of its wall.   The point of entrance of the tube into the intestine is buried by a few plicating sutures. The prosthesis is well covered with omentum.

In all such cases in which uncertain sutures are applied and doubtful attempts are made at bridging defects in the lower bile passages, the surroundings are carefully guarded by adequate drainage and packing against escaping bile.

D.   SECONDARY OPERATIONS ON THE BILIARY SYSTEM

1.   Operations for Recurrence of Gall-Stone Disease

In spite of the most careful technique, the complaints of patients with cholelithiasis are not relieved in all cases by the operations described.   In a certain percentage the same symptoms remain or they recur in a milder or an altered form, promptly or after months or years.   These "recurrences" in a clinical sense do not always mean the renewed presence of gall stones.

In a fraction of the cases the cause lies outside of the biliary tract in the form of organic disease of the stomach, the small intestine, the right kidney, the appendix, the pancreas, the female reproductive organs, etc.   In other cases the attacks are simulated by spasm of the bile passages, of the papilla of Vater or of the gastro-intestinal tract.   In still others it is a question of adhesions, which may have developed prior to operation as a result of inflammation, and stenoses arising in the biliary system (an urgent warning not to postpone operation too long) or the adhesions may have resulted from the operation itself.   At times an incisional hernia may lead to symptoms.   Sometimes not all the stones were found in the bile passages at the first operation and some were consequently left behind by mistake (a caution to examine the interior of the bile passages through a choledochotomy even in many apparently simple cases).   Only in a small fraction of the cases have new stones actually been formed, either in the lower bile passages or in the gall bladder, if the latter was not removed at the first operation.

It is extremely difficult and often impossible to determine clinically in a given case whether a stone or some other organic lesion is the cause of the renewed complaints.   The situation is only occasionally cleared up by the passage of calculi in the stool, by the appearance of continued or intermittent jaundice or by the results of cholecystography.

The reopening of the abdominal cavity after a gall-stone operation is always a dangerous matter and doubtful in its results.   The decision to re-operate is a serious one to make, and in such cases all conservative measures should first be given a thorough trial.   However, when the presence of stones or of an organic obstruction to bile flow has been established, an operation can no longer be avoided.   No binding rule can be laid down in such a case as to whether the incision should be made through the old scar or whether the old operative field should be approached by a different route (midline incision).   On the whole, a new area for the incision is to be preferred.

The operation often consists in a difficult anatomic dissection of the structures imbedded in the scar tissue, the under surface of the liver, the transverse colon, the duodenum, the stomach, and above all, the lower bile passages. This is fraught with great danger of injury to one of the structures. The individual therapeutic procedure is determined in each case by existing conditions. In view of the possible recurrence of the lesion, the surgeon should be particularly inclined to establish a wide internal biliary fistula if this is possible.

2. OPERATIONS FOR EXTERNAL BILIARY FISTULAE

The persistence or the development of a permanent biliary fistula after an operation on the biliary tract necessitates a secondary operation in most cases.

The first question to be decided is whether or not there is a free passage for the bile from the liver to the intestine. This question can be answered as a rule with fair certainty by the quantity of bile escaping from the fistula, by the temporary variations in the excretion, by the presence or absence of bile in the stool, by the stereoscopic Roentgen-ray picture or the fluoroscopic visualization of the bile passages filled with an opaque material injected through the fistulous opening.

If the passage between the liver and the intestine is patulous, the external biliary fistula is merely an unimportant lateral branch of the main stream and can probably be caused to close by simply damming it up.

The Closure of a Gall Bladder Fistula. If the fistula leads into the gall bladder, a frequent cause of its persistence lies in the formation of a lipped fistula. An incision is then made around the fistulous opening as described on page 250, under the treatment of lateral intestinal fistula. The fistula is followed to the surface of the fundus of the gall bladder. The opening is sutured after the removal of any stones present in the gall bladder and the suture line is buried by a second Lembert suture. The wound in the abdominal wall is closed, as far as possible by dissection and suture of the individual layers.

In view of the fact that the diseased gall bladder must be considered as the chief site of formation of gall stones, it is often better in such cases to remove the fistula-bearing gall bladder, provided always that there is a free passage for the bile from the liver to the intestine. This closes the bile fistula.

If a lateral fistula leads to the common duct or another of the deep bile passages, in the presence of a freely patulous common duct, it usually suffices to make an incision around the fistulous opening, follow it down for a few centimeters and ligate and amputate it at this point. If this simple procedure is not successful, the fistulous tract is followed down to its point of origin from the deep bile duct, is ligated at this point and cut off. The deep wound usually closes by granulation. The technique of following the fistula to its point of origin corresponds to the procedure described under the treatment of a tubular fistula of the intestine.

The removal of an external biliary fistula is much more difficult if the bile does not have an unobstructed passage from the liver to the intestine. The emphasis of the operation then lies on the reestablishment of this connection, while the closure of the fistula becomes a minor matter since it usually occurs of itself after the main objective has been reached.

The operation can be planned along two different lines.

The Reestablishment of the Normal Channel of the Bile from the Liver to the Intestine. For this purpose, the lower bile passages and the existing obstruction are dissected out through an abdominal incision made at a distance from the actual seat of trouble or through an incision excising the fistula. This may obviously be very difficult. Depending upon the conditions

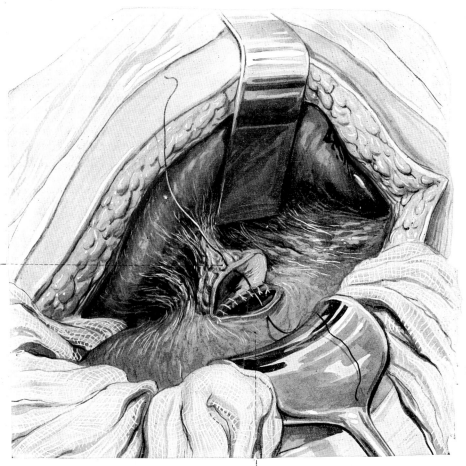

Fistulous tract

Anterior wall of the stomach

FIG. 378. Transplantation of an external biliary fistula into the stomach. The external biliary fistula has been freed from the skin and from its surroundings as far as the hilum of the liver. The fistulous opening is anastomosed to an opening made in the anterior wall of the stomach.

encountered, the drainage of the bile into the intestine is reestablished by the removal of a stone, by the relief of a stenosis, by an external or internal chole-dochoduodenostomy or by the plastic replacement of a defect in the common duct. If this is successful, the external biliary fistula usually closes of itself or it may be removed secondarily without difficulty by means of one of the procedures above described.

Transplantation of the Fistula. If the drainage of the bile through the fistula is permanently assured (lipped fistula), an attempt may also be made to conduct the bile into the intestine permanently through the fistula by anastomosing the fistulous opening to the intestine. In this procedure it is necessary to mobilize the fistulous tract sufficiently on the one hand and a suitable portion of the intestine on the other, so that the two strucures can be joined. The fistulous tract is colored by the injection of a methylene blue solution. An incision is made around the external opening of the fistula, and the tract, which is differentiated from its surroundings by its firmer consistency, is carefully dissected free. This is difficult because both the tract and any organs imbedded in the scar tissue may be injured. When the fistulous tract has been freed for a sufficient distance, a portion of the gastro-intestinal canal suitable for the anastomosis must be exposed. If it is possible to expose the stomach, it is to be preferred because its strong wall permits of a more dependable suture, because of the relative harmlessness of a gastric fistula should this develop, and because of the tolerance of the stomach to bile. Otherwise the duodenum which is less suitable must be used, or a jejunal loop brought up behind or in front of the transverse colon, after short-circuiting the loop on one side or performing an entero-enterostomy between its proximal and distal limbs.

The end of the fistulous tract with its narrow border of skin is sutured into a small opening in the wall of the viscus (Fig. 378). If sufficient material is available, this may be performed in the manner of a Witzel fistula. In every case the suture is insecure and there is always the possibility of a breaking down of the suture line with the formation of a new biliary fistula or of an intestinal fistula. These new fistulae are however usually temporary. The site of the anastomosis must always be drained.

E. EXAMPLES OF OPERATIONS ON THE BILIARY TRACT

The most important of the operations on the biliary tract which have thus far been described individually as to their indications and technique will now be illustrated in a connected form by a number of practical examples showing different variations and modifications.

Case 12. Example of the Removal of a Calculous Gall Bladder and the Examination of the Common Duct.

In a woman of 35, in whom a diagnosis of recurrent gall-stone attacks has been made, the operative treatment of the disease was decided upon. Jaundice has never been present.

The patient is given the girdle type of spinal anaesthesia. The operator stands at the left side of the patient, who is in the reversed Trendelenburg position with her left side lower than the right. The abdominal cavity is opened by a right lateral rectus incision which is continued to the ensiform process, and divides the right rectus and the highest intercostal nerve supplying it.

The liver is situated rather low, and beyond its edge projects a gall bladder the size of an average pear which externally shows little change. The liver edge can easily be tipped over the right costal margin without cutting the ligamentum teres. Numerous stones can be palpated within the gall bladder, which is not adherent.

The abdominal viscera, especially the stomach and the transverse colon with its mesentery, are packed off with moist compresses so that only the gall bladder and the adjacent part of the liver remain in the operative field.

The rather distended gall bladder is first evacuated because it obstructs the approach to the depths of the wound. After a careful walling-off of the surroundings so that only the dome of the gall bladder is visible, it is grasped with two Kocher hemostats. A trochar connected with an electric suction pump is plunged into the gall bladder between the two hemostats and the gall bladder is emptied of its fluid contents. The fundus of the gall bladder is then incised between the hemostats for a distance of about 3 cm. The contents of the gall bladder are evacuated with a gall-stone scoop. A great number of stones are found. A large stone situated in the neck of the gall bladder is purposely not removed in order to prevent the access of bile from the lower bile passages. The gall bladder is packed lightly with a dry strip of vioform gauze and its opening is loosely closed with a number of silk sutures. The sutures are left long and serve as a handle to elevate the gall bladder.

Traction on the fundus, however, does not suffice to put the cystic duct on stretch. It is therefore grasped well down near its neck with a curved forceps and made taut. While an assistant in this way pulls the cystic duct forward and straightens it, the operator splits its peritoneal covering with a sharp knife and then by blunt dissection pushes the two peritoneal edges back to either side with a sponge mounted on a forceps. This brings into view the cystic artery as it runs along the left side of the cystic duct, and it is picked up on an aneurysm needle, doubly ligated and divided. The aneurysm needle can now be passed beneath the cystic duct. A strong silk ligature is passed around it but is not tied. The cystic duct is lifted by the ligature and the forceps attached to the duct is removed.

The incision splitting the peritoneal covering of the cystic duct is extended in the direction of the common duct, the peritoneum being picked up with two surgical forceps, carefully split between them and then pushed to either side with a sponge mounted on a forceps. In this manner the junction of the cystic and common ducts is exposed. Toward the duodenum a number of transverse vessels belonging to the venous plexus of Zuckerkandl come into view on the anterior surface of the common duct. They are picked up on an aneurysm needle and doubly ligated before being divided. The anterior wall of the common duct then appears. It is not thickened and not distended. The operator introduces the index and middle fingers into the foramen of Winslow from the right and palpates the common duct between these fingers and the opposing thumb. This likewise discloses no abnormality.

In spite of the negative external findings and the negative previous history in this regard, the examination of the common duct from within is undertaken. Its anterior walls are picked up at an easily accessible point with two traction sutures, one on each side. After the surroundings have again carefully been walled off with compresses, and in particular after a gauze roll has been introduced into the foramen of Winslow, a small incision is made in the anterior wall of the common duct with a knife. A small amount of clear yellow bile escapes which is immediately aspirated with the electric pump. The interior of the duct is explored with a small gall-stone scoop. The right and left hepatic ducts can be entered with ease. In probing the retroduodenal portion of the common duct the spoon meets a slight obstruction and on its being withdrawn a small gall stone and some inspissated mucus escape. No additional stones can be found in spite of repeated search. However, it is impossible to pass the gall-stone scoop into the duodenum, but a probe slips through the papilla of Vater into the intestine, although with a certain amount of resistance. The injection test gives a positive result in that after the injection of hydrogen peroxide through a Nelaton catheter introduced into the common duct, the duodenum becomes considerably distended. Therefore, there can be only a slight obstruction at the papilla of Vater, obviously in the nature of a spasm. Consequently it is not considered necessary to expose the papilla. It is simply dilated by passing a graduated series of olive-tipped sounds up to the thickness of a lead pencil from the common duct opening through the papilla into the duodenum. This is easily done. The opening in the common duct is closed with fine catgut sutures, and this suture line is buried by suturing together the edges of the peritoneal covering.

The removal of the gall bladder follows. The cystic artery which was previously exposed is doubly ligated and divided. The ligature passed around the neck of the gall bladder is made taut. This puts on stretch a peritoneal reduplication between the liver and the cystic duct and gall bladder like the strands of a mesentery. It is picked up in segments on an aneurysm needle, doubly ligated and divided. The cystic duct which is clearly defined from the common duct is caught just above its junction with the latter with the two special clamps intended for this purpose and is divided between the clamps. The cystic duct is transfixed with a catgut suture just beneath the lower clamp and ligated on both sides. The clamp is removed. The stump of the cystic duct is buried by oversewing the adjacent peritoneal covering.

By means of gentle traction on the upper clamp closing its neck, the gall bladder almost frees itself from the liver. A few connecting strands are picked up on the liver side and are caught and ligated. The gall bladder is thus easily freed in a retrograde manner. The gall bladder bed in the liver is closed without difficulty by means of catgut sutures.

A small strip of vioform gauze is laid over the liver wound and a medium-sized drainage tube is carried to the site of the common duct suture. Gauze and drain are brought out through the upper angle of the wound. All compresses are removed, and the remainder of the abdominal wound is closed.

Case 13. Example of the removal of a shrunken gall bladder and an internal transduodenal choledochoduodenostomy in the case of a stone lodged at the papilla of Vater.

A woman of 44 has suffered from typical gall-stone attacks for 15 years. There have been repeated attacks of transient jaundice. For two weeks there has been a complete obstruction of the common duct.

The abdomen is opened with the patient in the position described in the previous operation and with the same type of anaesthesia and incision. The liver is small and hard. It cannot be brought forward or tipped, in spite of dividing the round ligament between ligatures and in spite of incising the falciform ligament. This greatly increases the difficulty of further procedure.

In the region of the gall bladder, which itself is at first not recognizable, there are numerous adhesions involving the great omentum, the transverse colon, the stomach and the transverse mesocolon. After the operative field has been walled off by moist sponges, a few highly vascular tissue strands running from the dome of the gall bladder to the colon are doubly ligated and divided. After this it is possible to separate the adhesions from the surface of the gall bladder for some distance by blunt dissection. Only at one point there are some unusually firm adhesions between the wall of the gall bladder and the stomach which demand sharp dissection. In the course of this, both the gall bladder and the stomach are opened, showing that a fistulous communication between the gall bladder and the stomach is present. Only a little purulent bile escapes from the perforation in the gall bladder since that organ has been converted into a hard, shrunken body tightly enclosing a few stones. The opening in the stomach is closed at once by a double-row suture. The opening in the gall bladder needs no special attention.

The exposure of the neck of the gall bladder and the cystic duct offers no particular difficulty. The operative field in the region of the gall bladder is walled off from the rest of the abdominal cavity with moist sponges in the manner described in the previous operation. After the peritoneal covering of the cystic duct has been split, the cystic artery is doubly ligated and divided and the cystic duct is picked up on a silk ligature.

The peritoneal incision over the cystic duct is continued onto the hepatoduodenal ligament. After doubly ligating and cutting numerous vessels of the venous plexus of Zuckerkandl running across it, there is exposed a thick cord-like structure that is obviously the obstructed common duct. In the interest of safety, the structure is first aspirated by means of a fine needle and a syringe. Cloudy purulent bile is obtained. The neighborhood is once more carefully walled off with packing and a gauze roll is introduced into the foramen of Winslow. The common duct is provided with two fine traction sutures and a small opening is made between the sutures. A large quantity of purulent bile gushes out and is promptly aspirated by the electric suction pump, held ready for the purpose. A number of small stones escape with the bile. After the flow of bile has abated somewhat, the common duct is scooped out with a gall-stone spoon, first in the direction of the liver, where a number of stones and thick purulent bile are evacuated, then toward the duodenum where a number of stones are likewise removed.

It is impossible, however, to pass the spoon into the duodenum, since an obstruction is encountered at the papilla of Vater. The duodenum is mobilized in order to gain access to this point. An incision is made through the peritoneum at its line of reflection from the posterior abdominal wall onto the lateral wall of the duodenum, and the duodenum is freed from the posterior abdominal wall by blunt dissection. When the retroduodenal portion of the common duct is grasped between the fingers of the left hand, a tightly lodged stone can easily be felt. After several unsuccessful attempts it is finally shoved upward toward the liver by milking manipulations and is removed through the opening in the common duct with the gall-stone spoon. Nevertheless it is still impossible to push the spoon or a probe into the interior of the duodenum. Palpation reveals a hard resistance in the region of the papilla of Vater which cannot be dislodged.

If it were proved that this resistance was the result of a cicatricial stenosis of the papilla of Vater, the simplest measure would be to short-circuit the cicatricial stenosis by a choledochoduodenostomy, by making a small anastomosis between the common duct and the duodenum at the point where the common duct, approaching the lateral border of the duodenum from the right, begins to disappear behind the gut.

In this case, however, a stone is tightly lodged in the papilla. There is consequently nothing else to do but expose the papilla transduodenally. After a further walling-off of the operative field, a longitudinal incision 3 cm long is made in the anterior wall of the duodenum at the level of the encountered obstacle with the electrosurgical knife. The escaping intestinal contents are removed by aspiration and sponging. Two sponges, tied together with a long thread, are inserted, one into each limb of the duodenum. The papilla of Vater is elevated by means of a slender Korn forceps introduced into the common duct through the supraduodenal opening. The tip of a stone the size of a cherry stone projects out of the papilla. An incision is made down on the stone with the electrosurgical knife so that it can easily be removed.

The wound edges of the duodenum and of the common duct resulting from the incision of the papilla of Vater are joined with interrupted catgut sutures to prevent subsequent stenosis. The sponges are removed from the duodenum and the opening in the anterior wall of the duodenum is closed in the usual manner by a double row of sutures. The duodenum, which has been freed from the posterior abdominal wall, is replaced and fastened into its original site with a few sutures.

The opening in the supraduodenal portion of the common duct is closed with interrupted catgut sutures and the suture line is buried by interrupted Lembert sutures. The duodenum and the common duct are then covered with moist compresses.

The gall bladder is then carefully exposed. In view of the obvious difficulties, the region of the gall bladder bed is first infiltrated with adrenalin solution by means of the high-pressure local anaesthesia apparatus in order to lessen the bleeding. The gall bladder is freed from the fundus toward the cystic duct. It is not possible to free the shrunken and thickened gall bladder from its bed in the liver by an anatomic dissection, since the boundary is broken through at a number of points and there are several abscesses in the adjacent part of the liver. The gall bladder is therefore actually excised from the liver with the electrosurgical knife. In so doing, the dividing plane between liver and gall bladder is frequently overstepped in both directions, so that it is often necessary to go back and trim off remaining bits of gall bladder wall. Not until the region of the neck of the gall bladder is reached is it possible to pick up and ligate a few strands of serosa stretching from the liver to the neck of the gall bladder before dividing them. Finally, the gall bladder remains attached to the common duct only by the cystic duct.

The cystic duct is divided between two clamps and its stump transfixed, ligated and buried in the manner previously described. No suture of the gall bladder bed in the liver is possible since this wall is rigid and unyielding. It is also impossible completely to control the bleeding since the parenchymatous vessels can not be caught. A vioform gauze pack is therefore placed in the gall bladder bed, and this is continued together with a drainage tube to the point of suture of the common duct and to the stump of the cystic duct. Drain and packing are brought out through the upper angle of the wound. The abdominal wound is then closed.

Case 14. Example of a cholecystgastrostomy in a case of inoperable carcinoma of the pancreas.

A man of 60 in the course of the last 6 weeks has gradually developed obstruction of the common duct. There has never been any pain. The gall bladder can be palpated as a large smooth swelling below the enlarged liver. The abdomen is opened by a "wave" incision under the girdle-type of spinal anaesthesia on a tentative diagnosis of carcinoma of the papilla of Vater. The smooth hugely distended gall bladder, large as a fist and nonadherent to its surroundings, extends quite a distance beyond the edge of the markedly congested liver. The gall bladder greatly obstructs the approach to the bile passages. Therefore, after careful walling-off of the surroundings, it is punctured at the apex of its fundus and emptied by a cannula attached to an electric suction pump. Since the viscid inspissated bile is not sufficiently evacuated by suction, the point of puncture is enlarged to a 3 cm. incision. The remaining fluid contents of the gall bladder are then sponged out. A gauze roll introduced into the gall bladder prevents the escape of the bile which continues to flow in through the cystic duct which is not obstructed. No stones can be felt in the gall bladder.

The empty gall bladder and the liver are forcibly retracted upward in order to examine the lower bile passages. It is then determined that the part of the common duct just above the duodenum, the duodenum, the head of the pancreas and the root of the transverse mesocolon are fused together by a hard tumor, concerning whose malignant nature and inoperability there is no doubt.

An anastomosis between the common duct and the duodenum is impossible because of the size of the growth and the changes in the involved structures. The flow of bile into the gastro-intestinal tract can be effected only by means of the gall bladder. In this case, the stomach, which is easily accessible, is used for the anastomosis. A fold of the anterior wall of the pyloric antrum is picked up in a clamp. The packing is removed from the gall bladder and its fundus which contains the aspiration opening is freed from the liver for a short distance and caught with an intestinal clamp. The clamped portions of the stomach and gall bladder are brought together side by side. A gauze roll is placed between them and the operative field properly isolated with sponges. The part of the gall bladder lying just above the clamp is turned upward with the aid of two Kocher forceps and attached to the anterior wall of the clamped fold of the pyloric antrum by interrupted silk Lembert sutures. The stomach is then incised at a distance of half a centimeter from the line of suture, the gall bladder having already been opened. The posterior three-layer suture is then applied as a running catgut suture. The anastomosis is completed by a running three-layer anterior Albert suture and by an anterior interrupted silk Lembert suture.

The compresses and the gauze roll lying beneath the anastomosis are removed. The abdomen is closed without drainage.

CHAPTER VII

OPERATIONS ON THE PARENCHYMATOUS ABDOMINAL ORGANS

A. OPERATIONS ON THE LIVER

The difficulties of liver surgery consist chiefly in the solution of two problems: the exposure of the lesion and the control of bleeding from the liver tissue.

1. The Exposure of the Liver

The normal liver is completely covered in the abdominal cavity by the costal arch. It is suspended from the diaphragm and attached to the posterior abdominal wall and can be displaced only very slightly. It consists of friable tissue and permits of no extensive attempts at changing its shape. An abdominal incision which goes only through soft tissues therefore affords a very limited view of the organ and makes practically only its lower surface accessible.

Conditions are somewhat more favorable if the liver as a result of enlargement or ptosis extends below the lower costal margin, if it may be drawn forward as a result of increased mobility, or if individual portions may be moved sufficiently because of a flaccidity of the organ.

The liver may be approached from in front, from behind, from the side or from above. It may be approached through incisions through soft tissues or by the removal of some of the ribs which cover it. The choice of the incision is determined by the site and the nature of the disease. As a result of the greater development of the right lobe and the right-sided position of the gall bladder and the hilum, the diseases of the right side of the liver preponderate considerably over those of the left side.

(a) In case of doubt as to the site of the lesion, a midline longitudinal incision extending downward from the xiphoid process is preferable for the exposure of the whole organ. This incision is also chosen in the case of most lesions of the left lobe of the liver. It is often necessary to enlarge a midline longitudinal incision by dividing the right or the left rectus. The left lobe of the liver is usually so mobile that it is possible to expose its convex surface from a midline incision by suitable traction. For every anterior abdominal incision the patient is placed in a position of marked lordosis of the lumbar spine.

(b) In case of lesions involving only the right lobe of the liver, the abdomen may also be opened by a right costal margin incision, which begins at the xiphoid process and runs parallel to and a few centimeters below the costal margin. From this incision a considerable part of the convex surface can be examined if the liver is flaccid and extends below the costal margin, as is often the case in chronic hepatic disease.

The liver is made more mobile by dividing the ligamentum teres between two ligatures and by nicking or incising the falciform ligament (Fig. 352). These measures are also used frequently in gall-stone operations for "tipping" the organ upward over the costal margin, and have already been described.

Nevertheless, the access provided by a midline or a right costal margin incision is in many cases inadequate, especially for reaching the dome of the liver on the right side. The lesion is better exposed if a part of the obstructing lower costal arch is removed. This can be carried out in the form of a temporary reflection of the costal margin according to Marwedel or by rib resection. In serious lesions which threaten life, permanent removal of the ribs is to be preferred, since this procedure gives more room and entails simpler conditions for healing. In both instances this preliminary operation is carried out essentially in the manner described and illustrated under the Marwedel operation on page 32. After dividing the (right) rectus, the upper triangular abdominal flap is split in the plane between the external oblique which is attached to the outer edge of the costal margin and the internal oblique which is attached to the inner edge of the costal margin. The ribs which are thereby exposed from in front are then resected or they are incised at both ends of the incision and reflected upward. As long as one is working below the 7th rib and between the sternal and the mammary line one is outside of the domain of the pleura. On the other hand, in the midaxillary line the pleural sac extends down as far as the 9th rib, and to the 12th rib at the side of the spine. In these regions any injury of the parietal pleura must carefully be avoided during the removal of the ribs. By resecting an appropriate number of ribs the dome of the right lobe of the liver can be made accessible from in front to a considerable extent.

(c) The right dome of the liver may also be reached by a transpleural exposure. This route is selected if an abscess has been located in the neighborhood of the posterior or the lateral convex surface of the right lobe of the liver and if lesions of other parts of the liver can be excluded. The transpleural exposure of the right lobe of the liver is carried out in the manner described on page 344, for the exposure of a right-sided subphrenic abscess. As a matter of fact, it usually remains in doubt in most cases whether pus aspirated in this region is situated within the liver as a liver abscess or whether it bathes the surface of the liver in the form of a subphrenic abscess.

(d) The posterior (dorsal) surface of the right lobe of the liver does not have a peritoneal covering but is attached directly to the posterior abdominal wall by means of connective tissue, and can therefore be reached from behind without opening the peritoneum. This approach is used chiefly in case of an abscess in the posterior part of the right lobe of the liver or in its neighborhood, as determined by aspiration. Here, too, the differential diagnosis between liver abscess and subphrenic abscess usually remains unsolved and the procedure is similar to that in case of a subphrenic abscess in this region. In cutting into the posterior surface of the liver exposed in this way, caution is necessary to avoid the thin-walled vena cava situated behind the liver at the inner wound angle of the operative field.

2. HEMOSTASIS AND THE TREATMENT OF INJURIES OF THE LIVER

General Considerations. Both in traumatic injuries of the liver as well as in intentional operative wounds inflicted by cutting the parenchyma, hemorrhage and hemostasis assume a dominant position. At the same time a large number of intrahepatic bile ducts are opened, so that the prevention of a further escape of bile likewise becomes a task in the management of wounds of the liver. The care for the bile passages, however, is made less important by the fact that the measures directed at the control of the bleeding, often a difficult matter, at the same time effect the more simple control of the escape of bile.

Hemostasis in traumatic as well as operative injury follows the same fundamental principles, so that the measures can be discussed together.

The diagnosis of a liver injury can often be made with ease from the position of the external wound or trauma and from the signs of peritoneal irritation and internal hemorrhage. In other cases, especially in blunt trauma of the abdomen, or when the position of an abdominal wound suggests various interpretations, the differentiation between a liver injury and shock or a perforative peritonitis is difficult. The opening of the abdominal cavity is indicated not only in every certain case of liver injury but also when such an injury is merely probable. Frequently the necessity for exposing the liver is of no greater importance than the necessity for examining the remainder of the abdominal cavity for injuries of other organs.

In case of such far-reaching indications, in which the inspection of the whole abdominal cavity must be reckoned with, it is best to open the abdomen in the midline above the umbilicus, in view of the varied problems with which the surgeon may find himself confronted. The access to the liver can be facilitated in case of necessity in the manner previously described by dividing the ligamentum teres, by incising the falciform ligament, by dividing the rectus muscle on one side or by rib resection. On the other hand if an examination of distant parts of the abdominal cavity seems unnecessary and if a fairly large external wound was made during the injury, one should gain access to the operative field in most cases by enlarging this wound.

The normal liver consists of a soft tissue rich in blood. In diseased states, its substance may become more firm and less vascular because of the increase in the connective tissue. This makes operative procedures in the liver tissue easier. The opening of the blood vessels of the liver may become dangerous not only because of the resultant loss of blood but also because air emboli may occur by way of the widely gaping liver veins, especially when the Trendelenburg position is used. This position should therefore be avoided in all liver operations.

A most valuable measure for lessening operative bleeding is to inject the operative field with adrenalin solution. For this purpose a solution of 20 drops of 1:1000 adrenalin in 100 cc. of saline solution or the usual local anaesthetic solution with added adrenalin is used. The liver tissue in the region of the incision or in the neighborhood of the operative field is so thoroughly infiltrated by means of a long thin needle that the tissue swells and assumes a whitish color. It is best to use the high-pressure local-anaesthesia apparatus for this purpose.

Bleeding may further be limited by the use of the electrosurgical knife. Adrenalin infiltration and the electric knife often make possible an almost bloodless procedure. However, one must not be deceived for the hemostasis effected in this way is only temporary, so that it is absolutely necessary in every case to carry out carefully the measures required for permanent hemo-

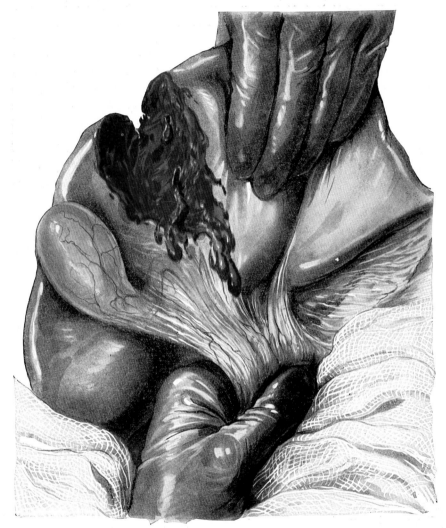

Fig. 379. Manual hemostasis in liver bleeding. The large vessels in the hepatoduodenal ligament are compressed with the left hand, the second to fifth fingers of which have been inserted into the foramen of Winslow.

stasis. While the use of the electrosurgical knife on the liver tissue does not produce disturbances in the healing of the wound, the use of the hot iron and the Paquelin cautery must be warned against, since the wounds so made show a lessened tendency to heal. Moreover, the actual cautery only slightly diminishes the bleeding from the larger vessels.

Permanent hemostasis is undertaken either in the region of the wound surface itself or at scme distance from it, in the manner later to be described.

Wedge-shaped biopsy specimens of liver tissue may be removed without bleeding if the area is surrounded by the injection of an adrenalin-saline solution. The resultant wound is closed by suture.

The arterial blood supply of the liver can be arrested by closure of the hepatic artery. For this purpose the surgeon reaches into the foramen of Winslow from right to left with the left hand and compresses the hepato-

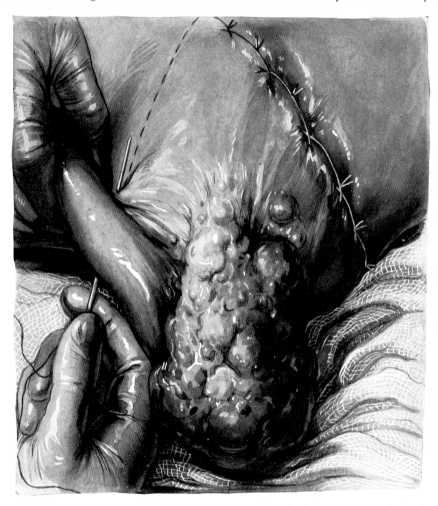

FIG. 380. Hemostasis in excision of a liver segment. The liver segment to be excised is being surrounded by overlapping sutures limiting the blood supply. They are passed through the whole thickness of the liver with a straight needle.

duodenal ligament with the fingers (Fig. 379), thereby interrupting the blood stream of the portal vein as well as the arterial supply. The retrograde entrance of venous blood by way of the hepatic vein is however not prevented by this maneuver. (Such a procedure is accompanied by a profound fall in the blood pressure and should be only rarely used since the patient is usually already shocked. I. S. R.) Finger pressure may be replaced by an intestinal clamp. The compression of the hepatoduodenal ligament, however, damages the intestine profoundly in a short time by the damming-back of the portal blood. It is said that the intestine can no longer recover after a quarter of an hour. The compression must therefore be restricted to the shortest possible time. This procedure may be used as a prophylactic measure before extensive liver operations as well as temporarily in the actual presence of hepatic hemorrhage.

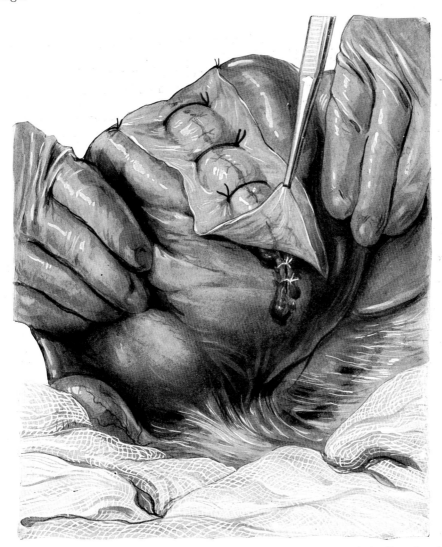

Fig. 381. Liver suture with fascial reenforcement. The capsule of the liver has been approximated with small sutures. A flap of fascia lata has been fastened over the suture line by large deep sutures and is attached at its edges to the liver surface with finer sutures.

In the resection of a lobe-shaped portion of the liver, the blood supply to the cut surface can be blocked by massive suture ligatures of catgut which grasp the whole thickness of the organ from its upper to its lower surface in a chain of overlapping interrupted sutures (Fig. 380). The sutures are passed through the liver substance by means of long straight round darning needles with blunted points. In view of the friable texture of the liver tissue the ligatures must not be pulled too tight, lest they cut through. They can be prevented from cutting through by interposing a more resistant material such as a free transplant of fascia or omentum (Fig. 381). The less clearly the operative field is defined against the rest of the liver, and the thicker the region of such an intended hemostatic suture is, the more difficult it is to carry out such a suture and the less effective is its hemostatic action. Temporary blocking of the blood supply to the operative field can often be effected more simply and suitably by manual compression, an assistant squeezing the liver with both his hands at the right and left of the operative site.

The surest control of bleeding from large liver vessels is by ligation of the vessels. They are caught with hemostats and tied off with catgut ligatures which are at times better mounted on needles.

The best way of handling a liver wound is suture, so that the peritoneal covering is again closed completely at the site of injury. The wound is drawn together with catgut sutures which are either passed through the full thickness of each side of the wound by means of long darning needles, or the superficial layers of each wound surface are merely picked up by means of curved needles (Fig. 381). Such a type of closure is possible only under aseptic conditions, and then only if the wound surfaces can be brought together, i.e., when there is no extensive loss of liver tissue or if the approximation of the wound edges is facilitated by great pliability of the liver tissue or by the wedge-shaped form of the defect. A supplementary suture of the capsule of the liver with fine catgut increases the dependability of the hemostasis effected in this manner.

Packing. If the bleeding can not be controlled in this way, as for example, in case of an irregular, ragged wound, the last resort is packing the wound. For this purpose I use vioform gauze, the gauze being packed firmly and systematically into the bleeding liver wound (Fig. 382). The gauze pack often has a great tendency to slip out. It may be fastened to the lower tissue by a few catgut sutures. If the gauze is removed too soon, secondary hemorrhage may occur; its removal should therefore not be started until it is entirely loose. After 5 to 6 days as a rule a cautious attempt may be made to see whether and how much of the gauze, moistened with hydrogen peroxide, will come out easily when light traction is made on it. The gauze is removed a little at a time.

The disadvantage of a partly open abdominal wound which packing entails can be avoided by using an absorbable packing material or a living graft. "Tabotamp" has been found useful as an absorbable form of packing. It is pressed into the liver wound in small pieces, which usually stick fairly tightly or else are fastened with catgut sutures. Living tampons are made of pedicled flaps of omentum, of free transplants of muscle or strips of fascia. The pieces of muscle may be taken from a rectus muscle, small strips of fascia from the anterior rectus sheath, and large strips from the fascia lata. They are packed into the cavity of the liver wound and are anchored with catgut sutures.

The management of free blood in the abdominal cavity. In every liver injury, clotted or fluid blood is present in the abdominal cavity. No attention should be paid to it for the time being, unless it impedes the view and the access to the liver, but the bleeding points should be located in order to stop the further escape of blood. A very free hemorrhage may be controlled successfully by the maneuver of compressing the hepatic artery for a short time as above described.

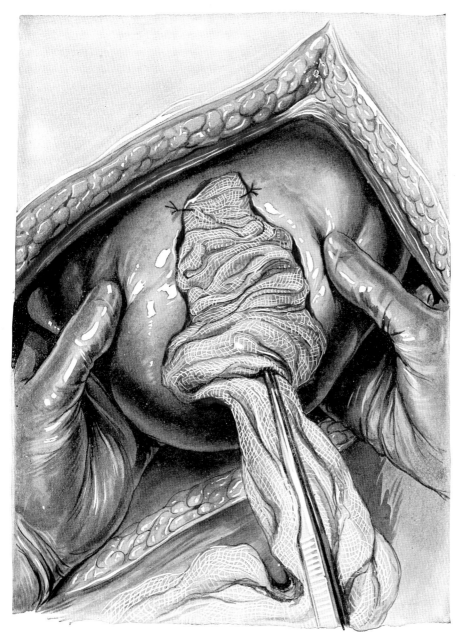

FIG. 382.   Packing a liver wound. The cavity of the liver wound has been packed with gauze which is fastened to the liver by sutures.

A few advocate that the blood found in the abdominal cavity be left there, on the ground that it is harmless locally and that it is of great value when it is quickly reabsorbed into the vascular system by the serous surfaces.   The generally accepted view, to which I also subscribe, favors the removal of the accumulated blood. Autotransfusion of the blood found in the abdominal cavity is of course permissible only when no bacterial contamination of the blood has occurred. This means that there must be no injury of the gastro-intestinal canal. However the blood which is present in the abdominal cavity as a result of a rupture of the liver may have a hemolytic effect when introduced into the circulation of the same individual, especially if it has been present in the abdominal cavity for more than 24 hours. It is uncertain whether this hemolytic action is due to the admixture of bile, or to other causes. At any rate, caution is necessary in autotransfusion. Some doubt can be removed by determining the absence of agglutination and hemolysis in a macroscopic test on a glass slide, but even here certain factors such as contamination cannot be ruled out.

The blood which has accumulated in the abdominal cavity is collected with a ladle or removed by suction. If the amount so recovered is considerable, if it is not contaminated, if there is no considerable admixture of bile, and if hemolysis is absent on testing, the blood can be citrated and immediately returned into a vein at the elbow by means of a gauze-covered funnel, in the manner described and illustrated in Vol. I, page 339.

Only in the rarest of instances will the hemostasis and the attendant closure of the intrahepatic bile ducts be so dependable that one can be sure that no further blood and bile will escape so that the abdomen may be closed without drainage. Even when the liver wound has been closed by suture, it is best to isolate it from the remainder of the abdominal cavity by a vioform gauze pack, carried to the surface through the abdominal incision.

3. Treatment of Neoplasms of the Liver

The resection of a portion of the liver containing a neoplasm is easy if the part to be removed is attached to the rest of the liver only by a narrow or thin bridge of liver tissue (Fig. 380). It is difficult if the tumor must be excised from the liver substance. It is advisable first to infiltrate the operative field with a solution containing adrenalin. The neighborhood of the region to be resected is blocked by a series of chain sutures (Fig. 380) or by manual compression. The diseased segment is best excised with the electrosurgical knife, if possible in the form of a wedge so that one flat wound surface can be joined to the other.

It is usually impossible to remove diseased portions which merge into the normal tissue of the liver without a clear-cut boundary. There is no point to such a resection since there can scarcely be any thought of a radical cure by the procedure. After the excision of a portion of the liver, the control of bleeding and the care of the wound are carried out in the manner already described.

4. Operations for Echinococcus Cysts of the Liver

The diagnosis of echinococcus disease of the liver, which formerly was based largely on palpation, is now made more certain by the complement fixation test. The establishment of the diagnosis calls for operation, in view of the possibility of suppuration and of extension by rupture of the cysts or by dissemination through the blood stream.

On inspection of the surface of the liver after opening the abdominal cavity the diagnosis sometimes seems uncertain because of the marked infiltration present and an inoperable neoplasm may be suspected. Aspiratory puncture with a large needle, which must never be omitted, or a deep diagnostic incision into the supposed tumor clarifies the situation.

After opening the abdomen, the general abdominal cavity must be protected carefully by packing against the entrance of cyst contents, since the fluid often contains bacteria or viable scolices whose spread can lead to peritonitis or to a dissemination of the echinococcus disease in the abdominal cavity. Every drop of escaping fluid is aspirated by an electrically driven suction apparatus or caught by sponges.

The action of a 1 per cent formalin solution is said to kill living echinococcus parasites within 5 minutes. It is therefore advised by some that the echinococcus cysts be punctured and filled with this fluid for 5 minutes. (Such a procedure is not without danger and should only rarely if ever be used. I.S.R.) The compresses used to isolate the operative field may be moistened with this solution. (The procedure should not be recommended because it is uncertain and dangerous. I.S.R.)

A solitary cyst which lies in an isolated lobe of the liver is best removed unopened like a malignant growth by resection of the liver lobe or treated by marsupialization.

One or more bulging vesicles lying just below the liver surface and which cannot be removed by liver resection are aspirated and emptied with a cannula connected with an electric suction apparatus and are then cautiously opened with the electrosurgical knife. The contents are carefully sponged away and the sac is packed with vioform gauze.

Cysts which are separated from the surface by a thick layer of liver tissue are also first evacuated by aspiration. Before incising the overlying layer of liver, it is infiltrated with an adrenalin solution and is then divided down to the interior of the cyst with the electrosurgical knife. Hemorrhage from the incision is controlled by ligation or by a chain of deep sutures, in the manner already described.

The further procedure after the opening of the cyst depends on whether the cyst wall can be peeled out of the liver, a maneuver which is often possible in young non-infected cysts, or whether the cyst has been anchored by firm adhesions.

If at all possible, the cyst should be dissected out of the liver. The wall of a cyst which can be shelled out is usually enclosed by a layer of fibrous tissue. The separation between the fibrous tissue and the cyst wall can generally be carried out by blunt dissection and without difficulty, the cyst wall being held taut with hemostats (Fig. 383). The few vessels which bleed are caught and ligated. The wound bed which remains after the removal of the cyst is carefully examined by sight, using an electric light in the interior, and by palpation for daughter cysts which are present in a considerable percentage of cases. Such secondary cysts must then also be removed.

If the cyst contents are not infected, which is indicated by clear fluid, and the absence of fever before operation, if there is no bleeding from the liver bed, if all the cysts present have surely been removed, and if the walls of the liver wound can be brought together fairly well, the liver wound is best closed by joining the surfaces and edges of the wound with catgut sutures. But even in such favorable cases the region of the liver wound is separated from the rest of the abdominal cavity by a strip of vioform gauze which together with a drainage tube are led out through the abdominal incision. The remainder of the abdominal incision is closed.

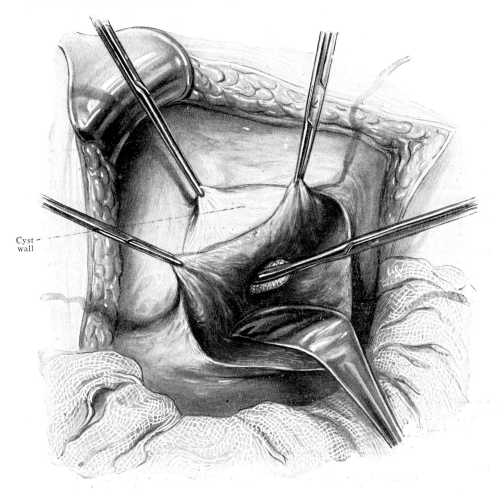

Cyst wall

FIG. 383. Single-stage enucleation of an echinococcus cyst of the liver. The smooth thin cyst wall has been put on stretch with hemostats and is freed by blunt dissection.

Occasionally it is possible to shell out an echinococcus cyst from the liver without preliminary aspiration or incision. This is always a risky procedure, since one cannot certainly prevent the rupture of the cyst during the dissection and since the resultant sudden flooding of the operative field with the cyst fluid entails the danger of dissemination of the echinococcus disease. On the other hand, the ease with which a cyst may be shelled out is not impaired by preliminary drainage and incision. The enucleation of an intact cyst should therefore be restricted to rare and particularly favorable cases.

If the cyst can not primarily be shelled out of the liver, and that is unfortunately the case in many instances, the edges of the opened cyst are sutured tightly to the edge of the abdominal incision which has been partly

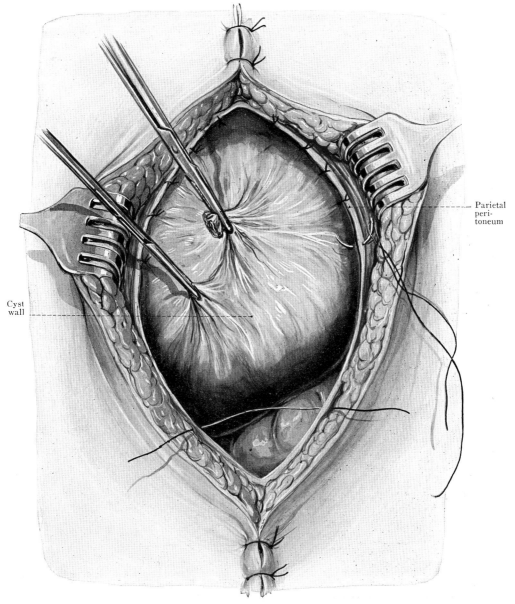

Parietal peritoneum

Cyst wall

FIG. 384. Marsupialization of an echinococcus cyst of the liver. The cyst has been emptied by aspiration and the puncture opening is closed with a clamp. The cyst wall is attached on all sides to the cut edge of the parietal peritoneum.

closed (Fig. 384). The cyst is provided with one or more thick drainage tubes and is packed with vioform gauze.

Such a marsupialized cyst wall frequently becomes free later, after suitable after-treatment consisting in dressings and irrigations with weak disinfectants, and it can later be removed with a forceps or can be shelled out by cautious blunt dissection with the finger or a sponge mounted on a forceps (Fig. 385). The cavity remaining in the liver after the removal of the sac as a rule closes gradually by granulation.

If the marsupialized cyst does not become free, healing frequently does not take place and a permanent fistula remains. The drainage fluid gradually

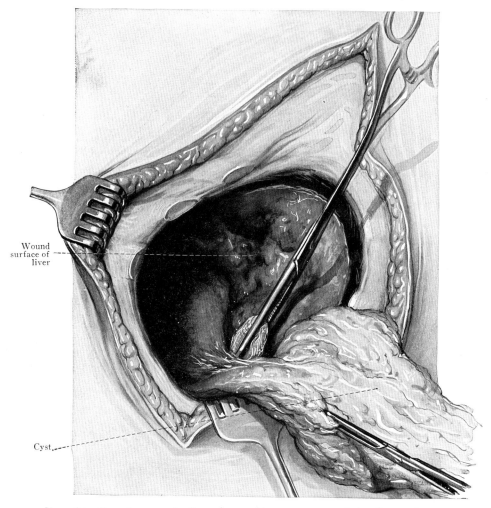

Fig. 385. Two-stage enucleation of an echinococcus cyst of the liver. Continuation of conditions of the preceding illustration. The thick irregular cyst wall, after a primary marsupialization of the cyst, is freed from the liver tissue which has become demarcated from the cyst by a wall of granulation tissue.

comes to consist chiefly of bile and may deprive the body of a large part of this secretion. The constant loss of bile and the chronic infection can assume threatening proportions. It has occasionally been possible in such cases to bring the opened cyst into communication with a large bile duct or with the intestine and eventually to effect a cure in this manner.

If primary enucleation of the echinococcus cyst cannot be counted upon, the opening of the cyst may be performed in two stages. At the first operation the cyst is sutured to the edge of the abdominal incision, or, since a thin cyst wall must not be punctured, it is brought into the wound which is held open around it by packing. The cyst is opened at a later operation after adhesions have formed.

5. Treatment of Liver Abscesses. Diagnostic Puncture of the Liver

Exploratory aspiration is at times unavoidable in the diagnosis and localization of liver abscesses. It is made through the liver substance with a long thick hollow needle and at a point where the liver lies as close as possible to the body wall and where the intestine cannot be injured. However it is frequently necessary to puncture the pleural sac as well. (I do not believe this is a justifiable procedure. It is better to do a laparotomy and then aspirate. I.S.R.) Since the entrance of echinococcus fluid into the serous cavities carries with it the danger of implantation, diagnostic puncture is not permissible if there is a possibility of the presence of an echinococcus cyst. In the presence of pus as well, a diagnostic puncture is not without danger, in view of the possibility of infecting the pleural and the peritoneal cavity. These dangers are lessened, in case the aspiration gives positive findings, by going on at once to the operative exposure of the abscess. In case echinococcus fluid is unexpectedly aspirated, the indication for immediate operation is even more urgent. If the aspirating needle is left in place for the time being, it will facilitate the finding of a small and hidden abscess at operation.

A liver abscess should be approached by the shortest direct route possible. This route frequently leads through the abdominal cavity below the costal margin from in front, or through the pleural space above the costal margin from in front, from the side or from behind after an appropriate rib resection. (The two-stage operation carries much less risk. At the first operation the ribs are excised and the costophrenic sinus of the pleura is obliterated by packing. At the second operation the exploratory puncture is made. I.S.R.) The localization and opening of the abscess are carried out in the manner described under the opening of subphrenic abscesses on page 343, and under the opening of echinococcus cysts on page 527. After isolation from the general abdominal or the pleural space, the abscess is either aspirated, evacuated, packed and drained at the first operation, or it is only walled off from the abdominal cavity or the pleural space by suturing it to the wound margins or by packing in the first operation and is drained and packed at the second operation. No attempt should be made to peel the abscess wall out of the liver.

6. Appendix: Treatment of Ascites

Among the various causes of ascites, the diffuse chronic diseases (cirrhoses) of the liver occupy a dominant place, together with the chronic diseases of the peritoneum. The operative treatment of ascites is limited chiefly to purely palliative measures. It consists either in the simple evacuation of the fluid or it may at the same time attempt to prevent the recurrence of the fluid accumulation by establishing new channels for drainage.

ABDOMINAL PARACENTESIS

Tapping is the simplest form of evacuation. While a **diagnostic** puncture of the abdominal cavity is not permissible for investigating doubtful lesions because of the danger of opening an infectious hollow viscus or an abscess, a **therapeutic** puncture is not dangerous in the presence of a large free collection of fluid.

For the puncture of the abdominal wall a site should be selected where there are no large vessels in the wall, and where no organ is attached to its inner side. These conditions are fulfilled in the midline between the umbilicus and the symphysis, so that this region is frequently preferred. After the bladder has been completely emptied, the patient is placed in a semi-sitting position so that the fluid collects below the umbilicus and the intestines float upward on its surface. The puncture site is anaesthetized. A small longitudinal incision, just large enough to admit the trochar, is made through the skin. The handle of the trochar, which must not be of too small a caliber, is braced against the palm of the hand; the tip of the index finger lies at the point up to which the tube is to be inserted (Vol. I, Fig. 271, page 280). With a twisting motion the trochar is pushed through the abdominal wall in a single thrust.

After the removal of the obturator the fluid is drawn off slowly, at times in stages. (Rapid decompression may be followed by circulatory collapse. I.S.R.) If the flow stops, it can frequently be started again by shifting the patient's position, by moving the cannula in a pendulum-like manner, by pressure on the abdomen or by inserting a sound or a Nelaton catheter. (Always use a cannula with lateral fenestrations. I. S. R.) If no further fluid can be obtained, the cannula is withdrawn and the skin wound is closed with a suture.

Frequently a portion of the abdominal wall thicker than the linea alba is preferred for the puncture, in an effort to prevent the subsequent leakage of fluid from the puncture site which is annoying and not without danger because of the possibility of infection, and also to insure a more dependable closure by scar tissue. Particular care must be taken to avoid the deep epigastric vessels and their branches coursing within the rectus sheath. The puncture is therefore made outside of the semilunar line of Spigelius, preferably at a point which lies a little to the outer side of the middle of the line connecting the umbilicus and the anterior superior spine of the ilium.

Evacuation of ascites by tapping is followed in most cases by a prompt reaccumulation of the fluid, so that further tappings become necessary at more or less frequent intervals. Unfortunately, most of the operative measures intended for permanent drainage of the ascites are only rarely successful. These operations have one of two objectives, to open new channels for venous return, thereby influencing the ascites indirectly, or to divert the newly formed fluid into the connective tissue by means of direct permanent drainage.

EVACUATION OF ASCITES BY LAPAROTOMY. TREATMENT OF TUBERCULOUS EXUDATIVE PERITONITIS

In spite of every effort, considerable amounts of fluid always remain in the abdominal cavity after tapping for diffuse ascites. If the fluid is to be removed completely, this can only be done by laparotomy. The procedure is used especially in those cases in which a favorable effect upon the underlying disease is expected from the opening of the abdomen, or in which the laparotomy also serves the purpose of another intraperitoneal operation, or of establishing the diagnosis. This is particularly the case in a tuberculous ascites. Just what the reason is for the favorable action frequently observed after such a laparotomy in tuberculosis of the abdominal cavity is as yet unknown. It may be due to the effect of light, air, mechanical, thermal or chemical irritation, the relief afforded by a single complete removal of the fluid, action on the blood vessels, formation of foreign protein, etc.

The abdomen is opened by a longitudinal incision in the midline below the umbilicus, with the patient preferably in the Trendelenburg position. The fluid encountered in the abdominal cavity is drawn off slowly, preferably by suction with an electric suction pump. By pushing back the bulging intestines, a little pool keeps forming out of which the fluid can be sucked or dipped. Loculated collections of fluid are freed with the hand. The remainder of the ascitic fluid is taken up with compresses or sponges. The last of the fluid tends to collect not only in the pouch of Douglas, but also beneath the diaphragm. Plenty of light, a certain amount of cooling and a mild mechanical irritation of the peritoneal covering of the intestines are considered advantageous.

At the end a disinfectant may be introduced into the abdominal cavity. I prefer to use iodoformosol, an iodine preparation with only a slight odor.

Any further operative measures which may be necessary should be carried out at the same laparotomy if at all possible. They are needed not infrequently in tuberculous peritonitis, for example, the freeing of intestinal adhesions, the short-circuiting of an intestinal stenosis by an entero-enterostomy, or the resection of a tuberculous intestinal loop, most frequently an ileocecal tumor.

At the conclusion of the operation the abdominal wound is completely and very carefully closed in order to prevent the subsequent leakage of fluid.

ESTABLISHMENT OF NEW VENOUS CHANNELS (TALMA OPERATION)

The object of this procedure is to produce highly vascular adhesions between the passively congested abdominal viscera and the abdominal walls, so that the visceral veins, avoiding the portal vein and the liver, shall be connected directly with the systemic venous bed.

The procedure most generally used is the Talma operation. The abdomen is opened by a midline incision above the umbilicus. The greater omentum is pulled out and its surface is freshened by rubbing it with a compress until it bleeds slightly. The parietal peritoneum on both sides of the abdominal wound is scarified over an area the size of the palm of the hand by scraping it with a knife. The scarified surface of the omentum is sutured to that of the parietal peritoneum with catgut (intraperitoneal attachment). The surface of the omentum may also be anchored extraperitoneally by suturing it into a pocket made on one side of the wound, either between the parietal peritoneum and the abdominal muscles (Fig. 386) or between the muscles and the skin (subcutaneous).

If the omentum is shrunken and therefore not suitable for the purpose, the freshened lower pole of the spleen may be sutured intra- or extraperitoneally in the same manner through an incision in the left flank.

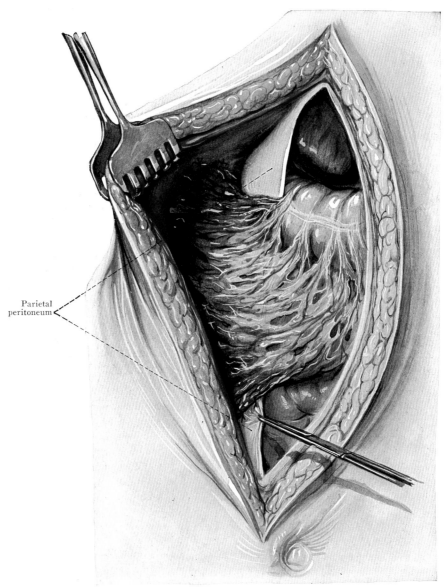

Parietal
peritoneum

FIG. 386. Talma operation for the treatment of ascites. Extraperitoneal transplantation of the omentum. The parietal peritoneum has been freed from the musculature on the right side of the abdominal wound. Into the pocket so formed the omentum has been placed and fastened with sutures, after having first been scarified.

"WINDOW" DRAINAGE

I have occasionally seen a satisfactory result after a subcutaneous drainage of the ascites in the manner proposed by Kalb. Its purpose is to form a wide permanent connection between the abdominal cavity and the subcutaneous connective tissue (Fig. 387), so that the fluid constantly being formed inside the abdomen is absorbed as in continuous hypodermoclysis.

The procedure is carried out as follows: The patient is placed in the Trendelenburg position and the side of the patient which is opposite the surgeon is elevated. The abdominal cavity is opened by a midline incision, a little more below than above the umbilicus. The ascitic fluid is completely removed. The side of the abdominal wound opposite the surgeon is forcibly retracted. While the intestines are held back, or in case of necessity after eventrating the intestines, the surgeon cuts a round opening the size of the palm of the hand through the abdominal wall from within the abdomen, with the exception of the skin. This is best done with the electrosurgical knife. The external muscle fascia must also be removed so that the subcutaneous fat

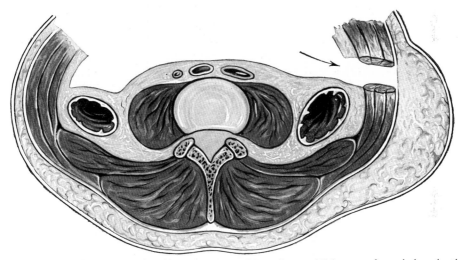

FIG. 387. "Winslow" drainage of ascites. After the establishment of a window in the abdominal wall, the fluid in the abdominal cavity can gain access in the direction of the arrow to the subcutaneous tissue and can there be absorbed.

and the uninjured skin are the only structures between the abdominal cavity and the exterior. The operator avoids injuring the skin by placing his left hand on the outside over the endangered area (Fig. 388). If visibility is limited by adhesions, caution is necessary to avoid injuring the ascending colon on the right side and the descending colon on the left. As a rule the muscle wound bleeds quite freely. Hemostasis may be quite difficult in the abdominal window which is hard to get at, and at times it must be controlled with a running suture. Finally, the midline incision is closed without drainage.

In a short time the skin over the window bulges hugely, and its neighborhood becomes infiltrated with fluid. The edema may spread extensively and may lead to a marked swelling of the scrotum or the labia majora. The more marked such an edema and the longer it lasts, the better is the result of the operation.

The operation may also be performed on both sides.

Other attempts at permanent drainage of the abdominal cavity into the subcutaneous connective tissue, for example the insertion of hardened calves' arteries or of silk threads, or of transplantation of the saphenous vein have not been successful.

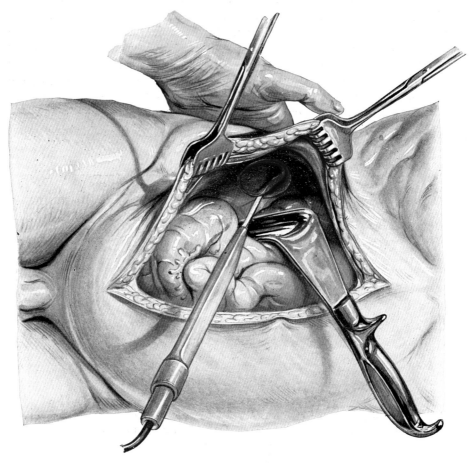

FIG. 388. "Window" drainage of ascites. The abdomen has been opened in the midline and the right side of the abdominal wall is being forcibly elevated. With the electrosurgical knife a section of the abdominal wall (except for the skin) the size of the palm of the hand is excised in the region of Petit's triangle. The surgeon's left hand placed on the outer surface guards the skin against injury.

B. OPERATIONS ON THE PANCREAS

1. THE EXPOSURE OF THE PANCREAS

Anatomic Considerations. The pancreas lies against the posterior wall of the abdominal cavity and forms a part of the posterior border of the lesser peritoneal cavity. It crosses in front of the body of the first or second lumbar vertebra, and is surrounded by the duodenum in the shape of a horseshoe open toward the left. Like the duodenum, it is clothed with peritoneum only on its anterior surface and therefore lies retroperitoneal. The major duct runs through the gland from left to right and empties into the descending limb of the duodenum together with the common bile duct through the papilla of Vater.

In exposing the pancreas and incising the glandular tissue great caution is necessary because of several large vessels in the neighborhood, some of them of vital importance (Fig. 389). Behind the pancreas in the long axis of the body are the superior mesenteric artery and vein which supply the whole small intestine. They are partly surrounded on the right by the head of the pancreas, the uncinate process, as it curves backward and thus they actually run through the gland. The artery gives off the inferior pancreaticoduodenal artery which runs around the head of the pancreas along the inner margin of the descending limb of the duodenum. Behind the head of the pancreas lies the

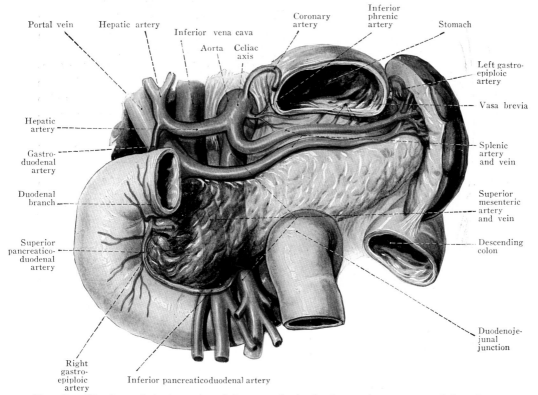

FIG. 389. Blood vessels in the region of the stomach, the duodenum, the pancreas and the spleen.

portal vein. It may also run through the pancreatic tissue. Along the upper border of the pancreas runs the splenic artery. It is the chief blood supply of the spleen. It may, however, be ligated without serious damage, according to the experience of von Mikulicz. Behind the pancreas lie the vena cava to the left and the aorta to the right of the spine.

The common bile duct runs through or posterior to the head of the pancreas to the papilla of Vater.

The pancreas itself receives its blood supply from the celiac axis by way of the pancreaticoduodenal artery and the splenic artery as well as from the superior mesenteric artery by way of the inferior pancreaticoduodenal artery. The veins of the pancreas empty into the portal vein.

The Approaches to the Pancreas (Fig. 390). In the majority of cases the pancreas is approached through a laparotomy. A midline incision just above the umbilicus is used. The incision may then be enlarged upward, downward or to the sides in case of a mistaken diagnosis or in the treatment of other abdominal organs.

(a) *The Approach through the Gastrocolic Omentum.* After opening the abdomen, the most suitable and most usual approach to the pancreas as it forms the floor of the lesser peritoneal cavity lies through the gastrocolic omentum which is divided to the necessary extent between ligatures (Figs. 106 and 391). The stomach is drawn upward with a broad spatula retractor and the transverse colon downward. This exposes the floor of the lesser peritoneal cavity and the pancreas. The pancreas lies parallel to and just above the origin of the transverse mesocolon.

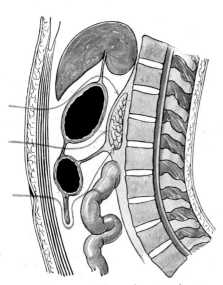

FIG. 390. The various anterior approaches to the pancreas. The cranial approach leads through the gastrohepatic omentum; the intermediate, shortest and most serviceable route is through the gastrocolic omentum; the caudal route is beneath the greater omentum through the root of the transverse mesocolon.

(b) *The Approach through the Gastrohepatic Omentum.* After opening the abdomen access to the pancreas may also be gained through the gastrohepatic omentum. In so doing, the stomach is forcibly retracted downward and the liver upward. This route, however, is less convenient and the exposure is less extensive, unless conditions are rendered more satisfactory by a very low position of the stomach.

In the course of gall-stone operations the head of the pancreas is occasionally exposed from the right by mobilizing and reflecting the duodenum.

(c) *The Approach through the Transverse Mesocolon.* In rare instances, an approach from the lower abdominal space through the transverse mesocolon is indicated. This route is not advisable because pancreatic juice can get among the loops of the small bowel through the communication with the lower abdomen which this procedure entails, and because the division of the mesenteric vessels endangers the nutrition of the transverse colon. In this operation the colon is drawn forward and turned upward, the transverse mesocolon is put on stretch and is partly divided at its base, with care to avoid the larger vessels supplying the transverse colon.

(d) *The Dorsal Approach.* Although the pancreas lies in direct contact with the posterior abdominal wall, the approach to it from behind is difficult, involved and dangerous, because the path is blocked by the spine, the great masses of muscle attached to it and the large vessels. The dorsal approach therefore comes into consideration only exceptionally in case of a posterior abscess. It is effected through a right- or left-sided incision just below and parallel to the 12th rib. The thick muscles are divided until an edematous infiltration of the tissue or escaping pus leads to the abscess. The upper pole of the kidney is pushed downward in case it comes into view.

General Considerations. The pancreas bleeds freely when incised. The thin-walled vessels are hard to catch and to ligate. Temporary packing usually controls the bleeding. The hemostatic qualities of the electrosurgical knife give it a great advantage for incising the pancreas.

Open pancreatic wound surfaces denuded of their peritoneal covering secrete a fluid which has a toxic action on serous-covered organs. Such wounds must therefore be closed if possible or else covered with omentum. Even then, it is absolutely necessary as a precautionary measure to place a drainage tube or packing at the threatened point in case of extensive injury of the pancreas. If it is impossible to cover large pancreatic wound surfaces, the drainage and packing of the pancreatic wound must be more thorough. Pancreatic juice also irritates and digests the skin. Therefore the skin in the neighborhood of a wound discharging pancreatic juice must be given a thick coating of zinc oxide ointment daily. (If the dressings used on the skin are saturated with any heavy metal the pancreatic ferments will be inactivated and excoriation will not occur. I.S.R.)

2. TREATMENT OF INJURIES OF THE PANCREAS

Injuries due to external trauma almost never involve the gland substance alone, nor, even if that is the case, are they operated upon on a diagnosis of pancreatic injury alone. They usually represent additional findings discovered during the treatment of abdominal injuries by blunt or sharp trauma involving other organs as well. In examining the abdominal cavity in such cases one must not forget to inspect the pancreas, in order that its injuries should not be overlooked.

The treatment of an injury of the pancreas includes first the control of the bleeding by catching and ligating or suturing the bleeding vessels. The next step is to seal the pancreatic wound thoroughly against the general abdominal cavity. This is done by means of deep sutures of the parenchyma with catgut, by superficial suture of the capsule and by applying and oversewing nearby peritoneal reduplications, especially the omentum. However, no such closures of large pancreatic wounds are dependable, and since the escaping pancreatic juice may seriously injure the abdominal organs, packing and drainage of the injured area must never be omitted.

Injuries of the pancreas are often produced at operation, especially in the course of a resection of an ulcerated or carcinomatous stomach. If these lesions have invaded the pancreas, the floor of the ulcer is formed by a deep greasy funnel of pancreatic tissue. If the stomach in the course of the resection is trimmed off from the edge of this crater with the electrosurgical knife, the ulcerated pancreatic surface is freely exposed. This surface which is open to the general abdominal cavity must be shaved away with the electrosurgical loop and covered by suture or by oversewing it with omentum. Such ulcerated wounds of the pancreas have a remarkably good capacity for healing, so that the abdomen may be closed without drainage after the procedure described.

In the course of the mobilization of ulcerated segments of the duodenum, tears of the capsule and the superficial gland tissue are almost always inflicted in dissecting free the head of the pancreas and in ligating the little vessels between the pancreas and the duodenal wall. Also during terminal closure of the duodenum, which has been divided as low as possible, it is often impossible to avoid pricking the head of the pancreas. Such minor injuries, however, have no serious consequences and do not prevent the closure of the abdomen without drainage.

3. Treatment of Neoplasms of the Pancreas

The total extirpation of the pancreas because of malignant neoplasms is extremely difficult, if not impossible. In attempting such a risk, the anatomic considerations already mentioned must be borne in mind.

In most instances only a partial removal of pancreatic tissue is undertaken. This is much easier and less dangerous in the tail of the organ than in the head, and is greatly facilitated by the use of the electrosurgical knife. After ligation of the duct of Wirsung the attached acinar portion of the gland atrophies while the island tissue hypertrophies. The wound resulting from the removal of parts of the gland must be closed by suture as well as possible and must be covered with peritoneum. For this purpose the omentum may be used to good advantage. Packing and drainage can usually not be avoided.

If the part of the pancreas adjacent to the duodenum was removed and if no excretory duct of the remaining portion of the pancreas is demonstrable, the cross-section of the pancreas is implanted into the duodenum, in doing which the suture of the serous covering of the pancreas to the serous covering of the duodenum must be absolutely tight.

Tumors of adjacent organs which have invaded the pancreas from without, e. g., carcinomata of the stomach, may frequently be excised in connection with the main tumor without any particular difficulty. Here, too, the electrosurgical knife is of the greatest value. The resulting raw surfaces of the gland are closed by suture, by peritoneal and omental plastic procedures and must be packed and drained if the closure is not complete.

(Adenomata of the islands of Langerhans may give rise to continued or intermittent hyperinsulinism with the resultant symptoms of hypoglycemia. The condition may prove fatal if the underlying cause is not removed surgically. The whole of the pancreas must be carefully inspected, since the adenoma may be only a centimeter in diameter and could easily be overlooked. I.S.R.)

4. Treatment of Cysts of the Pancreas

Cysts located within the pancreas are either sutured to the abdominal wound and drained, or they are excised.

Excision is the surer and shorter procedure and is therefore more to be recommended. It is however unduly dangerous for the moment because of the magnitude of the operation and because of the danger of hemorrhage and of unintentional injuries to adjacent structures. It should therefore be performed only under especially favorable circumstances, when the cyst can be shelled out easily and if the patient is in good condition. After opening the abdomen the question as to whether excision is possible must first be decided.

Extensive adhesions to the neighboring organs, the mesocolon, the transverse colon, the stomach and the great vessels, rule out primary removal.

If enucleation of the cyst is possible, the operative site is walled off in the usual manner. The peritoneum is carefully divided around the margins of the cyst and the cyst is dissected out by cutting between ligatures strands of tissue which are fixed to the cyst capsule by separating flat surfaces partly by blunt, partly by sharp dissection. This task is often made easier by a preliminary emptying of the cyst. Because of the harmful action of the pancreatic juice on the peritoneum, this should be done by aspiration and sponging, with the surrounding area carefully protected.

After the cyst has been completely removed, its bed is carefully searched for bleeding points. If hemostasis is complete and if the pancreatic tissue has not been otherwise injured, the edges of the wound bed are completely sutured together and the abdomen closed without drainage. In most instances the wound bed must be packed and drained, in which case the wound in the pancreas should be closed as well as possible around the packing in the form of a bag.

In the majority of cases the less dangerous procedure of suturing the cyst to the abdominal wound is undertaken. After the operative field has been carefully walled off, the cyst wall is sutured to the abdominal wound in as large a circumference as possible, visceral peritoneum to parietal peritoneum. If the needles pierce the thin cyst wall, it is better to empty the cyst first rather than risk contaminating the abdominal cavity with cyst fluid. After the cyst is opened it is thoroughly packed and drained. If it is possible to suture the closed cyst into the wound, the rest of the wound is closed and the cyst is opened immediately or in several days after the development of sufficient adhesions. The empty cavity is packed and drained. Healing takes place slowly by granulation. A permanent fistula often remains. (The recent recommendation of Cutler to use sclerosing solutions on these endothelial surfaces may be useful in lesions of this type. I.S.R.)

It has also been proposed that the cyst be drained into the intestine by establishing an anastomosis between the cyst and a loop of the small bowel according to the principles of entero-enterostomy. The danger of this procedure lies in the infection of the cyst by the intestinal bacteria and in the resultant suppuration. (This procedure is not based on sound surgical principles. I.S.R.)

5. Treatment of Acute Pancreatitis

Acute pancreatitis (necrosis of the pancreas, apoplexy of the pancreas) is often difficult or impossible to diagnose before the abdomen is opened and is particularly hard to differentiate from intestinal obstruction or peritonitis.

Obesity, previous attacks of gall stones, the sudden and intense onset of pain, abdominal distension, tympany, marked epigastric tenderness, radiation of the pain in a girdle around the left flank and back, between the shoulder blades and into the left shoulder, signs of collapse, severe vomiting, occasional hematemesis, labored breathing, slight cyanosis and a subicteric tint of the skin speak for an acute pancreatitis. Additional valuable diagnostic aids that have recently been evolved are the examination of the urine for diastase (Wohlgemuth test) and the estimation of the blood sugar.

Wohlgemuth test for the determinary of urinary diastase according to Baumann's modification. (a) A series of dilutions of the fluid to be examined is prepared in concentrations of 1:2, 1:4, 1:8, 1:16, etc. up to 1:4000 in the following manner: 1 cc. of physiologic salt solution is placed into each of 12 test tubes, 1 cc. of the fluid to be examined is added to tube No. 1 and shaken, 1 cc. of this mixture is added to tube No. 2 and shaken, 1 cc. of this mixture is added to tube No. 3 and shaken, and so on to the 12th tube.

(b) To each tube of this series is added 1 cc. of a phosphate buffer mixture, consisting of a freshly prepared mixture of equal part of $\frac{1}{15}$ molar solution of monopotassium phosphate (9.078 g. $KH_2 PO_4$ in 1 liter of water) and $\frac{1}{15}$ molar solution of disodium phosphate (11.876 g. $Na_2 H PO_4.2H_2O$ in 1 liter of water).

(c) To each tube is then added 1 cc. of a 0.2-per cent freshly prepared starch solution.

(d) The tubes are shaken, warmed in a water bath at $38°$ C for exactly 30 minutes, then cooled and to each is added 2 drops of $\frac{N}{50}$ iodine solution. A blue or violet color denotes the presence of unsplit starch.

(e) The test tube containing the highest dilution which has become completely starch-free, that is, the highest numbered tube with white contents, determines the computation of the diastase content. To determine the diastase value, the denominator of the dilution fraction of this tube is multiplied by 2. The resultant figure gives the number of milligrams of starch that have been split.

The following diastase values are therefore obtained for the individual test tubes: tube No. 1 = 4, tube No. 2 = 8, tube No. 3 = 16, and so on up to 8000.

If for example the contents of tubes 1 to 3 are colorless or opaque, whereas those of tubes 4 to 12 blue, then tube No. 3 is used in the computation and the diastase value is $3 \times 8 = 24$ mg. (The various methods for determining the urinary or serum amylase in acute and chronic pancreatic disease are not as yet absolutely reliable. They may however be of some help. I.S.R.)

Even if the diagnosis of acute pancreatitis is certain or probable, this is not necessarily an indication for immediate operation. When the disease manifestations are not stormy, an expectant policy is advised in most cases. Other patients come under treatment in so severe a state of collapse that operation is impossible for the moment.

Moderately severe cases and very severe cases in patients who are not too much weakened should be operated upon immediately. The opening of the abdomen is indicated all the more in such cases since it is often impossible to differentiate the condition from other diseases, especially intestinal obstruction, which in their further development will give rise to a suppurative peritonitis.

Care and speed are essential in the operation. Since local anaesthesia is inadequate for an operation involving the depths of the abdomen, and general anaesthesia is usually poorly borne by the greatly weakened patient, the girdle type of spinal anaesthesia is the method of choice.

The objectives of the operation are: (1) the aspiration of the fluid in the abdominal cavity which will inflict damage by its toxic and ferment action;

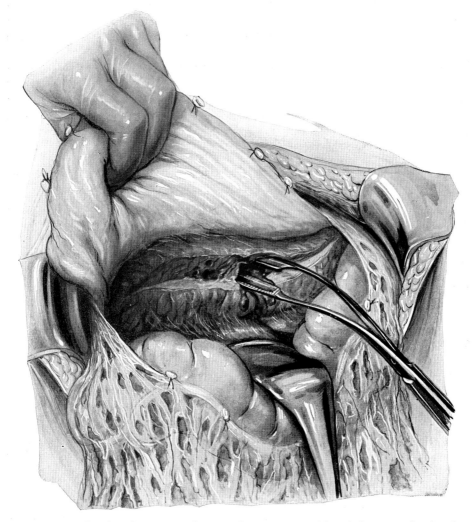

FIG. 391. Opening the pancreas in case of acute pancreatitis. A large opening has been made in the gastrocolic omentum and the stomach is retracted upward, the transverse colon with the mesocolon downward. The pancreas which lies in the bottom of the wound against the posterior abdominal wall has been slit open longitudinally with the electrosurgical knife. Isolated inflammatory foci are opened widely by inserting a forceps.

(2) the prevention if possible of further necrotizing of the pancreas, and (3) the protection of the neighborhood, both near and remote, from pancreatic ferments. There is the additional task of treating an underlying disease of the biliary tract.

On opening the abdomen the diagnosis can usually be made at once by the areas of fat necrosis which are recognizable by their sulphur-yellow color. Frequently a general peritonitis is already present. The neighborhood of the operative field is protected by moist sponges. The pancreas is exposed as a rule through the gastrocolic omentum. The lesser peritoneal cavity commonly contains a seropurulent or bloody exudate. This is sponged away. The pancreas is swollen, congested, at times softened, purulent or even necrotic. The peritoneal covering of the organ is split and the incision is carried into the gland substance. From this incision the surrounding tissue is explored (Fig. 391) in order to open necrotic foci or abscesses. If on splitting the pancreatic tissue a calculus is found, it is of course removed.

In view of the fact that acute pancreatitis in a high percentage of cases is caused and aggravated by diseases of the bile passages, an examination of the biliary system should be included, unless the poor general condition of the patient makes an early termination of the operation necessary. Any further harmful action upon the pancreas from this source should be checked by the simplest measures. In case gall-stone disease is encountered, no attempt should be made at its complete removal in view of the gravity of the general condition.

The most important point is to remove any obstruction to the bile in the common duct. If the common duct is distended and blocked, it should be opened supraduodenally. If stones are found in its interior, they are removed if possible.

In so doing, particular attention should be paid to possible stones lodged in the papilla of Vater. In that case the bile is drained externally through a T-tube in the common duct. If the condition of the patient permits the gall bladder should be examined, and if the gall bladder is found to contain stones, cholecystostomy should be performed.

The wound in the pancreas is packed and drained, and the neighborhood of the disease focus is also protected against a local spread of the toxic fluid by packing. The packing and drain are carried to the exterior through the abdominal wound which is only partly closed. In exceptional cases the drainage may be carried out through a special opening in the flank or in the posterior abdominal wall.

The packing should not be removed too soon. Large or small portions of necrotic pancreas are often discharged in the course of time.

6. Treatment of Chronic Pancreatitis

Chronic pancreatitis is usually the result of disease of the biliary tract. It is recognizable by the induration of the whole gland or of individual parts, especially frequently of the head. Our therapeutic measures are therefore directed primarily at the biliary tract. The local treatment of the pancreas is of secondary importance. It may consist only in splitting the capsule and packing the wound. The results of such a procedure, in itself by no means negligible and by no means without danger, are doubtful. (If jaundice is present internal drainage of the biliary passages should be established I.S.R.)

C. OPERATIONS ON THE SPLEEN

1. EXPOSURE OF THE SPLEEN

The normal spleen is about the size of the fist and lies against the posterior and lateral abdominal wall on the left side at the level of the 9th and 10th ribs. Its long axis runs parallel to the ribs. The spleen is therefore overlaid by the costal arch and by the pleura. Its convex surface is loosely attached to the diaphragm by connective tissue which can be stretched out into a band-like structure, the phrenicosplenic ligament (Fig. 392). The spleen is intimately connected with the stomach by the gastrosplenic ligament, a portion of the greater omentum, which contains the vasa brevia arteries. It adapts itself freely to changes of shape and position of the stomach incident to the state of filling of that organ, and to a large degree it follows traction made on the stomach, a matter of significance in the operative approach to the spleen. A special reduplication of peritoneum running to the splenic flexure of the colon is considered a part of the gastrocolic omentum and is occasionally called the colicosplenic ligament.

The blood supply of the spleen (Fig. 73) is the large splenic artery, which arises from the celiac axis, runs along the upper border of the pancreas and enters the spleen in a fan of branches at the hilum on its under surface. Fairly close to the spleen the splenic artery gives off the left gastro-epiploic artery and the vasa brevia. By the same route the splenic vein leaves the organ to empty the splenic blood into the portal vein which it forms with the superior mesenteric vein.

Since the blood supply of the spleen is concentrated in the vascular pedicle at the hilum, the blood supply can be interrupted at once by compressing the pedicle with the hand (Fig. 393) or with a clamp and can be reestablished by simply releasing it. Clamping the pedicle of the spleen, however, does not stop bleeding from the spleen by any means completely, since the spleen is filled with blood like a sponge and permits the accumulated blood to escape for quite some time. In the presence of disease, especially in case of marked enlargement of the organ, the three splenic ligaments mentioned, as well as adhesions which have formed, may contain large accessory vessels, particularly veins, at times as large as a thumb. These are frequently hard to get at, and their injury may cause the patient to bleed rapidly to death.

In the interior of the spleen the vessels are distributed at right angles to its long axis, a point to be remembered when incising the organ.

The operative approach to the spleen is through a laparotomy in most cases, only rarely through a thoracolaparotomy in case of an unusually situated injury.

In all diseases in which other parts of the abdominal cavity need to be examined, particularly in case of sharp or blunt abdominal trauma not limited with certainty to the left upper quadrant, the abdomen is opened through a midline incision above the umbilicus. To this, if necessary, may be added a transverse incision dividing the left rectus. In an operation on the spleen alone it is better to open the abdomen at a point much nearer to the spleen, either by a left costal margin incision (page 31) or by a left "wave"

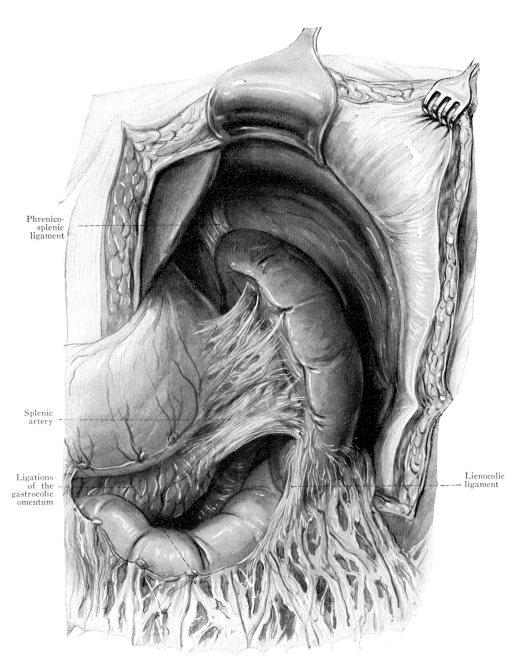

Phrenico-
splenic
ligament

Splenic
artery

Ligations
of the
gastrocolic
omentum

Lienocolic
ligament

FIG. 392. Position and attachments of the spleen. The spleen presents a broad surface to the left half of the diaphragm and is attached to it by connective tissue strands, the phrenico-splenic ligament. The gastrosplenic ligament contains numerous vascular connections with the stomach. The large vessels course to the spleen in the tail of the pancreas. The left side of the gastrocolic omentum which is connected with the spleen can be differentiated as the lienocolic ligament.

or "Z" incision (page 19). In particularly difficult cases it may become necessary to reflect the left costal margin (page 32).

In an operation on the spleen I stand at the right side of the patient since I can reach under the left costal margin more easily from that side than from the left. The spleen is exposed by pulling the stomach forward by its greater curvature. If the spleen is adherent to the abdominal wall, it can be reached by following the stomach to the left. In order to make it easier to deliver the spleen and to keep the intestines out of the way, the upper half and the left side of the patient are elevated, provided that the girdle type of spinal anaesthesia is not being used.

The extirpation of the whole spleen is compatible with life and health, in spite of the fact that the spleen is an unpaired organ. It is also claimed that the ligation of the splenic artery without removal of the spleen is not followed by necrosis or any systemic disturbances. On the basis of these experiences, surgeons were rather free for a time in the removal of the organ. More recently they have gradually adopted the more conservative principle of sacrificing this valuable structure only in case of necessity. On the other hand, the indications for splenectomy in certain blood diseases have been extended materially in the last few years.

2. Treatment of Injuries of the Spleen

Gun shot and stab wounds which penetrate the abdominal wall and blunt trauma of the abdomen in which an injury of an intra-abdominal organ cannot be excluded always demand an exploratory laparotomy. An injury of the spleen is probably present if trauma in the region of the spleen is followed by the signs of internal hemorrhage, pallor, weak, rapid pulse; and if dulness and muscular rigidity develop in the upper left posterior part of the abdomen.

Since the spleen lies beneath the left costal arch, the lower part of the left pleural space is pierced in many puncture wounds involving the spleen. In stab wounds and in small-caliber gun shot wounds, the injury of the pleural space and the frequently associated injury of the lower edge of the lung are usually of fairly little consequence so that they do not demand surgical intervention. Therefore, in such cases the path of the wound should not be followed through the pleural space and the diaphragm in order to reach the abdominal cavity. Aside from the greater limitation as well as the more involved nature of this approach, the opening of the pleural space entails a great danger of infection and imposes a considerable burden on the heart and lungs through the development of a pneumothorax. A direct laparotomy is therefore selected as the mode of approach.

If the type of trauma (stab with a sword, bullet wound, blunt trauma) makes it likely that more distant abdominal organs have been injured, the peritoneal cavity is opened by a midline incision above the umbilicus and this incision is enlarged in most instances by a transverse incision through the left rectus. If an involvement of distant organs seems unlikely, a left costal margin incision or a left lateral rectus incision extended to the ensiform process is used.

On the other hand, if there is a large gaping wound which opens wide the pleural space and if a traumatic pneumothorax is already present, a thoraco-laparotomy with division of the diaphragm is indicated, in which the fish-hook incision renders particularly good service. The type of incision, however, depends in the individual case largely on the wound which is present.

In every severe injury of the spleen considerable blood is found in the neighborhood of the organ within the abdominal cavity. It may be difficult to determine the source of the bleeding. If there is any suspicion that the hemorrhage is from the spleen, the surgeon standing at the right side of the patient, as soon as he has cleared the view sufficiently by removing some of the blood,

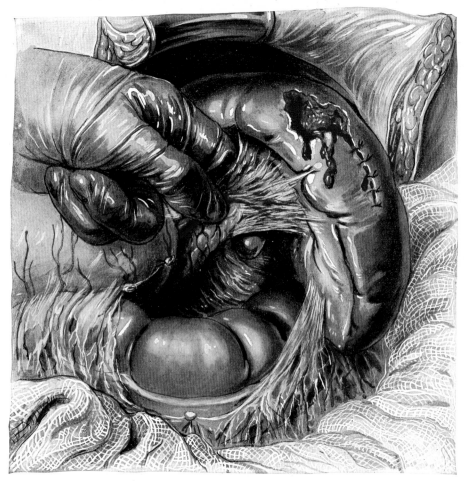

Fig. 393. Management of an injury of the spleen. While the blood supply of the spleen is interrupted by grasping the splenic pedicle with the fingers, the wound in the spleen is closed by suturing the delicate splenic capsule.

displaces the transverse colon downward and to the right, pulls the stomach to the right with the left hand, slips the right hand along the inner surface of the costal arch and reaches for the spleen to deliver it from the abdominal cavity. If the spleen is injured, the bleeding is temporarily checked by compressing the pedicle of the spleen first with the hand (Fig. 393) and then by a fairly stiff clamp. It is now possible to inspect the injury carefully to decide upon the type of procedure.

There are three possibilities: the spleen may be sutured, or packed, or removed. The choice is governed by the desire to preserve the injured organ and the extent of its injury. Its preservation, however, is possible only if the general condition of the patient is good enough to stand the suture of the spleen, which is time-consuming and always involves further bleeding, and if the injury of the organ is so slight that there is good reason to believe that the hemorrhage can be controlled by suture or packing. One must bear in mind the possibility of the so-called two-stage rupture of the spleen, in which as a result of continued bleeding into the soft splenic pulp there gradually develops a huge hematoma leading finally to a rupture of the spleen. The patient must not be exposed to this danger of massive secondary hemorrhage, a danger which is particularly great in splenic injuries and even after days may lead to marked blood loss, as a result of the delicate and exceedingly friable nature of the splenic tissue. In deciding whether the spleen should be removed or not, the surgeon should be guided not only by the changes on the concave side of the organ facing him, but before deciding in favor of preservation of the spleen he should also examine its convex surface which usually has suffered the greater damage. If the organ is to be removed, the pedicle is ligated and cut in the manner later to be described.

If the spleen can be preserved, its rupture is the procedure of choice. Any ragged portions are trimmed away with scissors or the electrosurgical knife so that the wound surfaces are fairly even. The suture of a deep wound consists in uniting the parenchyma by through-and-through sutures and the capsule by superficial sutures. The through-and-through sutures (Fig. 393) must not be pulled too tight because of the friability of the pulp. When the wound surfaces have been approximated in this manner, the edges of the fibrous capsule are separately joined and coapted by fine sutures.

If hemorrhage is not completely checked by suture, the bleeding point is packed. Since the spleen because of its mobility can easily evade the pressure of packing, it is often advantageous to fasten the packing to the spleen with catgut sutures.

Packing alone of a splenic injury is an unsafe and therefore usually an inadvisable procedure. It is to be considered only in particularly favorable cases. Here, too, it is generally advantageous to fasten the packing to the spleen by suture.

3. Aspiratory Puncture and Biopsy of the Spleen

Aspiratory puncture of the spleen, a procedure that is occasionally still employed, is fraught with considerable danger, especially because of the possibility of hemorrhage and of infection of the abdominal cavity. Even when the puncture can reach the spleen directly and with certain avoidance of the intestine and when a small-bore needle is used as recommended, there still remains the danger of an escape of pus or of echinococcus fluid into the abdominal cavity. This danger is not minimized by a laparotomy undertaken immediately in case the aspiratory puncture yields positive findings. In view of the vascularity, especially of a diseased spleen containing dilated veins as it often does, the danger of secondary hemorrhage from the puncture wound must not be underestimated. For these reasons the surgeon as a rule prefers an exploratory exposure and biopsy to exploratory puncture.

Excision of a biopsy specimen is undertaken if possible in the form of a wedge-shaped cut at the margin of the organ and perpendicular to its long axis.

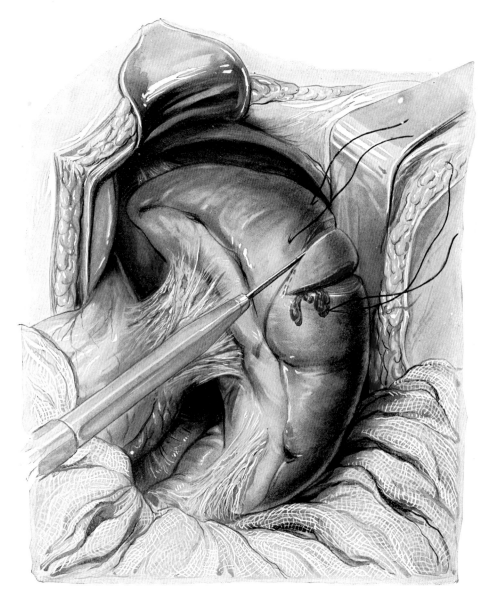

FIG. 394. Splenic biopsy. A wedge-shaped piece of tissue is removed from the splenic margin with an electrosurgical knife. Before the excision was begun the segment to be excised was surrounded by deep sutures which will be tied immediately after the excision is completed.

Bleeding can be limited materially, as in the liver, by a preliminary injection of adrenalin solution and by the use of the electrosurgical knife. In order to lessen the bleeding still more, deep sutures through the parenchyma may be placed around the site of resection before excising the wedge (Fig. 394), to be tied immediately after the excision. The wound in the capsule is always closed separately by fine sutures.

A prompt histologic diagnosis by frozen section makes it possible to await the result of the biopsy while the abdomen is still open and to undertake the necessary surgical measures at once.

4. TREATMENT OF CYSTS AND ABSCESSES OF THE SPLEEN

The diagnosis of cysts, echinococcus or other types, or of abscesses in the spleen is possible only after they have reached a considerable size. In view of the resultant disproportion between the small size of the spleen and the extensive lesion, a resection of the lesion is almost never to be considered. Splenectomy is the procedure of choice.

In some cases, however, the extensive adhesions, the undue size of the diseased spleen, or the poor general condition of the patient make this radical operation impossible. The cystic structure is then sutured into the abdominal wound to as large an extent as possible, the visceral peritoneum of the cyst being joined to the parietal peritoneum of the abdominal wall in the region of the abdominal wound. The cyst can then be opened primarily, or secondarily after the formation of adhesions.

If the wall of the cyst or abscess is so thin that the sutures will cut through and the fluid seep into the abdominal cavity, the abdominal cavity is carefully walled off by packing, and the cyst or abscess is emptied by aspiration, is opened widely, sponged dry and packed with vioform gauze. The abdominal wound is partly closed and the opening of the cyst or abscess is sutured to the remaining portion of the abdominal wound.

Cysts and echinococcus vesicles may at times be removed later from the splenic tissue by blunt dissection. Abscess cavities usually heal by granulation.

5. SPLENECTOMY

The diagnosis of malignant tumors of the spleen, of which practically only sarcomata come into consideration, is so difficult and is made so late, and the likelihood of local metastasis in view of the great vascularity of the spleen is so great, that only a complete removal of the organ should be considered, if any radical procedure is to be thought of at all. The conditions are similar in that extremely rare disease, tuberculosis of the spleen. When splenectomy is considered in blood diseases, the commonest indication, the organ is frequently greatly enlarged and in some cases may nearly fill the entire abdomen.

The danger in the removal of such a diseased spleen lies in hemorrhage, to a less extent from the greatly dilated vessels of the splenic pedicle, than from the accessory veins of the capsule of the spleen. Such vessels tend to form in the adhesions between the convex surface of the spleen, especially at its upper pole between the diaphragm and abdominal wall, and between the concave surface of the spleen and the stomach and the splenic flexure of the colon. Extensive vascular adhesions may make the removal of the organ impossible because of the danger of fatal hemorrhage.

If the splenic tumor extends beyond the midline, the abdomen should be opened by a midline incision which may be enlarged in case of necessity by a left transverse incision at the level of the umbilicus. In case of smaller tumors a left costal margin incision or a "wave" incision is used; the latter also gives a good approach in case of large tumors of the spleen. The patient is placed in a semi-oblique right lateral position.

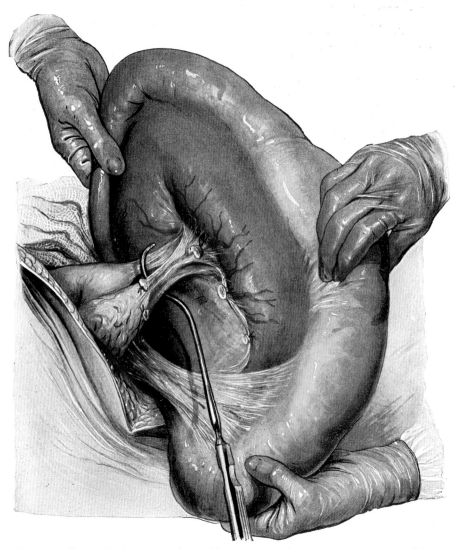

FIG. 395. Removal of a huge spleen. The spleen has been turned up over the left costal margin. The band-like vascular attachments are picked up in small segments on an aneurysm needle, doubly ligated and cut.

After opening the abdomen, the operator first palpates the convex surface of the spleen and its upper pole with the right hand to inform himself of the possible presence of adhesions. With the patient in a sufficiently marked right lateral position, if the left costal margin is elevated forcibly with a retractor, the spleen usually drops away from the anterior abdominal wall for an appreciable distance as a result of gravity, and in this cleft the operator can separate the existing peritoneal reduplications and adhesions under guidance of the eye, either by blunt dissection or with a scissors after double ligation. However, if the adhesions are extensive, vascular, difficult to free, if they cannot be stretched and if they cannot be approached without first tearing them, the attempt to remove the organ should be given up. Fortunately, this is only rarely the case.

When splenectomy has been decided upon, the pedicle is attacked as soon as possible. Adhesions which block the way are picked up on an aneurysm needle, doubly ligated and divided. The main vascular pedicle may also be divided between massive ligatures, carefully applied. In so doing, the surgeon must keep close to the spleen, as otherwise he runs the danger of including parts of the tail of the pancreas, the left gastro-epiploic artery or even the gastric wall in a ligature. The ligation of parts of the gastric wall or of the pancreas may lead to necrosis, while the ligation of the artery mentioned is without harmful results. (It has been proposed by Miller that the ligation of the left gastro-epiploic artery may lessen the likelihood of the gastric hemorrhage so often encountered in patients with splenic enlargements, especially in Banti's disease. It is certain that any attempts to prevent such bleeding must be made at the time of the splenectomy, for they are out of the question at a later time because of adhesions. I.S.R.) Experience has shown that ligatures easily slip off the splenic pedicle. Massive ligatures are therefore best applied in such a way that they pass through the tissue of the pedicle; they should not lie at the free end of the divided pedicle. However, every large vessel should also be ligated separately.

The better procedure is not to cut the splenic pedicle between massive ligatures, but to expose the artery and the vein singly and to ligate them separately. The artery is ligated first and then the vein so that the spleen may be emptied of blood as far as possible before it is removed. After the artery has been ligated and while the vein is still open a marked shrinking of the organ may be observed in many cases.

The further attachments are then divided close to the spleen after double ligation (Fig. 395). While the wound edges are widely retracted and the left costal margin is elevated, an attempt is made to stretch the flat adhesions of the convex surface so that their blood vessels may be ligated on the body side at least. Free bleeding which may arise during the separation of flat surfaces necessitates the temporary use of packing. The phrenicosplenic ligament is usually long enough so that it can be doubly ligated before being cut.

After the removal of the spleen the splenic bed is once more carefully examined for bleeding, and the bleeding points are ligated or caught by suture ligatures. If at all possible, the abdomen is closed without drainage.

If complete removal of the spleen in the manner described is impossible because of adhesions, the surgeon may be aided by the procedure recommended by Szendy. The pedicle of the spleen is ligated as close to the hilum as possible but is not divided. The spleen, for a considerable part of its surface, is sutured into the abdominal wound by joining the visceral peritoneum to the parietal peritoneum. The rest of the abdominal wound is closed. The capsule of the spleen is then split in the area sutured into the wound and the splenic pulp is shelled out with a large blunt scoop. In so doing, care must be taken not to injure the splenic capsule on the side of the abdominal cavity. The large wound cavity of the spleen is packed.

(When splenectomy is performed because of a blood disease, it is wiser to look for accessory spleens and if these are found to remove them. I.S.R.)

6. Treatment of Wandering Spleen

The inadequacy of its attachments, which consist of a few delicate peritoneal reduplications, makes it possible that the spleen, after its ligaments have become stretched, may shift to the dependent portions of the abdomen at some distance from its original position (wandering spleen). If this is only an individual part of a general enteroptosis and if it remains without marked symptoms, it does not require operative treatment. On the other hand, if the undue mobility of the spleen as an individual lesion gives rise to continued marked complaints, or if it leads to the acute picture of torsion of the spleen by twisting of the vascular pedicle, operation is indicated.

Here, too, the first therapeutic consideration is the preservation of the organ. In case of acute torsion of the spleen, the organ is returned to its proper position and it is watched to see whether and to what extent it recovers. If the bluish-red spleen, which may be enlarged to several times its original size, becomes small and brownish-red after the reposition, it may be left in the body.

Both a spleen whose pedicle has been sutured as well as an otherwise normal wandering spleen must be anchored securely. This is best done in the following manner: The parietal peritoneum on one side of the abdominal wound is dissected free until the resulting pocket is large enough to receive the organ. The spleen is inserted into this pocket and the opening of the pocket is then made smaller so that the spleen can not slip out again, but its vascular pedicle is not interfered with. The abdomen is closed without drainage.

If the spleen does not recover after being untwisted, or if the wandering spleen cannot be anchored securely in the manner described, it may be removed.

END

INDEX